Foundations of Orientation and Mobility

Richard L. Welsh, Ph.D.
Bruce B. Blasch, Ph.D.
Editors

American Foundation for the Blind
New York 1980

Foundations of Orientation and Mobility
Copyright 1987 by
American Foundation for the Blind
15 West 16th Street
New York, N.Y.   10011

For Barbara and Dolores

The American Foundation for the Blind (AFB) is a national nonprofit organization that advocates, develops and provides programs and services to help blind and visually impaired people achieve independence with dignity in all sectors of society.

Third printing, 1987

Library of Congress Cataloging in Publication Data
Foundations of orientation and mobility
Bibliography: p.
Includes Index.
1. Visually handicapped—Rehabilitation—Addresses, essays, lectures.
2. Orientation (Psychology)—Addresses, essays, lectures. 3. Space perception—Addresses, essays, lectures.
I.   Welsh Richard L.   II.   Blasch, Bruce B.
HV1626.F68   152.1'882   79-18782
ISBN 0-89128-093-6

PPM093
Printed in the United States of America

Contents

Preface

Russell C. Williams

Foundations of Orientation and Mobility is a presentation of the origins, history, and present state of a key discipline in the rehabilitation and education of blind people. Although this discipline has faced much opposition and misunderstanding over the years it has endured and finally flourished.

In the last 20 years much has been written about orientation and mobility needs and procedures, so there was a need to distil the basic elements of the subject from many articles into one book. Through the years a small number of dedicated people worked hard to give scientific validity to the art. This book is a monument to them and to the editors who brought them together.

From my ringside seat I had an exceptionally close view of how deeply effective orientation and mobility teaching is when it is taught by those who know what they are doing. It was my luck to be instantly blinded by enemy shellfire in war and to learn within a few days that my total blindness was permanent. This was a cruel blow as my satisfactions and reputation had been derived largely from sight-requiring competitive athletics, in which I was both a participant and a coach. Fortunately, I found that Richard Hoover and Warren Bledsoe, with the blessing of Army ophthalmology and sympathetic Army hospital administration, had a going program of instruction in foot travel, the embryo of the present orientation and mobility art.

I took well to the program, notwithstanding frequent mistakes, frustrations, and embarrassments. I had doubts too. Never as to whether I was being helped, because increasingly I was traveling farther by myself and keeping better track of my whereabouts. My doubts were those which most self-respecting students feel at times—that my teachers were not teaching me in the way that I thought I should be taught. However, my self-respect grew steadily from what I learned, as well as my respect for what I was taught and for the teaching environment. Realistic goals were beginning to bud in me shouldering aside the hopelessness with which I had entered the foot travel program.

I enjoyed an experience not always granted to pioneers when I read Welsh's chapter on psychosocial dimensions of orientation and mobility and realized that what was done for me at Valley Forge Hospital, and what we did for others at Hines, was based soundly on scientific principles of psychology, sociology, and education. Fortune favors the brave, and Vail, Randolph, Greear, Hoover, and Bledsoe were all brave in disregarding tradition and breaking new ground.

It was a real treat for me to read and re-read Bledsoe's chapter on the history of the development of the profession. I thought I knew its history, having lived much of it, but I recaptured much that had slipped away from me and learned about critical episodes and events of which I was unaware at the time.

During the 11 years I was associated with the orientation and mobility specialists at the Veterans Administration Hospital at Hines, I watched them practice their discipline as part of the personal and social adjustment program for blinded veterans which was carried out there. Their activity integrated a number of skills for which the orientation and mobility profession became well known. Indeed, they had in hand a burgeoning art based upon science, which was carried out in ways that soon gave them national and international acclaim. Much of the good report came from the testimony of veterans whose eagerness to meet life under blindness had been dramatically advanced by orientation and mobility training. The reputation of the teaching also spread because the hospital and community where they did their work was proud of it and said so. No less important was the fact that a few leaders in work for the blind understood orientation and mobility more than superficially. More than that, consistently, aggressively, and tenaciously they endorsed the pioneering skill at Hines and encouraged other agency personnel in work for the blind to come and see for themselves what was being done and why. As chief of the Blind Rehabilitation Center at Hines, I always knew I had the support of General Paul Hawley, Kathern Gruber, Father Thomas Carroll, Dr. Derrick Vail, Richard Hoover, and at a much later date, Dean George Mallinson, the indefatigable grant getter who made possible the establishment of the program at Western Michigan University.

Part of my role as Chief of the Blind Rehabilitation Center at Hines was to be sure that what I did was consistent with the scientific philosophy and standards of the large and prestigious general hospital of which we were a small part. We had a superlative medical administrator as manager of that hospital, Dr. Kelso Carroll, who left nothing to be desired in interpreting that philosophy to us in the blind center, and who also was superlative in interpreting the blind center to other hospital personnel.

Among other things, our work had to meet clinical recording standards of the hospital, by which what was done in orientation and mobility began to find its way into the written word. This was an immediate aid to me in talks with instructors about what was being done with blinded veterans in specific situations, and also with veterans about their progress and their future. It was thrilling to hear repeatedly from instructors reverberations of thoroughness, imagination, subtlety, and strong belief in the blinded persons with whom they worked. It was equally thrilling to get feedback from veterans that confirmed the meaningfulness of the program, as hopeless behavior and talk gave way to preoccupation with new vistas. Without self-scrutiny, I do not think we would have made the grade. Our recording of it was one of the real contributions our program made in the metamorphosis from trade to profession.

While I was at Hines, we had approximately 18 orientation and mobility specialists working in the program at one time. The number varied because some did not work out for the long haul, but they were comparatively few. Indeed, we had a remarkable record of retaining personnel, losing mainly those who were not up to the hard physical and emotional demands (and, I may add, peer discipline) that the unit required. Covering large areas on foot hour after hour, day after day, always in the right position to observe fine details of the blind person's performance is an exacting skill. The mere shadowing without inadvertently guiding is no mean achievement. It takes genuine emotional strength to teach and observe people who have uncommonly strong doubts about what you are teaching as well as their own ability to absorb it, and, in addition, to do this before an ever-present public who has stupendous doubts about the wisdom, safety, and validity of your efforts. This was the essence of the World War II period in work for the blind.

The poet, Clarence Day, in *Thoughts Without Words*, said,
> When eras die, their legacies
> Are left to strange police.
> Professors in New England guard
> The glory that was Greece.

Judging from this book, I do not believe that my era is in the hands of strange police. It was my privilege to be a part of a renewal and revitalization of concern for the blind in the United States. The most important trait of this concern is that it is not merely mechanical. It pays deep attention to feeling and the spirit, as did the founding fathers in work for the blind.

Thoughts Without Words © Alfred A. Knopf, Inc.

Foreword

Stanley Suterko

The appearance of the first, basic and comprehensive text in any field or discipline is of considerable symbolic importance. It is, indeed, a coming of age, a major milestone in the development of a body of knowledge or profession, signalling a field in readiness to consolidate and relate all the components that contribute to it and to begin viewing itself in more critical and sophisticated ways.

For this reason alone, I welcome the publication of *Foundations of Orientation and Mobility*. The very act of collecting together for the first time in one place and synthesizing the often highly technical information from the multitude of diverse disciplines that comprise mobility should help to deepen understanding of the process itself and of the complex relationships among the disciplines that contribute to it. By illuminating the ways in which visually impaired persons acquire control of space it should increase understanding of the intrinsic nature of the relationship between knowledge of space, movement and independence, an understanding that is crucial for the educator, the rehabilitation specialist, the program administrator, as well as for the mobility specialist, and the visually impaired person himself or herself.

Foundations of Orientation and Mobility should have immediate practical value too. A basic text eliminates a considerable part of the instructor's need to identify and pore through a multitude of books and journals from various subject areas with the hope that some little bit of information could be gleaned and effectively related to mobility. A difficult and not always productive task since the sensory processes aspects of most subjects as they relate to mobility for the blind are rarely treated. For example, in books and articles about audition, practical applications of echolocation are rarely discussed. Not only does a basic text such as this free the instructor for other tasks but it contributes substantially to the students' understanding not just of the individual topics but more importantly of how they relate to mobility.

A sound and comprehensive basic text can also influence the future of a field, be a powerful stimulant for change and the development of new knowledge. I would hope the availability of *Foundations of Orientation and Mobility* will encourage the identification and cataloguing of the various sensory tasks that contribute to mobility and that through such a cataloguing we could begin to set some minimum standards. For example: What should hearing do? What should touch do?

I would like to see it stimulate research into specific aspects of the process of mobility and encourage attempts to objectively validate the present empirically based practice. I especially hope that the book encourages sensory psychologists to become interested in mobility research.

Finally, I would like to suggest that the text's real contribution ultimately lies in the part it plays in providing better quality services to the visually impaired.

About the Editors

Richard L. Welsh is superintendent of the Maryland School for the Blind, Baltimore. Previously, he headed the mobility training program at Cleveland State University. He received a master's degree in mobility from Western Michigan University and a doctorate in rehabilitation counseling from the University of Pittsburgh. He has written many articles on mobility and on the psychosocial aspects of rehabilitation of the visually impaired and is co-editor of *Foundations of Orientation and Mobility*

Bruce B. Blasch heads a program to train mobility specialists to work with all handicaps at the University of Wisconsin, Madison. Previously, he was executive director of the American Association of Workers for the Blind and on the faculty at the University of Pittsburgh and Western Michigan University. He received a master's degree in mobility form Western Michigan University and a doctorate in special education from Michigan State University. He has written many articles on mobility and is co-editor of *Foundations of Orientation and Mobility*.

Acknowledgments

As instructors in training programs for mobility specialists, we were very much aware of the lack of a comprehensive textbook of information for orientation and mobility students, and the effect of this lack on the continuing improvement of services for clients. We wondered why such a book had not been done and, we naively set out to correct this deficiency.

The past five years have helped us to understand why such a book was not attempted by wiser individuals. Without the assistance of many people, this textbook would not have been completed.

Our wives (two) and our children (many), to whom we have dedicated this work, were always positive in their support of us, and they surrendered (reluctantly) their legitimate claim on our time. The children having grown up with our working on a book now have to adjust their images of us. Dee's spaghetti and Barb's Cheerios provided physical nourishment to go along with the intellectual stimulation of the task.

Many friends, family members, and innkeepers in various parts of the country provided meeting places, food, and lodging that enabled us to collaborate while living in different states.

The American Foundation for the Blind, under the leadership of Gene Apple, recognized the value of this project and provided generous and unqualifed support for us and the authors. The most significant contribution of AFB was the assignment of Mary Ellen Mulholland to work with us and direct our efforts. Mary Ellen helped us learn about editing, writing, thinking, and kvetching. She encouraged us when our spirits sagged, kept the project moving, and was the single most important person in bringing it to completion. Audrey Gilmour's expertise in technical copy editing and proofreading rescued us from embarrassment more than once.

We learned a lot from interacting with the authors, and we believe that the quality of their contributions will be evident to the readers. We greatly appreciate their willingness to become a part of this project and their patience with our efforts to relate their chapters to the overall thrust of the text.

Our employers at the American Association of Workers for the Blind, Cleveland State University, University of Wisconsin, and the Maryland School for the Blind have tolerated the diversion of our attention necessitated by the book and, seeing the value of the contribution, have encouraged our efforts. Our co-workers and staff, along with staff at AFB, have helped in many ways.

The project has demonstrated again that teaching and learning are inseparable processes. Our debt to both our teachers and our students is clear to us, even though it has been difficult to distinguish when we were teaching and when we were being taught.

Finally, our colleagues, other mobility specialists, have inspired us by their commitment to their profession, their interest in this project, and their willingness to discuss O&M any place any time. We particularly want to acknowledge Don Blasch who has served us and many mobility specialists as a model and sounding board, and who is, in our judgement, the primary stabilizing influence in a young, dynamic profession.

R.L.W. & B.B.B.

Illustrations

Tables

Introduction

Richard L. Welsh and Bruce B. Blasch

The ability to move independently, safely, and purposefully through the environment is a skill of primary importance in the development of each individual. Until confronted with temporary or permanent restrictions on this ability, people seem to take for granted a skill which occupies a central place in their growth and functioning. Orientation and mobility instruction, the task of helping visually impaired people to develop or reestablish this skill, has focused increased attention on its centrality in human development.

Foundations of Orientation and Mobility is one manifestation of the increased attention. Reflecting the growth and professionalization of orientation and mobility instruction, this volume draws together the diverse background knowledge considered necessary for mobility specialists.*

The custom of viewing success in mobility tasks as representative of significant stages in the development of the individual indicates the importance attached to the ability to move safely in a purposeful manner through the environment. The infant who learns to crawl, the toddler who takes his first steps, and the child who negotiates stairs by himself is each recognized as having accomplished important developmental tasks. When a young child is first allowed to cross a street, run an errand to the neighborhood store, or travel back and forth to school on her own, she is generally considered to have passed other developmental milestones. When an adolescent receives permission to travel alone to a complex downtown area or to drive a car, it is recognition of the fact that his skill and judgment in moving independently through the community have developed even further. Each of these accomplishments increases the status of the individual in the eyes of others and, in turn, has a positive impact on the individual's self-concept.

The tendency to consider success in mobility as significant reflects the essential role that movement plays in many facets of living. Movement is central to the entire process of psychomotor development. Independent mobility facilitates full participation in formal education programs. In many occupations, mobility is essential for job performance; and almost everyone finds it necessary to be able to get to and from work. The ability to travel is essential for meeting social needs and obligations. Without such competence, the number of social and recreational alternatives open to one are severely limited or can only be enjoyed at the whim or convenience of others. The inability to travel in the community limits a person's access to medical services and resources. In a more basic way, immobility itself can contribute to the onset of certain health problems or to the deterioration of various

---

*The term mobility specialist will be used throughout this text to refer to those who provide orientation and mobility instruction. They are referred to elsewhere as orientors, orientation and mobility instructors, and peripatologists.

aspects of the body, especially those related to circulatory and respiratory systems.

The ability to travel affects and is affected by all aspects of a person's life. Service providers who are mainly concerned with a visually impaired person's vocational success or social functioning will frequently encounter the need to know more about his ability to travel independently. In a similar way, a client's success in orientation and mobility will be affected by his success or difficulties in other aspects of his rehabilitation or education. The mobility specialist may find himself in the position of relying upon the understanding and skill of other professionals on a team to help a client overcome particular difficulties. At such times, the more other professionals understand about orientation and mobility, the greater the chances for effective collaboration.

The central role of independent mobility has both stimulated and supported efforts to clarify social policy in regard to the right to travel and to move independently through the community. Both state and federal legislation have been enacted requiring that buildings constructed with government funds be accessible to handicapped persons. The Federal Highway Safety Act contains provisions to make cities and transportation systems within cities accessible. Airlines have been refused permission for arbitrary restriction of the number of handicapped persons allowed on any one flight.

As people have become more aware of the ability to travel as a right of each individual which must be guaranteed and nourished by a democratic society, it has become more apparent that steps must be taken to provide whatever intervention is necessary to enable each member of society to avail himself of this right.

Integrating handicapped children into normal educational programs as much as possible will not lead to the desired benefits for such children or for society unless appropriate educational programs are available with the necessary supports. Children must be able to get to neighborhood schools each day, and, when there, they must be able to get from class to class. Without some type of mobility, handicapped students may be educated within the same system as nonhandicapped children, or within the same building, but they will not be integrated.

Similarly, policies have been changed to eliminate institutionalization as much as possible, especially for mentally retarded and mentally ill persons, and to provide community based programs for those who need such services. Unless these individuals possess the skills necessary for travel in the community so as to take advantage of community-based services, they are being set up for failure and for additional adjustment difficulties as institutions are closed.

Assisting disabled persons to become contributing members in society, the major thrust of vocational rehabilitation programs, must prepare those individuals to travel throughout the community so as to achieve their rehabilitation goals. Basic human rights guaranteed by various policies and laws will not be a fact unless the individuals affected receive the mobility training they need for full participation in community life.

KNOWLEDGE BASE

Formalized instruction in independent travel began first, and has been developed more extensively, for visually impaired people than for any other disability group. Efforts to provide orientation and mobility services to visually impaired persons sprang from the necessity of meeting their real needs in particular situations. As the practice-oriented profession grew and as the number and variety of clients served increased, the need for a comprehensive body of knowledge for the profession emerged with greater clarity. In recent years there were efforts by Foulke (1970), Kay (1974), and Krigman (1968) to present organized and coherent theories of independent mobility with impaired vision. But none seemed to be comprehensive enough to explain the total phenomenon. Implied in the organization of this text is the idea that the successful instruction of independent mobility with impaired vision should encompass an understanding of each of the knowledge areas represented herein. The diversity and dimension of the knowledge reflects the variety of components involved in the complexities of independent travel, as well as the great variety of individuals who may need such assistance. This book, therefore, will provide that comprehensive review of the state of knowledge considered essential to the mobility specialist, and a discussion of the particular application of this knowledge to orientation and mobility.

It is intended that mobility specialists in training will use the text as a starting point in their efforts to understand the current state of the art and to expand the body of knowledge. Such a compilation and integration of knowledge was not available before, and training programs for mobility specialists have had to draw information from a wide variety of sources to meet the needs of students.

In addition, all professionals, not just mobility specialists, should be more aware of psychological and social reactions to visual impairment, and should be informed about eye disease, visual functioning, general health and medical problems, and about the systems of services available to those who need them. Also, like all teachers, mobility specialists should have a thorough knowledge of the learning process and about child development. The ability to interact sensitively and effectively with people is another essential quality for professionals in human service settings. These topics and attributes are not dealt with as major topics in this text, but they are touched upon indirectly in a number of chapters.

Administrators in agencies as well as in schools can develop a more thorough understanding of the many and varied aspects of mobility training as a result of reading this text. Frequently, in the past, mobility training has been equated simply with teaching a person how to use a cane, and administrators did not appreciate the need for individualized instruction and for highly trained personnel. The text presents mobility training as a complex component of the rehabilitation and education of visually impaired persons.

One area of knowledge pertinent for mobility instructors, but not treated in this volume, is the body of techniques and teaching methodologies used by mobility specialists such as those in *Orientation and Mobility Techniques* (Hill & Ponder, 1976).

Review of the Text

The first few chapters present foundation knowledge necessary for mobility specialists relating to basic functions of the organism and their implications for independent movement with reduced vision. In Chapter 2, Hart presents a review of theories of psychomotor development and basic concepts of spatial orientation. It is important for mobility specialists to understand the effect of visual loss on this process of development and on the organization of concepts about space. Much of the assistance that students need to facilitate their psychomotor development and their concept development can be provided by special education teachers in traditional school programs, making the services of the mobility specialist more efficient.

The individual's ability to assume and maintain an upright posture and to move his body in a balanced manner represents an extremely important aspect of independent mobility. Aust, Chapter 3, discusses this component of the body's functioning and analyzes how visual loss may lead to certain posture and gait irregularities.

The next three chapters deal with the sensing systems that become very important to the visually impaired person. Through these other systems, the person attempts to receive from the environment and process information necessary for independent movement. Pick, in Chapter 4, deals with the vestibular and proprioceptive systems that supply a fundamental backdrop against which many other categories of information are interpreted. It is obvious from Pick's presentation that there is a close connection with the information presented earlier by Hart and by Aust. It is also clear that while the separation of these topic areas allows for the organization of the material, it does an injustice to the complex interrelation of the sensing systems.

In Chapter 5, Pick interprets the tactile and haptic sensing systems. The differentiation of these two processes is important for the mobility specialist to understand, and it becomes clear that much of what is casually referred to as tactual information and exploration, is more properly haptic perception.

Weiner, in Chapter 6, presents information related to the process of hearing and its significance for the person traveling with impaired vision. In addition to fundamental information about the hearing mechanism and auditory perception, he provides a review of the history of research efforts to isolate and understand the process of obstacle detection. Also presented are suggestions for auditory training activities that can be used in conjunction with orientation and mobility instruction.

Other professionals who work with visually impaired persons will find these three chapters useful. Much of knowledge about the sensing systems needed by mobility specialists is also needed by other disciplines, especially rehabilitation teachers, and to a lesser extent, physical and occupational therapists, work evaluators, training and placement specialists, classroom teachers, and other special educators.

As the majority of all clients served by mobility specialists have some useful vision, persons preparing for this profession must have an understanding of low vision evaluation and training. Blasch, Apple, and Apple, Chapter 7, review this critical area of knowledge as it relates to orientation and mobility.

As in all other areas of human functioning, a person's ability to move independently through the community is affected by psychological and social factors. In Chapter 8, Welsh discusses the impact of psychosocial factors on orientation and mobility, and draws out some of the implications of this information for the training situation. Rehabilitation counselors and social workers frequently interact with visually impaired clients in their participation in mobility training and will find this chapter of special interest. Many of the anticipated concerns of clients and some of the actual problems that arise in training are considered here.

In Chapter 9, Hill and Blasch focus specifically on concept formation by visually impaired persons and on the development of consistent terminology for the concepts most critical for orientation and mobility.

To help clients to conceptualize the environment through which they are going to travel, mobility specialists have relied on a variety of aids and equipment. Bentzen, Chapter 10, presents extensive information about orientation aids including practical information about their construction and availability as well as helpful suggestions on the use of some of these devices. Some of the ideas discussed here could be useful to classroom teachers in displaying certain information to students in non-visual media.

Mobility devices such as the long cane and electronic equipment are the most visible aids to mobility, and information about such devices is only one component of the body of knowledge that mobility specialists must possess. In Chapter 11, Farmer discusses a number of devices that have been suggested and developed over the years, each having their advantages and disadvantages when it comes to providing information that the visually impaired person needs for mobility. Mobility devices are a consideration in the employment of the visually impaired person and should be of interest to work evaluators and training and placement specialists.

Mobility specialists also need information concerning the special needs of clients whose visual loss is complicated by other factors, especially other disabilities. Chapter 12 consists of shorter contributions by various authors about the special needs of children and older persons who are visually impaired, as well as persons whose visual loss is combined with mental retardation, hearing impairment, cerebral palsy, diabetes, amputation, or other motor impairments. These sections do not deal with the additional problem areas in depth, but rather with some of the practical complications of providing mobility instruction to persons who combine these impairments with visual loss.

Medical personnel need to realize that maximum functioning of a visually impaired person's other body systems will contribute to success in independent mobility. A focus of the text on the ability of visually impaired persons to function even when other impairments are present, may help medical personnel to concentrate on the strengths and positive aspects of a patient's condition and make it easier to accept and deal with the negative results of a person's disease or disability.

Chapter 13 by Blasch and Welsh presents the most recent area of information recognized as necessary to practicing mobility specialists. It is becoming more common for mobility specialists to extend their services to persons with disabling conditions other than visual impairment. The authors present a rationale for this innovation as well as background information.

Wardell, Chapter 14, analyzes the effect of environmental variables on an individual's ability to travel with reduced vision. This is of concern to rehabilitation counselors as well as mobility specialists. Wardell's contribution on environmental modifications will also be of help to administrators facing the necessity of making such modifications in their schools and other facilities. At present environmental modifications for the most part accommodate physical and neurological impairments, with relatively little concern for the visually impaired. This is a controversial topic because on the surface it seems to conflict directly with one of the basic premises of orientation and mobility—that visually impaired persons can be helped to cope with whatever barriers exist, an approach that is generally preferred to any efforts to structure the environment to meet their needs.

LaDuke and Welsh discuss in Chapter 15 some of the implications of educational theory for mobility training. They review the literature on this point and discuss how various aspects of good teaching are reflected in the recommended methods of providing mobility instruction. This chapter will interest rehabilitation counselors because of the discussion of the assessment and evaluation procedures used by mobility specialists, which are related to the responsibilities of counselors to evaluate a client's needs and potential and to develop an appropriate rehabilitation plan.

Accompanying this treatment of the educational aspects of quality training, Crouse, in Chapter 16, presents information on the administrative concerns that must be considered when mobility services are offered. While mobility specialists will find this material helpful in knowing what kind of support to expect from administrators, administrators themselves will find in Crouse's chapter the elements of good programming that must be considered in establishing, monitoring, and reviewing mobility services. In addition, rehabilitation counselors should avail themselves of this knowledge area.

The educational and administrative procedures of a high quality mobility program as discussed in these last two chapters should be understood by classroom teachers and by educational administrators. These procedures may tend to upset the usual way of doing things in the school, so there is a need to appreciate individualized instruction and the amount of time necessary to provide the best service.

Some visually impaired persons over the years have chosen to use a specially trained dog to provide them with the information needed to safely move through the environment. While the training of these dogs is not the responsibility of mobility specialists, they should be well informed about the use of dog guides and able to advise clients about this alternative when appropriate. Rehabilitation counselors, work evaluators, and training and placement specialists should also be informed about dog guides as related to employment of the visually impaired person. Whitstock, Chapter 17, presents information about the training and use of dog guides from the perspective of the Seeing Eye experience.

The profession of orientation and mobility should also be considered within the historical context of its development. Bledsoe, in Chapter 18, tells of the early development of this service, presenting a view of the individuals involved in it and how their personalities molded the shape of things to come. As a member of the small cadre selected during World War II to develop the Army rehabilitation program for blind soldiers, Bledsoe was in a position to observe and record the development of orientation and mobility instruction. At the editors' request, Bledsoe has presented for the first time the critical role that he played in the development, preservation, and proliferation of orientation and mobility instruction.

Wiener and Welsh, in Chapter 19, continue the story of the development of the profession up to the present day, conceptualizing current issues and projecting future directions, including the necessity for mobility specialists to be concerned about the verification of existing information and the development of new knowledge through research. This chapter should also provide needed information to administrators related to the training and certification of mobility specialists and their code of ethics.

De l'Aune in Chapter 20 discusses the concept of research as it relates to a practice profession such as orientation and mobility. He reviews problems facing researchers in an area such as this, and some of the efforts made to develop a knowledge base. He encourages mobility specialists to be actively involved in the systematic development of knowledge about their profession. Administrators should be interested in comments here on proposing and developing research projects in order to demonstrate the effectiveness of their services and also to learn how to improve these services.

In summary, it will be helpful to the development of the field of orientation and mobility if this text is viewed as an effort to express in one volume much of the background information considered relevant to mobility training along with how this information is useful to mobility specialists. The publication of the information in one place is a step toward the critical review and analysis of the material with the intent of adding to it and modifying it where it is found lacking. It is hoped that the text will draw readership from members of other disciplines who will then realize the role of mobility in the habilitation or rehabilitation process and the role that they can play in helping a person to achieve independent mobility.

As in many other professions, orientation and mobility specialists draw upon information that is not their exclusive domain, but which they apply in a special way to the problems of independent mobility with impaired vision.

1

Bibliography

Foulke, E. The perceptual basis for mobility. American Foundation for the Blind Research Bulletin, 1970, **23,** 1-8.

Hill, E. & Ponder, P. *Orientation and mobility techniques: A guide for the practitioner.* New York: American Foundation for the Blind. 1976.

Kay, L. *Toward objective mobility evaluation: Some thoughts on a theory.* New York: American Foundation for the Blind, 1974.

Krigman, A. A mathematical model of blind mobility. *American Foundation for the Blind Research Bulletin,* 1968, **17,** 221-235.

Environmental Orientation and Human Mobility

Verna Hart

A newborn infant soon demonstrates skills that evidence a rudimentary environmental orientation. Prerequisite skills for independent orientation and mobility thus begin to develop early in the young infant's life. Emerging perceptual processes are carefully noted by parents as they observe the child. The motor aspects of development receive particular attention as they observe the sequence that the child goes through in preparation for walking. Although authors vary in the relative importance they place on the emergence of different development skills, Kephart (1960) is among those who place primary importance on the emergence of motor skills. He believes that the neurological system matures first in the motor area and that area becomes functional before the perceptual system is ready; also that the areas of motor activity and perception are then both operating before cognitive association develops. The motor system thus becomes the initial system in the hierarchy of development, and the more advanced systems are expansions and elaborations of those already existing. Piaget and Inhelder (1948) agree that the motor area develops first, and future learning is based upon the first motor learnings.

Theories of psychomotor development are a necessary component of the knowledge base of mobility specialists. The professional who specializes in helping visually impaired persons develop skills of independent travel should understand how oriented movement first develops, the problems that might arise in normal development, and how these deficiencies might be remedied. Some of the theories of psychomotor development also suggest that movement plays a central role in the total development of the individual. This provides additional justification for mobility services for visually impaired children at the earliest possible time in the child's development.

DEVELOPMENT OF MOTOR SKILLS

Before proceeding into the theoretical discussion that has evolved around the issues of early motor and cognitive learning, it is important to examine the early motor development of normal infants. Many of the developmental milestones found within the first year of life are necessary prerequisites for future development and of utmost necessity for the attainment of normal motor skills.

Some of these developmental milestones involve the appearance and fading of primitive reflexes. At birth the infant's body functions as a total unit without the ability of one segment to act independently of the others. The appearance and subsequent fading of primitive reflexes aid the young child in developing the necessary motor prerequisites for certain parts of the body to begin functioning without causing associated movement in the other parts of the body. Those who examine the newborn will observe the presence of various reflexes, but the pediatrician who follows the child continues to observe the reflexes to see that certain ones fade at the appropriate times and that others make their proper appearance to positively affect the development of the child's motor skills.

Reflexes

There are many reflexes that in some way give a general indication of the readiness of the infant's body to perform various skills. Among the ones that seem to have particular relevance to upright motor functioning are the asymmetric tonic neck reflex (ATNR), the symmetric tonic neck reflex, the downward parachute response, and the landau. Briefly, these reflexes can be demonstrated in the young child as follows; the ATNR is present in the newborn until around four months. When the child's head is moved or when the child begins to move his own head, there seems to be an inability for the head and arms to move independently of each other. When the head is moved to one side, the elbow on the side the child is facing bends or flexes less than the elbow at the back of the head, thus giving the appearance of a fencer in position. If the head is moved to the opposite side, the arms again change positions with the opposite elbow flexing. At around four months of age the ATNR fades and the symmetric tonic neck reflex appears. Up to this point the child has had the very typical unit movement that the ATNR demonstrates. With the appearance of the symmetric tonic neck reflex, the body begins to show some degree of segmentation. The child is then able to lift up his head when in the creeping position and also lower the tail at the same time, or the child can extend his legs while he lowers his head. Without this segmentation of the various parts of the body the child would be unable to make the movements necessary for crawling.

The downward parachute response is another indication that parts of the body can move independently of other parts. When a child is grasped under the arms and suspended vertically into a sudden downward movement, the presence of the downward parachute reaction will cause the legs to extend downward and rotate externally, evidencing readiness to bear weight. This reaction occurs after the ATNR has faded.

The landau is another indicator of the child's readiness to support himself against gravity. If you hold a child suspended in your hands on his stomach, presence of the landau will be indicated by a total extension of the body, thus forming a moon shaped curve.

If the ATNR fails to fade at the appropriate time, it becomes an abnormal reflex that affects the sequence in motor development and the child will be unable to develop a normal gait. Today, pediatricians observe the presence and absence of reflexes in their monitoring of a child's progress but knowledge of the effect of the ATNR upon the ability to walk is not new. Gesell, in 1938, made the statement that, "If the head cannot disengage itself from the tonic neck reflex pattern this becomes a prognostic sign that the child will never walk" (Barsch, 1968). In discussing persistent symmetric tonic neck reflex activity, Bender (1972) reported that the feedback from such movement is distorted and inconsistent and therefore inter- feres with sensory-motor integration and efficient information processing. It has long been recognized that the reflexes of the newborn must fade and the head must be disengaged from the reflex patterns in order for it to play the role as the key structure in building an erect posture. Barsch (1968) feels that the head must be liberated in order to scan the space field and to steer the organism while Gesell (1948) notes that the reflex patterns found during the first six months of life form the development of eye-hand coordination.

A normal gait demands not only the absence of abnormal reflexes, but also the development of righting reactions, balance, protective reactions, rotation, and normal muscle tone. Without these abilities the child is unable to develop and refine his walking, and progress to climbing and running.

Righting reactions are important in helping the infant to obtain an upright position in his world. The labyrinthine or vestibular righting reactions allow the head to remain in an upright position no matter how the pelvis is moved. The neck righting reactions then bring the lower parts of the body into line with the upright head. The optic righting reflexes are largely responsible for the orientation of the head and that orientation is controlled largely by vision. Howard and Templeton (1966) note that the head always returns to the vertical position through the mediation of the visual, vestibular, and tactile righting reflexes while the rest of the body is brought into line because of the neck righting, tactile body, and spinal reflexes.

Head Control

A young infant first has to attain head control before learning to control the rest of the body. Growth proceeds from general to specific, gross to refined, cephalo-caudal (head to tail) and proximo-distal (near to far). The infant, in learning to control for balance, follows all of these premises by first learning to control the head, then the body in a sitting position, then in standing, and finally in walking. At the same time that the child is learning to balance in various positions, he is learning self-protection from falling while sitting and standing. The child first, at about six months of age, learns to put his hands forward as a protection from tipping forward. At this stage, if he happens to tip in a side or backward direction, there will be no protection as yet and the child will fall. The forward direction is covered however, and the child will sit propped in a hands-on-knees position to keep from toppling over. At approximately eight months of age, the child has learned to extend these protective reactions to the side to keep from falling in that direction and by ten months of age, he has started to extend the hands to the back to keep from tipping backwards. By one year of age he can protect himself in all directions while sitting. As the child develops standing balance, the same types of protective reactions are developed in the standing position.

Body Rotation

Another factor mentioned as necessary for a normal gait is body rotation. As a very young infant, the child learns to turn over by following the direction of the head as it turns. However, at about five months of age, the ATNR has faded and segmentation begins as the child learns to roll over onto his side from the back position by rotating the upper part of the body, flexing the hips, and throwing a leg to the same side. Thus the child begins to be segmentally in control of his body and can manage the turn more readily than he could by relying on following the head turn. By eleven months of age the child learns to lead with his hips when turning over and the body is thus able to function by segments. It is important to point out that the child does not learn to walk normally until he has attained standing balance, has protective reactions both in standing and in sitting, and has hip rotation. These are all prerequisite skills and necessary for a well maintained gait. Developmentally these are accomplished before the twelve-to-fifteen-months age range that is the average age for a child to develop upright independent mobility.

Muscle Tone

Normal muscle tone is also a requirement for development of an upright normal gait. Too much tone results in rigid movements while too little results in flaccid motions, or perhaps in no movement at all if there is an absence of tone. The extremes in muscle tone are exhibited by children with cerebral palsy, where excessive tone results in the "leadpipe" characteristics of rigidity and the child with low tone demonstrates floppy characteristics.

Thus, a child who shows no abnormal reflexes, and has demonstrated the pres-

11

ence of righting reactions, attained good sitting, standing, and walking balance, developed good protective reactions and segmental rotation, and whose muscle tone is normal, has the requisites for a normal gait. While these factors lead to a normal gait, total physical development is composed of additional physical attributes such as:

1. Agility—the ability to move the body through space

2. Flexibility—the ability to increase the range of motion at a given point

3. Endurance—the capacity built by activity

4. Strength—the ability to move against or withstand resistance

5. Relaxation (Mosston, 1965)

6. Total body control and posture (Bentley, 1970).

These qualities are possessed in varying degrees, but everyone relies on them when they perform physically. The degree to which movement resulting from these activities can be affected may also be influenced by body build, reaction time, power, and the acuity of the senses (Broer, 1960).

A thorough understanding of the development of human movement must also consider the mechanical basis of movement.

Balance

A prerequisite to movement is balance, and can be defined as an ability to maintain or assume any body position against the force of gravity (Mosston, 1965). It has been found that balance measures are most predictive of scores in many tasks requiring large muscle control (Cratty, 1974). Posture becomes the basic pattern from which all other movement patterns develop and the center of gravity in one's posture is the point from which direction, space orientation, and movement must originate. Only when the child has determined the line, direction, and force of gravity can he proceed to the development of the coordinates of space around him (Chaney & Kephart, 1968). Gesell, Ilg, and Bullis (1949) state that posture may be either static or dynamic. Static posture is that which produces station, steadiness, and stance, and includes the muscle tone and balance discussed earlier. Dynamic posture translates into reactions such as locomotion, prehension, and inspection, and relates to movement. Posture thus becomes the embryology of behavior, determining the child's orientation to the world.

Posture

The study of posture has been an on-going effort since 1890. No other skill has commanded such attention for so long a period, along with great amounts of time and energy expended in testing its various aspects (Glassow & Broer, 1938). The position of the head, in particular, has been discussed as it relates to all movement patterns (Broer, 1960). According to Barsch (1968), the head must be properly aligned to the body with conformity to the supporting base. Thus, the body in proper alignment is designed to react to change and restore disturbed equilibrium (Freeman, 1948) to maintain posture and equilibrium. Posture thus results from the interacting motions of the head, torso, and limbs to maintain balance, orientation to gravity, and adjustment to acceleration. These interacting motions are affected by the vestibular, visual, tactual, and kinesthetic systems that aid in the positioning and dynamic stabilization of the body during active movement (Singer, 1972).

Howard and Templeton (1966) also believe that postural reflexes are concerned with the positions and relationships of various parts of the body. They state that the eyes, touch receptors in the skin, muscles, tendons, joints, and the vestibular apparatus all contribute to the total pattern or postural-reflex behavior. Therefore, spatial behavior is not only conditioned by ways in which the body is constructed and moves, but also by the nature of the physical world in which the body moves.

Equilibrium is an aspect of posture that is also important. Broer (1960) lists a number of principles of equilibrium among them: the larger the base, the more stable the body; and the nearer to the center of the base of support the line of gravity falls, the more stable the body. Thus, to increase the stability of the body when moving, the base must be enlarged but this must be done so that joint movement is not restricted or strained. Widening also must take into account the force of gravity. The center of gravity shifts with movement, but the lower this center of gravity, the more stable the body. The force of gravity must always be considered when a person is moving and equilibrium is developing.

Barsch (1968) reports that 75 to 85 percent of the adolescent population of this country have a significant postural deviation. This population includes all adolescents but the proportion among the blind is probably even greater because of several factors.

Posture is learned kinesthetically, but vision also plays a part in an appropriate postural stance. Because he cannot see possible danger, the blind child often uses a broad base of support to keep from falling when encountering unseen obstacles. Just as the young child places his feet in a widely separated position and stands in a flat-footed stance, taking tiny steps, so the blind child often attains a similar stance and maintains it into adulthood. Because balance is lost when one's center of gravity is changed and the body falls outside the base of support, the blind child learns early that the broad based stance will allow a broader based support and less likelihood of falling. Broer (1960) could well be describing a blind child when he described a child with poor posture, standing with the feet farther apart than the width of the hips and the body weight extended diagonally outward with the toes turned outward and the weight of the body falling on the arches, the inner border of the feet. A person standing consistently with the body weight falling diagonally across the arch, eventually flattens it and its function is lost.

The flat-footed stance of the blind child is a common sight. The "duck walk" often seen results from the wide stance because the body must shift its weight from side to side with each step and the resulting sideways movement of the entire body becomes immediately apparent. This broad based stance of the blind child fails to allow for quick movement, necessitates an awkward walk, and can result in joint restriction and strains. It also requires more energy than a normal gait.

PERCEPTUAL-MOTOR TRAINING

While psychomotor development usually emerges in a normal maturational sequence without intervention, specific training in the development of motor skills and perceptual orientation to the environment has been discussed by many theorists. The mobility specialist and others who concentrate on remediating deficiencies in normal development which might be caused by sensory loss, other types of impairments or experiential deprivation, are particularly concerned with the effect of training activities on these basic processes.

Lawther (1968) states that those factors developing phylogenetically (postural controls, eye coordination, reaching and grasping, crawling) do not seem to be greatly accelerated by short periods of special training, and that those factors of ontogenetic development (eating, toileting, buttoning, swimming) do seem to be dependent on training and experience. Mosston (1965) believes that for developmental purposes there must be an intentional development of those physical attributes which would remain undeveloped if left to chance.

Oxedine (Singer, 1972) states that research has overwhelmingly supported the concept of whole learning in developing motor skills while Cratty and Sams (1968) place emphasis on the extent to which the child is encouraged to think about what he is doing and why he is doing it. The four phases of Cratty and Sams's training sequences are from 2 to 5 years (body planes, parts, movements), from 5 to 7 years (left-right discrimination), from 6 to 8 years (complex judgments of the body and body object relationships), and 8 to 9 years (another person's reference system).

Mental practice and its effectiveness has also been discussed (Schmidt, 1975). Positive results have been shown in transferring mental to physical practice but as practice is continued, mental practice becomes less effective and eventually has no effect at advanced levels.

The effect of rhythmic accompaniment while teaching motor skills has been noted (Blane, 1975). The use of various types of rhythmics while teaching fundamental motor skills has resulted in improved performance over those where rhythmic accompaniment was not used.

Overlearning is another factor that has been studied as it relates to fine and gross motor skill retention. Studies indicate that overlearning to about 150 percent of the criterion is the most productive for retention, and practice above that level is not likely to produce a proportionate additional retention (Cratty, 1973).

Just as overlearning has been studied, so has spacing. Data indicate that spacing facilitates performance, particularly when plateaus have been reached (Cratty, 1973). Research reports that the optimal remediation of fine motor skills is achieved on a daily basis from 20 to 30 minutes, and that the training periods for gross motor activities should be from 30 minutes to an hour in length, and offered from 2 to 5 times a week (Cratty, 1974).

While Cratty and Sams (1968) emphasize that the child should be encouraged to think about an activity, Schmidt (1975) discusses the teaching of activities through verbal means. Schmidt believes that the verbal explanation may be the quickest way to teach a skill if the skill is made up of a number of units which the learner has already performed. Pictures or demonstrations of each act should accompany the verbal description. The nature of the skill and of the specific learner, and the nature and purpose of the verbal instruction are all variables which must be considered in verbal instruction of motor skills. Lawther (1968) adds to the discussion of verbal instruction by stating that one must distinguish between direct instruction that relates the how and why of performing the skill and verbal instruction that aims at focusing attention on the activity for motivating purposes.

Cratty (1973) contributes to the discussion by stating that, generally, the limited research on the topic finds that most extensive verbal instruction should be offered before or during the initial stages of learning a motor skill, and that it should be given between performance trials rather than during the performance. Not only verbal instruction but the use of sounds such as tone discrimination, localization and objective detection can be used in learning to move (Cratty, 1971). Bentley (1970) believes that language will develop through kinesthetic understanding of the meaning of the words that describe the movements. Meanings of such words as "back up" and "step under" take on added meaning for a child as he relates the words to actions.

Lawther (1968) summarizes the discussion well by stating that motor pattern learning involves the perception of the stimulus situation, selection of the movement, and integration of the selected movements into a unit of action. Much of this movement selection and integration is brought about by adjustment from the feedback of the results by proprioceptive facilitation. Mental practice, thinking rhythmic accompaniment, spacing, overlearning, verbal instruction and kinesthetic understanding may add to the integration. However, as the child's learning progresses, fewer clues from the stimulus situation are needed for a resulting adapted response.

Training Theories

The teaching of movement and the interaction of that movement with perceptual processes has consumed considerable interest among theorists and educators. The possibility that training in one area enhances the other has resulted in several training theories.

Piaget has long espoused the sensori-motor period as that time when motor skills interact with sensory input to become the basis for cognitive development. Other authors have examined motor development as it relates to academic skills and still others as it relates to intelligence.

The basic movement patterns that the child exhibits are of particular importance to those who believe that movement is the basis for cognitive learning. Theoretically, the various advocates can be divided into four groups with emphasis on different aspects of motor development theories as they relate to learning and conceptual development (Cratty, Ikeda, Martin, Jennett & Morris, 1970). The first group believes that all learning stems from motor functioning which contributes to perceptual development, which in turn forms the basis of intelligence. A second group espouses a central cognitive theory where the movement activities that provoke thought may improve intelligence. The third group bases their programs on a dynamic theory where improvement in academic and intellectual processes are derived indirectly because successful experiences in play heighten self-concept and thus create a willingness to try harder to attain academic and motor tasks. The fourth group advocates a theory of cortical integration where movement at various developmental levels somehow improves the functioning of different parts of the central nervous system which influences other peripheral processes.

Researchers have based studies on each of these theoretical foundations. Basically, the research findings relative to motor activities increasing cognitive functioning are of three primary types: correlative studies in which comparisons are made between mental, academic, perceptual, and motor scores; experimental studies in which programs of perceptual motor education are evaluated by the extent to which they change other attributes; and studies of the development of perceptual-motor capacities in infants (Cratty & Martin, 1969). The findings themselves have been open to criticisms on the basis of confused methods, too short training periods, lack of controls of the variables, small numbers of subjects, undifferentiated samples, inadequate statistical techniques, inadequate reporting, and over-interpretation and over-generalization of findings (Cratty & Martin, 1969; Goodman & Hammill, 1973; Hallahan & Cruickshank, 1973; Halliwell & Solan, 1972; Keogh, 1974; and Saphier, 1973). However faulty the research findings, the theories are being used across the country as the basis for various curricula.

Specific theorists representing various schools of thought will be discussed separately as to their specific beliefs and related research findings. In so doing, it can also be demonstrated that some of the theories are built on more than one school of thought.

Newell C. Kephart

Kephart believes that perceptual-motor training can increase a child's academic potential and remediate learning disabilities. His basic premise is that sensori-motor skills are the foundation upon which all learning takes place, and that the earliest generalizations to be concerned with in a child's training are motor generalizations (Chaney & Kephart, 1968). He states that later complex learning is built upon initial learning in a hierarchal fashion of development. The seven stages through which the child moves in his learning experiences are defined as:

1. The motor stage

2. The motor-perceptual stage

3. The perceptual-motor stage

4. The perceptual stage

5. The perceptual-conceptual stage

6. The conceptual stage

7. The conceptual-perceptual stage (Singer, 1972).

Kephart has developed a survey to determine weaknesses in these stages in the perceptual-motor development of children. Skills are assessed in his *Purdue Perceptual-Motor Survey* (Roach & Kephart, 1966). A major problem arises with the interpretation of data, however, because criteria are lacking for interpretation of scores in terms of perceptual-motor functioning and classroom performance (Arnheim & Sinclair, 1975).

Training activities are divided into four major areas: chalkboard training, sensory-motor training, training for ocular control, and training in form perception (Kephart, 1960, 1971). Many school systems have undertaken Kephart-type training programs "to prevent reading problems." While much has been written about the Kephart training and its effectiveness, the results can be summarized by concluding that, although the results of training reflect positive improvement in certain perceptual-motor characteristics which are inherent in the training, it has exerted little or no effect upon dependent variables such as reading proficiency (Cratty & Martin, 1969; Goodman & Hammill, 1973).

Rather than throw out all of the training because data have not shown that it prevents reading problems, it is important to remember that positive gains have been made in those areas inherent in the training. Such training can be of use for children with specific identified problems in perceptual-motor skill areas.

Gerald N. Getman

An optometrist who worked closely with Gesell, Getman believes that perception, primarily visual perception, can be developed through motor training. He believes that the child's growth, intellectual achievement, and behavior are all directly related to a sequence that has visual development as its base. His program is based on the sequences and associations within the first five years of life, with six interrelated stages:

1. General motor patterns that allow the child to learn when he moves

2. Specific movement patterns that synchronize the use of body parts

3. Eye movement patterns

4. Visual language patterns formed when words assist in verifying visual discrimination

5. Visualization patterns when visual memory skills can be substituted for action, speech, and/or time

6. Visual-perceptual organization that occurs with the ability to interchange memories of the original and interrelate them with the environment (Arnheim & Sinclair, 1975; Getman, 1965; Singer, 1972).

The perceptual model is based on four premises: that academic performance in today's schools depends heavily upon form and symbol recognition and interpretation, that there are some perceptual skills which can be trained and developed, that the development of these perceptual skills is in relation to the levels of coordination of the body system, and that the child whose perceptual skills have been developed is the one who is free to profit from instruction and to learn independence (Singer, 1972). Getman is less concerned with the use of movement for total development than is Kephart. His emphasis is mainly training the eye and his program has the basic components of general coordination activities, balance, eye-hand coordination, eye movement, form recognition, and visual memory (Gearheart, 1973). The criticisms of the Kephart programs have also been applied to the Getman program in that the few well-controlled studies fail to demonstrate that motor training leads to an increase in academic skills (Goodman & Hammill, 1973). However, the program with its emphasis on developing the use of vision can be used validly with children who have such a need. Misuse comes in assuming that developing such use of vision will also increase academic skills.

Raymond H. Barsch

Barsch has drawn from the work of several theorists and has formed a movement theory known as Movigenics, a learning system based on the efficiency of movement. Barsch considers movement as basic to learning, and thinks these skills should be sequentially learned. As with Kephart and Getman, vision takes precedence over other sensory channels, although Barsch includes not only the visual channels, but also the auditory, kinesthetic, and tactual as the primary functional channels of reception and expression. Movement efficiency has as its primary objective the economical promotion of the survival of the organism. Movement efficiency is derived from the information the organism processes from its surroundings, and is developed in a climate of stress and within a spatial terrain. Barsch carefully delineates this spatial terrain in terms of direction (right, left, front, up, etc.), with near-space defined as that 2 ft (0.6 m) from the midline, mid-space as 2 ft to 16 ft (0.6 m to 4.8 m), far-space as 17 ft to 30 ft (5.1 m to 9 m), and remote-space as 30 ft (9 m) and beyond (Barsch, 1968). A percepto-cognitive system is formed through normal developmental sequences with movement efficiency also occurring in segments of sequential expansion. An adequate feedback system is critical to develop movement efficiency and is communicated through language.

The Barsch curriculum places emphasis on the fact that all movement must be cognitively oriented. Patterns of movement of increasing complexity explore muscle relationships, positions of balance, involve all parts of the body, all positions of space, and vary in relation to time. All perceptual modes are utilized. Exposure to multiple variations when performing learned tasks is an integral part. The components of movement efficiency are muscular strength, which allows the body to maintain an erect position in gravity; dynamic balance, which allows the movement of muscle to support motion; body awareness, which permits strength and balance in the pattern of motion; and spatial awareness, which synchronizes movement for survival (Barsch, 1968). Barsch also places a child in one of four groups according to the child's functioning: integrated function, when the child performs adequately under stress; organized function, which indicates an otherwise organized performance but which breaks down under stress; organized immature function, which reflects behavior that is quantitatively inadequate; and disorganized or unorganized level of performance, which is so inadequate that it prohibits learning, checks skill acquisition, and keeps the child a poor adapter. Barsch views his program as just one dimension of the whole curriculum

(Singer, 1972). Because Barsch believes it is but one dimension, advocates have not been as eager to claim it as a single cure-all for academic problems and researchers have not been as interested in testing its effectiveness as a single variable in academic success.

Carl H. Delecato

Of all the programs using psychomotor development, the Doman-Delecato approach is the most controversial. The program is based on the theory that "ontogeny recapitulates phylogeny" or that individual human development repeats the pattern of man's evolutionary development. Procedures are based on the premise that certain brain levels have separate, consecutive responses in terms of mobility and, therefore, treatment begins at the level of the neurological development at which the child fails. In direct opposition to the theorists previously mentioned, Delecato (Myers & Hammill, 1969) states that the remedial techniques treat the brain directly, rather than the peripheral areas. The theory encompasses several aspects. The major one is that the child's central nervous system develops in a definite pattern from conception to about eight years of age, with the rate of development varying widely among individual children. This neurological growth can be slowed down or enhanced by different methods of child rearing, slowed considerably by depriving a child of necessary environmental stimulation, or stopped completely by brain damage. The child can thus range from close to death to very superior in mental and physical development (in terms of neurological development), with a slow child being delayed because of a delay in neural development. A child with reading problems is considered to have a disorganization of neurological growth. By stimulating the development of the central nervous system. Delecato believes it is possible to push the child up the ladder of neurological development and help him to perform at normal and sometimes better than normal levels. In the same manner it is possible to increase the mental ability of normal children.

Delecato evaluates each child on a scale of neurological organization that includes the six areas of mobility, language, manual, visual, auditory, and tactile competencies. After the children who are to undergo treatment are evaluated on this profile, they are given a specific prescriptive program based on the findings. The child must master each successive level before advancing to the next one (Singer, 1972; Arnheim & Sinclair, 1975). Patterning manipulation is used when adults physically put the child through various movements. Additional techniques used may include rebreathing of expired air (to increase vital capacity and to stimulate cerebral blood flow); sensory stimulation; and the restriction of fluid, salt and sugar intake (to decrease cerebrospinal fluid production and cortical irritability). The American Academy of Pediatrics, the American Academy for Cerebral Palsy, the United Cerebral Palsy Association of Texas, and the Canadian Association for Retarded Children have all published statements expressing concern about the effectiveness of such therapy (Silver, 1975). Other areas of controversy that have been raised in addition to whether patterning affects the brain directly are the exclusion of the child from normal activities, the lack of research to back up the claims, the parents acting as therapists, and the validity of the Doman-Delecato neurological developmental profile (Gearheart, 1973).

Marianne Frostig

Frostig has been a pioneer among those interested in the development of psychomotor skills. The development of the Frostig Movement Skills Test Battery in 1972 added to her program of visual perception assessment and training. The movement test was constructed on the premise that sensory-motor competence is highly differentiated. Attributes of movement are tested; coordination, flexibility, strength, and balance. The assessment instrument requires very little special training and takes approximately 20 to 25 minutes to administer. Since the sample used in establishing norms consisted of 744 white elementary school children in Southern California, caution is advocated in its use in any other geographical location, and with children of different racial origins or socioeconomic levels (Arnheim and Sinclair, 1975).

Several common variables are found among the perceptual-motor programs of Barsch, Delecato, Frostig, Getman, and Kephart. All use gross motor activities and incorporate awareness of the necessary body movements. All are structured and use action activities in programmed procedures. All use training to improve basic sensory skills such as vision, hearing, and touch, as well as motor skills. Each of the programs seems to be similar relative to the importance and emphasis that is placed on the perceptual-motor areas in relation to academic learning and/or gains. Differences appear to stem from the theoretical modes on which they base their programs, the areas of major emphasis in remediation, and the claims linked to the specific programs and procedures (Singer, 1972).

Various investigators have studied the effectiveness of some of the programs. These studies are summarized by Hallihan and Cruickshank (1973) in their analysis of programs using a variety of perceptual, motor, and perceptual-motor training when they state, "Little may be concluded concerning the effectiveness of perceptual motor training, in general, let alone particular programs" (p. 212).

Taken individually or as a group, research evidence fails to support the validity of the previously listed theories of perceptual motor training. Most studies show no significant differences in academic achievement and in reading (Cratty et al., 1970). Also, there is little justification for the idea that motor learning is the basis for all learning or that movement is the basis of the intellect if one considers the corrective studies (Cratty & Martin, 1969). It is also difficult to locate definitive research studies that demonstrate the manner in which motor activities cause change in any other component of a child's perceptual or intellectual make-up (Cratty & Martin, 1969). Thus, the state of the art can best be summarized by stating: programs of perceptual-motor education are likely to elicit change only in those attributes that are trained for, and are unlikely to result in marked changes in academic success; not all children have a need for large doses of perceptual-motor training; individual needs should be examined when choosing a perceptual-motor program; practice should include those tasks leading toward skills essential for success; motor activities can be used to quiet children; exact impact on behavior is unknown; and games are an effective way to learn (Cratty & Martin, 1969). Rather consistent research findings indicate that training or changing a few simple movements are highly unlikely to modify academic or perceptual abilities or to modify total movement abilities (Cratty, 1974). Certainly more research is called for, particularly well-conceived research designs that can study the influence of the various components of the training programs and can isolate and study the variables. Studies undertaken by other theorists continue to add to the controversy of motor development and its relationship to the development of cognitive skills.

While the questions raised about much of the research and many of the claims related to the increase of cognitive skills, through the development of perceptual motor skills have been disappointing to teachers, the fact that during the research it was found that the training could contribute to the motor-skill attainment of individual children should be encouraging to mobility specialists. Thus in considering any of the programs, it is important to remember that individual programs may be very appropriate to the motor needs of specific children.

Jean Piaget

Although Piaget does not have a perceptual-motor program by which he trains children, he believes that sensori-motor development is the basis of all learning. Piaget and Inhelder (1948) offer a developmental theory supported by limited clinical experimentation. Thus, there is a need for empirical verification of a more scientifically controlled nature before justifying a general acceptance of the theory. Piaget states, ". . . there can be no movement occurring in any conceivable type of behavior which does not rest on perception. Neither can there be a perception taking place without activity which involves motor elements. It is the total 'sensori-motor schema' which must constitute the starting point for the analysis of behavior, and not perception or movement considered in isolation" (Piaget & Inhelder, 1948, p. 14). Thus, while others may interpret and relate a motor base to cognitive growth in a narrow manner, Piaget and Inhelder interpret it very broadly, allowing that movement contributes to knowledge of the effects of movement, which is the basis for spatial understanding and orientation, a major concern of mobility specialists.

Ausubel (1966) accepts the part that normal reflexive behavior plays in the development of motor skills and takes issue with Piaget's theory. He states that Piaget ignores the fundamental distinction between reflexive and nonreflexive activity. He believes that Piaget's description and explanation of early motor development obscures basic differences in rate, patterning, and regulation characteristic of reflexive as compared with nonreflexive behavior. Ausubel expresses surprise at the acceptance, in the United States, of Piaget's views concerning the ontogenesis of motor behavior, especially since the distinction between reflexive and nonreflexive behavior has traditionally prevailed among American psychologists and students of early motor development. He states that there is little resemblance in the behaviors involved on the subcortical or reflex level and the cortical or voluntary stage that follows. Since there is little controlled data to substantiate Piaget's theory, it remains another area where carefully designed and implemented studies are needed.

Bryant J. Cratty

Cratty has been vocal about claims made by advocates of the perceptual-motor training programs. He is particularly critical of the idea that reading or learning improvements made through the use of various perceptual programs are panaceas for enhancing the child's cognitive domain. Athough he does believe that participation in games and sports can help the child in gaining personal control, increase the arousal level, and lengthen the attention span, he fails to agree with other theorists that movement is the primary basis for mental, social, and emotional development. He considers it only one facet in the child's total development and not a central core from which all social, intellectual, perceptual, and academic skills spring (Cratty, 1974). In 1974, Cratty noted that the early measures of competency which are primarily motor in nature are poor predictors of later intelligence. He noted one longitudinal study where it was found that the silent, contemplative, relatively passive male infants were more intelligent in their later years than the more active infants (Arnheim & Sinclair, 1975).

In addition to the effect of motor development on cognitive functioning, Cratty has also reported the effects of poor motor development on the child's self concept. He states that boys with motor problems, as a group, seemed to avoid participation in the more vigorous games compared to a matched group of normal children, that girls with motor problems seemed more likely to answer questions with a negative self-concept type of answer, and that boys with movement problems gave negative answers, which reflected concerns about their social relationships (Cratty, et al., 1970).

Following his interest, Cratty carried out research in several areas of motor development. He states that ideational and ideomotor apraxias, the inability to deal with figures and numbers in a cognitive manner, and disorders that are more conceptual in nature are all related to left hemisphere lesions. He relates that visual-spatial disorders arise from right-sided lesions so that those with this type of lesion exhibit disorders of body image and spatial information (Cratty, 1969). Cratty carried out studies with blind subjects to resolve questions that could not be resolved with sighted subjects, even though blindfolded, and became interested in the motor development of blind children. Also, through such research, Cratty has evolved a theory of perceptual-motor behavior that deals with task specific, perceptual-motor ability traits, and general supports of behavior (Singer, 1972).

Jean Ayres

Ayres, an occupational therapist, proposes a theory of sensory integration therapy. Drawing heavily from neuropsychological research, she believes that disordered sensory integration is the primary cause of learning disorders and that by improving sensory integration learning can be facilitated. Ayres contends that integrated processing results in perception and that the ability to synthesize these data helps the individual to interact efficiently with the environment. Differing from the other perceptual-motor programs, she does not instruct the child in specific skills. Instead, Ayres' concern is to assist the brain in functioning optimally by modifying the neurological dysfunction that interferes with the child's ability to learn. Unlike the Doman-Delecato system, the integrative therapy does not try to eliminate the cause of the neurological organization, but attempts to eliminate some of the neurological conditions that interfere with learning. Sensory integration therapy is mainly concerned with the lower brain, particularly the brain stem which ultimately affects the functioning of the higher brain levels (Arnheim & Sinclair, 1975). Ayres believes that most cognitive functioning begins in the spinal cord, is aided by the brain stem and other subcortical structures, and that the cortex mediates the total effort (Ayres, 1961, 1963, 1972a, 1972b, 1972c).

Unlike some other theorists who believe that all children can benefit from their training programs, Ayres thinks that sensory integrative therapy is appropriate for only some types of neurological dysfunctions. She lists five types of disorders found in children who have learning problems: disorders in postural, ocular and bilateral integration; apraxia; disorder in form and space perception; auditory-language problems; and tactile defensiveness. She tentatively identifies a sixth disorder as unilateral disregard and notes that a child seldom has only one of these disorders. Ayres attempts to overcome abnormal reflex patterns which interfere with the integration of sensory information (1972c).

Activities which are used in the Ayres program for sensory integration consist of spinning in a swing or net hammock, scooter board activities, rolling on a large ball, rolling on a rug, and rolling in several inner tubes tied together. If the body schema is disturbed, Ayres recommends that a child develop a conscious knowledge of the body and its movement by using verbalization while movements are being executed (1961).

Thus, Ayres has taken a slightly different approach to training children with problems. She recognizes the presence of abnormal reflex patterns and her training attempts to overcome the effects of such patterns, not by eliminating the cause, but by teaching the remaining system as a method of integrating incoming information.

Although the major theorists have been discussed, others have also been engaged in developing perceptual-motor programs. However, all of the published effectiveness studies of the psychomotor programs can be summarized as long in theory and short on carefully documented research efforts to verify results, although recent findings seem to be more supportive of a central-cognitive theory of learning through movement (Cratty et al., 1970). This is the training of task specific traits which result in changes of specific ability traits.

The popularity of the programs across the country can vouch for a perceived need to accomplish something in the perceptual-motor area. Future defined studies will be able to give direction as to the most appropriate programs to use with particular children. However, past and present studies, although not proven effective in preventing academic problems or in enhancing academic skills, can be helpful as aids in developing specific motor skills, which is the primary concern of the mobility specialist.

THE PSYCHOMOTOR DOMAIN

The interest in the area of psychomotor development has resulted in a need to analyze exactly what it is that makes up the psychomotor domain. Recognizing that cognitive, affective, and psychomotor skills are inter-related in many areas, it has sometimes become necessary to emphasize one area to the exclusion of the others in order to measure achievement of desired skills in that area.

Benjamin Bloom (1956) and his committee published a taxonomy of educational objectives in the cognitive domain. The function of a taxonomy is to arrange the components of a topic area in a hierarchical order to facilitate the assessment of an individual's functioning in that area and the development of training activities to remediate deficiencies. While the Bloom committee found it difficult to duplicate its efforts and to determine a hierarchy in the affective domain, a taxonomy was determined and the results were published in 1964. The third domain, the psychomotor, presented even more difficulties. The educational literature contained few objectives in the psychomotor domain and so the committee decided that it would wait for more attention to be directed in this area before working on a taxonomy.

Ragsdale, in 1950, had developed one of the first models to help teachers and curriculum specialists classify behaviors in the psychomotor domain. Believing that every class subject included elements of the motor domain, he divided his classification into object-motor, language-motor, and feeling-motor categories. In 1958; Guilford identified six primary psychomotor abilities: strength, impulsion, speed, precision, coordination, and flexibility (Singer, 1972). Kibler, Barker and Miles (1970), viewing a need for a systematic classification of the various identified psychomotor behaviors, formulated a set of subclassifications in that domain. Not meant as a taxonomy, these classifications were meant to provide a framework for examining a variety of psychomotor objectives and to provide initial definitions for classes of psychomotor behavior. Kibler, et al. (1970) also developed a nontaxonomical classification in which movements were divided into gross bodily movements, finely coordinated movements, nonverbal communication behaviors, and speech behaviors.

Elizabeth Simpson

Recognizing that a taxonomy in the psychomotor domain was needed but would not be forthcoming from the authors of the cognitive and affective domains, in 1964 Elizabeth Simpson and her students began developing a taxonomy with seven major levels in the psychomotor domain:

1. Perception

2. Set

3. Guided response

4. Mechanism

5. Complex overt response

6. Adaption

7. Origination (Singer, 1972).

Because this taxonomy has been relatively inaccessible, these levels will be briefly reviewed.

Perception is viewed as the first step in performing a motor act. It is an awareness of the objects, qualities or relations and is basic to motor activity. Sensory stimulation, using one or more of the sense organs, is a part of this level. Also a part of this level is cue selection, when the child must decide what cues he will respond to in order to satisfy the particular requirements of task performance. Translations within the individual then relate perception to action in performing the motor act. Translation is a mental process and determines the meaning of the cues received for action. The next level, *set,* or readiness to perform a particular motor act, can involve mental or physical aspects. *Guided response* is an early step in the development of a particular skill in a motor act. Emphasis is on the abilities that are components of the more complex skills. Imitation and trial and error aid in the selection of response. At the *mechanism* level, the learned response becomes habitual. Thus the learner has achieved a certain confidence and a degree of proficiency. At the *complex overt response* level, skill has been attained, and the act can be carried out smoothly and efficiently with a minimum expenditure of time and energy. Here there is a resolution of uncertainty and performance becomes automatic. *Adaptation* alters motor activities to meet the demands of new situations, and *origination* creates new motor acts or ways of manipulating materials of other understandings, abilities, and skills already developed in the psychomotor area.

Because of the relative inaccessibility, there have been few attempts to assess the usefulness of this taxonomy. Simpson admits that the objectives are complex and include not only a psychomotor component but also affective and cognitive components. However, each of the objectives has some motor performance as its primary focus and the total taxonomy shows promise as a framework for planning motor programs.

In 1972, Ely, Urback, Singer, Simpson, Fleishman, Greer, Hitt, Sitterly, and Slebodnick attended a consortium of higher education institutions to work on a project of national interest, a seminar devoted to the psychomotor area. The group discussed such factors as the classification of educational implications of the structure and measurement of psychomotor abilities; the examination of environmental stresses such as temperature, noise, altitude, and vibration; time and work efforts; toxic and drug effects; and task loading as a way of viewing systematic operation performance.

Harrow's Classification

Anita Harrow (1972) published classification levels in her taxonomy of the psychomotor domain. The six levels included reflex movements, basic-fundamental movements, perceptual abilities, physical abilities, skilled movements, and nondiscursive communication. Because this taxonomy includes each of the prerequisite skills mentioned previously in this chapter as necessary for normal gait, an outline follows. The taxonomy holds definite promise for developing and evaluating comprehensive programs in the psychomotor domain.

I. Reflex movements, involuntary in nature

A. Segmental reflexes, reflex movements that involve one spinal segment
   1. Flexion reflex involves the limbs, arms, or legs
   2. Myotatic reflex, a fine balancing mechanism
   3. Extensor reflex, a reaction of a limb
   4. Crossed extension reactions, causes an extension of the opposite leg
B. Intersegmental reflexes involve more than one spinal segment
   1. Cooperative reflex, two or more reflexes aid or follow in a smooth pattern
   2. Competitive reflex, inhibition of one reflex by another
   3. Successive induction, antagonistic reflexes follow each other in pattern
   4. Reflex figure, interactions of reflexes in all four limbs
C. Suprasegmental reflexes require participation of the brain centers
   1. Extensor rigidity, contraction of all the antigravity muscles of the limbs
   2. Plasticity reactions bring about lengthening and shortening
   3. Postural reflexes cause varying amounts of tone
      a. Supporting reactions, postural adjustments to maintain position
      b. Shifting reactions help to maintain balance during shifts
      c. Tonic-attitudinal reflexes increase overall muscle tone
      d. Righting reactions help to regain balance
      e. Grasp reflex, an involuntary hand grasp
      f. Placing and hopping reactions establish better base of support

II. Basic fundamental movement, the basis for specialized complex skilled movements
   1. Locomotor movements change position from stationary to ambulatory
   2. Non-locomotor movements, those of the body in motion around axis
   3. Manipulative movements, the coordinated movements of the extremities
   4. Prehension combines reflexes with visual perceptual abilities
   5. Dexterity, a quick precise movement

III. Perceptual abilities include all perceptual modalities
A. Kinesthetic discrimination, accurate concepts of the body
   1. Body awareness, the ability to recognize and control the body
      a. Bilaterality—movements performed by both sides of the body
      b. Laterality—movement performed by one side of the body
      c. Sidedness—dominant side takes the lead
      d. Balance—postural adjustments to remain upright
   2. Body image, an awareness of the body
   3. Body relationship to surrounding objects in space (directional concepts)
B. Visual discrimination has five dimensions
   1. Visual acuity, the capacity to distinguish form and fine details
   2. Visual tracking, the ability to follow symbols or objects with coordinated eye movements
   3. Visual memory, the ability to recall from memory past visual experiences
   4. Figure-ground differentiation, the ability to select the dominant figure from the surrounding background
   5. Perceptual consistency when viewing the same type of object
C. Auditory discrimination has three divisions
   1. Auditory acuity, the ability to receive and differentiate between sounds
   2. Auditory tracking, the ability to distinguish direction of sound and follow it

  3. Auditory memory, the ability to recognize and reproduce past auditory experiences

 D. Tactile discrimination, the ability to differentiate between varying textures

 E. Coordinated abilities that involve two or more perceptual abilities and movements
  1. Eye-hand coordination, the selection of an object from the background coordinated with a manipulative movement
  2. Eye-foot coordination, the ability to differentiate from background coordinated with lower limb movement

IV. Physical abilities characteristic of organic vigor
 A. Endurance, ability to continue activity
  1. Muscular endurance, the ability of muscles to sustain their tone for a long period
  2. Cardiovascular endurance, the ability to continue strenuous activity
 B. Strength, the ability to exert tension against resistance
 C. Flexibility, the range of motion in the joints
 D. Agility, the ability to move quickly, such as
  1. Change direction, the ability to alter direction in a movement without stopping
  2. Stops and starts, the ability to initiate and terminate a movement with little hesitation
  3. Reaction-response time, the time occurring between initiation of a stimulus and initiation of the response
  4. Dexterity, deftness of manipulative activities

V. Skilled movements, degree of efficiency in performing a complex movement
 A. Simple adaptive skill, adaptation of the manipulative movement found in Level II
  1. Beginner
  2. Intermediate
  3. Advanced
  4. Highly skilled
 B. Compound adaptive skill, efficiency in basic skill plus management of an implement or tool
  1. Beginner
  2. Intermediate
  3. Advanced
  4. Highly skilled
 C. Complex adaptive skill, performer must judge space and estimate time necessary to complete skills
  1. Beginner
  2. Intermediate
  3. Advanced
  4. Highly skilled

VI. Non-discursive communication, behaviors which communicate
 A. Expressive movement, communicative movements used in everyday life
  1. Posture and carriage
  2. Gestures
  3. Facial expression
 B. Interpretive movement, aesthetic movement and creative movement
  1. Aesthetic movement, skilled movements, effortless beautiful motion

2. Creative movement, performed to communicate a message.

A taxonomy is a framework to be used by educators who are concerned with developing and structuring meaningful sequential curricula for their students. Harrow has provided such a framework so that relevant observable movement behaviors can be identified. Since the stages reflect a hierarchy of development, the progressive neuromuscular maturation of an individual can be observed. Thus, three kinds of responses: reflexes, maturational, and acquired, can be observed (Harrow, 1972).

Validation Need

Validation studies of Harrow's hierarchy need to be carried out with carefully controlled research studies. As a comprehensive list that contains all of the physical and developmental attributes that are found in the orientation and motor development literature, the taxonomy should become a helpful guide in developing psychomotor programs.

One hypothesis about the development of motor skills learning is that the basic repertoire of skills is developed by about four years of age. These basic movements then form a basis for more complex movements and skills. Thus, new skills are simply a combination of old skills that have been combined in some new way. Although there seems to be popular support for this theory, as evidenced in the motor development literature, it is very difficult to prove that it is correct, and there has been very little research evidence to support it. There is, however, evidence that the greatest amount of perceptual-motor change occurs in children before seven years of age (Cratty & Martin, 1969). Certainly a validation of Harrow's psychomotor taxonomy would deny or support the existence of such a basic repertoire of skills, for these skills are attained in the first four levels of the taxonomy and refined in the fifth and sixth.

An additional reason for validating the taxonomy is the placement of the perceptual abilities within the hierarchy. Of particular interest is the placement of the visual and auditory discrimination and the part they play in the hierarchical development of psychomotor skills.

A valid taxonomy of the psychomotor domain would be of particular value to mobility specialists in their efforts to assess the level of psychomotor development of a particular individual, to specify the deficiencies that may be evident, and to plan training activities to extend the individual's abilities in this area.

VISION AND DEVELOPING PERCEPTUAL-MOTOR SKILLS

Mobility specialists are particularly concerned with the psychomotor development of those with impairments, especially visual impairments. Many studies have investigated the role of vision in development. Hebb, Riesen, Senden, Ronchi, Harmon, and Gesell have reported work in the areas of optics; visual psychology; photochemical processes; evolution; interwoven developmental sequences of organismic performance; sensory integration; dynamic theory; and the biology, physiology, function, and perception of vision (Barsch, 1968). Of all of these, the work that relates best to the development and use of vision in developing perceptual-motor skills is that of Gesell, who had based his theories on actual experiences observing and evaluating both normal and blind children.

Gesell, Ilg, and Bullis (1949) studied the development of vision in infants and young children and their observations have withstood the passage of time. They describe three functional parts of vision: fixation, focus, and fusion. *Fixation* is defined as that part of vision which seeks and holds an image. *Focus* enables the viewer to discriminate and define an image. *Fusion* unifies and interprets the image on a cortical level. In addition to these, Gesell lists four additional factors which are involved in the development of vision: coordination, reaching, scope, and drift. *Coordination* correlates the two eyes; *reaching* determines the distance at which the visual system operates; *scope* determines whether the plane of regard is central or peripheral; and *drift* reflects the growth trends of the visual system. Gesell states that the actual visual apparatus and functioning are also affected by such action system factors as age, sex, maturity, metabolism, experience, education, acculturation, constitutional traits, and personality make-up (Gesell et al., 1949). The use of vision, then, is not a simple, single developing action, but a complex activity affected by multiple factors.

Incorporating all of the above factors, Gesell et al. (1949) have developed age norms for children from four weeks to nine years of age and believe it possible to interpret the visual maturity level of a given child by determining five distinguishable functions: eye-hand coordination, postural orientation, fixation, retinal response, and projection. It is noted that the child, during the first year, has acquired all the functions of adult vision but that those functions alone will not totally explain the development of vision. This development is pictured as a growing complex of structured functions which change with the developing and advancing organism.

Neonatal Development

Since visual behavior patterns are among the first and the most complex to assume form and function, vision has a preeminent place in neonatal development. In essence, the child is born with a pair of eyes, but not with a visual world. The child must, throughout infancy and childhood, learn to interpret that which is viewed and to organize it in relation to itself and other objects in the environment. Therefore, the child's psychosomatic maturity influences all visual phenomena, because the visual cues do not automatically report to the child the position he occupies in space, but the visual mechanism undergoes changes which serve to reorient the ever-changing and growing individual (Gesell et al., 1949).

The young infant begins at an early age to stare into faraway space, but the meaning of the visual world begins close to the child's eyes and develops in conjunction with body needs and satisfactions. It helps the child to become oriented in space. "No other sense tells us so constantly and instantaneously where we are" (Gesell et al., 1949, p. 269). If the eye movements fail to take the lead in organizing the child's world, it denotes the possibility of visual complications.

Spatial Concepts

Other authors have discussed the role of vision in the development of spatial concepts. Howard and Templeton (1966) noted that there are three main tasks of the human visual system as far as orientation is concerned:

1. To provide information so as to know where a seen object is in relation to the body; stimulating other senses so that they can determine whether or not the object is moving

2. To maintain accurate functioning and position in space in spite of changes in the position of the eyes, head, and body

3. To judge relative directions and distances.

Such tasks involve the retina, eye movements, visual direction, kinesthetic judgments, the vestibular apparatus, and auditory location. Since man lives in an environment surrounded by visible objects and surfaces which usually maintain a constant relation to gravity, such objects can provide a visible frame of reference. In fact, Witkin and Asch conclude that this visual frame is more important than postural factors in judgments of verticality (Howard & Templeton, 1966). Broer

(1960) also states that the eyes give a point of reference and are important in the maintenance of body balance.

Motor Aspects

Cratty states that vision seems critical to the learning and performance of most motor skills. He believes that motor aspects of vision have far-reaching implications in developmental optics, for he interprets the growth of visual functioning in terms of basic motor maturation, and thinks that it is influenced by current as well as previous motor factors (Cratty et al., 1970). He holds that visual training is an ancillary part of many motor education programs because children observe and are visually involved in the activities (Cratty & Martin, 1969).

Howard and Templeton (1966) note that man has four sources of sensory information which can serve to preserve postural stability: vision, vestibular inputs, proprioception, and touch. Of these, the visual system can process exact information about space more efficiently than the other sensory modalities (Cratty & Sams, 1968). Gesell reports that knowledge to be gained of any point or interval in space depends upon its position in the visual field, and upon the developmental maturity of the organism at the given time (1948).

While many authors believe that vision and movement must go together to form a knowledge of spatial relationships, studies have been carried out with subjects who do not have the ability to move through space but do have vision. Some authors support the contention that it is the observation of movement rather than the movement itself that is critical for the development of perceptual and conceptual abilities (Frostig & Maslow, 1970). Athetoid cerebral palsied children have scored as well in the intellectual and perceptual areas as children who have had normal movement from birth. The ability to process visual information normally has been cited as the critical variable in attaining perceptual and intellectual development if body movement has been affected. However, congenital bilateral upper limb amputees who could not reach their body midline were significantly deficient in spatial ability, even though they tested normal or above in intelligence tests (Kershner, 1974). Cratty (1973) concludes that not all children must use the visual mode for learning and relates that research has shown that some individuals seem to learn best by movement rather than by means of visual or verbal directions.

The question has not yet been settled but is waiting for research to demonstrate the actual extent that vision and movement play in psychomotor development, and especially in orientation. Certainly the answers to these questions have critical significance for mobility specialists.

BASIC ORIENTATION PROCESSES

It is not vision but gravity that Howard and Templeton (1966) believe is the most significant of all the factors in the environment that man uses for orientation to the world. They relate that the eye judges body orientation and relates it to something viewed in the environment as well as determines the body's orientation with respect to gravity. Cratty (1973) reports instructional methods combining several approaches for transmitting information are more effective than the use of only one method. He does not advocate using only vision, or gravity, or some other means of information input as a sole means of orientation, but reports a multi-sensory approach as more effective. Cratty and Sams (1968) see a marked relationship between movement and body perceptions and relate that unless a child can perceive his body parts, it would be unlikely that he could move them very effectively.

Cognition in Kinesthesia

Barsch states, "cognition in kinesthesia is the crux of all motor learning" (1968,

p. 227), and believes that necessary modifications to improve efficiency can only be made if the child can perceive his own movements. Such perception begins early, and the early stimulation and environment of a child has much to do with later perceptions. The exploration that a child carries out aids in obtaining and storing information regarding the surrounding environment. This eventually leads to body image and laterality, which is the directional differentiation that forms the lateral dimension of space (Chaney & Kephart, 1968). Thus, the infant's first crawling helps in later orientation development.

There is a typical pattern of prone progression or crawling in infants. The emergence of the typical pattern depends on adequate and very early body stimulation (Freedman & Cannady, 1970). If the child is missing this vital ingredient, later orientation can be defective or ill formed. Initial stimulation gives feedback to an egocentric organism with no reference to any point or plane outside the observer (Howard & Templeton, 1966).

Geographic Orientation

Geographic orientation of a person that relates to the direction a person is facing in respect to objects on the earth's surface (Howard & Templeton, 1966), takes place later and assumes many forms. The ability to walk in a straight line, maintain a sense of direction when rotated or moved, and draw a map or point to a distant place all involve a different complex of modalities, movements, and conceptual skills (Howard & Templeton, 1966). Geographical orientation skills fall into two classes: those tasks that require intellectual knowledge such as pointing to the North, and those which do not require prior knowledge of the spatial position, such as the ability to maintain a sense of direction when moving about in a strange environment.

Blasch, Welsh, and Davidson (1973) have further subdivided geographic orientation into three components: topocentric, cartographic, and polarcentric orientation. Topocentric orientation refers to the individual's ability to relate his position in space to a particular dominant clue in an environment. In visual terms this type of orientation is frequently used in large cities where individuals might relate their position in the city to the location of a dominant building that can be seen from many parts of the city or to a body of water or a visible land mass. This was also the type of orientation that was of considerable value to astronauts walking on the moon's surface. For the visually impaired child, this type of orientation is demonstrated by maintaining an awareness of his relationship to a dominant auditory or visual source in the environment such as a radio or television sound, the noise from the street in front of the house, or the motor noise from the refrigerator air conditioner.

Cartographic orientation refers to a person's ability to relate his position to other objects on the earth's surface by means of geometric patterns that are reflected in the structure of buildings and city environments. This type of orientation is reflected in a person's ability to understand that a particular building is shaped as a rectangle and that a particular objective can be located by traveling along the sides of the rectangle in a particular manner. This type of geographic orientation is also implied in a person's ability to pinpoint an objective by describing its location as being on a particular side of a certain street between two intersecting streets.

Polarcentric orientation, as defined by Blasch, Welsh, and Davidson (1973), refers to a person's ability to be oriented on the earth's surface through the use of compass directions. But most people rely on a combination of modes of orientation. One might consider an objective as being located on the north side of a particular east-west street, three doors east of an intersecting north-south street.

Another person might designate a location as being northwest of a particular visual or auditory landmark.

Cratty (1971) lists several indications of spatial orientation: rotary movement while standing, perceptions of the pathway linearity and distance while walking, walking straight and correcting the veer, position relocation and distance estimation and underestimations along a line, linear distance estimates, conformation of curved pathways walked, position relocation after a person is led away, perception of gradients while walking, and geographical orientation where a fourth direction can be found if three are known.

Body Awareness

Thus, basic orientation relates to the knowledge of space and the relation of objects to each other and to the person (Bentley, 1970). Kephart says that body image is the point of origin of all spatial relationships to objects outside of the body, and the motor activities of the child are what teach him an awareness of his body in space (Lawther, 1968). This body awareness becomes a critical factor in helping a child relate to his environment. Cratty (1971) offers some basic principles and assumptions concerning how children learn about space. He believes that children learn body space because of the way the child's body parts move in relation to the central body mass, and the child learns that there are relatively stable spatial landmarks on its body that do not move even though the body may move in space. Knowledge of that space generalizes from the body to more distant obstacles and events, and children learn that things can change position in relation to themselves.

Distance concepts must be learned as things that can exist without being heard. Gravity and the concept of falling must be taught. Also as part of space, children must learn that two things can be the same shape but differ in size (Cratty, 1971).

Cratty and Martin (1969) list guidelines that are helpful in evaluating and training body image: initial body-image training that includes parts of the face and names of the limbs; simple object to body relationships; simple directions involving body movements, directions that are chained together; body-image activities (at about age 6) that enhance knowledge of left and right, teaching that space has left-right dimensions corresponding to body parts and transferring from the body to space; at age 8 to 9 teaching judgments of left and right of another person.

Left-Right Discrimination

Knowledge of left and right has received considerable attention in some of the perceptual-motor training programs. Deemed an important factor, much research has been conducted on the time and sequence of emergent left-right cognition. The ability to disassociate the body from left-right judgments in space seems to be an attribute of age. Most children cannot correctly identify their left and right body parts and sides consistently until about seven years of age, although by using methods of classical conditioning, Spionnek produced associations between the names of limbs, their movements, and the visual stimulus preceding movements two years before children could normally be expected to make these kinds of judgments (Cratty & Sams, 1968). Blane (1975) noted that discrimination of right-left followed the developmental course of discrimination of the child's own body parts, other persons opposite the subject, and objects in relation to the environment (which becomes stabilized at age 11). The fact that right-left discrimination of body parts occurs at an earlier age than clearly-established handedness, suggests that these two functions are independent (Blane, 1975). It has been suggested that the children's organization of space, particularly left and right dimensions, is related to the ability to identify their own left and right body parts.

However, Ayres (1965) found that there was no significant correlation between a test of body-image emphasizing laterality and the test score of how well children organized left and right in visual space. Lord attempted to establish norms for a number of tasks contributing to mobility and to daily living in and around the home, and found that there was no relation between measures of directionality and measure of left-right discrimination of body parts (Cratty & Sams, 1968).

Several factors have been discussed so far as they relate to the development of skills that aid in orientation and mobility training. The facts presented indicate the importance of the prerequisites leading to the attainment of normal developmental milestones which lead to the ability to orient and move. Certainly posture and equilibrium are significant aspects and the effects of training cannot be overlooked.

A review of the literature on the effectiveness of current studies in perceptual-motor training indicates changes only in those attributes that have been directly trained. Therefore, instruction should be given in those areas leading to success in developing psychomotor skills. These instructions should be given only after careful planning. The use of some type of taxonomy is indicated as a means of hierarchically planning for such activities and two of the more recent psycho-motor taxonomies have been presented for consideration.

The importance of vision, as a major factor leading to the development of perceptual-motor skills and spatial concepts, cannot be overlooked. However certain non-visual processes also contribute to the development of spatial orientation. Thus, with all of the factors considered, the problems that visually impaired children have in developing orientation and mobility can be readily understood, as well as the skills and abilities that make orientation possible without vision.

PROBLEMS IN ORIENTATION PROCESSES

McGraw related nine phases in the evolution of crawling and creeping in a cephalo-caudal sequence (Freedman & Cannady, 1971). Freedman and Cannady studied the phases that handicapped infants go through and compared them with McGraw's. They found that a critical stage in the normal blind children seemed to be their learning to use hearing cues to indicate the existence of something "out there." Although the blind children could discriminate their mother's voice from all others at ten weeks, it was not until approximately 10 months of age that the children were likely to use sound for cognitive purposes and to reach out for sound-making objects. Once the substitution of the auditory channel was completed, the children were able to respond appropriately with search and/or locomotive behavior (Freedman & Cannady, 1971).

Congenital blindness in otherwise intact infants resulted in minor delays in the development of prone locomotion, crawling and creeping. Despite the absence of visual stimuli, the blind infants were within the range of the 82 normal subjects or only slightly behind it. The study lends support to the concept of a relatively fixed developmental sequence in prone locomotion with blindness itself not a significant factor of delay. In fact, the most striking delays in the emergence of crawling patterns occurred in children who showed no evidence of congenital somatic disease but had suffered severe environmental deprivation (Freedman & Cannady, 1971). In another study, Freedman (1971) relates that the lack of handling probably results in a lack of awareness of body parts.

Sound Cues

Lord (1967) notes that sighted persons are able to survey both near and distant space visually, but blind children limit their surveys to objects that they can reach and to those nearby objects providing distinguishing cues, such as sounds that can be used for identification and localization. While sighted children probably copy the movement patterns of their peers, blind children are not able to do this. Piaget and Inhelder (1967) note that poor depth perception or peripheral vision, inferior hearing or ineffective proprioceptive activity provide error-filled information. In discussing the sighted child, the implications would seem to be that the world of the child who lacks vision would be filled with inconsistencies and errors. Some factors can be compensated for, as illustrated by Bitterman and Worchel's blindfolding seeing subjects and comparing them with congenitally blind subjects to demonstrate the effect of tilt, because it was presumed subjects had relied on vision and were therefore less practiced in using postural cues than the blind subjects (Howard & Templeton, 1966).

Space Concepts

Piaget states that there are differences between perceptual and intellectual space concepts. Perceptual space is much more limited in scope than intellectual space and is ego centered or tied to the person's location relative to an object. Szatlocky (1974) demonstrated that children with a vision loss and normal children develop these spatial concepts in the same manner.

Also using Piagetian theory, Simpkins and Stephens (1974) found that blind subjects exhibited a four to eight year delay in cognitive development. They particularly note the unsuccessful performance by the blind students on tasks involving spatial orientation. Although blind children lack the vision to imitate by seeing, Gesell (1948) notes that such a capacity to imitate by seeing is self-limited and that a child can imitate only those movements which are already in his repertoire due to maturation.

Lord (1967) found that there was a 15 percent difference in functioning between the children who were totally blind and those who had light perception; those with light perception scored higher. Gesell (1948) states that all sense of place, space, position, distance, contour, size, solidity, substance, texture, and surface had to come through the gross muscles of locomotion, prehension, and manipulation for the blind child and, therefore, even a slight vestige of vision is of priceless value.

Barsch (1968) summarizes several authors in discussing the use of vision and relates that it is a dynamic, persistent ongoing behavior in a light-sensitive organism seeking information and directing movement, localizing space, identifying significance, and unifying data from other sources. While some tasks require a great deal of vision others do not. It has been found that the blind perform less capably in some tasks and score at about the same level as those with vision in others. Also, the totally blind perform less well in some physical tasks than do those with low vision. One area where the lack of vision restricts children is in vigorous movement, and this lack is likely to diminish motor ability scores (Singer, 1972).

Sequencing

In teaching blind children, Cratty and Sams (1968) state that blind children should be carefully sequenced through the task and accompanied by explicit instruction so they might gain insight into the nature of space. Cratty (1974) believes that there are marked deficiencies in two areas when considering the total education program for blind children. These are in pre-primary preparation for the complexities of classroom learning and in the preparation that will enable the children to become mobile and self-sufficient in their environment. Poor posture and faulty carriage have been noted among the inefficiencies of movement (Harrow, 1972). The reasons for posture problems of blind children are probably due to a number of subtle factors. Such things as a tendency to place the head on the chest, or to drop the head, result from the fact that there is no need to look anyone in the face; but it also may be due to the fact that balance is easier. So, by correcting the posture, it may add to the balance problems or create such a problem (Cratty, 1971). The lack of visual points of reference to determine an upright position is another problem. The inability to interpret such commands as "stand up straight" accurately, which have no conceptual basis for the congenitally blind, probably adds to the problem (Cratty, 1971).

Kephart, Kephart, and Schwartz (1974) developed a concept scale and noted that the results showed that the body image of blind children was constructed, and that they retained little knowledge of body parts across age levels when contrasted with sighted children. They also noted that half as many blind as sighted children were able to give information about the street. The authors state that the experiences of the children may account for the differences between the blind and sighted groups because the results seem to indicate that the blind children did not understand what they encountered. This supports the data collected by Buell who suggests that there is a relationship between parental restrictions upon movement, fitness, and motor performance scores (Cratty, 1971). Groups of blind children who have had the opportunity for vigorous physical activities evidenced reasonably good fitness scores (Singer, 1972).

Developmental Freedom

Motor ineptitude in some blind children has been traced to the amount of freedom that had been given to the maturing child, with those children who were inordinately restricted performing less capably than those who were allowed more freedom (Singer, 1972). Some parents feel a need for restrictions because of the lack of vision. Parental guidance is needed so they can help their children to develop as normally as possible.

Cratty reports that these scores of blind children can be affected by the fact that what is expected of them is not made clear, and this lack of understanding can diminish the scores (Singer, 1972). This and other factors need research to determine how attitude can influence mobility; and how such things as independence, interest in exploration, self esteem, anxiety, auditory cues, and others, relate to good movement in blind children (Lord, 1967).

Orientation and mobility preparation must begin early. A blind person's faulty perception can lead to inaccurate organization of the home, neighborhood and school environment (Cratty & Sams, 1968). Lydon (1973) relates that one of the main problems of those he works with can be described as experiential deprivation. He asks for a well-planned educational enrichment program stressing concept development. Cratty (1971) discusses how the children learn about space, integrating the sensory information collected during movement, and evaluating the sounds and echoes. The blind child learns that spatial objects and sounds change positions relative to him when he moves in space. He learns that sound cues have meaning, and that sounds get louder or softer and still may not be moving.

Hapeman (1967) lists concepts that the blind child needs for understanding the true nature of the environment: body image; the nature of fixed, movable, and moving objects; the terrain; and sounds and odors. The latter has been cited by Barsch (1968) as one that assists the young blind child in acquiring a spatial orientation. Even though olfaction is a primitive mode, it offers clues necessary for survival. Hapeman (1967) also lists concepts for achieving and maintaining orientation: the path of moving objects, the position of objects in space, directions, and sound localization. He goes on to relate that concepts of distance and time are needed for efficient mobility as are an awareness of the meaning of words; the following of a sequence of fixed objects or the fact that one comes before the other; turning, detouring and moving with and against moving objects. All are important and children must begin developing these concepts early. Hapeman omits the tactual modality and its role in orientation. As Howard and Templeton relate, "The tactual modality has been omitted, as its role in orientation is of minor importance" (1966, p. 1).

Lord (1967) includes those factors included in Hapeman as well as others; he bases his mobility model upon environmental control. The environmental types of stimulus are noted as fixed objects; moving objects; spatial relation between objects; variations in textures, temperatures, moisture, air currents, sound; time as a sequence of events and duration; and psychological stimulation.

Schlitz (1974) in discussing pre-mobility skills notes that body image, basic concepts and abilities, motor coordination, sensory modalities (including vision), audition, tactile, olfactory and gustatory, and pre-cane skills must all be developed. The basic-concepts checklist includes sizes; shape; texture; color; weight; location; use; position, movement; time; sounds; taste; odor; the ability to identify, describe, label, group, sort, order, copy, pattern; and to contrast each of the above as being necessary for good travel.

Hart (1974) has grouped the teaching of these concepts together, and called them "Communication." The words are not taught in a meaningless way that might lead to the well-known blind verbalisms, but are taught by putting the students through simple activities at the same time that the verbal label is given. Only by repeated activities will the child learn true concepts. "Up" refers not only to a direction on a map, but can also mean the movement sensed in an elevator, the sensation of an ascending escalator, the feeling when a plane takes off, the climb into a tree, and the simple movement of changing from a sitting to a standing position. The child must also learn that when you "put *up* with something" there is no movement involved.

Cratty (1971) notes that the children in his study who benefited most from training were the children in the lower grades. Teaching very young blind children the basics of environmental orientation and basic mobility could very well mean serving those who will benefit most from training. Many mistakes could be avoided and many benefits gained. With very early training perhaps there would be no old habits to be unlearned. New habits would have a firm foundation and time could be spent building on pre-existing skills rather than in developing them. It is never too young to begin.

The implications are clear. Authors have clearly defined the concepts that need emphasis. Taxonomies have been developed to give guidance to the sequence for introducing and developing such concepts. Data show that specific instruction in particular skill areas is beneficial. For well-developed orientation and mobility skills, education should begin early, be well-planned and sequenced, and well-taught.

Bibliography

Abercrombie, M. & Tyson, M. Body image and draw-a-man test in cerebral palsy. *Developmental Medicine and Child Neurology*, 1966, **8,** 9-15.

Arnheim, D. & Sinclair, W. *The clumsy child*. St. Louis: C. V. Mosby, 1975.

Ausubel, D. A critique of Piaget's theory of the ontogenesis of motor behavior. *Journal of Psychology*, 1966, **109,** 119-122.

Ayres, A. J. Development of the body scheme in children. *The American Journal of Occupational Therapy*, 1961, **XV,** (3), 99-102.

Ayres, A. J. The development of perceptual-motor abilities: A theoretical basis for treatment of dysfunction. *The American Journal of Occupational Therapy*, 1963, **XVII,** (6), 221-225.

Ayres, A. J. Improving academic scores through sensory integration. *Journal of Learning Disabilities*, June/July, 1972a, **5,** (6).

Ayres, A. J. *Sensory integration and learning disorders.* Los Angeles: Western Psychological Services, 1972b.

Ayres, A. J. Types of sensory integrative dysfunction among disabled learners. *The American Journal of Occupational Therapy,* 1972c, **26,** (1), 13-18.

Ayres, A. J. Patterns of perceptual-motor dysfunction in children: Factor analytic study. *Monograph Supplement Journal of Perceptual and Motor Skills,* 1-V20; 335-368, (1965).

Barsch, R. *Enriching perception and cognition.* Vol. II. Seattle: Special Child Publications, 1968.

Bender, M. *The relationship between abnormal activity of the symmetric tonic reflex and learning disabilities in children.* Lafayette, Indiana: Purdue University Achievement Center for Children, 1972.

Bentley, W. *Learning to move and moving to learn.* New York: Citation Press, 1970, p. 13.

Blane, L. (Ed.) *Development of psycho-motor competence.* New York: MSS Information Corporation, 1975.

Blasch, B., Welsh, R., & Davidson, T. Auditory maps: An orientation aid for visually handicapped persons. *The New Outlook for the Blind,* 1973, **4,** 145-158.

Bloom, B. (Ed.) *Taxonomy of educational objectives: Handbook I: Cognitive domain.* New York: David McKay Company, 1956.

Broer, M. *Efficiency of human movement.* Philadelphia: W. B. Saunders Company, 1960.

Chaney, C. & Kephart, N. *Motoric aids to perceptual training.* Columbus, Ohio: Charles E. Merrill Publishing Company, 1968.

Chess, S. & Thomas A. (Eds.) *Annual progress in child psychiatry and child development 1973.* New York: Brunner/Mazel, 1974.

Cratty, B. *Developmental games for physically handicapped children.* Palo Alto, California: Peek Publications, 1969.

Cratty, B. *Movement and spatial awareness in blind children and youth.* Springfield, Illinois: Charles C Thomas, 1971.

Cratty, B. *Perceptual-motor behavior and educational processes.* Springfield, Illinois: Charles C Thomas, 1969.

Cratty, B. *Psycho-motor behavior in education and sports.* Springfield, Illinois: Charles C Thomas, 1974.

Cratty, B. *Teaching motor skills.* Englewood Cliffs, New Jersey: Prentice-Hall, 1973.

Cratty, B., Ikida,N., Martin, M., Jennett, C., & Morris, M. *Movement activities, motor ability and the education of children.* Springfield, Illinois: Charles C Thomas, 1970.

Cratty, B. & Martin, M. *Perceptual-motor efficiency in children.* Philadelphia: Lea & Febiger, 1969.

Cratty, B. & Sams, T. *The body-image of blind children.* New York: American Foundation for the Blind, 1968.

Freedman, D. Congenital and perinatal sensory deprivation: Some studies in early development. *American Journal of Psychiatry* 1971, **127,** (11), 115-121.

Freedman, D. & Cannady, Delayed emergence of prone locomotion. *Journal of Nervous and Mental Diseases.* 1971, **153,** 108-117.

Freeman, G. L. *The energetics of human behavior.* Ithaca, New York: Cornell University Press, 1948.

Frostig, M. & Maslow, P. *Learning problems in the classroom.* New York: Grune and Stratton, 1973.

Frostig, M. & Maslow P. *Movement education: Theory and practice.* Chicago: Follett Educational Corporation, 1970.

Gearheart, B. *Learning disabilities: Educational strategies.* St. Louis: C. V. Mosby, 1973.

Gesell, A. *The embryology of behavior.* New York: Harper, 1945.

Gesell, A. *Studies in child development.* New York: Harper 1948. Reprinted Westport, Conn.: Greenwood Press, 1972.

Gesell, A., Ilg, F., & Bullis, G. *Vision —its development in infant and child.* New York: Harper & Brothers, 1949.

Getman, G. The visuomotor complex in the acquisition of learning skills. In Hellmuth, J. (Ed.), *Learning Disorders,* Vol. I. Seattle: Special Child Publications, 1965.

Getman, G., Halgren, E., & McKee, P. *Teacher manual—developing learning readiness: A visual-motor-tactile skills program.* New York: Webster Division, McGraw-Hill, 1966.

Glassow, R. & Broer, M. *Measuring achievement in physical education.* Philadelphia: W. B. Saunders Company, 1938.

Goodman, L. & Hammill, D. The effectiveness of the Kephart-Getman activities in developing perceptual-motor and cognitive skills. *Focus on Exceptional Children.* February, 1973, **4,** (9), 1-9.

Hallihan, D. & Cruickshank, W. *Psychological foundations of learning diasabilities.* Englewood

Cliffs, New Jersey: Prentice-Hall, Inc., 1973.

Halliwell, J. & Solan, H. The effects of a supplemental perceptual training program on reading achievement. *Exceptional Children.* April, 1972, 613-620.

Hapeman, L. Developmental concepts of blind children between the ages of three and six as they relate to orientation and mobility. *International Journal for the Education of the Blind* December, 1967, **XVIII**, 41-48.

Harrow, A. *A taxonomy of the psychomotor domain.* New York: David McKay Company, 1972.

Hart, V. *Beginning with the handicapped.* Springfield, Ill.: Charles C Thomas, 1974.

Howard, I. & Templeton, W. *Human spatial orientation.* New York: John Wiley and Sons, 1966.

Keogh, B. Optometric vision training programs for children with learning disabilities: Review of issues and research. *Journal of Learning Disabilities,* 1974, **7**, 219-231.

Kephart, J., Kephart, C., & Schwartz G. A journey into the world of the blind child. *Exceptional Children.* March, 1974, **40**, (6), 421-427.

Kephart, N. *The slow learner in the classroom.* Columbus: Charles E. Merrill, 1960.

Kephart, N. *The slow learner in the classroom (2nd ed.).* Columbus: Charles E. Merrill, 1971.

Kershner, J. Relationship of motor development to visual-spatial cognitive growth. *Journal of Special Education.* 1974, **8**, (1).

Kibler, R., Barker, L., & Miles D. *Behavioral objectives and instruction.* Boston: Allyn and Bacon, Inc., 1970.

Lawther, J. D. *The learning of physical skills.* Englewood Cliffs, New Jersey: Prentice-Hall, 1968.

Lord, F. *Preliminary standardization of a scale of orientation and mobility skills in young blind children.* Washington, D.C.: HEW (OE), 1967.

Lydon, W. Two little, too late. *DVH Newsletter,* Council for Exceptional Children, 18, **2**, Fall 1973.

Mosston, M. *Developmental movement.* Columbus, Ohio: Charles E. Merrill Publishing Company, 1965.

Mueller, C. *Sensory psychology,* Englewood Cliffs, New Jersey: Prentice-Hall, 1965.

Myers, P. & Hammill, D. *Methods for learning disorders.* New York: John Wiley & Sons, 1969.

Piaget, J. & Inhelder, B. *The child's conception of space.* New York: W. W. Norton and Company, 1967.

Roach, E. & Kephart, N. *Purdue perceptual-motor survey.* Columbus: Charles E. Merrill, 1966.

Saphier, J. The relation of perceptual-motor skills to learning and school success. *Journal of Learning Disabilities.* November 1973, **6**, (9).

Schlitz, C. (Ed.) *A curriculum guide for the development of body and sensory awareness for the visually impaired.* Springfield, Illinois: Illinois Office of Education, 1974.

Schmidt, R. *Motor skills.* New York: Harper & Row, 1975.

Silver, L. Acceptable and controversial approaches to treating the child with learning disabilities. *Pediatrics.* March 1975, **55**, (3) 406-415.

Simpkins, K. & Stephens, B. Cognitive development of blind subjects. *Selected Papers, 52nd Biennial Conference.* Philadelphia: Association for Education of the Visually Handicapped, 1974.

Singer, R. (Ed.). *The psychomotor domain: Movement behaviors.* Philadelphia: Lea & Febiger, 1972.

Szatlocky, K. Assessment of spatial concepts of visually impaired children. *Selected Papers, 52nd Biennial Conference.* Philadelphia: Association for Education of the Visually Handicapped, 1974.

Kinesiology

Adrienne M. DiFrancesco Aust

Kinesiology is the study of human motion and the mobility specialist, as implied by his title, deals with motion. Whether he is teaching a basic body motion related to a concept such as "forward" or emphasizing a technique of independent travel, his client is actively engaged in body motions of one type or another. A mobility specialist should have a basic understanding of kinesiology in order to understand the principles that lead to efficient patterns of posture and gait.

Those body motions, primarily related to the acquisition and maintenance of good posture and gait, are emphasized in this chapter. This is done through a brief introduction of the anatomy and physiology of the skeletal and neuromuscular systems, and the mechanics of human motion, posture and gait, so that the mobility specialist can recognize those posture and gait deviations common to the blind and visually impaired population more readily, and have a better understanding of why they occur and how they may be corrected. Efficiency, expediency, and comfort during mobility depend on a well-integrated skeletal-neuromuscular system.

SKELETAL PHYSIOLOGY

The skeleton consists primarily of bone, except in its earliest stages of fetal development when it is comprised of cartilage. Cartilage is characteristically nonvascular, fibrous connective tissue. It can be either "temporary," which upon ossification (a process of bone formation) becomes bone, or "permanent," such as the white fibrocartilage found in the hip, knee, and shoulder joints. White fibrocartilage is also located between the vertebrae where it is commonly referred to as an intervertebral disk.

Variations in the structure and composition of cartilage account for its classification into three types: hyaline cartilage, white fibrocartilage, and yellow fibrocartilage. Hyaline cartilage is very smooth, white, and shiny in appearance and may or may not ossify. The xiphoid process, which is the "tail-like" distal end of the sternum, is comprised of hyaline cartilage. White fibrocartilage is found in many of the major joint areas. It is tough, strong and flexible but not usually resilient in nature except where associated with yellow cartilage between the lamina of the vertebrae. Yellow fibrocartilage, such as that found in the epiglottis, is known for its great elasticity.

Bone growth occurs as a result of the ossification of cartilage. In the process of bone formation, blood vessels invade this nonvascular fibrous tissue and bone components such as calcium salts are deposited.

Bone is comprised of two kinds of tissue: compact and cancellous. Compact tissue is dense in structure as opposed to the more spongy latticed texture of cancellous tissue. Spaces or pores are present in both types, the difference occurring between the number and size of the spaces and the amount of solid material between them. In compact tissue the spaces are small and the amount of solid material more prevalent than in cancellous tissue. Blood vessels are located throughout bone tissue, with the larger but more sparsely distributed vessels located in cancellous tissues and the smaller, more dense network of vessels found in compact tissue.

The exterior fibrous membrane of bone is the periosteum. Numerous blood vessels and fine nerves penetrate the periosteum and pass into compact tissue. Larger but less numerous blood vessels penetrate cancellous tissue. Openings or foramina can be found in the periosteum of long bone through which pass nutrient arteries and veins. These vessels join with the arteries of compact and cancellous tissue. Foramina are also located in the shorter, more flat bones through which vessels similar to the nutrient arteries and veins of long bones pass and anastomose (join) with arteries of compact and cancellous tissue.

The blood vessels in bone pass through a network of canals referred to as haversian canals. These canals extend to the surface of the bone as minute orifices. Each canal contains, in addition to fine nerve filaments, one or two blood vessels. Some canals also contain osteoblasts (bone forming cells) and lymphatic vessels.

Marrow, a soft yellow or red material, fills the interior cavities of bone. Yellow marrow, found in the more cylindrical long bones, consists primarily of fatty tissue and a few blood vessels. Red marrow is the site of blood formation and is found in short flat bones such as the ribs and vertebrae, and in the ends of long bone. Mature blood cells pass from red bone marrow into the blood stream.

Inorganic components such as calcium and phosphate account for the rigidity of bone, and organic components such as collagen (protein) account for its tenacity (toughness).

Joints or articulations are those areas where two or more bones of the skeleton unite. There are three classifications of joints, based on the amount of movement each permits:

1. Immovable joints, called synarthrosis, such as those found in the skull

2. Slightly movable joints, amphiarthrosis, such as those found in the vertebral column

3. Freely movable joints, diarthrosis, which comprise most of the joints in the body, also referred to as true or synovial joints.

Characteristically, synovial joints have a closed capsule-like space between the bones lined with a synovial membrane that secretes an egg-white-like substance, synovial fluid, to lubricate the joint space.

True joints (diarthrosis) can be further classified according to movement:

1. Hinged or ginglymus joints, which permit movement in one plane such as flexion (bending) and extension (returning from flexion) of the elbow

2. Condyloid joints permit excursion about two axes, such as flexion, extension, abduction (movement away from the midline), and adduction (movement toward the midline). The wrist is a condyloid joint

3. The ball and socket or spheroidal joint is that in which motion occurs about an indefinite number of axes having one common center, such as the hip joint.

Also included in this classification of joints, although less directly related to body movement as emphasized here, are the trochoid, saddle, and arthroidil joints.

The range of motion through which a bone passes is determined at the joint site. Limitation of motion of a joint inhibits the range through which a part can pass. For example, if a client has an ankylosed (fused) wrist, which limits or prevents wrist range of motion, he may be unable to flex or hyperextend his wrist sufficiently for adequate arc coverage in using the long cane. Forearm movement may be a necessary substitute for the lack of sufficient range of motion of the wrist. All joints have a determined "normal" range of motion through which they can be expected to pass.

FUNCTIONS OF THE SKELETAL SYSTEM

The skeletal system has numerous functions. It is a highly structured, multi-purpose framework which supports, protects, furnishes surfaces for attachments, and functions as a system of levers in providing movement. Each function, whether supportive, such as the pelvis in supporting various reproductive and excretory viscera; protective, such as the skull in protecting the organs of the head and face; providing for the attachment of muscles, tendons, etc.; or acting as a system of levers by means of which all joint motion occurs, is essential to the total structure and function of the human body. The functions of furnishing surfaces for attachments, and the system of bony levers, through which energy is transmitted in providing body movement, will be emphasized, as these two functions are imperative to a basic understanding of human locomotion.

There are 206 bones in the adult skeleton. A basic knowledge of their location as shown in Fig. 1-3 is necessary, in order for the mobility specialist to understand the skeletal system's relation to human locomotion.

Before analyzing the skeleton and its functions in furnishing surfaces for the attachment of muscle, differentiation of the various types of muscle is necessary because not all muscle attaches to the skeleton.

Muscle can be classified into three groups: *cardiac muscle; visceral or smooth muscle;* and *striated muscle.* Cardiac muscle is the muscle of the heart. Although it resembles striated muscle, it is not included in this particular classification of striated muscle. Visceral muscle, or smooth muscle, is found in the internal organs such as the intestine and stomach. Visceral and cardiac muscle are generally slow moving and contract involuntarily, that is, without conscious effort. These two divisions of muscle differ from striated muscle, which is generally quick to contract upon stimulation, and functions voluntarily (with conscious effort) or involuntarily on a reflex basis. Striated muscle is strandlike in appearance and is found in some visceral locations such as the pharynx. However, it is more commonly known as the contractile component of skeletal muscle. Skeletal muscle attaches to bone and its contraction causes movement. Skeletal muscle can be directly attached to bony surfaces by way of muscle fibers or tendons. Tendons are fibrous (threadlike) cords which can be located at either end of skeletal muscle.

Muscle is comprised of numerous muscle fibers. The outer membrane of a muscle fiber is called the *sarcolemma.* Within the sarcolemma is the cytoplasm, the life-giving substance of the fiber, called *sarcoplasm. Myofibrils,* threadlike structures that can be microscopically observed within muscle fibers, are composed of alternating dark and light bands responsible for the striated appearance of skeletal muscle. Each myofibril is composed of myofilaments. The thicker filaments are composed of protein myosin and the thinner ones of protein actin. The actin and myosin associated as actomyosin make up the contractile elements of muscle.

Upon close observation of skeletal muscle, the striations are composed of numerous multinucleated cells referred to as fibers and are arranged in bundles called fasciculi. The sarcolemma of these fibers has an elastic quality that allows muscle lengthening (eccentric contraction) and shortening (concentric contraction). A specialized region of the sarcolemma is electrically polarized. Depolarization of this region causes muscle fiber to contract. Impulses, stimuli received from the central nervous system, transmitted to muscle, induced depolarization. For a more comprehensive analysis of muscle contractility see *Textbook of Physiology* (Tuttle & Schottelius 1969).

SKELETAL MUSCLE

Every skeletal muscle has two points of attachment, the *origin*, its proximal attachment to the bony surface, and the *insertion*, the point of distal attachment. In discussing movement of the skeletal system, in reference to levers, it is important to remember that the proximal attachment of the muscle is more fixed than the distal attachment, and primarily provides stability of the part during movement.

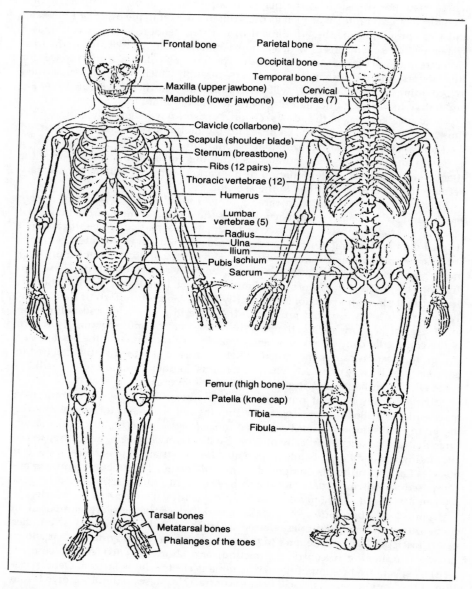

Frontal bone
Parietal bone
Occipital bone
Temporal bone
Maxilla (upper jawbone)
Mandible (lower jawbone)
Cervical vertebrae (7)
Clavicle (collarbone)
Scapula (shoulder blade)
Sternum (breastbone)
Ribs (12 pairs)
Thoracic vertebrae (12)
Humerus
Lumbar vertebrae (5)
Radius
Ulna
Ilium
Pubis Ischium
Sacrum
Femur (thigh bone)
Patella (knee cap)
Tibia
Fibula
Tarsal bones
Metatarsal bones
Phalanges of the toes

Figure 1-3. Skeletal system.

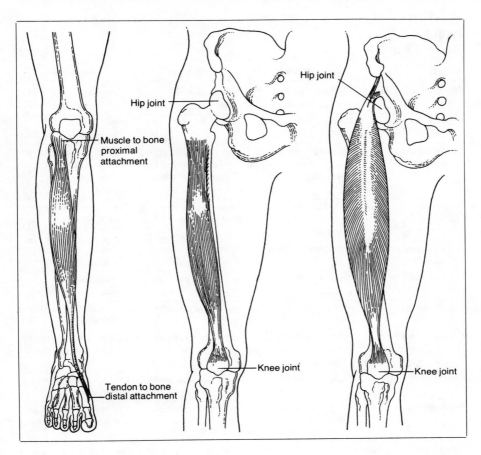

Figure 2-3. Proximal and distal attachments of tibialis anterior. (Drawn by Margaret Pulis.)

Figure 3-3. One-joint muscle, vastus intermedius. (Drawn by Margaret Pulis.)

Figure 4-3. Two-joint muscle, rectus femoris. (Drawn by Margaret Pulis.)

The distal attachment allows for movement of the part above the joint (Fig. 2-3). Depending on the location of the proximal and distal attachments of the muscle, the muscle can be referred to as either a one-joint muscle, one which acts upon one joint, or a two-joint muscle, one which acts upon two joints. In Fig 3-3 the vastus intermedius, a one joint muscle, passes over the knee joint only. In Fig 4-3 the rectus femoris, a two-joint muscle, passes over the hip and knee joints.

Skeletal muscles vary in size and shape. The larger muscles attach to longer bones (lever arms) and are responsible for gross joint movement such as movement of the limbs. Shorter muscles, such as the palmar interossei, which are responsible for finger adduction, are the smaller in size, attached to smaller bones, and are generally associated with the more coordinated, fine movements required of the fingers.

Table 1-3 lists the major sets of muscles, their origins and insertions, and the primary functions of each. The origins and insertions listed are general and not precise. Exact landmarks are provided in *Gray's Anatomy* (Gross, 1962).

TABLE 1-3.
Muscle Chart

Muscle	Action	Origin	Insertion
Sternocleidomastoid	Cervical flexion; head rotation	Sternum and clavicle	Mastoid process and occipital bone
Deltoid (anterior fibers)	Shoulder flexion to 90°	External 1/3 of clavicle	External side of humerus
Latissimus dorsi	Shoulder extension; adduction; internal rotation	Lower 6 thoracic vertebrae; lumbar and sacral vertebrae; iliac crest	Bottom of intertubercular groove of humerus
Teres major	Shoulder extension; adduction; internal rotation	Posterior surface of scapula	Below lesser tuberosity of humerus
Deltoid (posterior fibers)	Shoulder extension	Posterior border of scapula	External side of humerus
Deltoid (middle fibers)	Shoulder abduction to 90°	Acromion process	External side of humerus
Suprascapular	Shoulder abduction to 90°	Supraspinatus fossa	Greater tuberosity of humerus
Pectoralis major (hugging muscle)	Horizontal shoulder adduction; internal rotation	Clavicle, sternum, first 6 ribs	Below greater tuberosity of humerus
Infraspinatus	Shoulder external rotation	Infraspinatus fossa	Greater tubercle of humerus
Teres minor	Shoulder external rotation	Axillary border of posterior scapula	Greater tubercle of humerus and area below
Biceps	Arm and forearm flexion; forearm supination	*Short head:* Apex of coracoid process *Long head:* supraglenoid tuberosity of scapula	Posterior tuberosity of radius
Brachialis	Forearm flexion	Distal portion of humerus	Tuberosity of ulna anterior surface of coronoid process
Brachioradialis	Forearm flexion	Distal portion of humerus	External surface of radius
Pronator teres	Forearm pronation	Above internal epicondyle of humerus internal side of coronoid process of ulna	External surface of radius
Supinator	Forearm supination	External surface of humerus	External surface of radius
Triceps (3 heads) (Long head)	Extends forearm, extends adducts arm	Infraglenoid tuberosity of scapula	
(External head)	Extends forearm	Posterior surface of humerus	Olecranon process of ulna

TABLE 1-3, Continued

Muscle	Action	Origin	Insertion
(Internal head)	Extends forearm	Posterior surface of humerus	
Flexor carpi radialis	Wrist flexion, assists in wrist abduction	Internal epicondyle of humerus	Base of second meta-carpal
Flexor carpi ulnaris	Wrist flexion ad-duction	Internal epicondyle of humerus, olecra-non process and proximal, dorsal border of ulna	Pisiform; base of 5th metacarpal
Extensor carpi Radialis longus	Extends and abducts hand	External supracondy-lar ridge of humerus	Radial side of base of 2nd metacarpal-posterior surface
Extensor carpi Radialis brevis	Extends and abducts hand	External epicondyle of humerus	Radial side of base of 3rd metacarpal-posterior surface
Extensor carpi ulnaris	Extends and adducts hand	External epicondyle of humerus	Ulnar side of base of 5th metacarpal
Psoas major	Hip flexion internal rotation	Transverse processes of lumbar, and sides of bodies of last thoracic and all lumbar vertebrae	Lesser trochanter of femur
Iliacus	Hip flexion and internal rotation	Iliac fossa and crest base of sacrum	Femur—below lesser trochanter
Sartorius	Hip flexion and ab-duction, *external* rotation, *with* knee flexion	Anterior superior iliac spine	Anteromed, surface of tibia
Gluteus maximus	Extends and external-ly rotates thigh	Posterior gluteal line of ilium	Posterior surface of femur and iliotibial band
Gluteus medius	Hip abduction and internal rotation	Outer surface of ilium	External surface of greater trochanter
Gluteus minimus	Hip internal rotation	Outer surface of ilium	Femur, at the anterior aspect of greater tro-chanter
Adductor magnus Adductor brevis Adductor longus	Hip adduction	Inferior ramus of ischium and ante-rior surface of pubis	Internal surface of femur
Biceps femoris	Knee flexion	Ischial tuberosity	External side of head of fibula and exter-nal condyle of tibia
Semitendinosus		Ischial tuberosity	Anteromedial surface of tibia
Semimenbranosus		Ischial tuberosity	Posteromedial surface of tibia
Rectus femoris	Knee extension hip flexion	Interior, inferior spine of ilium	Base of patella
Vastus intermedius	Knee extension	Upper shaft of femur	Base of patella

TABLE 1-3, Continued

Muscle	Action	Origin	Insertion
Vastus medialis	Knee extension	Upper shaft of femur	Medial border of patella
Vastus	Knee extension	Upper shaft of femur	External border of patella
Gastrocnemius	Plantar flexion of foot at ankle, flexes the leg	Posterior surface of external and interior condyles of femur	Tendo calcaneus and into posterior surface of calcaneus
Soleus	Plantar flexion of foot at ankle	Posterior surface of tibia and fibula	Tendo calcaneus
Tibialis anterior	Foot dorsiflexion and inversion	Upper ⅔ of external surface of tibia	Internal surface of first cuneiform bone; base of first metatarsal
Peroneus longus	Foot eversion from plantar flexion	Proximal ⅔ of external surface of fibula	External side of base of 1st metatarsal and first cuneiform bones
Peroneus brevis		Distal ⅔ of internal surface of fibula	Internal side of base of 5th metatarsal

Having been introduced to the skeleton's role as providing places of attachment for muscles, a brief review of its role as a leverage system is appropriate. Considering a lever as an object built for either force or speed, we can construct the following analogies relating bones to levers. A lever is a bar moving about a fixed point called a fulcrum (Δ), which utilizes force (F) applied to a second point to move a third point (R). In the body, a bone serves as the bar, moving about a joint which serves as the fulcrum. The force is provided by a muscle contraction which is applied to the distal insertion of the muscle, which in turn moves the bone.

Generally levers are classified according to the relative positions of the force, the fulcrum and the resistance. In a *first class lever,* the fulcrum lies between the force and resistance. In a *second class lever,* the resistance lies between the fulcrum and the force. In a *third class lever,* the force is applied between the fulcrum and the resistance points.

Figure 5-3 is an example of a third class lever in the body. The weight arm (R) is longer than the force arm, giving distance and speed the mechanical advantage over force. Examples of third class levers within the body are found in the upper and lower extremities where movement of the legs and arms through range of motion and at sufficient speed for performance is optimal, such as pitching a baseball or kicking a football.

A first class lever demonstrates the seesaw principle. In Fig 6-3 the sternocleidomastoid muscle functions as the prime mover (agonist) muscle of cervical spine flexion, acting against the tension of the posterior neck muscles (antagonist). In a second class lever, force, having the longer leverage arm, has the mechanical advantage over weight. It is debatable whether examples of a second class lever can definitely be found acting within the body, but a wheelbarrow is the most common example of a second class lever.

The amount of energy exerted through movement depends on the number of motor units activated in the agonist, the prime muscle or muscles producing the desired movement. Again, the muscle eliciting opposite tension or contraction to

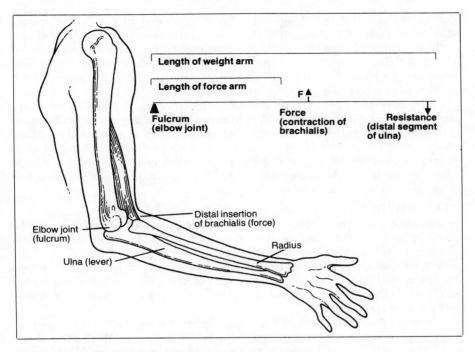

Figure 5-3. Third-class lever. (Drawn by Margaret Pulis.)

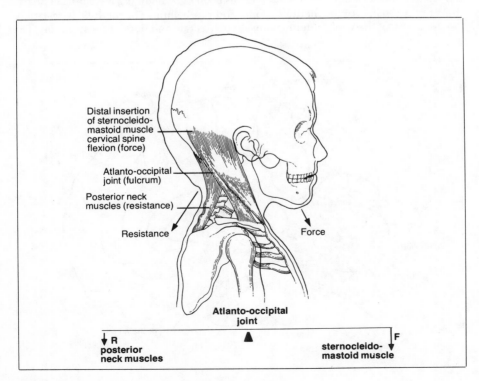

Figure 6-3. First-class lever. (Drawn by Margaret Pulis.)

the agonist is called the antagonist. This is illustrated in Fig. 6-3 where the sternocleidomastoid is the agonist in cervical spine flexion, and neck extensors, such as the semispinalis capitis, are the antagonists, those muscles whose contraction elicits movement or tension opposite head flexion. The amount of force necessary for normal movement to occur is influenced by the action of the antagonist counteracting the action of the agonist.

Nervous control of muscles can be graded from exceedingly small contractions to the muscle's maximal potential of contraction. The degree of gradation of contraction is provided by the number of muscle fibers in a motor unit. Finer, more precise movements occur where muscle fibers per-motor-unit are fewer in number, such as in the fingers. In the muscles of the trunk, the number of muscle fibers per-motor-unit are more numerous and, therefore, gradation of contraction is less than in the finger muscles.

NEUROPHYSIOLOGY

The following review of the central and peripheral nervous systems is presented in order to show the relationship that exists between impulse transmissions, muscles, bones, and movement.

The central nervous system is composed of two defined parts: the brain and the spinal cord (Fig. 7-3). The brain is a mass of nerve tissue divided and further subdivided, and directly integrated with the spinal cord in its function to receive and transmit impulses.

There are three main parts of the brain, the brain stem, the interbrain and the forebrain. The brain stem, comprised of the hindbrain and midbrain, serves as a conduction pathway for impulse transmission to and from the cerebrum. It also serves as a reflex center where vital reflexes such as swallowing are controlled. The hindbrain consists of the medulla, pons, and cerebellum. The medulla is responsible for many of the vital center responses such as rate and depth of respiration. The

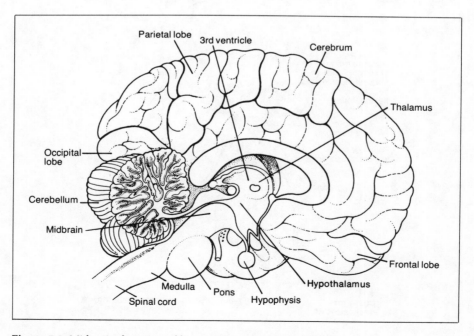

Figure 7-3. Midsagittal section of brain. (Drawn by Margaret Pulis.)

pons is partially a continuation of the medulla. The cerebellum is the primary center involved with posture and balance control as well as smooth and coordinated movement of voluntary muscle. The midbrain, among several functions, contains centers for righting and postural reflexes. Also, as its name implies, it connects the hindbrain with the forebrain (cerebrum).

The interbrain, comprised of the thalmus, hypothalamus, and third ventricle, is located just above the midbrain. Here regulation and control of body metabolism, visceral activities, and the autonomic nervous system occur.

The forebrain (cerebrum) is the upper frontal section of the brain. Its lobal divisions are named according to the overlying protective cranial bones: frontal lobe, parietal lobe, temporal lobe and occipital lobe. Numerous sensory and motor areas lie within the cerebral cortex, the surface layer of the cerebrum. Electrical stimulation of various parts of the cerebral cortex elicits various responses, not the least of which is contraction of skeletal muscle.

The external layer of the cerebrum is composed of gray matter; white matter and nerve fibers are located internally. In the spinal cord, the distal extension of the brain, the gray matter is located in the interior and the nerve fibers are located in the exterior.

The spinal cord is an elongated mass of nerve tissue protected by the vertebral column and extending from the base of the skull distally to the level of the intervertebral disc between the first and second lumbar vertebrae in the adult. It gives rise to 31 pairs of nerves called spinal nerves, which are part of the peripheral nervous system.

The peripheral nervous system is comprised of cranial, spinal, and visceral nerves. The visceral nerves, as their name implies, are those concerned with visceral activity such as movement of the digestive tract and contraction of the heart. The cranial nerves transmit impulses between the central nervous system and facial and head musculature. They are also associated with sensory reception including information from auditory, olfactory, and visual senses.

The spinal nerves function primarily in movement of the limbs and trunk. There are eight cervical, twelve thoracic, five lumbar, five sacral and one coccygeal spinal nerves . . . one for every vertebra. Each has its own posterior and anterior root. It is by way of these roots that the spinal nerve is connected to the spinal cord. Each spinal nerve has two roots: the posterior (dorsal) nerve root, called the sensory root and containing afferent nerve fibers (dendrites) responsible for transmitting nerve impulses to the spinal cord, and the anterior (ventral) nerve root, referred to as the motor root, containing efferent fibers (axons) and carrying or conducting impulses away from the spinal cord.

The cell bodies, located in the gray matter of the spinal cord, consist of a nucleus surrounded by cytoplasm. The cell body plus extended nerve fibers is called a neuron. Neurons conduct impulses. As previously mentioned, those fibers that carry impulses to the cell body are called afferent fibers or dendrites, and those carrying impulses away from the cell body are called efferent fibers or axons. Physically, the axons differ from dendrites in length and number. A neuron rarely has more than one axon, which is long and thin, as opposed to having several dendrites which are thicker than an axon. Dendrites also have more branches.

A synapse is the point of impulse transmission or contact from axon to dendrite. In the gray matter of the spinal cord are internuncial neurons through which impulses from the anterior root synapse with the dorsal nerve root.

A motor unit is a neuron plus the muscle fiber it innervates. Muscle fibers are innervated by nerve fibers. Following stimulation of nerve or muscle fiber, the action potential travels over the entire fiber or not at all. This is known as the "all or none principle." The force with which a muscle may contract can vary, depending upon the existing contractile state of the muscle fibers. For example, a muscle in a state of partial fatigue may elicit a weak contraction. Even at rest there exists an amount of muscle tautness (a degree of contraction) in skeletal muscle known as tone.

Muscle contractions are most commonly referred to as isometric or isotonic contractions. During an *isometric* contraction, the muscle does not shorten significantly nor is there any significant joint movement observed as in pushing against an immovable object. An isometric contraction is more of a measure of force. During an *isotonic* contraction, the muscle lengthens or shortens, and movement is observed as in flexing the arm at the elbow.

It is important to remember that each muscle has thousands of muscle fibers, and that muscle fibers are innervated by nerve fibers. The endings of nerve fibers are called receptors. Receptors are sense organs located on the distal ends of dendrites. When excited (stimulated) the impulse is transmitted over the neuron to the central nervous system. Receptors are specialized, responding specifically to the demands called for by their location. Those receptors located in the eye respond to light, and those located in the ear respond to sound. Receptors located in muscles, tendons, and joints are referred to as proprioceptors and respond to movement. While receptors located on the ends of dendrites carry impulses to the central nervous system, the effectors located at the end of the axon transmit impulses away from the central nervous system to muscle and glands. The path of travel of a nerve impulse from receptor to effector is called the *reflex arc* (Fig. 8-3).

Movement can be impaired as a result of a number of problems that affect neurophysiological functioning. Diseases may be specific to just one part of the motor unit, such as the axon in diabetic neuropathy, or the anterior horn cell in paralytic poliomyelitis. The entire motor unit may be functioning but muscle fibers may be diseased, as in muscular dystrophy where degeneration of muscle fibers occurs.

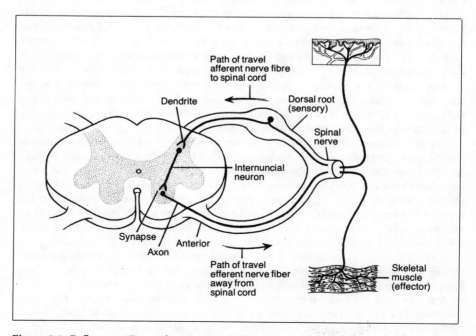

Figure 8-3. Reflex arc. (Drawn by Margaret Pulis.)

Impulses can spread from one neuron to another. This is known as irradiation. Negative irradiation can occur and thereby elicit undesirable movement as commonly noted in cerebral palsy, or in a tense, anxious client. When a client is fearful, anticipating falling, stepping into objects, or being hit by a car, there may ensue an increased spread of excitation irradiation throughout the central nervous system. This spread can result in two factors that inhibit good mobility. First, with a general increase of excitation within the central nervous system additional body movements may occur which are unrelated to the desired activity. For example, during gait, excessive head, arm, or leg movements may be observed which are otherwise nonexistent in a more relaxed, confident client. Second, and equally important, the greater the spread of excitation or activity within the central nervous system, the greater the expenditure of energy. This variable may result in two states: fatigue and/or a decrease of accuracy in movement, which are adverse to good mobility.

THE MECHANICS OF HUMAN MOTION

During any vertical state, whether at ease or rest, some force, such as the pull of gravity, is exerted on the body. During stance and physical activity, a system of checks and balances occurs between the internal and external forces acting upon the body. Internal body forces are those derived from muscle contraction and external forces are those attributed to gravity and friction. (External forces can also include atmospheric pressure, manually produced forces such as the assistance of or resistance to movement offered by a second party—a push or pull, or mechanically produced forces such as that of weights added to the body.)

The sum total of all the forces acting upon the body, internal and external, when permitting no displacement of the body, is equal to zero. When this occurs, the resultant state is referred to as that of static equilibrium (a body in standing balance), or that state of the body during which no one force is out-charging or overpowering another. It is not a state of inactivity, though it is a state of immobility. For the state of static equilibrium to exist, the skeletal and neuromuscular systems are responding to various forces such as those being exerted on the dorsal (bottom) surfaces of the feet.

During stance, when the center of gravity is properly positioned, if the body parts are segmentally aligned with the line of gravity falling in the center of the base of support, it is the body's weight not excessive muscular contraction that is responsible for maintaining the state of static equilibrium. Several factors disrupt the state of static equilibrium and produce movement. Displacement of the center of gravity from over the base of support will result in movement. The direction in which the body will move depends on the direction from which the force is applied. Newton's Third Law states: "Action and reaction are equal in magnitude, but opposite in direction." A force exerted posteriorly upon the body, such as a push, will propel the body forward. In lifting the right lower extremity the pelvis shifts laterally to the left with compensatory upper trunk movement to the right in order to maintain balance, a state of proportioned distribution of the body's weight.

The center of gravity is that point about which all the parts of the body can be said to balance each other exactly, or where body weight is equally distributed. If this point were accessible, the body could be freely rotated about it, as the body parts and forces are symmetrically arranged around it.

At the center of gravity, during the state of static equilibrium there is no displacement of the body in any of the three cardinal planes. The three cardinal planes consist of the cardinal sagittal plane which divides the body into right and left halves; the frontal plane, which divides the body into front and back halves;

49

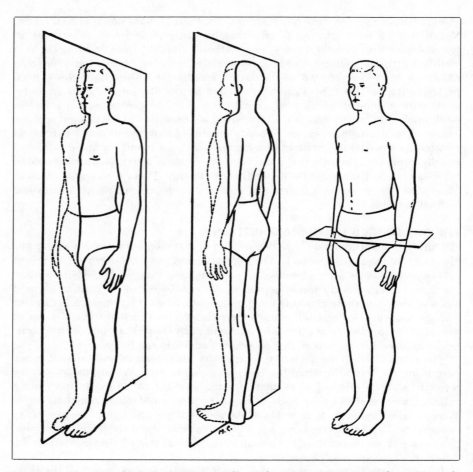

Figure 9-3. The planes of the body. (From Wells, Katharine F. & Luttgens, Kathryn, *Kinesiology*, 6th ed. Copyright © 1976, by W. B. Saunders Company. With permission of authors and publisher.)

and the horizontal or transverse plane which divides the body into upper and lower parts (Fig. 9-3).

The center of gravity can also be referred to as that point at which the three cardinal planes of the body intersect one another. The location of the center of gravity depends on posture and body movement. Generally, in the anatomical position (closely approximating the facing skeletal view seen in Fig. 1-3) the center of gravity during stance is located in the upper sacral region of the pelvis, approximately in front of the second sacral vertebra. "In the normal erect standing position with the arms hanging at the sides, the center of gravity of adult males is approximately 56 to 57 percent of their total height from the floor. The center of gravity of adult females is somewhat lower, being about 55 percent of their standing height" (Rasch & Burke, 1965).

The line of gravity is an imaginary line which vertically passes through the center of gravity. In order for balance to be maintained, the line of gravity must remain within the limits of the base of support—the feet; and the center of gravity must be located at some point directly above the base of support. The nearer the line of gravity and center of gravity are to the base of support, the greater one's stability. In order for balance to be maintained, the center and line of gravity must be more precisely located, for balance depends on a "proportioned" distribution of the body's weight. During a state of body balance, the exact location of the center of gravity will vary from one individual to another as body weight distribution varies from person to person. However, in speaking of "stability" the prerequisite of a precisely proportioned distribution of body weight is no longer necessary. Rather, the center and line of gravity must remain within certain limits and the degree to which these limits vary will increase or decrease stability, a state of resistance to undesired movement. Body balance depends on the equalization of forces acting on the body. Body stability is greatly influenced by the degree of equalization existing among those forces acting upon the body.

The vertical position of man during stance does not afford maximum stability. Greater stability can be gained by kneeling on hands and knees because of a lowering of the center of gravity in the quadraped position. When a child begins to crawl he falls less often than when he is learning to walk. Yet his desire to rise to his feet from the more stable quadraped position is persistent. Eventually the child learns to maintain a functional level of stability in the upright position which permits him to experience the full benefits of the development of the species and leads to the maximum use of his hands, increased use of his vision, and greater freedom of movement.

FACTORS INFLUENCING BODY STABILITY

Several factors influence body stability and thereby influence body movement: width of the base of support, friction, degree of deviation from the "horizontal" travel surface, texture variances, and body weight.

The width of one's base of support, that is the distance between the feet during stance, can either increase or decrease stability. Generally, the wider the base of support the greater the stability. Observing a child beginning to walk illustrates this point. As the toddler strives to maintain the biped position during the first weeks of ambulation, the base of support is wide in order to increase stability. Progressively, as the child becomes more experienced and with practice in standing and in ambulating, the base of support narrows. One's base of support can increase not only by positioning of the feet, but also with the addition of another point of support. For some people the use of a standard orthopedic cane serves as another point of support to gain additional stability during stance and gait.

External forces, such as friction, and the travel surface's degree of deviation from the "horizontal" directly affect stability. Friction is that force exerted between the feet and their surface of contact. A dry, gritty cement sidewalk affords greater friction beneath one's feet than wet, smooth asphalt. A horizontal plane, as opposed to a parallel surface deviation such as a slanting driveway or ramp, and firm textured surfaces such as concrete and asphalt, as opposed to soft shoulders, dirt, and gravel roads afford greater stability to the body during stance and gait. The heavier the body's weight, the greater the force exerted between the foot and the surface of contact, and the greater the stability. Heavier bodies afford greater resistance to loss of stability. Where there are uncontrolled, involuntary body movements, as in various neurological diseases such as spastic cerebral palsy, stability of the body becomes more of a premium than a constant.

KINETICS AND KINEMATICS

Kinetics is the study of those internal and external forces acting on the body which either serve to disrupt body equilibrium or return the body to a state of

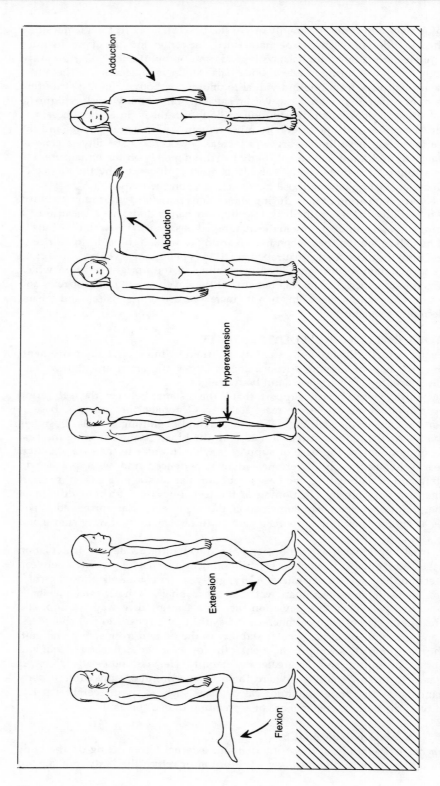

Figure 10-3. Flexion, extension, hyperextension, abduction, and adduction. (Drawn by Margaret Pulis.)

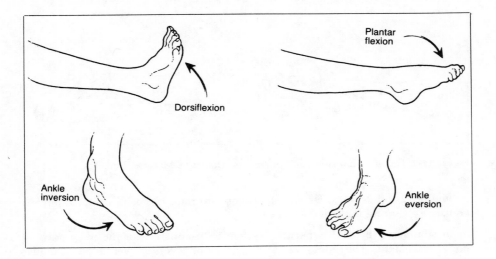

Figure 11-3. Dorsiflexion, plantar flexion, ankle inversion, and ankle eversion. (Drawn by Margaret Pulis.)

equilibrium. It is the study of bodies in motion as related to the forces acting on them. *Kinematics* is the study of bodies in motion without reference to the forces acting on them. In kinematics, for the purposes of this presentation, the observer is concerned with the position and range of joint motion, or location of other parts of the body, such as the knee joint during movement. For example, the observer is concerned with the position and range of motion of the knee joint at heel-off in a kinematic study, as opposed to interest in the forces acting upon the knee joint at that same moment in a kinetic study. The mobility specialist is likely to identify more readily those problems related to position change and joint range of motion, such as the presence of a joint contracture (fixed position) which impedes normal range of motion of a part, as opposed to problems directly related to forces acting upon body parts. In kinematics, surface body landmarks may be plotted on the subject and, by various methods of observation and photography, angular changes of the joints or paths of movement of body landmarks, such as the path of movement of the head during gait, can be recorded and studied.

The integration of the above components is necessary for the understanding of movement. In addition to these components, several terms are essential to analyze and describe various movements of particular interest to the mobility specialist. They are dynamic terms of motion as indicated by the direction of the arrows in Figs. 10-3 through 12-3. When the movement is stopped and the part held within a particular range, the term becomes static—a nonmoving, position term. For example, in the sentence, "The elbow is flexed," the word flexed denotes a position, as opposed to the word "flexion" which implies a state of motion.

Figure 10-3 illustrates: *flexion*—the angle of the joint decreases; *extension*—return from flexion; *hyper-extension*—extension beyond the neutral position; *abduction*—movement away from the midline of the body; *adduction*—movement toward the midline of the body.

Figure 11-3 illustrates: *dorsiflexion*—upward flexion of the foot; *plantar flexion*—downward movement of the foot (also referred to as foot extension); *ankle inversion*—turning the foot inward toward the midline; *ankle eversion*—turning the foot outward away from the midline.

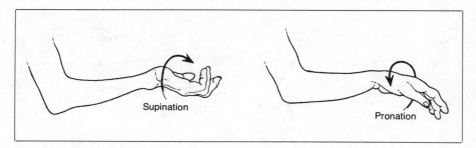

Figure 12-3. Forearm supination and pronation. (Drawn by Margaret Pulis.)

Figure 12-3 illustrates: *forearm supination*—turning the palm upward; *forearm pronation*—turning the palm downward.

In summary, the central nervous system is responsible for the integration of body movement. The bones act as a system of levers powered by muscular contractions which cause movement of bones about the joints. All body movements revolve about joints as previously described: about one axis as in the hinge joint; two axes as in the condyloid joint, or about three main axes as found in the ball and socket joints of the hips and shoulders. All of these joints have a normal range of motion through which they are expected to pass, the limitation of which will impede function of the body part involved.

THE MECHANICS OF GOOD POSTURE

The body in good segmental alignment provides for a more efficient maintenance of static equilibrium and aids efficiency in mobility. Posture, whether dynamic as observed with the body in motion, or static as observed with the body at rest, is an attitude involving an arrangement of the body parts. Before gait or stance some form of vertical, skeletal alignment must occur in order for man to advance from the quadraped to biped position. For the purposes of knowledgeable observation and evaluation, the mechanical aspects of good posture will be presented.

Good posture involves proper, segmental alignment of the body parts (Figs. 13-3 and 14-3). The line superimposed on the illustration is a plumb line, suspended from above the head and weighted distally. Note the vertical arrangement of the given body landmarks. The arrangement of body landmarks in relation to a plumb line provides more objectivity in comparing a given posture to the "norms" of good posture than through simple observation alone. For good posture to be maintained in all body states, whether dynamic or static, there must be a balance of those forces acting upon the body, a proper distribution of the body's weight about the joints, adequate joint range of motion, and the presence or absence of certain reflexes appropriate or inappropriate to the assumed state. In addition, the subject must possess adequate kinesthetic and body image awareness and accurate concepts relevant to the postural state being assumed.

During a state of "static-stance," which by true definition of the word "static" would be impossible to obtain or maintain as some body movement is generally observed during any state, good posture is more dependent upon the external forces acting upon the body, and balanced distribution of the body's weight, than by internal forces elicited by excessive muscle contractions. When the center of gravity is maintained over the base of support during stance, then it is the body's weight in response to external forces such as gravity and friction, and not excessive contraction of the muscles of the back, hip, and knees which maintain these parts in

54

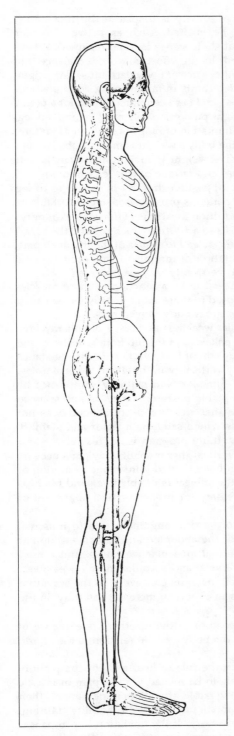

Figure 13-3. Anatomical structures that coincide with line of reference.

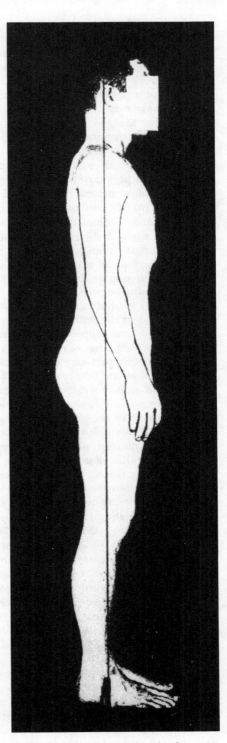

Figure 14-3. Surface landmarks that coincide with line of reference.

good segmental alignment. If the center of gravity is displaced during "static" stance, then compensatory forces must be elicited, such as active muscular contractions (internal forces), if the state of static stance is to be regained. Where muscle activity is compensatory, elicited in an effort to counterbalance the excessive or incomplete functioning of another force or body part, muscular fatigue or undue joint stress may occur that are deterrents in maintaining good posture.

A person who sustains a fractured right leg and has been immobilized for a period of time is not likely to distribute body weight proportionately over the injured leg, either due to pain, muscular weakness, or limitation of range of motion. Therefore, during stance, shift in the distribution of the body's weight is made to the left leg, which disrupts body verticality. If excessive weight is maintained over the left lower leg for a period of time, undue stress and fatigue of this leg can occur.

Compensatory muscular activity of the opposite extremity in instances of leg amputation may be continuous where the patient's prosthesis is uncomfortable or malfunctioning. General body fatigue, in addition to fatigue of the good extremity, is common, particularly if the patient persists in activities which require the biped position. Persistent fatigue, stress and pain can lead to disuse of the involved part, and further result in atrophy, and/or limitation of motion. If this occurs, one's ability to even assume, let alone maintain, verticality may be hindered.

Postural adjustments are generally believed to be a function of those muscles more centrally located in the body, as opposed to those more distally located such as the muscles of the limbs responsible for gross body movements.

In multiply handicapped clients a muscular weakness as a result of poliomyelitis; a limitation of joint range of motion such as ankelosis of the hip from arthritis; or the absence of a body part may result in disruption of body verticality during stance and/or gait. In attempting to establish body verticality in these and like examples, function and stability may be inhibited. Function and stability should not be sacrificed in pursuit of a cosmetically acceptable posture. It may be necessary to settle for less than the "norm," as long as that accepted postural state does not interfere with safety in travel. In instances where safety is a factor and stability cannot be maintained, a comprehensive mobility program is not feasible.

Figure 15-3 illustrates the disruption of vertical alignment of body parts because of hip and knee flexion contractures which have limited joint range of motion of hip and knee extension. In this instance, the subject is unable to extend his hips and knees to the degree of extension necessary for proper vertical alignment of these parts in relation to the upper trunk.

Figure 16-3 illustrates the disruption of vertical alignment due to muscular weakness. In this photograph protrusion of the abdomen and associated lumbar lordosis, which are associated with abdominal muscular weakness, and a mild dorsal kyphosis, associated with dorsal, cervical and scapular muscle weakness, are evident. Lumbar lordosis is an abnormal increase, concavely, in the curvature of the lumbar spine, and dorsal kyphosis is an abnormal increase, convexly, in the curvature of the thoracic spine.

Figure 17-3 illustrates fairly standard posture. Although there is evidence of mild dorsal kyphosis and lumbar lordosis, the body parts in relation to the plumb line are closely accurate.

Generally it is the exception rather than the rule to hear a client complain of poor posture. Rather, his complaint is likely to be related to joint pain or muscle fatigue. If the complaint is due to a reversible (functional) deviation, then correction certainly should be considered in conjunction with mobility training, providing that the deviation is not compensatory. If the deviation is compensatory, even though reversible, correction may pose more difficulties than there are in allowing the deviation to persist. The experience and the input of physical

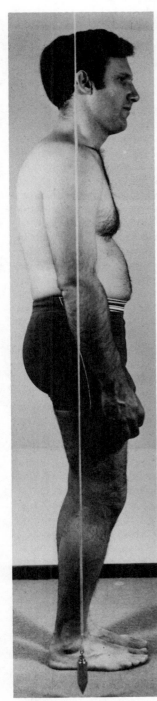

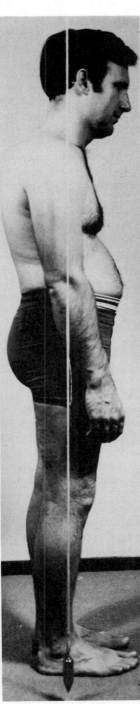

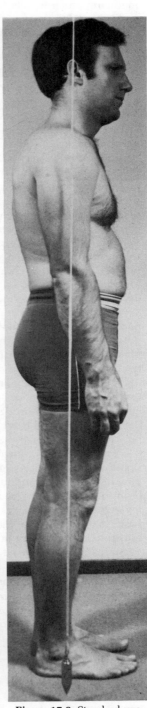

Figure 15-3. Disruption of alignment because of hip and knee flexion.

Figure 16-3. Disruption of alignment because of muscular weakness.

Figure 17-3. Standard posture.

medicine professionals serves best in evaluating such situations.

Miller (1967) states that treating functional postural deviations as isolated conditions is a disservice to the visually impaired person if the deviation is compensatory to his visual loss.

ROLE OF THE REFLEXES IN POSTURE

In rising to his feet, the biped position, man passes through various stages of development. He progresses from the prone (stomach lying) and supine (back lying) apedal, infant positions, through the creeping/crawling, quadraped position to that of vertical alignment or biped stance. To pass from one stage to another, specific reflex development occurs in conjunction with motor development and the maturation of the central nervous system. Fiorentino (1974) lists three levels of reflexive development and the corresponding levels of central nervous system maturation and motor development. She emphasizes the importance of the presence or absence of specific reflexes during motor development. Positive reactions, movements characteristic of a given reflex, if persistent beyond the corresponding level of central nervous system maturation (that area in the central nervous system "housing" the reflex) are regarded as abnormal and can result in the inhibition of normal sequential motor development. For example, if primitive reflexes housed at the brain stem level, such as the asymmetrical tonic neck reflex, are persistent beyond six months of age, this may be an indication of an arrest or delay in motor development at brain stem level. Therefore, at one period, the first six months of life, the presence of the asymmetrical tonic neck reflex is considered normal, but beyond that point, it is regarded as abnormal and inhibitory to progressive motor growth and development. The asymmetrical tonic neck reflex is illustrated in Fig. 18-3. Upon the head being turned to one side, the child extends the arm and leg on the side to which the face is turned and flexes the arm and leg on the opposite side. Fiorentino (1974) referred to the brain stem reflexes as "static" postural reflexes, because they effect changes in body position at the apedal level, either through proprioceptive stimulation in the cervical area, such as the turning of one's head, or through stimulation of the vestibular apparatus—the network of canals making up the inner ear.

Postural reflexes contribute to muscle tone throughout the body and respond to vestibular stimulation. Such reflexes are responsive to changes of head and body positions in space, and to proprioceptive stimulation such as the turning of one's head in relation to the body which stimulates the neck proprioceptors. Siegel (1970) reviews postural reflexes, citing various studies which "link" tonic neck and vestibular reflexes to the regulation of trunk and head movement to motor coordination necessary in dynamic posture.

Spinal reflexes housed in the distal area of the pons are also primitive reflexes, coordinating flexion and extension patterns of the lower extremities. Fiorentino (1974) points out that complete domination by either the spinal or brain stem reflexes results in a permanent apedal position. Diminution and consequent extinction of these reflexes must occur if man is to progress to the next area of postural development, that of the quadraped, successfully.

Briefly, the righting reactions, the development of which are imperative to the quadraped position, are convened at the midbrain level. They are the reflexes essentially responsible for head-to-body relationship in space and to each other as a functional mobile unit. As opposed to the primitive reflexes, it is imperative to normal sequential motor development that some of these reflexes (reactions) persist throughout life. For instance, if it were not for the persistence of the labyrinth righting reflex responsible for righting the head when body position is changed, such as when the body is tilted forward or laterally, one might completely

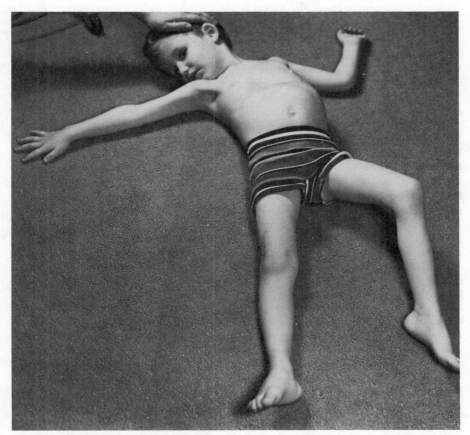

Figure 18-3. Asymmetric tonic neck reflex.

lose balance in sudden contact of a decline underfoot disrupting vertical alignment. This is also an illustration of the role reflexes play in the "reestablishment"
of good posture.

Finally, the development of the equilibrium reflexes advances man to the biped
position. Once developed, positive reaction to these reflexes should persist
throughout life. Without their persistence, static equilibrium could not be
achieved or maintained, nor could any state of body balance or stability be
maintained in response to changes of position.

The development of the equilibrium reactions corresponds with motor development resulting in stance and gait. Equilibrium reflexes are associated with
the development of the cerebellum. A lesion at any one of the previously
mentioned levels of the central nervous system can either delay or inhibit
corresponding reflex and motor development, or, the corresponding reflex, once
diminished through the development of a higher cortical area, may again manifest
itself and produce undesired reflex reactions that inhibit or prevent functional
body movement or maintenance of good posture, if indeed the attitude of good
posture can even be assumed.

Kinesthetic awareness plays a vital role in the development and maintenance of
good posture. An accurate concept of position, whether it be "verticality"
(referring to the state of being perpendicular to a horizontal component, such as

the ground), or the displacement of verticality in either of the body planes, is essential if functional postural deviations are to be improved upon or corrected.

A "functional" deviation is one observed during a given function or position, such as stance or gait, but not otherwise present when a change of that given function or position occurs. For example, during stance a functional scoliosis (abnormal S-shaped lateral curvature of the spine) may be evident in a subject, but is no longer evident when the subject hangs from an overhead trapeze without support.

A structural deviation differs from that of a functional deviation in that it involves a deviation in the normal arrangement of the anatomical parts, such as a bony deformity of the spinal column, which is evident despite a change in function or position. In the previously cited example, the scoliosis, if structural in nature, will remain evident even though the subject is hanging from a trapeze. Surgical intervention is often necessary in the correction of a structural deviation, whereas education and exercise may be adequate in the treatment of a functional deviation.

Accurate perception of verticality is a function of visual and kinesthetic awareness. Inability to discern "vertical" as being different from other positions is at best difficult when one cannot accurately assess his position in space, and lacks the visual cues that readily illustrate verticality for the sighted. In hemiplegia, following a cerebral vascular accident (stroke), visual perception problems are common, not only in regard to the discrimination of vertical planes; depth and horizonal perception may also be lost or impaired. Also, where the visual field is affected (homonymous hemianipia), the patient is required to turn his head on a vertical plane in order to see where he is going, which disrupts vertical alignment of the head in relation to the rest of the body. Siegel (1970) emphasizes the importance of head and body position in the assessment of verticality in the absence of visual cues. He states that minor changes in head and body posture from the upright position in the absence of vision ". . . had very disturbing effects on the subject's ability to orient to the vertical . . ." (p. 17). Miller (1967) relates poor posture in blind subjects to neurological disintegration, which would include the vision and position senses. She stated that neurological integration is greatly maintained by vision, and that blindness significantly disrupts neurological integration as revealed in the posture and mobility of the blind.

In the sensory area, neurological integration involves vision, position, and motion senses among others. Relative to the long cane as a prosthetic device, ". . . an extension of the index finger . . .," Miller (1967) views the long cane as an aid through which kinesthetic and visual losses are compensated for in part. With proper use of the long cane, the blind client can establish the distance between himself and his cane, and is aware of changes in the terrain, whether they are depth changes or changes in the horizontal component of surfaces, in time to react appropriately. Allowing "reaction time," and supplying information to assist in kinesthetic awareness are two of the greatest assets of the long cane, which in turn give a client increased confidence and security resulting in an attitude or emotional state optimal not only for good posture but also for good gait patterns.

The image one has of his body is believed to influence his perception of verticality, together with his image of the space around him. If a client has little or no conscious awareness of the relationship of his parts, such as his head to the whole of his body, he cannot be expected to align his body parts properly in an attempt to gain and maintain accurate vertical alignment. Also, void of an accurate understanding of concepts pertinent to good posture and gait, such as knowledge of self (self-concept), and non-self (concepts of space and objects external to self), it should not be surprising that a visually impaired or blind client is unable to position and move himself accurately in relation to space.

BODY IMAGE AND ATTITUDE

An inaccurate assessment of body image can be debilitating as a lack of body image. If one's idea of himself is thwarted, frustrated, insignificant, and small, these feelings may well be reflected in the postural states he assumes. That one's posture reflects his attitude is certainly a valid consideration. For example, one's emotional state, such as fear and tenseness, may be revealed through a rigid type posture, with isometric muscular contractions such as the persistent clenched fist. Brunnstrom (1972) notes that higher tension values exist in isometric than in isotonic contractions. Fatigue is an end product of tension and can result in poor posture.

What is considered good posture at one age may not necessarily be acceptable at another age. The posture of a toddler, the wide base of support, body inclined forward, protruding abdomen, knock knees and flat feet, should not be noted in the posture of an older child, adolescent, or young adult. However, some of the postural characteristics of the toddler may be observed in the elderly, such as the reappearance of the wide base of support and the forward leaning of the body.

Regardless of one's body type, mesomorphic, muscular, athletic type; ectomorphic, more slender type; endomorphic, heavier, but less muscular type, with particular enlargement of the trunk and thighs, the given landmarks for correct posture (Fig. 14-3) should be applied. In the extreme endomorphic subject, these landmarks may be more difficult to observe, and one may have to rely on body curvatures, such as in approximating the location of the hip joint, to assess the alignment of the body part to the plumb line.

Both a lateral observation and an anterior-posterior observation of the client using the plumb line, are beneficial in assessing posture. In the anterior-posterior plumb line observation, the existence or absence of body symmetry, such as the height of the hips and shoulders, should be noted. Additional analyses of the observations to be made in the anterior-posterior and lateral positions can be obtained from sources such as Bennett (1969).

Good posture is flexible in that it can be maintained regardless of the state, dynamic or static, of the body. It meets the demands of temporary position change required in the performance of various physical activities, or brought about by emotional states and attitudes, without yielding to them. Posture can be more objectively and accurately assessed through comparative photography, yet the experienced and/or trained eye of the observer familiar with the standards of good posture, in addition to being familiar with the frequently noted deviations in the population he is serving, may prove to be quite accurate.

ANALYSIS OF GAIT

For the mobility specialist, gait deviations are relevant when they interfere with efficient, safe, and independent mobility, or lead to cosmetic problems. This section presents what is considered normal, efficient gait, and several pathological gaits (those caused by muscular weakness) for comparison through observation and evaluation.

The structure and state (diseased or healthy) of the skeletal and neuromuscular systems influence the efficiency and quality of gait. Bone length and weight and the number of muscle fibers and the presence of tone in muscle vary in the following examples. A short, stout body requires more muscular energy to move through space, as opposed to the tall, more lean body. Although the shorter, more stout body usually affords greater stability due to its wider base of support, the tall, leaner body, with its longer system of levers, and relatively linear relation to the ground results in longer, less labored strides which yield greater facility in movement. The shorter, more stout body may require additional body movements, such as pelvic and shoulder rotation, together with those movements linear in nature, such as flexion and extension, during gait. The additional rotary movements require an increased expenditure of body energy, which can result in decreased efficiency. Generally, the taller, leaner person is able to walk faster, expending less energy than the shorter, stouter person.

A well-developed, well-nourished muscle is able to elicit a quicker, more vigorous and stronger contraction, as opposed to the sluggish, slower contraction of a muscle in a relatively inactive, poorly nourished, overweight body, where muscle may even be in a state of atrophy. Muscle tone, the degree of firmness or tension of a muscle, is influenced by nutrition. Exercise alone is not sufficient to develop good muscle tone. As cited previously, the contractile mechanism of muscle is comprised primarily of protein. Thus, a diet consistently low in protein may significantly influence the quality of the contractile mechanism of muscle.

In analyzing gait, it is important to consider the state of the client's total physical condition, not just his degree of vision loss. Is there a structural or functional postural deviation evident? Is an additional handicap present, such as an existing neuromuscular disease or a history of one? What is his general state of health?

Normal gait consists of numerous tasks, beginning with the forward progression of the body due to displacement of the center of gravity anteriorly, and including numerous balance and counterbalance activities, leg-length variances, and shifting of weight to various body segments. All of this is done in order to accomplish what might be viewed as the simple task of taking one step followed by another.

Stance and Swing Phases

The two phases of gait are the stance phase and the swing phase. Each phase is distinct in itself, but in order for the normal gait cycle to be completed the two phases must function synchronously. While one limb is involved with the components of stance, the opposite limb is involved with the components of swing. Stance phase begins at heel-strike, which is that point of body weight acceptance by the limb. From heel-strike, stance phase proceeds through flat foot, mid-stance, heel-off and then toe-off of the same limb. Mid-stance occurs from the position of flat foot to heel-off. It is during this phase of stance, mid-stance, that the body's weight is immediately over the flat foot limb. Figure 19-3 (*a* through *e*) follows the stance phase from heel-strike through toe-off.

Swing phase begins with toe-off and ends at the moment of heel-strike of the same extremity, Figure 19-3 (*e* through *g*). Between toe-off, when acceleration of the body begins, and just before heel-strike, when internal and external forces are acting to decelerate the body, mid-swing occurs. Mid-swing (*f*) is that time during which the limb is passing just beneath the pelvis. At this point, the knee is flexed (leg-length adjustment) in order that the limb may pass beneath the body.

There are several norms to be followed when observing what is considered to be normal gait in a sighted male adult. The width of the base of support during gait is approximately 7.5 cm (3 in.) measured from mid-heel to mid-heel, give or take a few centimeters in either direction (Fig. 20-3). Measuring from heel-strike to heel-strike, the length of a normal step measures approximately 65 cm (26 in.). The average number of steps taken per minute, at a moderate pace, is approximately 96.

Center of Gravity Shift

During mid-stance, (Fig. 19-3) the body's weight shifts from one leg to the

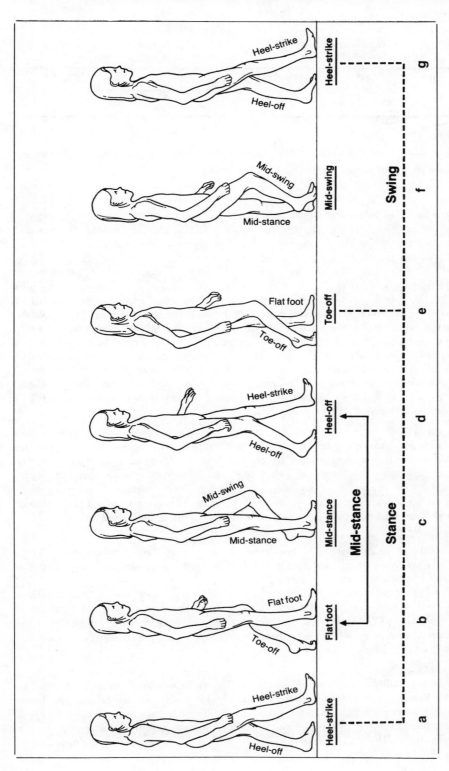

Figure 19-3. Normal gait cycle. (Drawn by Margaret Pulis.)

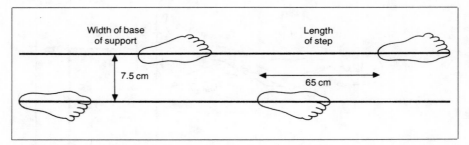

Figure 20-3. Gait norms. (Drawn by Margaret Pulis.)

other, and the pelvis and trunk also shift to the weight bearing side. The center of gravity, at this time also moves from side to side, and is referred to as *lateral displacement of the center of gravity*. The movement of the center of gravity from side to side is generally within a 5-cm (2-in.) range.

Vertical displacement, the upward and downward movement of the center of gravity during gait, is also within a 5-cm (2-in.) range, with the highest point occurring during mid-stance, and the lowest point occurring at the moment of double support—that time when both feet touch the ground (Fig. 21-3). Where vertical and lateral displacement are excessive, increased body movements, which are disruptive to smooth and efficient gait, may be observed.

The text following emphasizes the significance of adequate joint range of motion and muscular strength in the mechanics of normal gait. Note the normal joint positions of the ankle, knee, and hip at various phases during the gait cycle. A brief discussion of some commonly observed deviations from normal gait due to muscular weakness will be presented.

Slapping Gait

Between mid-swing and heel-strike the ankle must progress from the neutral position through approximately 10° of dorsiflexion, otherwise a slapping gait may occur. Foot drop, resulting in a slapping gait, is frequently observed because of weakness or paralysis of the ankle dorsiflexors after a stroke. A slapping gait, sometimes referred to as an "echo" gait, may be observed in a blind client where there is no evidence of weak ankle dorsiflexors. This is discussed later.

Genu Recurvatum

Excessive knee extension, resulting in back-knee, "genu recurvatum," (Fig. 10-3), observed during heel-strike, flat-foot, or mid-stance can cause undue stress on the knee joint resulting in pain.

The angle of the hip joint during single-limb balance, mid-stance, at which time the body's total weight is being supported by the foot in ground contact, is approximately 0°. A deviation from this position of extension may be due to a hip-flexion contracture, which is frequently accompanied by a knee-flexion contracture (See Fig. 15-3).

Plantar Flexion

During heel-off, sufficient strength in the calf musculature must be exerted to allow the ankle to plantarflex approximately 15° to 20° in accelerating the body forward and upward through toe-off. If this ankle movement is prevented, due to a limitation of motion in the ankle or weakness or paralysis of calf musculature, the pelvis on the affected side will not elevate sufficiently for smooth, rhythmic, linear gait.

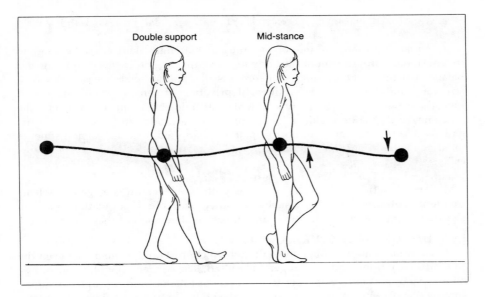

Double support   Mid-stance

Figure 21-3. Vertical displacement of center of gravity while walking. (Drawn by Margaret Pulis.)

Limb Length Adjustment

At toe-off, the knee joint must flex sufficiently for the extremity to pass smoothly beneath the body. This shortening of the extremity caused by knee flexion is called limb length adjustment. (Limb length adjustment may also occur in the reverse motion, extension, as seen at heel-strike when the knee is extended at that point of deceleration.) If sufficient knee flexion is absent at toe-off, preventing limb length adjustment to occur adequately for the limb to pass beneath the body, the client may compensate for this lack of movement by circumducting the affected limb at the hip joint in order to advance the limb forward. This is readily noted in a patient wearing a long leg cast which prevents both knee and ankle movement. To advance the affected extremity forward, the patient will circumduct the limb at the hip, that is, he will extend, abduct, flex, and adduct the limb at the hip in order to advance it forward.

As the heel leaves the ground during toe-off, the hip should hyperextend approximately 15° to 20°. Where paralysis or weakness of the gluteus maximus (agonist muscle of hip extension) occurs, the compensatory movement of lurching backward may be observed.

Referrals

Where a gait deviation is suspected, allowing the client to run or speed up his normal pace is likely to cause the deviation to become more evident and thus facilitate observation, because it is more difficult to compensate for an existing weakness when body movements are increased.

Where linear movement during gait is disrupted due to muscular weakness, paralysis, or where limitation of joint range of motion occurs, increased symmetrical or asymmetrical body movements may be observed. The degree of deviation from the linear path of travel, and the treatment program necessary to correct or improve upon gait where function (mobility) is impeded is, primarily, the duty of allied professionals such as a physiatrist, a physician or a physical therapist.

Observation of deviations, and referrals to the proper allied professional, is within the realm of the mobility specialist.

Adequate joint range of motion and muscular strength alone are not enough to insure smooth progression of the body forward during gait. Delayed righting and balance reactions, the presence of neuromuscular and skeletal disease processes, structural and functional deformities, deprivation of sensory input, degree of kinesthetic awareness, body type, mental attitude, etc., can all influence the efficiency and quality of gait. Like posture, one's attitude can be reflected in his gait. Where the mechanics of normal gait are disrupted, mechanical adjustments must be made. Miller (1967) indicated that loss of vision affects the gait mechanically in three ways: loss of sensory data necessary for timing the step; impoverished balance; deficiency of protective reflexes.

The final section in this chapter deals with those posture and gait problems frequently observed in the visually impaired and blind population and the significance of the use of the long cane in partial alleviation of these problems.

EVALUATION OF POSTURE AND GAIT

In an evaluation of posture and gait, a distinction should be made between the adventitiously blind and the congenitally blind. The congenitally blind client has no reserve or recall of visual cues to rely upon or to refer to in concept formation, such as that of "verticality." He also lacks the ability to use vision in modeling the posture and gait of others. Therefore, in the attempt to correct posture and gait deviations, or in offering suggestions whereby improvements in these areas may be made, the mobility specialist may have to begin with basic concept formation and body awareness. Obviously, requesting a client to stand or walk "straight" is likely to be ineffectual if "straight" is merely a word rather than a functional or accurate concept to the client.

The adventitiously blind client, in contrast, may have an accurate reserve of information acquired through vision that he can recall and apply where the need exists. His program, therefore, may not necessitate training in the areas of basic concept formation, body awareness, etc., prior to instruction geared toward improving posture and gait. The instructor and client must have a like understanding of terms and concepts being used in the training program.

There are a number of posture and gait deviations that occur with a higher incidence in the blind population. These are to be differentiated from posture and gait deviations with pathological or physiological explanations that are in no way attributed to poor habits resulting from visual loss. Pathological or physiological reasons should be considered where the instructor has been unsuccessful in his attempts to assist the client in correcting postural or gait deviations. Referral to the client's physician and/or his past medical history may be appropriate where gait and posture problems persist.

POSTURAL DEVIATIONS

In good segmental alignment there are natural curves characteristic of the vertebral column. It is the exaggeration of these curves that is of concern. Proceeding from head to foot, anterior head tilt and dorsal kyphosis are two of the more commonly observed postural deviations in the blind (Fig. 16-3). There are several possible conclusions as to why one assumes anterior head displacement, ranging from protecting oneself from a "face-on" collision with objects such as doors and walls, to Miller's (1967) explanation that anterior head tilt develops as a compensatory position to counteract the backward leaning of one's trunk during gait. Rounded shoulders can easily be related to dorsal kyphosis because of the association of the shoulders with the thoracic spine. As the thoracic spine rests in forward flexion the shoulders are likely to follow. Dorsal kyphosis may also

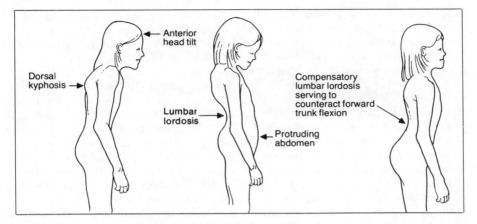

Figure 22-3. Postural deviations. (Drawn by Margaret Pulis.)

develop compensatory to lumbar lordosis.

Lumbar lordosis is commonly associated with weak, flaccid, abdominal musculature. Where lack of physical activity persists and excessive weight is accrued about the midline, lumbar lordosis is frequently evidenced. Lumbar lordosis may also be compensatory in counteracting forward flexion of the trunk (Fig. 22-3).

Chest deformities may develop secondary to other postural deviations, such as the hollow chest. The hollow chest, similar in appearance to the chest during exhalation, is often associated with dorsal kyphosis and rounded shoulders.

Mild to moderate hip and knee flexion (Fig. 15-3) may be evident in visually impaired people simply because of long periods of sitting. This deviation may also be related to the client's reluctance to extend his knees during stance or extend his hips during the swing phase of gait in an attempt to increase his stability by way of decreasing limb motion, or as a defensive reaction to unexpected drop-offs.

Both Siegel (1970) and Miller (1967) note instances of flat feet, *pes planus,* in the blind. This may be related to out-toeing, as excessive out-toeing places additional weight on the medial surface of the feet. If excessive out-toeing persists, it is likely that the long and transverse arches of the feet will flatten. The combination of knee flexion and foot eversion may present the appearance of having knocked knees.

Siegel (1970) suggests various ways of treating postural problems, such as use of "reminder splints." An example of a reminder splint would be the use of a soft cervical collar as a reminder to avoid anterior head tilt. Siegel further states the importance of noting structural orthopedic problems where definitive treatment such as surgery may be necessary for the correction of postural faults.

GAIT DEVIATIONS

In review, Miller (1967) states that loss of vision affects gait mechanically because of the loss of sensory data necessary for timing the steps, impoverished balance, and deficiency of protective reflexes. Therefore, it should not be surprising that various gait deviations occur where there is a visual loss, regardless of the existence or nonexistence of other pathological or physiological problems.

Out-toeing is commonly noted in the gait patterns of the congenitally blind. Out-toeing may develop as a source of increased tactual input. In this instance the feet are used as feelers, particularly during indoor travel where "runners" or "trail strips" are placed along hallways, or during outdoor travel when the client is looking for shorelines. Within limits, out-toeing can also increase the base of one's support. However, if it is excessive, linear travel may be impeded, and stability decreased. Most individuals exhibit some degree of out-toeing during gait, with the majority ranging somewhere between 7° to 8° for each foot. Out-toeing beyond these limits is not necessarily abnormal, with 20° of out-toeing falling within what is described as normal limits (Rasch-Burke, 1965).

A wide-based gait is probably the easiest and most commonly observed gait deviation characteristic of the blind. The reasons are obvious, as this type of gait is assumed in an effort to increase stability. A blind person may exhibit a shuffling gait, either to examine surfaces underfoot, or to increase stability. The "normal" heel-toe gait requires one to lift the feet, thereby shifting weight from one foot to the other, during which time single limb balance is necessary for a moment. Single limb balance does not occur when one shuffles the feet forward, rather than picking them up in advancing forward. Also, the shuffle gait reduces body momentum and thereby requires less use of equilibrium reactions. A shuffle gait is generally a slow gait in which limited hip, knee, and ankle movements are observed. The factor of "reduced speed" during gait may be desirable for the client who is reluctant or fearful of "stepping out" because of lack of or insufficient travel techniques.

A slapping gait, whereby the client over-exaggerates the force of dorsiflexion at heel-strike, may be a bother to one who is listening to the client walk. However, this type of gait may provide the client with auditory help, as his feet act as sound generators and the echoes produced are used to locate intersecting hallways, for example. This gait is sometimes known as the "echo gait."

A shortened, guarded stride may be seen in a client who is fearful of walking into objects, or who is unable to maintain sufficient balance during gait. A shortened stride may disrupt linear travel, because as one's speed during gait increases, the tendency to veer is modified; whereas a shortened stride, which tends to decrease speed during gait, may serve to increase veering.

In an attempt to avoid loss of balance or to be ready for an immediate stop, a visually impaired person may lean the trunk backward during gait. In doing so, an increase in pelvic motion may be observed when advancing forward.

Lack of contra-lateral arm movement during gait, commonly associated with tenseness, is often observed. Overconcern with posture and gait deviations where they do not interfere with comfort and safety during mobility may produce problems where none exist. If anterior head tilt and posterior trunk lean are not excessive, concentration on their correction may increase tenseness in the client and interfere with an already established, functional gait pattern. "Need" is a prerequisite to any remediation program.

VEERING

Numerous tests have been devised to support the evidence that there is a high incidence of the veering tendency in the absence of vision.

Fleharty (1968) conducted a study which concluded that the veering tendency depends more on perceptual organization than upon structural measures, such as posture or leg length. He stated that learning played a more important role than structure in determining the amount of veer evidenced.

Kimbrough (1966) studied the prescribed changes in individual characteristics of walking and standing on the veering tendency. He found that increasing the speed of gait and informing the walker of the direction in which he veered would modify the veering tendency. Kimbrough stated that it might be possible to teach a person not to veer by changing certain characteristics of the stride or stance.

Lund (1930), after measuring leg length, found that 80 percent of his 125 subjects continually veered to the side of the shorter leg. Lund concluded that his results were indicative of a high degree of interdependence between structural and functional asymmetrics since 80 percent of the subjects showed correspondence between structural and functional dominance. Several of Lund's critics contended that no significant correlation was made between physical asymmetry, veering, and leg length differences in this study.

B. J. Cratty (1967) found that no significant correlation existed between leg length and amount of veer. He stated that in spite of the findings of Lund, Cratty's own data tended to swing the weight of evidence concerning the causality of the direction and pattern of veer toward perceptual rather than structural forces. Cratty concluded that a significant difference did not exist between the tendency to veer and stride length, leg length difference, head torque, and hand and leg dominance.

OTHER FACTORS AFFECTING POSTURE AND GAIT

Tension, fear, and anxiety may influence one's gait significantly. Neuromuscular tension impedes quality of motion. During a state of tension, muscular fatigue can occur. Attempting to improve posture and gait in a client who is fearful of standing erect and moving forward is futile if he is unable to respond accurately due to existing fears and tensions. A client under tension must be encouraged to relax, for muscles in a state of isometric contraction, such as in the sustained clenched fist, rigid posture and rigid, guarded gait, over a period of time will eventually cause fatigue. Where muscle fatigue occurs, optimal contraction will not occur before recovery from the state of fatigue. Weak musculature, pain, fatigue, and the client's emotional state are all important factors to consider where the mobility specialist observes disruption of the smooth, rhythmic gait cycle or where postural deviations are observed. All of the above can contribute to undesirable movements and it is important for the observer to consider whether or not the etiology of such movements is emotional, pathological, or physiological in nature.

Posture and gait patterns vary with age. For example, where a wide-based gait may be considered a deviation from normal in a 21-year-old, it certainly is not in a toddler. Many of the common orthopedic concerns of parents of young children beginning to walk, such as flat feet or out-toeing, diminish or disappear as the child grows older. The "deviations" were not pathological in nature at all, but merely characteristic of that period in his development, that is, physiological in nature.

The elderly frequently exhibit mild dorsal kyphosis and anterior head tilt, in addition to mild degrees of hip and knee flexion, particularly if they spend a good amount of time sitting. Also, their gait may decrease in speed, and stride length may shorten, in addition to an increase in base of support. Where instability persists, the use of a standard cane may be necessary for additional support.

To ignore the client who passively sits at home all day is not only resigning him to a state of mental deterioration but also physical deterioration. A child left in the confines of his crib or playpen for the first several years of his life is likely to experience delayed or permanent loss of the righting and balance reflexes, in addition to delayed walking skills and loss of spatial perception. In addition, the child may also exhibit joint-flexion contractures and underdeveloped musculature, particularly of the legs. The list of delayed or permanently lost responses or skills of an individual confined to a limited environment is endless.

CONCLUSION

A rehabilitation program for visually impaired and blind persons should employ a team approach. The guidelines given for observations of posture and gait deviations in this chapter are simply guidelines and are not intended for any diagnostic or prognostic purpose. The mobility specialist should have knowledge of where to seek professional answers to questions which he feels are imperative to the total physical, mental, and vocational rehabilitation of the client, and how to refer clients to these sources.

Siegel (1970) introduced exercises geared toward the elimination of given postural faults. Before the initiation of any exercise program, the client's medical history should be reviewed and the physician's consent obtained. The reasons for these precautions are obvious in view of the physiological effects of exercise, such as increase in heart rate, blood pressure, and rate of respiration. These effects can be compounded and more severe where exercise is prolonged beyond a person's tolerance. In the event that an exercise program is contra-indicated, fatigue, pain and muscle soreness would be minor considerations compared to possible hyperventilation, rapid pulse rate, and elevation of blood pressure. These possibilities should not be overlooked in the multiply handicapped, diabetic, or geriatric client in an exercise program geared toward improving posture and/or gait deviations, as an uncontrolled increase in heart rate and blood pressure might lead to cardiac arrest or cerebral vascular accident (stroke).

Good posture and efficient gait should be habitual not functional. They should persist throughout all activities of daily living, not simply within a structured situation, such as when the instructor is present. To expect a client to maintain optimal posture and gait patterns without providing him with techniques in the use of a suitable "prosthesis" (Miller, 1967) that will adequately assist in providing him with sensory input deprived him by a visual loss, would be a disservice. As a client steps off without the aid of a mobility device, his posture and gait problems may immediately or soon again manifest themselves.

There is no question as to which comes first, mobility training or posture and gait training, for one without the other may be ineffectual. The question is rather what the client's combined needs are and/or how can they best be served in obtaining independent, safe, and efficient mobility with the least expenditure of energy.

Bibliography

Bennett, W. Principles of therapeutic exercise. In S. Licht (Ed.) *Therapeutic exercise*. Baltimore: Waverly Press, 1969.

Brunnstrom, S. *Clinical kinesiology*. Philadelphia: F. A. Davis, 1972.

Chaffee, E. & Greisheimer, E. *Basic physiology and anatomy*. Philadelphia: J. B. Lippincott, 1964.

Chusid, J. & McDonald, J. *Correlative neuroanatomy and functional neurology*. Los Altos, California: Lange Medical Publications, 1962.

Cooper, J. & Glassow, R. *Kinesiology*. Saint Louis: C. V. Mosby, 1972.

Cratty, B. J. The perception of gradient and the veering tendency while walking without vision. *Research Bulletin, American Foundation for the Blind*, 1967, **14**, 31-51.

Cratty, B. Perceptual thresholds of non-visual locomotion, Part I: Veering tendency perception of gradient, and of curvature in pathways: Inter-relationships, norms, group comparisons and a mobility orientation test. U. S. Dept. of HEW, Public Health Services, Grant No. NB05577-0251. Los Angeles: University of California, August, 1965.

Cratty, B., Peterson, C., Harris, J., & Schoner, R. The development of perceptual-motor abilities in blind children and adolescents. *The New Outlook for the Blind*, 1968, **62** 111-116.

Cratty, B. & Williams, H. Perceptual thresholds of non-visual locomotion, Part II: The effects of brief practice upon veering, upon accuracy of facing movements and upon position relocation: The perception of lateral tilt in pathways walked and of curvature. Department of Physical Education, Monograph 1966. Los Angeles: University of Caifornia, NIH Grant No. NB05577-0251.

Daniels, L., Williams, M., & Worthingham, C. *Muscle testing*. (2nd ed.) Philadelphia: W. B. Saunders, 1961.

Ducroquet, R., Ducroquet, J., & Ducroquet, P. *Walking and limping*. Philadelphia: J. B. Lippincott, 1968.

Fiorentino, M. *Reflex testing methods for evaluating C. N. S. development.* Springfield, Illinois: Charles C. Thomas, 1974.

Fleharty, D. R. An analysis of the relationship between walking speed and veering. Unpublished M.A. dissertation, School of Graduate Studies, Western Michigan University. Kalamazoo, Michigan, 1966.

Gross, C. (Ed.) *Gray's Anatomy.* Philadelphia: Lea & Febiger, 1962.

Greenspan, K. Receptors and effectors. In E. E. Selkurt (Ed.), *Physiology.* Boston: Little, Brown, 1966.

Guyton, A. *Textbook of medical physiology.* (2nd ed.) Philadelphia: W. B. Saunders, 1964.

Hines, T. Posture. In S. Licht (Ed.) *Therapeutic exercise.* (Rev. ed.) Baltimore: Waverly Press, 1969.

Hooper, B. *The mechanics of human movement.* New York: American Elsevier Publishing Company, 1973.

Johnson, E. Electrodiagnosis. In Frank Krusen (Ed.), *Physical medicine and rehabilitation.* (2nd ed.) Philadelphia: W. B. Saunders, 1971.

Kendall, H., Kendall, F., & Boynton, D. *Posture and pain.* Baltimore: Williams and Wilkins, 1952.

Kimbrough, J. The effects of prescribed changes in individual characteristics of walking and standing on the veering tendency in blind persons. Unpublished MA dissertation, School of Graduate Studies, Western Michigan University. Kalamazoo, Michigan, 1966.

Kottke, F. Therapeutic exercise. In Frank Krusen (Ed.), *Physical medicine and rehabilitation.* (2nd ed.) Philadelphia: W. B. Saunders, 1971.

Long, Charles, II, Pathological gait. A discussion of pathological gait due to muscular weakness. Institute of Physical Medicine and Rehabilitation, New York. (No date.)

Lund, F. H. Physical asymmetries and disorientations. *American Journal of Psychology*, 1930, **42,** 51-62.

MacConaill, M. Mechanical anatomy of motion and posture. In S. Licht (Ed.), *Therapeutic exercise.* (Rev. ed.) Baltimore: Waverly Press, 1969.

Miller, J. Vision a component of locomotion. *Physiotherapy*, October, 1967.

Northrip, J., Logan, G., & McKinney, W. *Introduction to biomechanic analysis of sport.* Dubuque, Iowa: Wm. Brown, 1974.

Pesczynski, M. Gait and gait retraining. In S. Licht (Ed.), *Therapeutic exercise.* (Rev. ed.) Baltimore: Waverly Press, 1969.

Raney, R. & Brashear, H. *Shands' handbook of orthopaedic surgery.* Saint Louis: Mosby Company, 1971.

Rasch, P. & Burke, R. *Kinesiology and applied anatomy.* (2nd ed.) Philadelphia: Lea and Febiger, 1965.

Reith, E., & Ross, M. *Atlas of descriptive histology.* New York: Harper and Row, 1967.

Romanes, G. (Ed.) *Cunningham's textbook of anatomy.* London: Oxford University Press, 1972.

Salter, R. *Textbook of disorders and injuries of the musculoskeletal system.* Baltimore: Williams and Wilkins, 1970.

Selker, L. Methods of measurement in Soviet gait analysis research. *Journal of the American Physical Therapy Association*, 1976, **56**(2), 163-167.

Siegel, I. *Postural determinants in the blind.* Springfield, Ill.: Charles C Thomas Publisher, 1970.

Turek, S. *Orthopaedic principles and their application.* Philadelphia: J. B. Lippincott, 1959.

Tuttle, W. & Schottelius, B. *Textbook of physiology.* (16th ed.) Saint Louis: C. V. Mosby, 1969.

Wells, K. F. *Kinesiology,* Philadelphia: W. B. Saunders, 1967.

Williams, M. & Worthingham, C. *Therapeutic exercise.* Philadelphia: W. B. Saunders, 1962.

Perception, Locomotion, and Orientation*

Herbert L. Pick, Jr.

Many of the traditional sense modalities contribute to man's ability to maintain posture and to locomote through the environment. Vision, of course, typically plays a dominant role. It enables one to find and traverse desired clear pathways as well as to anticipate and avoid obstacles in locomoting. On the basis of vision, we can also maintain our posture with respect to the up-down dimension since most environments include horizontal and/or vertical lines which can act as frames of reference. Audition may also play a role in locomotion although it is unlikely that it is important for postural maintenance. We can localize sound emitting objects with an accuracy of a degree or two in direction. Sound emitting objects which are approaching and receding produce the well-known Doppler effect (an increasing pitch as the object approaches, shifting instantaneously to a decreasing pitch as it passes and begins to recede from us). In addition audition can operate through echolocation. The classical studies of Dallenbach and his colleagues (Cotzin & Dallenbach, 1950; Supa, Cotzin, & Dallenbach, 1944) and more recent studies of Rice (1967), discussed by Wiener in Chapter 6, have demonstrated considerable acuity in detection of distance of objects and even some ability to identify the nature of objects.

The presence of some objects can be detected by odor so it is possible to get some information about where one is or about where particular objects are if they emit distinctive odors. Our ability to detect the presence of odors is relatively good but our ability to localize the direction of their source is relatively poor. And the number of objects in our environment which provide us with clear distinct odors is rather small. Similarly the presence of some objects in our environment can be detected by radiant heat energy. The presence of an overhang occluding the sun, for example, or the warm temperature near the open door of a bakery may provide us with information about where we are and in a general way the direction of particular objects. However, there are again relatively few objects in our environment which give rise to such sharp temperature gradients.

All the previously mentioned modalities provide us with information about the environment at some distance from us. The haptic sense system, on the other hand, will only provide us with information through quite proximal contact. The long cane, of course, extends this haptic contact distance slightly. Haptic perception can provide us with information about where we are in the environment when we make contact with objects with our limbs, body, or some instrument such as the long cane. A particular aspect of the environment with which we are

*Preparation of this chapter was supported by grants from the National Institute of Child Health and Human Development to the University of Minnesota: Institute of Child Development (HD 05027), and Center for Research in Human Learning (HD 01136), and by a grant from the National Science Foundation also to the Center for Research in Human Learning (GB-17590).

always in contact while locomoting is the ground surface. On the basis of haptic perception we are able to get information about the texture of the ground surface—its roughness, smoothness, regularity, etc., and about the slope of the surface. This, of course, can provide us some information about where we are in the environment. Through haptic perception we are also able to obtain information about posture, by the direction of pressure on our feet and perhaps by the pressure of clothing on our body.

Classical proprioception provides us with an important source of information about body posture. This information is based mainly on sensitivity to position at the body joints. (See Chapter 5 on tactual and haptic perception.) We know the position of our joints with respect to each other and hence are sensitive to whether we are leaning, our head is cocked or turned, etc.

The major nonvisual sensory system, however, for maintaining orientation with respect to gravity and for perceiving change of position in the environment is the vestibular system. This system is localized in the inner ear and provides information about the orientation of the head with respect to gravity, and, in addition, information about linear and angular acceleration of the head which occurs with any change of body position.

The first section of this chapter will focus on the structure and operation of the vestibular system. The second section will focus on a different source of information which helps us stay oriented in our environment—efference or motor outflow. Very briefly, we know where we are because we gave motor commands through our nervous system to get our body or limbs to a particular position. The third section will discuss the way spatial information about where we are is encoded or represented in our minds.

THE VESTIBULAR SYSTEM

This section is based mainly on sources by Gernandt (1959), Gibson (1966), and Howard and Templeton (1966). The interested reader is referred to them for more detail.

Structure and Function

The vestibular system is composed of a labyrinthine structure in the inner ear. The term labyrinth is well chosen as the system consists in each inner ear of three interconnected canals, the semicircular canals, and two membranous sacs called the *utricle* and *saccule* (Fig. 1-4). This structure is well suited to detect the mechanical forces created by changes in linear and rotary velocity. In short, it detects the initiation and cessation of movements of all kinds as well as changes in rate of movement. It is not well suited to detect steady-state motion.

The part of the system primarily responsible for detection of linear acceleration is in the utricle sac. The sensory cells in this sac are embedded in a receptor organ called the *macula*. Hairs from these cells project upward in the sac into a gelatinous endolymph. In this endolymph are small bony-like particles called *otoliths*. These particles are heavier than the surrounding gelatinous substance. Thus when the body, and naturally the head, is subjected to acceleration the inertia of the heavier particles causes them to lag slightly. Stimulation is caused by the otoliths bending the hairs projecting from the sensory cells. This stimulation thus provides the basis for sensitivity to linear acceleration. When acceleration ceases and we are in constant velocity motion, as in a car or an airplane, the otoliths assume their normal positions and the hairs are no longer bent. The sensory cells are no longer stimulated. When we start to slow down, the inertia of the otoliths again bends the hairs and we can detect the change in velocity by means of the vestibular system.

The utricle mechanism (sac, otoliths, hair cells) also seems to provide information about the direction of gravity. When the head is in a tilted position the macula

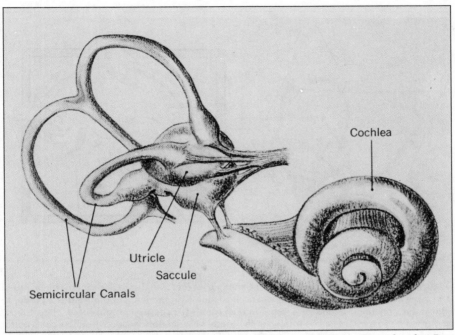

Figure 1-4. The labyrinth or inner ear. (From James J. Gibson, *The Sensus Considered as Perceptual Systems*, p. 64. Copyright © 1966 by J. J. Gibson. Reprinted by permission of Houghton Mifflin Company.)

is tilted with respect to its normal (horizontal) position and the relatively heavy otoliths again bend the hairs projecting from the cells. Electrophysiological recordings from these cells indicate that they adapt very slowly. That is they maintain their firing rate for long periods at any particular head orientation. This means that information about posture of the head is continuously signaled to the brain. It is important to note that the stimulation in the utricle is ambiguous: the same stimulation could arise from a static head tilt and from a linear acceleration. In order to eliminate that ambiguity, additional information is necessary, e.g., from pressure on the skin when accelerating, from visual input, or from knowledge that one has actively tilted her head.

The part of the system primarily responsible for sensitivity to turning is the set of three semicircular canals in each inner ear. These canals are filled with fluid and actually form a continuous loop beginning and ending in the utricle. As depicted in Fig. 1-4 the canals are approximately at right angles to each other and hence are able to detect components of turns around the three spatial dimensions in the sagittal, frontal, and transverse planes. In the end of each semicircular canal there is a swelling known as the *ampulla*, which contains the sensory mechanism. This mechanism consists of hair cells originating in ridges or cristae in the bases of the ampulla and projecting up into a gelatinous mass called the cupula. The cupula in each canal is free to move back and forth in the ampulla like a swinging door. It moves that way with (components of) head movement in the plane of each canal. That is, when the head turns in a particular direction, the inertia of the fluid in the corresponding semicircular canal pushes the cupula in the opposite direction (Fig. 2-4). The movement of the cupula stimulates the hair cells. The pattern of

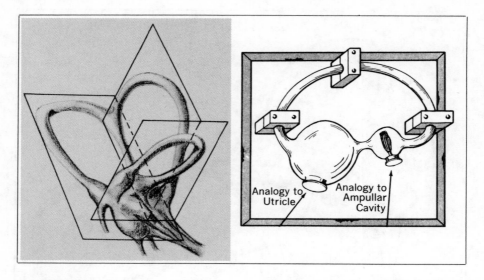

Figure 2-4. The semicircular canals and Exner's model of a semicircular canal. The layout of the three canals in the three planes of space is shown on the left. On the right is a model to show the presumed action of a semicircular canal. It consists of fluid-filled glass tubing mounted on a base that can be rotated at the center. The flexible brush (cupula) in the smaller chamber bends and then recovers when the model is turned through any angle. (From E. B. Titchener, *A Textbook of Psychology*, The Macmillan Company, 1928, by permission of the publisher.)

stimulation from the different semicircular canals provides information about the exact direction of turning. As with linear motion and the utricle, if a constant velocity turn is achieved, the cupula will return to its normal position and stimulation will cease. Then when the movement starts to slow down, the inertia of the fluid will cause the cupula to move in the same direction as the motion. Thus the semicircular canal system also provides information about the initiation and termination of movement (primarily turns), but not steady-state turning.

Neural Pathways

The sensory cells of the vestibular system feed mainly into four vestibular neural nuclei. From two of these, fibers ascend to higher neural centers, some to oculomotor centers and some to the cortex. The fibers to oculomotor centers control vestibular nystagmus. These are slow eye movements opposite the direction of head turning followed by a rapid flick back to straight ahead. The function of such eye movements is to permit a person to maintain visual fixation during head rotation. Measurement of such nystagmatic eye movements in sighted persons must be carried out without vision because the visual stimulation resulting from rotation itself produces a similar (optokinetic) nystagmus. That is, a stationary subject viewing a moving visual field will also show a nystagmus, in their case slow movements in direction of the motion followed by the rapid saccade to straight ahead. Under rotation with vision the nystagmus involves both visual and vestibular stimulation. Blind persons or sighted persons rotated in the dark will evince purely vestibular nystagmus.

The fibers projecting to the cortex from the vestibular nuclei presumably mediate conscious awareness of linear motion, rotation, and posture. From the other two vestibular nuclei, fibers descend to motor neurons in the spinal cord. These control righting reflexes, which occur, for example, when one starts to fall.

Psychophysics of Vestibular Perception

The traditional way of measuring vestibular perception in humans is to assess sensitivity to rotary and linear acceleration, and to orientation with respect to gravity (i.e., posture). For rotary acceleration the technique employs a rotating (Barany) chair or a torsion swing. The Barany chair is something like a motor driven dental chair whose rate of acceleration can be accurately controlled. Unfortunately, in addition to vestibular stimulation such devices also produce tactual and proprioceptive stimulation. For small accelerations this extraneous stimulation may not play an important role. Thresholds for rotary acceleration have been determined with such devices. Using as an index initial reports of rotation, thresholds for detection have been found ranging from $0.12°/sec^2$ to $2°/sec^2$ (Dodge, 1923; Clark & Stewart, 1962). The occurrence of vestibular nystagmus has also been used as an index of detection of rotation and threshold accelerations of $0.8°/sec^2$ to $1.0°/sec^2$ have been reported (Dohlman, 1935; Montandon & Russbach, 1953).

The same difficulties of extraneous tactual and proprioceptive stimulation interfere with measurement of vestibular perception of linear acceleration and orientation to gravity. One of the more effective ways of assessing sensitivity to linear acceleration has been to swing a subject systematically back and forth. In doing this, frequency of oscillation, amplitude, velocity, and acceleration of motion all play a role in detection of motion and change of direction of motion. Peak acceleration thresholds of 6 to 10 cm/sec^2 (2.75 to 4 in./sec^2) have been reported for swing frequencies of 0.1 to 0.3 cycles/sec (Walsh, 1962). That is, when each cycle of swing takes about three seconds acceleration has to reach 6 to 10 cm/sec^2 (2.75 to 4 in./sec^2) to be detected.

For assessing sensitivity to orientation to gravity, subjects in various postures have been asked to set a visual line to vertical, or to point upward. To reduce tactual and proprioceptive information, subjects sometimes have been immersed in water. Brown (1961), for example, found that subjects immersed in water and passively rotated to a randomly assigned orientation were very poor at judging the direction of "up." Their errors ranged up to 180°. They improved considerably if permitted to nod their heads. The maximum error in that case was 112°. The perception of up-down direction in the absence of vestibular and visual or tactual input is very poor or completely missing. Thus people with bilateral loss of vestibular input when swimming under water are reported to become so disoriented that they are as likely to swim downward as upward.

SENSORY COMBINATION AND MOTOR OUTFLOW

In the discussion above it was repeatedly noted that it was difficult even in the laboratory to investigate vestibular perception in isolation from other sensory input. That fact is even all the more true outside the laboratory where the norm in moving around the environment and maintaining posture involves information from several sense modalities and from knowledge about our own actions, so-called motor outflow information. How are these combinations of sensory input handled? How does information as to our own actions affect our perception of our posture and orientation?

Sensory Combinations

In order to study how combinations of sensory input are processed, the usual procedure has been to provide a subject with conflicting sensory input from two or more sense modalities and see how the conflict is resolved. A common example of such conflict occurs in railroad stations when trains adjacent to us start forward.

We often feel like we are moving backward. We are responding to misleading visual stimulation in conflict with veridical (correct) vestibular and proprioceptive stimulation which should inform us that we are stationary. A recent experimental example of this phenomenon has been provided by Lee and Lishman (1975). Subjects were provided conflicting visual and vestibular and proprioceptive information for being upright. This was done by placing them in a four-walled cubicle suspended just off the floor of a room. The cubicle could be moved back and forth as subjects standing on the stationary floor viewed a wall. Consider what happens if the wall sways slowly away from a subject. The proprioceptive and vestibular information does not change; on its basis the subject should perceive herself as being stationary in a normal upright posture. On the other hand, the visual stimulation would suggest that the subject is falling backward; in order to maintain her balance she should sway forward. To which information does the subject respond? The answer is to the visual—people will sway in the direction of movement of the room. Young children who have just learned to stand will sway so far as to topple over (Lee & Aronson, 1974).

In considering perception by the blind it is of more interest to know how conflicts of nonvisual sensory information are resolved. There is not a great deal of research on this question. One study (Pick, Warren, & Hay, 1969) pitted proprioceptive and auditory information against one another. Subjects were asked to indicate the position of an object that felt like it was in one place and sounded like it was in a somewhat different position. The situation was created by having subjects place one finger on a small loudspeaker which was emitting clicks. By means of a pseudophone the clicks were made to sound displaced a few degrees to the right or left. (A pseudophone is a device which functionally shifts the position of our ears and hence shifts the apparent positions of sounds. For example, if our ears are rotated to the right, a sound straight ahead will be heard as if it comes from the left.) Subjects were asked to point with the other hand at the source of the sound. The results indicated a compromise between the proprioceptive and auditory positions. Subjects pointed in between the two positions but somewhat closer to the proprioceptive position. The conflict is resolved more in favor of proprioception but the auditory information does have an effect. A similar proprioceptive bias over audition occurs in both blind and sighted subjects (Warren & Pick, 1970). Strangely enough, with adventitiously blind persons the more visual experience they have had, the weaker the bias seems to be. Somehow visual experience appears to influence the resolution of this nonvisual sensory conflict. These results indicating proprioceptive dominance over audition in both sighted and blind subjects confirmed an earlier study by Fisher (1964).

Fisher also provided direct normative data for perception of auditory and proprioceptive position or direction. Two measures of accuracy are typically used to characterize performance in such tasks. Actually they are measures of inaccuracy, i.e., error: constant error and variable error. Constant error refers to the fact that in judging a characteristic like the direction of a sound or the position of a limb a person might show a constant bias in one direction or another. For example, if I am asked to point with one hand at the position of my other hand (with eyes closed) I might perhaps always point 2 in. (5 cm) to the right of the true position. Thus I would have a constant error of 2 in. (5 cm) to the right. That, of course, would be very valuable to know. That is, if I knew I made such a constant error, I could always correct my pointing and hit the location exactly correctly. Such a constant error would be much less harmful to my performance than if I simply averaged 2 in. (5 cm) to the right over a series of trials. On some trials I might be 4 or 5 in. (10 or 13 cm) to the right, on others I might be exactly correct or even in error to the left. This variation in performance is understandably called a variable error. Fisher found that under some conditions blind subjects made larger constant errors than sighted subjects. However, the pattern of variable errors was more interesting. When subjects were matching the positions of two sounds or matching two proprioceptive positions, there was no difference between sighted and blind subjects. However, when the task was to match a sound to a proprioceptive position the variable error was considerably greater for the blind than for the sighted. Again, somehow, visual experience was playing a role in this nonvisual sensory combination task. That is, the fact of having had visual experience affects the way one performs nonvisual sensory integration tasks.

Motor Outflow or Efference

An often neglected source of information about our posture including the relative positions of parts of our body and about where we are in the environment is information derived from our intentional acts. For example, if we *initiated* movement of our head to the right we would presumably be able to judge on that basis alone that our head was turned to the right. We might not need to use proprioceptive or vestibular (or other) feedback information at all. To take another example if we stood up and moved forward and sat down we might well know where we were on the basis of the fact that our brain programmed and initiated and carried out such an action and not on the basis of vestibular or other stimulation from these movements. Of course in such natural situations there is the programmed motor outflow information, also called *efference,* and there are various kinds of sensory feedback information from visual, vestibular, and proprioceptive stimulation. However, in the laboratory it is possible to eliminate the sensory feedback and see if the motor outflow information is sufficient. An often cited experiment by Merton (1964) indicates that in principle motor outflow information can be sufficient for judging positions of parts of our body. Merton anesthetized the thumb joint of a subject so that without vision he could not tell when the thumb was passively moved back and forth. The muscles which control bending of the thumb are somewhat removed from the joint and were unaffected by the anesthesia. When the subject actively bent or straightened his thumb he could report its position. Interestingly, if the thumb were passively held in one position against the subject's active flexing of his thumb muscle he nevertheless reported the thumb as being in the intended position. This demonstrates that motor outflow information can serve as sufficient basis for judging position of a body part. Eye movements can also provide an example of using motor outflow information for judging position. We do not seem to be aware of proprioceptive feedback from the eye muscles although there are some sensory fibers in the eye muscles. How do we know where our eyes are pointed? Apparently, at least partially, we know where our eyes are pointed because we directed our eyes to move to a given position. This fact is used to explain a paradoxical perceptual phenomenon. When a visual object moves across our field of vision we experience it as moving presumably because its image moves across our retina. However when we move our eyes the image of the whole visual field moves across our retina but we don't experience the world as moving. Apparently, when we actively move our eyes the ensuing image movement on our retina is discounted or canceled out. In other words, motor outflow information not only tells us where our eyes are pointed but also tells us how to interpret image movement on our retina.

There are a number of other types of experiments which support the idea that motor outflow information is sufficient to help us regulate our movements (and if we know how to move to accomplish something we presumably know where our limbs are or where we are). One of the other types of experiments has involved "de-efferenting" monkeys (Taub & Berman, 1966). They operated on monkeys, surgically cutting off all relevant proprioceptive and tactual feedback, yet the monkeys were able to learn to make a new motor response even when visual feedback was also precluded. For present purposes there are two problems with the evidence showing the sufficiency of motor outflow information. One is the fact that practically all the experimental evidence pertains to the judgment of relative positions of parts of our body and none pertains to the judgment of where we are in our environment. The other is the fact that the evidence shows motor outflow is sufficient when sensory information is eliminated but the evidence has not shown whether motor outflow information is typically used when other sources of information are available. With respect to the first problem, what is needed are experiments with subjects *actively* traversing routes while blindfolded. Some of the subjects should be patients who lack labyrinthine function while others should have intact labyrinths. We know from the work of Beritov (1965) that patients without functioning labyrinths (and the consequent lack of vestibular information) are unable to traverse simple routes along which they have been passively taken, but we don't know about their performance on routes which they have actively traversed.

The second problem concerning whether motor outflow information normally plays a role in maintaining orientation or only does so when other information is missing could be approached through sensory conflict experiments. If it could be arranged that efference indicates one thing and sensory information something else we could see how a person resolves this conflict. If motor outflow information dominated, it would suggest (but not prove) that such information normally played an important role. Some observations on eye movements suggest that at least with the eye movement system motor outflow information is important. Helmholtz (1962) reported that if a subject's eye muscle is paralyzed so he cannot move his eye, but nevertheless tries to do so, the visual field appears to move. In this case, motor outflow information (the attempt to move the eye) indicates that the eye is being moved. The stationary visual-image information (from the nonmoving eye) indicates that no eye movement has taken place. How is this discrepancy resolved? The subject reports that the visual field has moved. That is, the subject's perception accepts that the eye has moved, and since the image didn't move, the visual field must have moved at the same time. There is no general systematic evidence about resolution of conflict between motor outflow and nonvisual information.

ENCODING OF SPATIAL INFORMATION

Maintaining orientation, that is knowing where objects are in relation to each other and in relation to ourselves, is a *vital* function of mobile organisms. In fact, in recent years there has been considerable evidence to the effect that even within the visual system (Trevarthen, 1968) and within the auditory system (Evans, 1974) there are anatomically and functionally specialized subsystems that subserve orientation as opposed to identification. In the case of vestibular sensitivity, the whole function of the system appears to be orientation. However, the sensory information relevant to spatial orientation is transduced by receptor mechanisms, that is, no matter how the receptors work, sensory stimulation is only the beginning of maintaining orientation. Whether the stimulation is vestibular or proprioceptive, visual or auditory, that stimulation must be used appropriately if we are to stay oriented to the environment. But what are the relevant aspects of the environment to which we stay oriented?

Frames of Reference

In discussing the work of Lee and Lishman (1975) above, it was noted that visual stimulation provided one kind of orienting information and vestibular stimulation provided different orienting information. That was a case of two sources of stimulation providing different orienting information. In many cases the *same* source of stimulation can provide different kinds of orienting information depending on what frame of reference is effective. Consider the following situation: a person without vision is standing upright and a vertical line is traced on his forehead. He is told to call that "a" and a similarly traced horizontal line is to be called "b." Now the person is asked to lie horizontally on his side and the same two lines are traced on his forehead. Which will he call "a" and which will he call "b?" The line which is up-down with respect to gravity is now horizontal with respect to his forehead and vice versa. His answer will depend on whether he perceived the original lines when he was upright in relation to an egocentric or geographic reference system. An experiment of just this sort was carried out by Rieser and Pick (1976). In that experiment the reclining subjects called the line "a" when it was up-down on their forehead. That is, the judgment of the orientation of the line was based on an egocentric or body-axis frame of reference and not a geographic or gravity based frame of reference. In another condition of the same study, upright subjects were given to feel a vertical bar identified as "a" and a horizontal bar identified as "b." When these subjects felt the bars while reclining on their side they used a geographic frame of reference. Apparently the type of reference system used depends on the task of the subject. When the task is identifying a tactual stimulus traced on the skin an egocentric reference system is used. When the task is haptically identifying an object or bar, a geographic reference is used. But note that the use of a geographic reference system requires coordination between haptic and vestibular perception. The orientation of the hand doing the feeling must be integrated with vestibular (or other) information about the direction of gravity.

An even more complex problem of the same nature relevant to the blind is how to interpret a route traced on one's skin. If indeed there is a natural tendency to refer tracings on the skin to a body reference system this should be taken into account when someone provides routes by skin tracing. It must be very clear to the student or receiver of information what directions of the body or body part correspond to what directions of space. Little is known about the ability of blind subjects to use or transform such directional correspondences.

Another example of the same source of stimulation providing different orienting information depending on frame of reference can be taken from Attneave and Benson (1969). They asked subjects to place each hand on one of two bars arranged in the form of a "T." Thus one hand was horizontal and the other was vertical. Underneath each finger of each hand were individual vibrators. The subjects learned to associate an arbitrary letter of the alphabet with stimulation by each vibrator. For example, when the middle finger of the right hand was stimulated they might have to report "d" and when the pointer finger of the left hand was stimulated they might have to report "b." After a set number of learning trials the positions of the hands were interchanged, and the subjects were to continue responding with the same associated letters. Did they continue to respond with the same letter when the same finger was stimulated even though that finger was in a new spatial position? Or did they continue to respond with the same letter to stimulation of the same spatial position even though that position was occupied by a finger on the other hand? Four times as many responses were made with the same letter to the same spatial position as with the same letter to the same finger. In other words there seemed to be a strong bias towards using a geographically defined frame of reference rather than an egocentric or body-relevant frame of reference. In that experiment subjects had their eyes open although they couldn't actually see the vibrators which were hidden by the fingers and the bars. In a supplementary experiment of the same study, subjects performed the task with eyes closed and the geographical bias was eliminated. Responding was about equally determined by egocentric and geographic frames of reference.

From this study it might be concluded that the presence of a visual space encouraged use of a geographic over an egocentric frame of reference. Extrapolating from such a conclusion it would be possible to go on and infer that blind subjects with relatively little visual experience at all would be very likely to use an egocentric reference system in such a task. While that particular experiment was not carried out with blind subjects, one very similar in principle was conducted by Hermelin and O'Connor (1971) comparing the performance of blind children and sighted children, with and without vision. The children held their fingers in the configuration depicted in Fig. 3-4. They learned to associate touch of each finger with an arbitrary word: "run," "sit," "walk," and "stand." After they learned to respond with the appropriate word each time a finger was touched, the position of the hands was interchanged. As in the Attneave and Benson study the children were asked to continue responding when their fingers were touched. The sighted children with vision responded overwhelmingly in terms of the geographic position while both the blind children and the blindfolded sighted children responded in terms of an egocentric frame of reference, i.e., the finger which was stimulated. Another study, by McKinney (1964) demonstrated that blind children would use a body-relevant frame of reference while sighted children even though

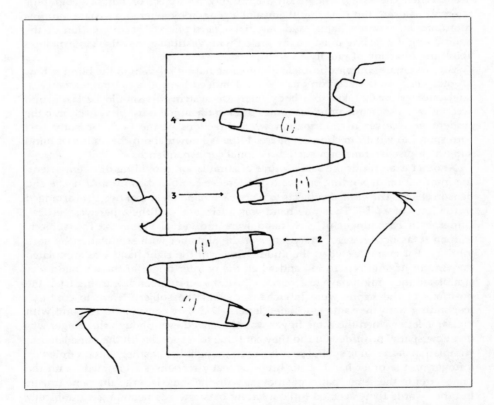

Figure 3-4. Position of subject's hands during stimulation. (From B. Hermelin & N. O'Connor. Spatial coding in normal, autistic, and blind children, *Perceptual and Motor Skills*, 1971, 33, 127-132. Reprinted with permission from authors and publisher.)

blindfolded used a geographic frame of reference. In his study, children held their hand palm up on a table and one of their fingers was touched. The children were asked to turn their hands upside down on the table and after a three-second delay, to point to that *finger* which had been touched. Blindfolded sighted children made a large number of mirror-image-type errors since they responded to the same position in space. The (congenitally) blind children made fewer such errors, either responding to the correct finger or simply forgetting during the delay and making random errors.

These studies support the idea that the presence of a visual field encourages the use of a geographic reference system in the various tasks. The absence of vision during the task and/or the lack of visual experience due to blindness encourages the use of an egocentric reference system. This is not to say that blind subjects or, in some of the tasks, blindfolded sighted subjects could not respond geographically. In none of the studies using blind subjects were they required to respond geographically. However, the results do suggest that when the situation imposes no particular requirement blind subjects and sighted subjects without vision may tend to use a body-relevant frame of reference.

So far this discussion of frames of reference has centered around experimental tasks that mostly involve identification of positions and objects close to a person's body or of parts of his body itself. While these tasks are quite relevant to maintaining orientation in the sense of knowing one's own posture and the relative position of one's limbs, they don't have much to do with maintaining orientation in the sense of knowing where in the world one is. However, the concept of frame of reference is relevant to this environmental sense of orientation. For example, suppose you learn to get to work by turning left from your house heading down the street towards a gas station and then turning right towards the just visible supermarket. You could be traveling in terms of either an egocentric or a geographic reference system or both. Turning left then right would be egocentric; heading towards a gas station and then a supermarket would be geographic. Which sort of reference system do we use? When vision is available it is quite likely that people use geographic reference systems in simple situations. Acredolo (1976), for example, brought children of various ages into a small relatively uniform room with a single table on one side. She led a child up to the table, blindfolded her, and led her back to the door. The blindfold was taken off and the child was requested to return to the same *place* in the room where she had first come and been blindfolded. Unknown to the child, while she was blindfolded the table was moved to the opposite side of the room. Children tended to go to the table rather than to make the same right or left turn as they had when they entered the room. That is, they were responding geographically rather than egocentrically. (The walls of the room provided no distinctive geographical cues.)

Again, just as with the Attneave and Benson study described above, it is reasonable to ask whether the availability of vision encourages the use of geographic as opposed to egocentric frames of reference. In order to begin to answer this question, Goldsmith, Mohr, and Pick (1977) taught subjects a set of locations in a small reaching space. Subjects were taught to reach to each of three positions on a horizontal shelf. Over the shelf was a table top blocking sight of the locations and the subject's own hands. That is, the subjects reached under the table top and pointed to the locations on the shelf. After learning to reach to the locations from one side of the table they moved around to the opposite side and again pointed to the location. It was possible to infer from their pointing from the opposite side whether they had learned initially geographic positions or egocentric positions. For example, suppose on the first side a particular position was to the subject's right towards the wall of the room. When the subject got to the opposite side and was asked to point to that position would she point to the right or towards the wall? All subjects pointed geographically. Thus, in this experiment even though subjects couldn't see their hands or the locations, they responded in terms of a geographic frame of reference. Of course there was a visual space available to which proprioceptive and motor outflow information might be referred. If that visual space were eliminated would subjects still respond geographically? The experiment was repeated with blindfolded subjects. Without the visual space available, some subjects, but still a minority, responded egocentrically. Thus, in this example of a very simple and small-scale space, we have evidence of a strong tendency to use geographic frames of reference, but this tendency was weakened but not eliminated by absence of vision during the task. It is possible that the tendency would be further weakened by a more general absence of vision as with blindness. That possibility has not been tested. Again, it must be stressed that this particular study showed that people tend to use a geographical reference system when given a choice. It did not show that people could not use an egocentric frame of reference if that were required.

Cognitive Maps

Part of the way spatial orientation is maintained depends on the use of frames of reference to which incoming stimulation is referred. However, an important part of maintaining orientation involves organization of spatial information. This idea is captured by Foulke (1971) in discussing mobility of the blind:

As an individual's knowledge of a terrain increases through repeated contact with it, he gradually acquired information about it, and this information is organized into a schema. This schema is abstract in character. The information in it is a selection from the potential supply of information about that terrain. The selection of information for inclusion in the schema is governed by the individual's needs, and these needs are determined by the nature of his interaction with his environment.

Cognitive maps, a term used by Tolman (1948) refers to a concept-like schema but it more directly connotes the organized information relevant to getting around the environment. A number of investigators, Siegel and White (1975), Piaget and Inhelder (1971), have suggested that as we become acquainted with a spatial layout our cognitive map changes from being fragmented route knowledge relevant for getting from one particular place to another to knowledge of the layout, integrated and coordinated reflecting the spatial relations among all the locations of the environment.

What does it mean to have such integrated knowledge of a spatial layout? It should mean that one knows how to get from any location in a space to any other. It should mean that one can take detours when the way is blocked. A strong test of such integrated knowledge would be that one could infer spatial relations among locations that one had not traveled directly between. For example, if one had traveled from point A to point B, and from point B to point C, one should be able to go directly from A to C. The study described above by Goldsmith, Mohr, and Pick (1977) in which subjects learned to point to three locations on a shelf, was designed to test such spatial inferences. The reader will recall that in that study, sight of the hand and the locations was occluded by a table top. Subjects learned to point to the three locations from a "home base." They pointed at location A from the home base and then moved their hand back to the starting position. This was repeated until they were accurate at locating A, then they learned to move from home base to location B, and then from home base to location C. Only after these three locations were learned relative to home base were they tested on their ability to move directly from A to B to C. All subjects were quite accurate at this. Apparently, people do induce spatial relations without direct experience. A study by Kosslyn,

Pick, and Fariello (1974) demonstrated this capacity in children in a larger walking space. However, in this larger space the subjects were permitted sight of the locations.

How would blind subjects compare with sighted on such a task? Worchel (1951) devised a task that, although simpler, did require spatial inference. He led subjects along two legs of a path that was laid out in the form of a right triangle and then asked them to return directly to the starting point, i.e., along the hypotenuse. He also led subjects conversely along the hypotenuse and asked them to walk back along the legs of the right-triangular path. Blind subjects made considerably greater errors than blindfolded sighted subjects under both conditions. In a task requiring actual walking as the performance measure, it is possible that the differences between blind and sighted do not reflect the differences in their knowledge of the path but rather differences in their ability to walk with precision. Rieser, Lockman, and Pick (1976) employed a method of assessing spatial organization which overcame that difficulty of interpretation. In their method, subjects were asked to compare the distance between every pair of locations in a space with the distance between every other pair. For four locations, A, B, C, D, for example, subjects were asked if the distance AB was greater than AC, if the distance AB was greater than AD, if AB was greater than BC, if AB was greater than CD, if AC was greater than CD, etc. The comparative judgments can be analyzed using a computer program developed by Kruskel and Carmone (1970) based on nonmetric scaling techniques developed by Shepard (1962) to show the simplest spatial organization which could have given rise to the subjects' comparative judgments. That is, a simplest spatial organization can be derived from rank order data. This derived spatial organization or cognitive map can be compared to an actual map of the spatial layout. In particular, it is possible to determine whether a Euclidean metric is the best way of describing the spatial organization of the knowledge. For example, if subjects are asked to make comparative judgments about a complex indoor space such as the layout of a building, their judgments might reflect the direct Euclidean distance between points not taking into account the walls or other barriers separating locations, or the judgments might reflect the functional distance between locations, that is how far apart locations are in terms of walking distance from one to another. It would seem reasonable that blind subjects might have more difficulty in integrating their spatial knowledge in an Euclidean form than would sighted subjects. Rieser et al. examined the derived cognitive maps of blind and sighted subjects for the layout of the floor of a building which they all knew very well. The maps of blind as well as sighted subjects reflected an Euclidean organization although the sighted subjects were slightly more accurate. These results were obtained with neutral instructions to the subjects, that is they simply were asked to compare pairs of distances. Subsequently, the same subjects were asked specifically to make Euclidean judgments and to make functional distance judgments. When this was done the sighted subjects showed more flexibility in adapting their spatial judgments to the task. In particular, they were able to make considerably more precise Euclidean judgments. This technique of assessing spatial knowledge is quite a powerful one and it could be used to track the cognitive maps of individuals as they learn a space. It might be a valuable diagnostic technique during mobility training.

Once a person has a cognitive map at whatever level of organization, she is often confronted with manipulating or transforming it. For example, you have always approached a neighborhood from one direction and now you are approaching it from another. You are looking at or feeling a map in one orientation but you are moving through space in the opposite direction. There is some research in certain of the factors involved in the accomplishment of such mental transformation of spatial information. One well-used technique that originated with Piaget involves asking subjects how a spatial array appears from someone else's point of view, or how a spatial array would appear after it has been rotated. Millar (1976) examined the performance of blind and blindfolded sighted children on several such tasks. Her basic experimental situation was quite simple. She used a matchstick glued on a square cardboard card. Subjects had to judge the orientation of the matchstick under the several conditions. In one condition, a simple recognition task, children were asked to feel the matchstick on a table placed in front of them at various orientations. That is, the matchstick would be lying left-right or toward-away or at an oblique angle. They then had to find a matchstick in the same orientation in a set of several displayed below. In a second condition, a perspective-taking task, the matchstick to be judged always lay on the table running toward and away from the child. The child was to indicate how that matchstick would appear from different positions around the table by selecting the appropriate matchstick from the display. For example, the toward-away matchstick would appear as lying left-right if viewed from the side of the table. Quite reasonably the older children performed better than the younger, the perspective-taking task was more difficult than the recognition task, and oblique orientations caused more errors than horizontal or vertical orientations. There was no difference between sighted and blind children. In these two conditions subjects could feel the matchstick lying in front of them while making their choice. In two other conditions a major memory component was added to the task. In one of these new conditions, a rotation task, the child always felt the matchstick in a toward-away orientation on the table in front of him. Then he felt the card on which the matchstick was mounted being rotated by some amount between 0° and 360°. When the rotation was complete the child was asked to draw how the matchstick would appear from where he was sitting. In the other condition, another perspective-taking task, the child felt the toward-away matchstick then walked to various positions around the table. He then had to draw how the matchstick would appear from his new position. In these tasks involving memory and transformations in memory, the sighted performed better than the blind. The blind children had particular difficulty with oblique views and with the greater amounts of rotation and larger changes of position. The contrast between the results of the first two conditions and the latter two suggest that the lack of visual experience may cause difficulty with tasks involving mental transformation of spatial information particularly when there is a heavy memory load.

The tasks used by Millar involve recognition of an object at various orientations rather than perceptions of spatial layout. However, this type of task as originally used by Piaget and in many subsequent studies, involved models of spatial layouts rather than objects such as matchsticks. Modifications of the task have also been used to study cognitive maps of real spatial layouts. Hardwick, McIntyre, and Pick (1976) asked subjects to imagine themselves at different station points within a space. From each of these imagined station points, subjects were asked to point to certain target locations. The directions of their pointing responses were used to triangulate locations on a map of the space. That is, the locations determined by the intersection of their pointing directions were used to construct a subject's cognitive map. These tasks involving model or real spatial layouts have not been exploited for use in studying spatial orientation of the blind.

SUMMARY AND CONCLUSION

Conceptually this chapter has moved a long way—from otoliths to cognitive maps—in an attempt to describe how stimulation relevant to maintaining spatial orientation is detected, processed, and used by people. First the mechanisms of perception of spatial information were described paying particular attention to the vestibular system. However the vestibular system does not operate in isolation and it was important to indicate how information obtained through that system was integrated with other spatial information as well as to examine the role of motor-outflow information in maintaining orientation. In many cases spatial information by its very nature is defined with respect to frames of reference. To understand the use of spatial information it was necessary to see how the stimulation was related to reference systems. Finally the spatial information is organized and transformed, and in recent years interesting techniques have been developed for studying the course and products of such information processing. These techniques, by and large, have not been used with the blind but they present intriguing possibilities for use as a basic research tool with the blind and as an aid in mobility training both for assessment of spatial knowledge and as components of training exercises. To take one example of where such techniques might be used consider two very general ways a blind person can get information about spatial layout. One is through actual experience in a space with or without the various mobility aids available. Another is through maps, tactual (Berla & Murr, 1974) or auditory (Blasch, Welsh, & Davidson, 1973). We know very little about the organization of spatial knowledge obtained through these different methods of exposure. Some of the cognitive mapping techniques would lend themselves very nicely to assessing that spatial knowledge.

Bibliography

Acredolo, L.P. Frames of reference used by children for orientation in unfamiliar spaces. In G. Moore and R. Golledge (Eds.) *Environmental knowing.* Stroudsburg, Pa.: Dowden, Hutchinson, and Ross, 1976.

Attneave, F., & Benson, B. Spatial coding of tactual stimulation. *Journal of Experimental Psychology,* 1969, **81,** 216-222.

Beritov, I. S. *Neural mechanisms of higher vertebrate behavior.* Boston: Little, Brown, and Company, 1965.

Berla, E. P., & Murr, M. J. Searching tactual space. *Education of the Visually Handicapped,* 1974, **4** (May), 49-58.

Blasch, B. B., Welsh, R. L., & Davidson, T. Auditory maps: An orientation aid for visually handicapped persons. *New Outlook for the Blind,* 1973, **67,** 145-158.

Brown, J. L. Orientation to the vertical during water immersion. *Aerospace Medicine,* 1961, **32,** 209-217.

Clark, B., & Stewart, J. P. Perception of angular acceleration about the yaw axis of a flight simulator. *Aerospace Medicine,* 1962, **33,** 1426-1432.

Cotzin, M., & Dallenbach, K. M. Facial vision: The role of pitch and loudness in the perception of obstacles by the blind. *American Journal of Psychology,* 1950, **63,** 485-515.

Dodge, R. Thresholds of rotation. *Journal of Experimental Psychology,* 1923, **6,** 107-137.

Dohlman, G. Towards a method for quantitative measurement of the functional capacity of the vestibular apparatus. *Acta oto-laryngology, Stockholm,* 1935, **23,** 50-62.

Evans, E. F. Neural processes for the detection of acoustic patterns and for sound localization. In F. O. Schmitt and F. G. Worden (Eds.), *The neurosciences third study program.* Cambridge, Mass.: MIT Press, 1974.

Fisher, G. H. Spatial localization by the blind. *American Journal of Psychology,* 1964, **77,** 2014.

Foulke, E. The perceptual basis for mobility. *Research Bulletin* No. 23. New York: American Foundation for the Blind, 1971.

Gernandt, B. E. Vestibular mechanisms. In J. Field, H. W. Magoun, and V. E. Hall (Eds.) *Handbook of Physiology* Section 1: *Neurophysiology,* Volume 1. Washington, D.C.: American Physiological Society, 1959.

Gibson, J. J. *The senses considered as perceptual systems.* Boston: Houghton Mifflin Company, 1966.

Goldsmith, L. T., Mohr, D. M., & Pick, H. L., Jr. Cognitive maps in children and adults: Inferences about spatial relations after rotation. Paper presented at Eastern Psychological Association Meetings, Boston, April, 1977.

Hardwick, D. A., McIntyre, C. W., & Pick, H. L., Jr. Content and manipulation of cognitive maps in children and adults. *Monographs of the Society for Research in Child Development,* 1976, **41**(3), Serial No. 166.

Helmholtz, H. von *Treatise on physiological optics.* New York: Dover, 1962.

Hermelin, B., & O'Connor, N. Spatial coding in normal, autistic, and blind children. *Perceptual and Motor Skills,* 1971, **33,** 127-132.

Howard, I. P., & Templeton, W. B. *Human spatial orientation.* New York: Wiley, 1966.

Kosslyn, S. M., Pick, H. L., Jr., & Fariello, G. R. Cognitive maps in children and man. *Child Development,* 1974, **45,** 707-716.

Kruskal, J. P., & Carmone, F. *How to use M-D SCAL (Version 5M) and other useful information.* Cambridge: Marketing Science Institute, 1970.

Lee, D. N., & Aronson, E. Visual proprioceptive control of standing in human infants. *Perception and Psychophysics,* 1974, **15,** 529-532.

Lee, D. N., & Lishman, J. R. Visual proprioceptive control of stance. *Journal of Human Movement Studies,* 1975, **1,** 87-95.

McKinney, J. P. Hand schema in children. *Psychonomic Science,* 1964, **1,** 99-100.

Merton, P. A. Human position sense and sense of effort. Society of Experimental Biology Symposium XVHI *Homeostasis and Feedback Mechanisms.* Cambridge: Cambridge University Press, 1964, **18,** 387-400.

Millar, S. Spatial representation by blind and sighted children. *Journal of Experimental Child Psychology,* 1976, **21,** 460-479.

Montandon, A., & Russbach, A. L'epreuve giratoire liminaire. *Pract. oto-rhino-laryng.,* 1955, **17,** 224-236.

Piaget, J., & Inhelder, B. *Mental imagery in the child.* New York: Basic Books, 1971.

Pick, H. L., Jr., Warren, D. H., & Hay, J. C. The resolution of sensory conflict between vision proprioception and audition. *Perception and Psychophysics,* 1969, **6,** 203-206.

Rice, C. E. Human echo perception. *Science,* 1967, **155,** 656-664.

Rieser, J., Lockman, J., & Pick, H. L., Jr. The role of visual experience in spatial representation. Paper presented at meetings of the Psychonomic Society, St. Louis, Missouri, November, 1976.

Rieser, J. J., & Pick, H. L., Jr. Reference systems and the perception of tactual and haptic orientation. *Perception and Psychophysics,* 1976, **19,** 117-121.

Shepard, R. N. The analysis of proximities: Multi dimensional scaling with an unknown distance function. I. *Psychometrika,* 1962, **27,** 125-140; II. *Psychometrika,* 1962, **27,** 219-246.

Siegel, A. W., & White, S. H. The development of spatial representations of large-scale environments. In H. W. Reese (Ed.), *Advances in Child Development and Behavior,* Volume 10, New York: Academic Press, 1975.

Supa, M., Cotzin, M., & Dallenbach, K. M. "Facial vision": The perception of obstacles by the blind. *American Journal of Psychology,* 1944, **57,** 133-183.

Taub, E., & Berman, A. J. Movement and learning in the absence of sensory feedback. In Freedman, S. J. (Ed.), *The neuropsychology of spatially oriented behavior.* Homewood, Ill.: Dorsey Press 1966.

Tolman, E. C. Cognitive maps in rats and men. *Psychological Review,* 1948, **55,** 189-208.

Trevarthen, C. B. Two mechanisms of vision in primates. *Psychologische Forshung,* 1968, **31,** 299-337.

Walsh, E. G., The perception of rhythmically repeated linear motion in the horizontal plane. *British Journal of Psychology,* 1962, **53,** 439-445.

Warren, D. H., & Pick, H. L., Jr. Developmental study of sensory conflict in sighted and blind Ss. *Perception and Psychophysics,* 1970, **8,** 430-432.

Worchel, P. Space perception and orientation in the blind. *Psychological Monographs,* 1951, **65,** 1-28.

Tactual and Haptic Perception*

Herbert L. Pick, Jr.

This chapter deals with haptic perception. However, as will be pointed out in detail below, haptic perception is hard to define in a precise way. A working definition for the chapter topic will, following Gibson (1966), stress what the layman means by *touch*. It will include both perception as it occurs when stimulation is imposed on a person's skin (when a person reports he feels something touching him) and perception when a person actively touches something else (when he says he is feeling something). The term *haptic perception* will be used to refer to this latter active perceptual process and it will receive the major emphasis of the discussion. *Tactual perception* will refer to the former more passive process. Occasionally, in particular situations the distinction becomes blurred.

The plan of this chapter is to focus on how object identification and pattern recognition can be accomplished by tactual and haptic perception. In the first section, haptic perception of shape and pattern will be directly examined to see what in the way of perception can be accomplished and how these perceptual processes can be studied. In the second section, the discussion will become more analytic and a psychophysical approach to haptic perception will be considered. The third section will focus on the physiological and behavioral mechanisms of tactual and haptic perception. In the fourth section, there will be consideration of the processing and encoding of tactual and haptic information.

It is important for the mobility specialist to understand these aspects of haptic perception since haptic perception is one of the most important modes of information input available to blind persons. Haptic perception is implicated directly in the mobility of blind persons when they are reading braille maps or identifying objects in order to orient themselves in spaces such as rooms. It is also implicated more directly in general strategies blind persons might use for perceiving, processing, and storing spatial information.

SHAPE AND PATTERN PERCEPTION
An Empirical Approach

One of the early systematic studies of nonvisual pattern recognition was undertaken under the pressures of World War II. Control of military aircraft was becoming increasingly complex. Pilots were being required to process more and more information under greater and greater time pressure. They had to make decisions and position controls appropriately. Often pilots were positioning controls manually according to information they were obtaining visually. Some-

*Preparation of this chapter was supported by grants from the National Institute of Child Health and Human Development to the University of Minnesota: Institute of Child Development (HD 05027), and Center for Research in Human Learning (HD 01136); and by a grant from the National Science Foundation also to the Center for Research in Human Learning (GB-17590).

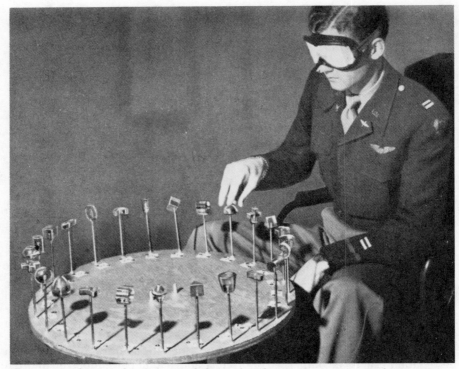

Figure 1-5. Subject performing tactual shape identification experiment. (Jenkins, 1947.)

times confusion would occur when pilots would move the incorrect control lever. While the spatial location of control levers is often a useful nonvisual cue for recognition, different planes had the same control handles in different positions. W. O. Jenkins (1947) undertook an investigation to determine a set of control-handle shapes which would not be confused when felt by pilots. He surveyed a large set of possible shapes and chose 25 for systematic experimentation. In one experiment, he placed the 25 shapes on a turntable (Fig. 1-5) and asked blindfolded pilot-subjects to feel a shape and then to recognize that shape from the set of 25 after the turntable had been rotated to a new position. This procedure was repeated for each of the 25 different shapes. A confusion matrix (Fig. 2-5) recorded results in terms of confusions among the various shapes and in terms of hesitation in making recognition judgments. Some of the shapes were highly confusable with others. A subset of 11 shapes (shown in Fig. 3-5) were never or rarely confused with each other. These could serve as a very distinctive set for coding control levers. A secondary finding was that performance did not markedly deteriorate if the pilots were wearing light flying gloves.

This investigation was undertaken with a very specific pragmatic goal in mind—to find a small set of unconfusable three-dimensional shapes. The study did not report any general principles about what properties of shapes made them very distinctive or how the pilots went about exploring the shapes in the recognition task. As can be seen in Figs. 1-5 and 3-5, the shapes used tended to be geometric forms or at least fairly regular forms and in many cases, quite readily

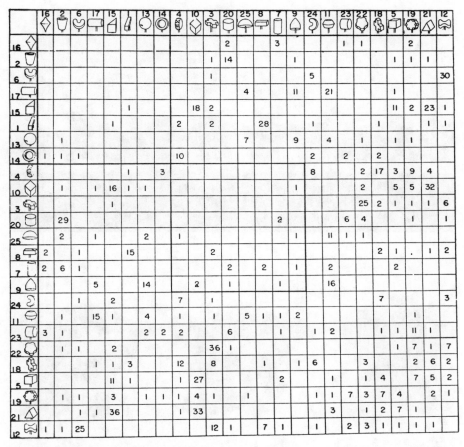

	16	2	6	17	15	1	13	14	4	10	3	20	25	8	7	9	24	11	23	22	18	5	19	21	12
16												2			3				1	1		2			
2											1	14			1							1	1	1	
6											1					5									30
17											4				11			21				1			
15					1				18		2											11	2	23	1
1			1						2		2			28		1					1			1	1
13		1										7				9		4		1		1	1		
14	1	1	1							10						2			2	2					
4					1		3									8				2	17	3	9	4	
10		1	1	16	1	1									1						2	5	5	32	
3				1																25	2	1	1	1	6
20		29														2			6	4		1			1
25		2	1				2				1					1			11	1	1				
8	2		1		15						2									2	1	.		1	2
7	2	6	1								2		2			1		2				2			
9			5				14				1				1			16							
24			1	2					7		1									7					3
11		1	15	1			4		1		1		5	1	1	2						1			
23	3	1					2	2	2		6				1		1	2			1	1	11	1	
22		1	1	2							36	1									1	7	1		7
18			1	1	3				12		8			1		1		6		3		2	6		2
5				11	1					1	27					2		1		1		4	7	5	2
19		1	1	3			1	1	1	4	1					1		1	7	3	7	4		2	1
21		1	1	36					1	1	33									3		1	2	7	1
12	1	1	25							12	1			7	1		1		2	3	1	1	1	1	

Figure 2-5. Confusion matrix: number of times shape in vertical column was erroneously selected for stimulus in horizontal row. (Jenkins, 1947.)

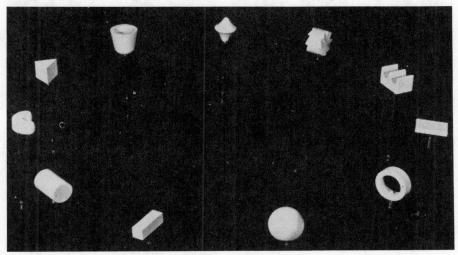

Figure 3-5. Eleven highly distinct shapes. (Jenkins, 1947.)

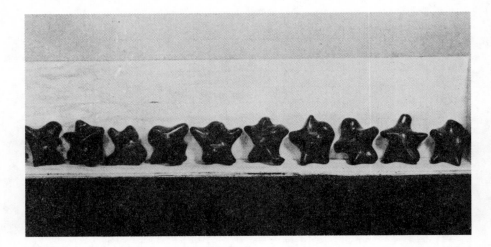

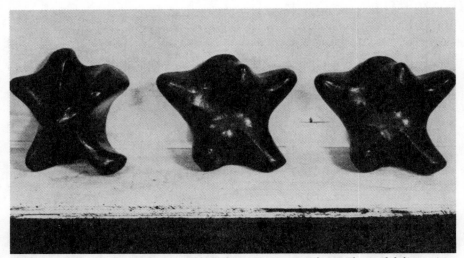

Figure 4-5. Irregular shapes developed by Gibson. (From J. J. Gibson, The useful dimensions of sensitivity, *American Psychologist*, 18(1), 1963, 1-15. Copyright © 1963 by the American Psychological Association, Inc. Reprinted by permission.)

nameable. Those characteristics were quite appropriate for the task at hand. However, they are probably just the characteristics which should be missing if one wanted a difficult object recognition task to find out how people extracted the perceptual information in such tactual shapes.

Nature of Haptic Exploration of Objects

James Gibson and his colleagues (Gibson, 1963) generated a set of irregular solid shapes which at first glance were highly confusable (Fig. 4-5). These shapes all had six protuberances with various sized convexities and concavities on the front side and a smooth convex back side. The distinctive parts of these shapes were not easily countable or nameable. They were presented to subjects (college students) to explore for subsequent recognition. One major purpose of the investigation was to observe just how the perceptual exploration was carried out.

Gibson (1966, p. 125) reports that an observer given such a shape to feel behind a curtain typically does the following:

1. He curves his fingers around its face, using all fingers and fitting them into the cavities.

2. He moves his fingers in a way that can only be called exploratory, since the movements do not seem to become stereotyped, or to occur in any fixed sequence, or even to be clearly repeated.

3. He uses oppositions of thumb and finger, but with different fingers; he rubs with one or more fingers, and occasionally he seems to trace a curvature with a single finger. The activity seems to be aimed principally at obtaining a set of touch-positions, the movement as such being incidental to this aim . . . the tracing out of the surface with one finger, as if the observer were trying to draw a model of it or reproduce the shape, did not occur often enough to be typical . . . the manual activity mght be called scanning but it is not the same as visual scanning.

Gibson means that subjects do not trace out the contours of objects with their fingers nor do they scan systematically left to right across objects or jump from one side to another as they might do visually. Subjects can learn to discriminate these forms within an hour or so of nonvisual training. They can then identify the objects as soon as they are placed in the hand.

Another investigation with the aim of ascertaining how people actually go about perceiving haptically was conducted by a group of Soviet investigators, Ananev, Lomov, Vekker, and Yarmolenko (1959). In this research, time motion analyses of hand movements during haptic exploration were described. Subjects were given cutout forms to explore and then to reproduce by drawing. Their hand movements were filmed during the haptic exploration and subjected to a frame-by-frame analysis. Three general stages of exploration were distinguished: an orienting phase, a first groping phase, and a second groping phase. The orienting phase involved movements of both hands in the air or on the table on which the form rested; movements away from the body until the form was contacted. Then the hands typically skimmed along the form until its distant edge was reached. At that edge there is a pause in movement for 0.2 to 1.5 seconds. Thus the relative location of the body is fixed. In the first groping stage, the two hands circumscribe the object apparently to get a general idea of the form. A drawing of the form at this stage demonstrates general knowledge of the form but little detail or relations between details. Subsequent exploration in the second groping phase provides more detailed knowledge. In this stage the movements of the two hands are coordinated so that they tend to move in succession, one hand seeming to act as a reference point while the other hand is in motion. Sometimes this detailed exploration is carried out with one hand. In that case, typically, the finger movements are coordinated. Again, a single finger will remain fixed while the others move as if to establish a reference point.

These studies by Gibson and the Soviets are provocative in that they suggest what the active haptic perceptual behavior is like. They are not as informative as they might be because it is difficult to tell in any detail what information a subject has gotten from his particular kind of perceptual behavior. To study that question in detail requires that the stimuli to be perceived vary systematically, and that changes in perception be carefully related to that systematic variation in the stimuli. Unfortunately, there are practically no studies which both examine the perceptual behavior and relate that behavior to how changes in stimuli are reflected in change of perception.

Systematic Variation of Object Characteristics

In relating stimulus variation to perception, two slightly different approaches have been taken. One involves analysis of complex patterns or objects which are changed in systematic ways. (Jenkins' study, described above, varied complex objects but not in systematic ways.) The second involves varying pure physical dimensions and seeing how perception changes. This is essentially the approach of traditional psychophysics.

Let us see how an investigation involving systematic variation of complex objects would work. Pick and Pick (1966) presented to blindfolded subjects for discrimination, pairs of forms consisting of raised lines on a metal background. The shapes were letter-like forms prepared for an earlier study of visual perception (Gibson, Gibson, Pick & Osser, 1962). The forms were nonsense line drawings made with straight and curved line segments (Fig. 5-5). For any given pair the shapes differed in one of four ways: a rotation or reversal of the other, curved or straight line(s) in one were changed to the opposite in the other, a size or perspective transformation (a non-uniform compression or expansion) of the other, a topological transformation of the other (continuous line segments in one were disrupted in the other). The two stimuli were explored simultaneously by a subject using one hand for each. Subjects simply judged whether the two forms were exactly the same or were different.

The perspective transformations were most difficult to discriminate, line-to-curve changes were second in difficulty, while rotations and reversals, and topological transformations were equally easy. In the visual discrimination study by Gibson et al. (1962), perspective transformations and line-to-curve changes were also very difficult to discriminate. However, rotations and reversals were harder than topological transformations. The relative ease in discriminating both the latter two types of transformation by touch probably reflects the nature of the subjects' simultaneous explorations of the pairs of shapes. A subject would typically place his finger at corresponding points on the two shapes and move them in unison across the form. When a point was reached where the two forms did not match, a judgment of *different* could be made. With such exploration, rotations and reversals produced distinct mismatches in the same manner as the topological transformations.

Another example of perception of systematically varying complex objects involves the use of irregular "random" shapes. These shapes are generated by interconnecting a set of points related at random from a matrix. For example, starting with a 20 x 20 matrix, 8 points might be chosen at random and a polygon constructed by interconnecting these. Then a second polygon would be constructed from another set of 8 points, etc. That is, in terms of information theory it requires the same amount of information to specify all polygons constructed from the same number of points from a given size matrix. Brumaghim and Brown (1968) asked subjects to judge the complexity of such shapes and found that complexity was linearly related to number of sides. In a subsequent study, Owen and Brown (1970) correlated a large number of physical measures of shapes of this general type with judgments of complexity and with reaction time in making such judgments. They found (by factor analysis) that four factors accounted for 90 percent of the variance of complexity judgments. The single best factor described as "jagged-ness" was almost as good by itself as the four factors. This jaggedness factor was highly correlated with number of sides, perimeter, length, and variability of interior angle.

These sample studies of nonvisual perception of complex objects are a little disappointing insofar as they do not provide any general rules or description of how nonvisual object perception operates. Part of the difficulty appears to be that

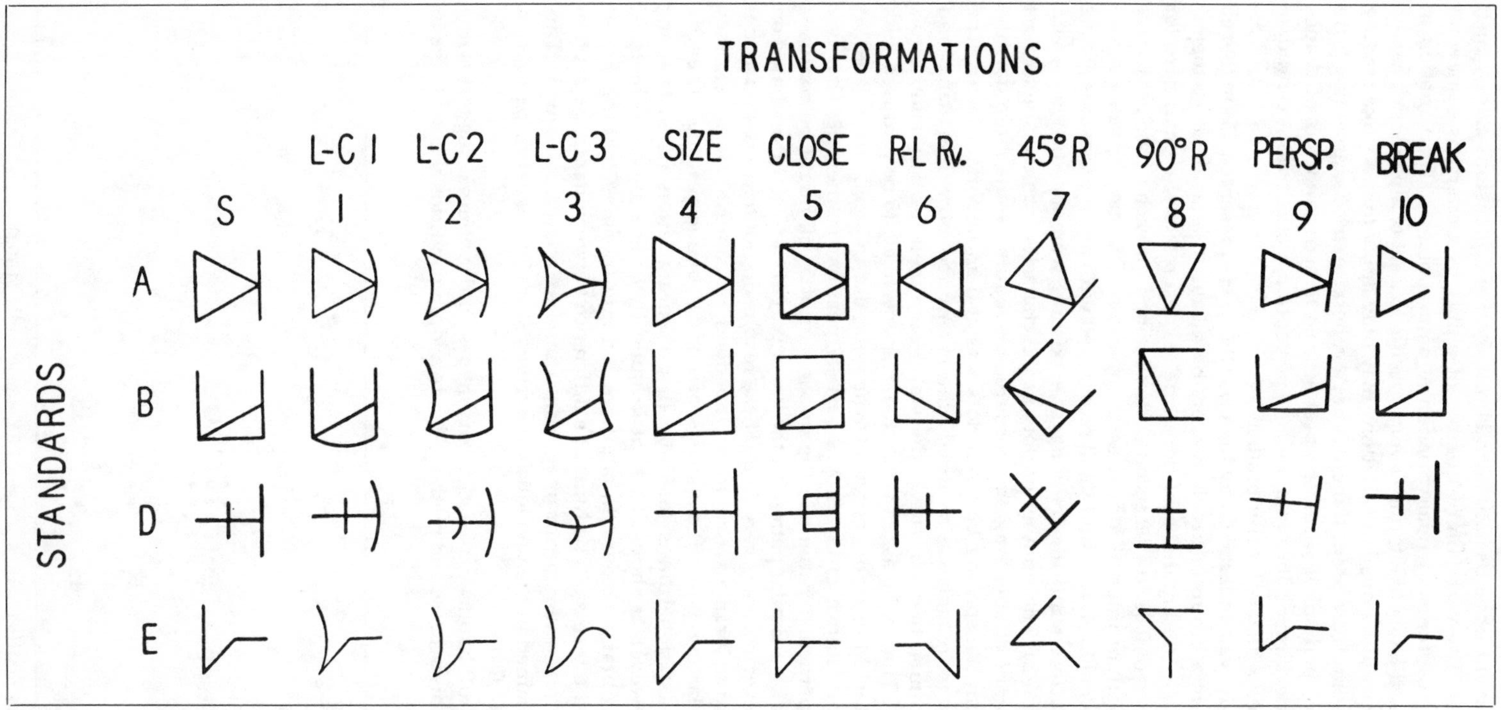

Figure 5-5. Standards (prototypes) and transformations used by Pick (1965). Some children had only standards (S) A and B and two types of their transformations in training. Other children had in training only standards D and E and two types of their transformation. After learning, they were tested on new standards and/or new transformations. (S refers to standard form: L-C1, L-C2, L-C3 refer to line-to-curve changes of 1, 2, and 3 segments respectively; BREAK and CLOSE refer to topological transformations; R-L RV. refers to right-left reversal; 45°R and 90°R refer to 45° and 90° rotations respectively; PERSP. refers to perspective transformation, and SIZE refers to size transformation.) (From A. D. Pick. Improvement of visual and tactual form discrimination. *Journal of Experimental Psychology*, 69(4), 1965, 331-339. Copyright © 1965 by the American Psychological Association, Inc. Reprinted by permission.)

there does not exist any obvious natural and limited set of dimensions along which to vary the objects. The variation of number of points in a matrix is somewhat arbitrary and only captures a trivial variation of natural objects. The variation in the case of the raised letter-like forms is very specific to a set of alphabetic shapes. Understanding perception of such variations may only apply to tasks like reading where that set of stimuli are used. If there is not a general metric for assessing form or shape variation, perhaps it would be best at least to start with sets of shapes which are of practical importance in nonvisual perception. One obvious candidate is the set of shapes which comprise braille.

Just such a study was undertaken by Kederis (1963). He presented 55 single-cell braille characters to a group of braille readers by means of a tachistotactometer. This device enabled presentations of very brief exposures of the characters for controlled durations of 0.01 to 1.00 second. He obtained for each of the characters the minimum length of interval for correct recognition. The most quickly recognized characters were *E, A, I, C,* and *K,* all recognized with mean exposures of 0.02 second. The characters requiring the longest exposures were *for*—0.19 sec., and *Q*—0.18 sec. (Fig. 6-5). The number of dots in the character was the single most important determiner of how long an exposure was required—the more dots the longer. In addition, the spacing between dots was also an important factor. The closer the dots, the more time was required, thus *H* required more time than *U* and *dis* required more time than *sh,* etc. Kederis also examined the confusion errors which were made. That is, he asked what character was likely to be confused with any given character. Most errors occurred when one dot in a cell was missed. A relatively secondary source of errors was vertical position in the cell. That is a character with a particular pattern in the upper part of a cell might be confused with a character with a similar pattern in the lower part of the cell. Errors based on added dots and reversals were very rare. These results do not necessarily account for errors in reading braille when it is embedded in context. However, they suggest a good starting point for analysis of normal braille reading. They do suggest perhaps a rational basis for order of presenting letters when teaching initial braille. However, it should be kept in mind that the subjects in Kederis' study were skilled braille readers. In addition, it might be noted that the lack of confusion errors of a reversal type hints at a difference between haptic perception and visual perception where mirror image confusions are relatively frequent. This result was also obtained in the previously described study of the haptic perception of raised letter-like forms.

These studies of haptic exploration of shapes and patterns suggest some characteristics of this process and methods for developing additional knowledge in this area.

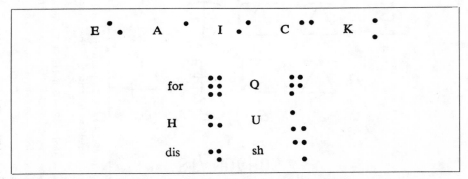

Figure 6-5. Exemplar braille characters used in Kederis study (1963).

5

PSYCHOPHYSICS OF HAPTIC PERCEPTION
Weber's Law

The traditional psychophysical approach is to determine how perception changes with variation in "pure" stimulus dimensions. These pure dimensions are also relatively simple ones and the emphasis of research is, by definition, not on complex or meaningful objects but on objects simply as carriers of the dimension of interest. The hope is that if the perception of simple pure dimensions is well understood, that understanding can be applied to complex shapes and objects made up of combinations of values of the pure dimensions. Size is such a simple dimension and will be used to illustrate the traditional psychophysical approach. One way to measure the way perception changes with variations in the dimension of size is to examine how much an object must be changed in size before the change is detected. The amount of change required for such detection depends on the initial size. Thus small objects require small changes and large objects require larger changes. In fact the ratio of amount of change required for detection to the initial size is roughly a constant. This statement has come to be known as Weber's Law and the constant ratio is known as the Weber Fraction. For a variety of experiments on haptic size judgments, the Weber Fraction was found to be around 0.10 (Berlá & Murr, 1975; Gaydos, 1958; Duran & Tufenkjian, 1969; Kelvin, 1954; Ringel, Saxman, & Brooks, 1967). Berlá and Murr, for example, asked blind subjects to run their fingertip along a standard raised line, attending to the line's *width*. They were then asked to feel a comparison line and judge which one was wider. The standard line was compared with a set of different comparison lines which were both wider and narrower than the standard. Thus a standard line 0.08 in. (0.2 cm) in width was compared with comparison lines ranging from 0.05 in. (0.13 cm) in width to 0.11 in. (0.28 cm) in width in 0.005-in. (0.12-cm) steps. A set of different standard lines was also used. Thus after a subject finished the comparisons with the 0.10-in. (0.25-cm) standard he would repeat the procedure with a different standard, e.g., 0.04 in. (0.10 cm) wide, etc. For each standard the width of comparison line detectable as wider 50 percent of the time was determined. For most of the standards that width had to be about 10 percent wider than the standard. Hence the Weber Fraction of 0.10.*

Stevens' Power Function

Another way of assessing how perception changes with variations in a single dimension is simply to see how perception on that dimension increases with increase of values on the corresponding physical dimension. In the case of size, for example, how does our perception of size increase with increases in physical size? S. S. Stevens has demonstrated that for many dimensions perceived magnitude is proportional to physical magnitude raised to some power. Formally: Perceptual judgment $\sim$ (Physical Value) n where $\sim$ means "is proportional to." The exponent n differs for different dimensions. When n is greater than 1, perception is increasing faster than the physical dimension. That is, small physical changes produce large perceptual changes. Judging the intensity of electric shock, for example, produces psychophysical functions with n greater than 1. Where n is less than 1, large physical changes produce small perceptual changes. Judging the intensity of light, for example, produces psychophysical functions with n less than 1. Stevens and Stone (1959) asked blindfolded subjects to estimate the thickness of blocks held between the fingers of one hand. They found that the judged size was

---

*In this experiment the standard stimuli were very small, between 0.08 and 0.11 in. (0.2 and 0.28 cm). However, similar results have been obtained with larger stimuli up to 4 in. (10.2 cm) (Gaydos, 1958) and 12 in. (30.5 cm) (Duran & Tufenkjian, 1969). The Weber Fraction was about 0.04 in. (0.10 cm) in the former case and 0.10 in. (0.25 cm) in the latter case.

equal to the physical size raised to the 1.3 power. In general, other experiments on haptic perception of size have also found the exponent of the power function to be about 1.0.*

Although an original aim of experiments like those on the Weber Fraction and on Stevens' Power Function was to be able to predict perception of complex objects, perception psychologists have rarely followed through on the goal. (In fact that goal may really be unobtainable because the perception of complex objects often depends on the relations *between* the simple dimensions and, of course, these relations are not captured when dimensions are studied in isolation.) Does this mean that such psychophysical experiments are useless? Not so; they can be valuable in their own right. Consider a case where one wants to represent different kinds of information for a blind person on a map. For example, one might want to represent the outline of countries with wide lines, the outline of states with narrower lines, and the outline of counties with still narrower lines. How wide should the lines of these three different political subdivisions be made? The information collected by Berlá and Murr (1975) would be most valuable. They found changes in line width of 0.10 or 10 percent would be detectable 50 percent of the time. Of course, 50 percent detectability would not be good enough for most people to read the maps. However, they also went ahead and found what change was detectable 90 percent of the time. It turned out to be a change of 25 to 30 percent. Ninety percent detectability is probably high enough to be useful and armed with that data a map maker would be in position to at least start to use line width for encoding political boundaries.

To illustrate a possible use of the Stevens' Power Function for haptic size perception, consider the following: If one wanted to represent for blind people the relative sizes of objects, using scale models, would one building which is twice as big as another, in reality be twice the size in the model? No, doubling the width of the model would be too much. If the judged size is equal to the physical size raised to the 1.3 power as described above, then doubling the actual size would more than double the perceived size. This can be demonstrated formally by remembering that Perceived width = (Physical width)$^{1.3}$ or Original perceived width = (Original physical width)$^{1.3}$ If the physical width is doubled we have New perceived width = (2 original physical width)$^{1.3}$ which equals $2^{1.3}$ (Original physical width)$^{1.3}$ which is approximately 2.5 times the original perceived width. So if we want to double the perceived size we should increase the physical size by a factor somewhat less than two.

Other Haptic Psychophysical Dimensions

It is hoped that by this time the reader is convinced, at least in a general way, of the usefulness of these psychophysical techniques of measuring or characterizing our perception of various pure dimensions. Assuming that is true, a few other dimensions for which Weber Fractions and/or power functions have been determined will be briefly mentioned. Such dimensions as weight, hardness, viscosity, and geometric properties of straightness and curvature can be important for identification of objects and for precise estimation of object properties. In addition there are certain haptic illusions which could mislead blind persons, particularly where precise metric or quantitative judgments are necessary. Weight was one of the first stimulus dimensions to be investigated psychophysically. In fact, Weber himself developed the concept of his constant fraction on the basis of experiments

---

*Again stimuli which can be held between the fingers of one hand are quite small. However, similar results have been obtained with larger stimuli. Estimates of distances between the hands up to 33 in. (84 cm) yielded power functions with exponents of 0.94 for empty space and 0.98 and 1.05 for length of rods held between the hands (Stanley, 1966; Teghtsoonian & Teghtsoonian, 1965).

on lifted weights. Subjects were asked to lift a series of weights and compare them to a standard weight, in each case saying which is heavier or lighter. He obtained a Weber Fraction of about 1/40 or 0.025 and in subsequent research Weber Fractions between 0.05 and 0.10 have usually been obtained (Woodworth, 1938). This would mean according to the definition of the Weber Fraction that 5 to 10 grams would have to be added to a 100-gram weight for it to be discriminated.

Harper and Stevens (1948) determined a power function for lifted weights. They used a ratio scaling procedure to generate this function. Their particular method involved simply asking subjects to find a weight perceived as half a given standard weight. Plotting these results revealed that the perceived weight could be related to the real weight by a power function with exponent of 1.45. In terms of the previous analysis, this would indicate that perceived weight is increasing faster than physical weight.

In analogous fashion, power functions have been obtained for a variety of other haptic dimensions: Perceived hardness is a power function of physical hardness, as measured by the ratio of force divided by indentation, with an exponent of 0.7 (Harper & Stevens, 1964). Perceived viscosity (the relative stickiness of liquids like water, oil, gasoline, etc.) is a power function of physical viscosity, measured in centipoises, with an exponent of 0.4 (Stevens & Guirao, 1964). Perceived roughness and smoothness of emery grit paper are power functions of physical roughness measured by grit size or coefficient of friction, with exponents ranging between 0.90 and 1.85 for different experiments (Stevens & Harris, 1962; Eckman, Hosman, & Lindstrom, 1965; Stone, 1967).

There are other physically simple dimensions which have not been explored systematically using the psychophysical measures under discussion. Some of these have been investigated with less sophisticated techniques. In a classic study, von Skramlik (1937) examined haptic perception of straight lines, parallel lines, right angles, and circles. For example, in the case of straight lines he determined that the direction of motion of the exploring organ's surface biased the perception of the direction of the line in space. Thus if a subject moved the upper surface of his hand along a frontal-parallel horizontal edge and the hand motion had a transverse vector in its motion, the edge was perceived as having a tilt and not being horizontal. Again, if a subject ran his finger along a surface pivoting the entire movement at a single joint such as the elbow, a curve is obviously traced out. However, if the arc is not too long there is the illusory perception of a straight line. (For example, if a person moved his fully extended hand horizontally from left to right in front of himself pivoting it at the shoulder his finger would trace out a slight arc rather than a perfectly straight line. However if the left right movement is not too great his impression is that his hand or finger has moved in a straight line.) A similar observation was more systematically explored by Rubin (1935). He also found that an edge concave toward a person was perceived as straight. In his study, subjects ran their fingers along the edge of a piece of steel 24 cm (9.5 in.) in length. Different amounts of curvature were perceived as straight depending on whether movement was made from the elbow or shoulder. This error, as well as thresholds for detecting curvature, was slightly less for movements of exploration that involved only the shoulder joint than if involving only the elbow joint. The constant error, i.e., perceiving a curved line as straight, might be interpreted in the following way: A line is perceived as straight if the exploring organ maintains contact with it during movement pivoted around a given joint. Thus, fingers exploring with movement around an elbow trace out a sharper curve than movement around a shoulder joint. The presence of such a constant error was confirmed by Blumenfeld (1937), Crewdson and Zangwell (1940), and Hunter (1954). Crewdson and Zangwell also verified the greater precision of movements involving the shoulder joint. This discovery has implications for the use of the cane and arm in exploring the curvature of curves or the shape of objects used in establishing orientation.

Parallelism represents another example of an important geometric property investigated by von Skramlik. He studied the precision with which a rod could be set haptically so that it was parallel to a given standard rod. Previous work had shown a rather high degree of precision when the rods were placed on the same plane surface and hence had only one degree of freedom. He showed that the error was considerable when the task was such that the rods were not on the same surface, i.e., they could be rotated in three dimensions. Errors ranged from 15' to 6° of arc depending on the particular orientation of the standard and on the plane in which errors were measured as well as which hand was used and the distance from the person. In general, the farther away the comparison was made, the greater the error.

As noted before, the existence of such errors has implications for precise perception by blind persons when it is directed toward metric or quantitative judgments. Probably for ordinary object perception by blind persons such precision is not necessary. Objects are distinguished from each other by multiple cues, even some which have distinctive arbitrary features. For example, coins differ along the dimensions of size, thickness, weight, and radius of curvature. In addition, they have different distinctive markings. Nevertheless it might be helpful to at least call attention to such constant errors as can occur.

Haptic Perception of Geometric Form

Another type of constant error which occurs in haptic perception is the geometric illusion. It turns out that at least two of the classical visual geometric illusions have haptic counterparts: the Müller-Lyer illusion and the horizontal-vertical illusion. The Müller-Lyer illusion is the well-known illusion in which a line segment terminated by arrowheads is perceived as shorter than an objectively equal line segment terminated by arrow tails. This occurs haptically when the forms are presented as raised lines, Over (1966). The horizontal-vertical illusion consists of an overestimation of vertical lines in comparison with horizontal lines. This occurs haptically when a person without sight moves a stylus medially toward and away from himself the same subjective distance that he previously moved it in the frontal parallel plane (i.e., right-left). The medial movement is made too short (Reid, 1954). Further work on this illusion by Davidon and Cheng (1964) indicated that it was not so much the direction of movement that produced the illusion but whether the movement was flexion-extension as was involved in the medial movement or abduction-adduction which was involved in the frontal parallel movement. At first it was thought that these illusions might be due to the effects of visual experience because the illusions were first discovered visually and the original haptic experiments were conducted using blindfolded sighted subjects. However, congenitally blind subjects were also found susceptible to both these illusions (Hatwell, 1960; Tsai, 1967).

A final illusion to be mentioned is the size-weight illusion. This occurs when two equal weights of *different* sizes are compared, for example, by picking one up in each hand. The smaller weight feels heavier. This illusion was also first discovered when the procedure was carried out with vision. However, it works just as well if the weights are presented without vision (Pick & Pick, 1967), that is, if blindfolded subjects compare the weights when they are perceiving both the size and weight information haptically. It is possible to measure the magnitude of this illusion by increasing the weight of the larger object until it is judged as heavy as the smaller object. It was found with one set of objects that the weight of the larger object had to be increased by as much as 40 to 50 percent to reach this point of equilibrium.

Again, it may be that the size-weight illusion and the geometric illusions do not matter a great deal for ordinary perception by blind persons but one can imagine cases where a blind person might want to compare the weight of two different sized objects or to feel if a shape is approximately square. In both such cases, the existence of these illusions is likely to lead to an error. The horizontal-vertical and the Müller-Lyer illusions, for example, might well cause errors in reading braille maps. In cases where a blind person might want to compare the weight of two different sized objects, the size-weight illusion would produce an error. Since these errors are substantial, blind persons should certainly be warned of their existence.

Constancy

Paradoxically, illusions where perception is not as good as one would like seem to be closely related to the so-called constancies where perception appears to be better than it ought to be. Perceptual constancy in visual perception refers to the fact that perception remains constant and valid in spite of changes in the image on the retina of the eye. Thus, size constancy refers to the fact that the perception of the size of an object is constant even when viewed from very different distances from which, of course, the size of the image projected to the eye would be very different. In some way or other that variation in retinal image size does not produce errors in our perception. Similar constancy occurs for shape: we perceive the same object shape in spite of great differences in the shape of the retinal image from the same object when it is viewed from different angles. Constancy occurs too for brightness: we see objects as white or dark in spite of gross changes in illumination. Generally speaking, constancy refers to the fact that our perception is faithful to the distal object and not to the varying proximal image in our eye.

With haptic perception the phenomenon of constancy also exists but it is not as obvious as with visual perception. If one thinks back to Gibson's description of haptic exploration quoted early in this chapter, it will be recalled that his subjects felt around those peculiar shapes in a non-stereotypic way. In fact, if the hand exploration were to be photographed from trial to trial, we would see that each exploration would be quite different. These different patterns of exploration obviously would give rise to different patterns of stimulation on the skin. Yet the perception remains the same—a haptic shape constancy. The reason this is not so obvious a phenomenon for haptic exploration as for vision is probably due to the fact that it is much more difficult to measure the haptic pattern of stimulation than it is to measure the visual retinal image.

There are two examples of weight perception which do seem quite analogous to the visual constancies. In one, Fischel (1926) studied the perception of lifted weights. He found that perception of weights was remarkably constant in spite of natural or artificial changes in the weight of the body member doing the lifting. In a second, Torrey (1963) studied the effect of torque on perception of weight. Weights were fastened at different distances along a horizontal rod and blindfolded subjects lifted the weights by grasping the end of the rod and applying a lifting torque (much as one might do when lifting an egg with a spatula). Results indicated that the perceived weight was a compromise between that predicted on the basis of true weight and that predicted on the basis of torque applied.

One other type of constancy will be briefly mentioned here. That is object constancy or conservation. This is a concept discovered by Piaget which refers to the fact that at a certain age infants appear to realize that an object continues to exist even when it goes out of sight. Before this critical age, infants act as if out of sight means out of mind. If they drop something or it is hidden they appear to have forgotten completely about it and appear to be surprised when it reappears. After this age they will search for objects which are dropped or hidden and show little surprise when they reappear. Blind infants are generally slow to develop such object constancy (Fraiberg, 1968; Fraiberg, Siegel, & Gibson, 1966). At a much later age than sighted infants they will ignore dropped objects. They will attend an object that makes a noise, but if it is silent they will cease to be interested in it—long after the age when a sighted child shows object constancy.

Recently Bower (1977) has reported that the Sonic Torch when worn by a blind infant seems to accelerate the development of object constancy. The head-mounted echo device seems to provide the infant with a way of actually controlling stimulation from objects at a distance. This cannot be done by touch because of the distance and cannot be done by passive listening if the object does not generate sound.

MECHANISMS OF TACTUAL AND HAPTIC PERCEPTION

How are the tactual and haptic receptor systems stimulated? Tactual perception occurs when something touches our skin directly or indirectly through a covering such as clothing. This, of course, occurs when routes are conveyed to blind persons by drawing on the hand or back. Haptic perception occurs when we actively explore an object, usually with our hands, although such exploration is possible with almost any part of our body. We are concerned in this chapter with object identification and pattern recognition.

What can we learn about objects and patterns from the stimulation which occurs when they touch our skin? One of the very first things we know when something touches the skin is where it is happening. Traditionally this aspect of our experience was described by saying that all parts of our skin had a *local sign* so that we knew we had been touched in one place rather than another. Local signs have been carefully mapped out. Generally speaking there are two procedures for determining tactual local signs. One is to touch a particular place on the skin of a subject without letting him see it and then have the subject point to that place with or without vision. This procedure has been carried out, for example, by Renshaw, Wherry, & Newlin (1930). They compared congenitally blind and sighted children and adults in their ability to localize a point on the skin by moving a stylus quickly to that point. Sighted children were better than blind children at this but blind adults were better than sighted adults. It seems that the blind improved in accuracy with age whereas the performance of the sighted became worse.

A second procedure for investigating local signs is to touch one place on the skin and then to touch the same or another place close by. The goal is to determine how small a change in position can be detected as different. A measure of the smallest difference which can be detected is often called the two-point threshold or two-point limen. These aspects of local sign are important in object identification and pattern recognition inasmuch as they bear on whether a person can tell if there are one or more objects touching him, and how extensive an object is. For example, the number of objects or points being touched would be very important for communication through the skin by patterns of vibrations.

When something touches the skin we can also tell about its intensity. If the stimulation at the skin involves higher force we experience intensity. It was discovered long ago that the linear size or extent of the stimulation rather than the area is closely related to experienced intensity (Boring, 1942). We can also tell to some extent if the force is being applied to a point or across a region. When the force increases too much we experience pain. Observers are able to distinguish whether this is a sharp pain such as from pricking or a dull pain as from a very heavy weight. From the point of view of objects and patterns these aspects of intensity discrimination by themselves or in collaboration with local sign information can tell us about whether surfaces of objects or edges or corners are touching us.

If an object touches us repeatedly at low repetition rates we experience a series of discrete impacts. As the repetition rate or frequency increases we experience a tactual flutter and with further rate increases a tactual vibration or hum (Mountcastle, 1968). We are very sensitive to such repetitive or vibrating stimuli. For example, at a frequency of 300 Hz (cycles-per-second) a change of pressure which results in a depression of the skin of one micron or 0.0001 cm can be detected! At lower frequencies our sensitivity decreases and a depression of the skin of 100 times as much is required for detectability at a vibratory frequency of 10 Hz. However, with low frequencies of vibration we can detect *changes* in frequency much better than with high-frequency stimuli. For example, at 10 Hz a change of 3 Hz may be detectable while at 200 Hz a change of 60 Hz may be required. What is the relevance of vibratory sensitivity for mobility training? When actively exploring a surface, our skin passes over a series of minute indentations and protuberances. It is likely that we experience the roughness and smoothness of the surface because of the alternations in pressure produced by them. (Recall from the previous discussion of psychophysical functions that roughness and smoothness of emery paper is a function of grit size or coefficient of friction.) Our sensitivity to vibration may be the mechanism for our ability to distinguish among objects on the basis of surface texture. The touch and slide technique in the use of the long cane provides information about surfaces by means of vibratory stimulation. Our sensitivity to vibration again would be an important factor in artificial devices for communication through the skin. A convenient way for presenting graphic information through the skin is by means of vibrators as in the Optacon (Bliss, 1973).

In haptic perception, all of the above local sign, intensity, and vibratory information is available. In addition two further kinds of information are available to the perceiver. One is proprioceptive information about the position and movement of parts of the body particularly those doing the active exploration of objects. For example, if one picks up an object with caliper-like movements of the fingers and is sensitive to the position of the fingers or the distance between them it would be possible to make a size judgment about the object. Similarly, sensitivity to position and movement of the hand in exploring around an object should potentially provide information about the shape of an object. How sensitive are we to this sort of position information? In determining sensitivity to limb position, the usual procedure is to determine the smallest detectable passive change in position. That is, when a limb is passively moved a small amount by the experimenter, and the subject reports whether he noticed a change in position of different body joints, the smallest detectable movement ranges from about one-third to about 2° of angle (Howard & Templeton, 1966). An alternative method of determining limb sensitivity is to measure how accurately subjects can localize one body part with another. For example, subjects are asked to point with one hand at the locus of a finger on the other hand. Such procedures have also indicated an accuracy of about ±1° to ±2° (Paillard & Brouchon, 1968; Smothergill, 1973).

A second kind of additional information available to the perceiver in haptic perception is efferent or outflow information. This, in contrast to proprioceptive information, does not depend on sensory information from the senses but rather is information available to the perceiver because he knows how he "signaled" his exploring limbs to move. Consider the case again of a person picking up an object with caliper-like finger movements. As before, if he can sense how far his fingers are separated he will know something about the size of the object. But he will also know something about the size from knowing how far he decided to open his fingers. Physiologists and psychologists have been able to show that these two sources of information are distinct. Proprioceptive information without outflow or efferent information is available when the limb is passively moved to a position. Efferent information without proprioception is available when sensory information can be cut off without hurting the motor system. Such a procedure works for certain joints. In a classic experiment Merton (1964) was able to anesthetize the thumb joint without affecting muscular control. Subjects reported the position of the thumb on the basis of the motor commands that they issued to it. Other analogous procedures have yielded similar conclusions (Taub, Ellman, & Berman, 1966; Lazlo, 1968). This sort of limb position awareness based on outflow information just as that based on proprioceptive or sensory information is obviously potentially useful in object shape and size perception.

Outflow information is seemingly also useful in a variety of other activities that we engage in when we explore something. These are activities like thumping, squeezing, rubbing, palpating. They are hard to measure and hence investigate in a systematic way. Yet it seems apparent that they are important, and that they involve *correlating* sensory information with outflow information. For example, a soft surface would be one where our experience of pressure (sensory information) does not increase very much as we move (outflow) our finger into the surface. A springy surface may well be one where our experience of pressure increases as we penetrate into the surface farther.

Physiology of Tactual and Haptic Perception

It is clear from all of the foregoing that haptic and tactual perception have considerable capacity for processing information. But what is the mechanism of this mode of perception? Classically, since the time of Johannes Müller in the nineteenth century when physiologists and psychologists considered sensory systems, they tried to find a distinctive sensory mechanism for each distinctive quality of sensation. Very grossly, of course, the visual system mediated sensations arising from light, the auditory system mediated sensations arising from sound, the gustatory system from taste, and so on. Touch, however, seemed to pose a problem. Was it one sense or several? People have different qualities of tactual experience: pressure, temperature, pain, itch, slipperiness, etc. Are these simply aspects of one sensory experience or do they reflect different sense modalities? To some, the differences between pressure, temperature, and pain seemed to be more distinctive than other differences within one sense modality such as differences in color of light, or differences in pitch of sound, or differences in taste. Such observations led some investigators to hypothesize that touch was actually a group of senses rather than a single sense. This group of senses together with other types of experience, like vascular-motor sensations, nausea, thirst, and hunger are often referred to as the somatic senses. The interested reader is referred to Boring (1942) for a historical review of the research on the somatic senses. The following discussion is based primarily on Mountcastle (1968) and Mountcastle and Darian-Smith (1968).

If there were different senses underlying some of these tactual and haptic sensory experiences, ideally, they should be identifiable by anatomically distinct neural mechanisms. For the somatic senses there are no grossly distinctive receptor organs like the eye, ear, tongue, nose, but perhaps there are distinctive neural receptors embedded in the body. A careful mapping of the skin by stimulators which controlled pressure, size of area, temperature, etc., indicated that there are small areas which differentially give rise to very specific sensations no matter how they are stimulated. Thus, some spots give rise to pressure sensations but not temperature sensations and conversely. Indeed, some spots give rise to a sensation of cold even though stimulated by a warm probe, a phenomenon referred to as "paradoxical cold." Are these areas of selective sensitivity correlated with distinctive receptors? Histological examination of various layers of the skin did yield a variety of neural endings of three types: free nerve endings; endings with expanded tips also called Markel's discs; and encapsulated endings of a variety of specific shapes known as Meissner corpuscles, Golgi-end organs, Kraus-end bulbs, Ruffini cylinders (Fig. 7-5). However, unfortunately these nerve endings bore little or no relation to the selective sensitivity shown by the skin mapping. Spots that were highly selective were often served by a variety of neural endings. Also the variations in endings probably do not reflect a set of distinct types but a continuum of variation.

Given that the receptor endings themselves do little to explain the sensory selectivity of the skin, can anything be learned from the functioning of the nerve fibers innervating them? The development of techniques for single-unit recording from nerve fibers provided the possibility for answering this question. Single nerve fibers can be separated and the electric activity of neural impulses measured when a stimulus is applied to the skin. The relation between the nature of the stimulus and the characteristics of the neural impulse activity can be investigated. One aspect of this relation is the receptive field of the fiber or cell. The receptive field refers to the *area* on the skin which when stimulated gives rise to activity in the fiber. It is, of course, related to the concept of local sign discussed above. Another aspect of the relation between stimulus and neural activity is the temporal course (variation over time) of neural activity consequent upon stimulation. Does initiation and cessation of stimulation produce a high frequency of neural impulses? Is this activity sustained or transient? These questions are related to issues of intensity and vibrations discrimination discussed above. For example, if the onset and cessation of stimulation produces a great deal of neural activity, that is, a high frequency of neural impulses as compared with steady stimulation, the system would be especially sensitive to changes in stimulation. Such a system might be especially responsive to vibratory stimulation and not to steady pressures of particular intensities.

Such electrophysiological recording indicated that functionally neural fibers innervating receptor endings in the skin can be divided into two groups. One group of fibers adapts quickly to stimulation but fires rapidly at initiation and termination of stimulation. These fibers thus transmit information about start and stop of contact, but not steady state. This first group might be more sensitive to movement because of its firing at both onset and offset of stimulation. The receptive fields of this group overlap extensively, thus local sign information could only be provided by the patterning of firing from several fibers. The second group adapts slowly. Fibers of this group show a burst of activity upon onset of a stimulus, and then a sustained but lower rate of activity with continued exposure to the stimulus. These fibers innervate very specific receptive fields. In terms of perception, this second group of fibers can signal contact with an object and intensity of contact, position of the object on the skin, and perhaps something about the quality of the contacted surface, its hardness, springiness, etc.

The nerve fibers from a specific region of the skin join into nerve bundles and enter the spinal cord at the cervical roots. At the point of entry into the spinal cord, all the sensory nerves from a given region of skin are in one group. A lesion at that point disrupts sensitivity of all qualities to that skin area. (There are overlapping sensory fibers, however, that enter other dorsal roots.) After entering the spinal

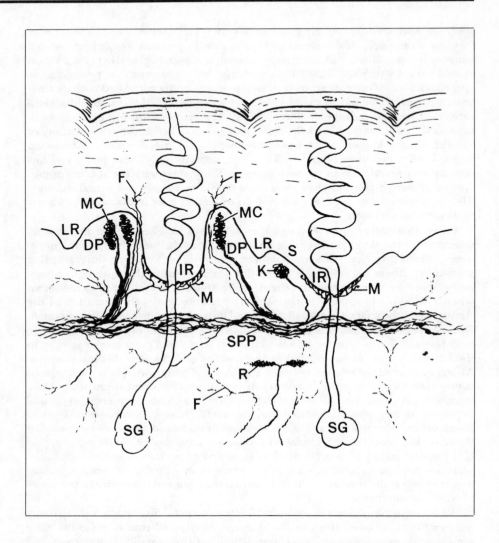

Figure 7-5. Diagrammatic vertical section of epidermis and underlying dermis and associated nerve endings in human fingertip. Two papillary ridges are shown. Two sweat glands **SG** are shown in dermis. Their ducts proceed toward skin surface and enter base of intermediate epidermal ridge, **IR.** Coiled sweat-gland duct progresses upward through epidermal strata and opens in central portion of papillary ridge. Epidermis extends most deeply into dermis in region of intermediate ridge, **IR.** At lateral edge of papillary ridge is another epidermal ridge projecting into dermis, the limiting, **LR,** or anchoring ridge. Upward dermal projections between intermediate and lateral ridges form dermal papillae, **DP.** A dermal papilla is seen on each side of intermediate ridge of left papillary ridge. Dividing papillary dermis transversely are septa, **S,** connecting intermediate and limiting ridges. Partitions may further subdivide papillae. Ruffini's endings, **R,** are found in dermis. Free nerve endings, **F,** are encountered in dermis, dermal papillae, and epidermis. Krause's end bulbs, **K,** are usually located just under epidermis. Meissner's corpuscles, **MC** occur in dermal papillae. Merkel's discs, **M,** are closely associated with lowermost layer of cells of epidermis in region of intermediate ridge, **IR,** and septa, **S-SPP** is subpapillary plexus. (From Vernon B. Mountcastle, Physiology of sensory receptors: Introduction to sensory processes. In Vernon B. Mountcastle, (Ed.) *Medical Physiology*, ed. 12, St. Louis, 1968, The C. V. Mosby Co.; courtesy Dr. M. R. Miller.)

cord the fibers divide into two systems. One called the *lemniscal system* is composed of the larger myelinated fibers. It ascends the same side of the spinal cord and after synapsing crosses over to the opposite side of the cord and ascends to the thalamus. This system preserves spatial specificity to receptive field and modal quality specificity. That is, activity of fibers at the thalamus is just as specific to particular areas of the skin and just as specific to the type of stimulation as are the fibers before they enter the spinal cord. The other system called the *anterolateral* is composed of smaller myelinated and unmyelinated fibers which cross over to the opposite side of the spinal cord immediately and ascend the spinal cord to the thalamus. This system is not nearly as specific as the lemniscal and seems to mediate pain and temperature stimulation. It is phylogenetically an older system and apparently serves a general arousal and vegetative function.

Position Awareness

Kinesthetic information about the position of limbs is derived from receptors in the joints. These receptors are of the encapsulated ending type and are found in large numbers in the joint capsule tissue and around the ligaments. There are sensory receptors in the muscles but these play little role in providing information about the position of the limbs. Their function is presumably to help regulate muscle contraction and extension in motor behavior. Recordings from fibers innervating joint receptors indicate that they are very sensitive to position of joint and to change of position. Typically a given fiber will fire at a great frequency upon initiation of an appropriate limb movement. The rate of firing is proportional to the rate of movement. Then it will settle down to a steady state firing rate which is characteristic of the particular joint angle. Different fibers have different ranges of joint angles to which they are sensitive. When movement exceeds these ranges the fibers do not increase their firing rate. These fibers adapt very slowly and will continue to fire at this steady-state rate for hours. Thus, these fibers serve beautifully to transmit information both about movement and absolute position of joints. These fibers join either muscle nerves or nerves of the other skin senses and enter the spinal cord. They are represented in the lemniscal system and like the other fibers preserve spatial specificity.

The lemniscal and anterolateral systems both project to the thalamus and thence to the cortex. The lemniscal system preserves in both places a topographical and functional correspondence with the peripheral sensory systems. That is, it is possible to map out an orderly continuous representation of the body surface in the thalamus and cortex by recording activity of neural cells when the skin is stimulated. The representation in the brain reflects the density of peripheral innervation. So areas of the body like the ends of fingers, face, etc., which have a high density of neural receptors are represented by large numbers of cells in the thalamus. The central neurons are not only specific as to place on the skin stimulated but also as to type of stimulation. In the cortex there are two somatic projection areas, one of which also preserves a topographic mapping of the body as well as specificity for quality and quantity of stimulation. The central nervous system specificity is illustrated by the possibility of recording activity of neural cells in the thalamus during rotation of a knee joint of a monkey. Cells can be found where each movement of flexion of the joint produces a large neural discharge which then settles down to a steady-state charateristic of the joint angle. As with peripheral fibers the central neurons have preferred joint angles. The central neurons are maximally responsive to the preferred angles and show decreased firing for larger and smaller joint angles.

A great deal is known about the details of central neural activity particularly with respect to the relation between peripheral stimulation of the skin and joints and neural activity in the projection areas of the cortex. The total picture is quite complicated. But the picture is even more complex when we try to go beyond the initial projection of the peripheral nerves to the central nervous system. There is very little known about the mechanisms of the interaction of somatic sensory information with other sensory information and with information in memory or with information about planned activity. That is, there is little efferent or outflow information discussed above. There is some behavioral information about these complex interactions which will be discussed in terms of the encoding of tactual and haptic informaton.

PROCESSING OF TACTUAL AND HAPTIC INFORMATION

In the sections above on the psychophysics and mechanism of tactual and haptic perception the emphasis was on perception of simple or pure dimensions of stimulation. In the research discussed, the stimuli typically varied in only one dimension. Even in the first section on object identification and pattern recognition the stimuli were treated mainly as simple units and the emphasis was on input-output relations. In this section the focus will be on the complexities of tactual and haptic perception. In particular, the modification and transformation of stimulation from the time it impinges on the person till it results in useful behavior will be considered. There is not a large body of literature concerned with this aspect of tactual and haptic perception. Rather than to try to review the spotty state of the art, the present approach will be to discuss particular topics in the context of illustrative experiments.

Selective Attention in Tactual and Haptic Perception

The simplest kind of processing of information can occur in terms of selection of certain aspects of stimulation to which to pay attention. Any real object or pattern is very complex. When we feel it do we pay attention to all its aspects—its size, shape, texture, hardness, temperature, etc.? Obviously most adults could pay attention to any of these characteristics. However, the fact that in ordinary circumstances we are also simultaneously perceiving auditory information, perhaps sensing the ambient temperature of the environment, noting the presence or absence of unusual odors, adjusting our posture to gravity, it is unlikely that we pay attention to all the detail characteristics of an object that we are feeling. Certainly, those characteristics we pay attention to depend to some extent on our purpose. If we were searching for an object to use as a paper weight we would probably pay more attention to the weight and size than we would if we were looking for something to use as a guide in drawing a straight line.

However, given a relatively neutral task such as telling a set of objects apart, is it possible to make generalizations about the aspects of the objects to which people attend? One experimental procedure for doing this is to teach people to discriminate between objects that vary in two (or more) aspects. After they have learned to make the discrimination they are presented with another pair of objects in which the relation between the original aspects has been changed. Consider the following example. A person is presented a pair of objects for haptic exploration—a fat smooth ellipse and a narrow rough ellipse. The fat smooth ellipse is arbitrarily designated as correct. The person learns, over a series of presentations, to choose that one no matter in what order they are presented or no matter what the relative position of the two objects. Now the person might have learned to choose the ellipse that was fat or the ellipse that was smooth or the combination as a whole. That is, the person could have attended to shape, or texture, or the combination of both. In order to find out which of these possibilities is correct, a new pair of objects could be presented: a fat rough object and a narrow smooth object. If the person unhesitatingly and reliably chooses the fat rough object it would be reasonable to infer that initially the shape dimension of fat-narrow was being attended to. If, instead, with the new pair of objects, the narrow smooth object were selected, the reasonable inference would be that, initially, the texture dimension of smooth-rough was being attended to. If the person hesitated and vacillated in his selection of the new pair, one would infer that initially the combination of dimensions was the basis of his selection.

Gliner, Pick, Pick, and Hales (1969) carried out just such an experiment with kindergarteners and third grade children. It was found that the younger children on the whole were selectively attending to texture and the older children to shape. In addition, it was found that it was fairly easy to bias the younger children toward using shape by making the shape differences very large and the texture differences very small. It was quite difficult, however, to bias the older children to use texture. Although it is now known how general these results might be with respect to types of texture and varieties of shape as well as general situations, the message is one of caution. In teaching people to identify complex objects haptically, they may learn easily but may be relying on aspects of the objects that are not crucial. The particular aspects relied upon may change as a function of age as well as from individual to individual.

In a study of discrimination of more complex shapes than the ellipses just considered, Pick (1965) asked the question whether children taught to discriminate between pairs of shapes would learn what the individual shapes themselves were like or whether they would just learn how the shapes differed from one another. She used the letter-like forms made of raised lines on a metal background illustrated in Fig. 5-5. Children felt pairs of shapes simultaneously, one with each hand, and learned to tell in each case whether the two shapes were the same or different. As before, the shapes might differ in one being a perspective or size transformation of the other, one being a rotation or reversal of the other, one having a straight line where the other had a curved line or vice versa, or one being a topological transformation (break or close) of the other. (A topological transformation signified by a break or close is one in which a segment is added to a standard form, or part of a segment is deleted.)

The children learned to make these discriminations with a small number of prototypic or standard shapes. That is, for several pairs the same basic shapes were transformed. They also learned to do this with only two of the four kinds of transformations. After learning to make the discrimination they were presented with new pairs. For some of the children the new pairs were the same prototypic shapes but new kinds of transformations. For other children the new pairs had new prototypic shapes but the same kind of transformations as in the original learning. There were relatively few errors in this latter group where the same transformations and new prototypes were given, and relatively more errors in the first group which had the new transformations but the same prototype. Apparently in this haptic task children had learned to attend to the distinctive features—the features which were critical for discriminating among the shapes and they had not attended to what the particular prototypic shapes were like.

In a companion experiment, Pick had children feel the members of each pair of shapes successively. Otherwise the experiment was essentially the same. In the transfer experiment, when new pairs were presented, the two groups were approximately the same. With this successive presentation the children had learned both what the particular prototypes were like *and* how the shapes differed from each other. Again we do not know how far these results may be generalized but the suggestion is that in haptic perception simultaneous and successive exploration of objects may have somewhat different effects. If the detection of differences or distinctive features is of primary importance, simultaneous presentation of objects would be efficient. If perception of the nature of the objects themselves is important, it may be facilitated by successive presentation. Indeed, to the extent that much of haptic and tactual perception is successive, people in general may be learning about the objects they explore rather than focusing on how the objects differ among themselves.

However, it should also be emphasized as it was in the first section that haptic exploration of all but the smallest patterns is successive. That is, it occurs over time for larger patterns and the stimulation must be somehow integrated over time in order to achieve configurational knowledge of an object. There is little known about how such achievements occur. One intriguing observation was made by Vekker (personal communication, 1960). He observed that if people were asked to draw the shape of an object immediately after haptically exploring it, their reproduction would begin at the same point of the object at which their exploration had begun. However, if the reproduction were delayed for several days, the starting point might be anywhere. His interpretation was that during a long delay between exploration and reproduction a successive image of the object was being transformed into a simultaneous image. This possibility leads directly to the next major topic of this section.

Encoding of Tactual and Haptic Information

Directly relevant to the question of encoding of information is the unit in which information is perceived. When exploring the contour of an object haptically do we take in information about the successive points or do we take in information about segments of a line or edge? Introspection and observations such as the one by James Gibson quoted early in this chapter suggest that it is larger units which are perceived. Yet to the extent that *successive* is a correct characterization of haptic perception, we should expect larger units to be integrated from smaller ones. One observation that suggested that the obvious units were not always the ones used came from a study of braille reading (Pick, Thomas, & Pick, 1966). The hypothesis was that since haptic perception is successive, braille reading would proceed character by character unlike print reading which had been shown to proceed using letter cluster units called grapheme-phoneme correspondences (Gibson, Pick, Osser, & Hammond, 1963). If reading goes letter by letter, a pronounceable nonsense word like "bleasks" would be read as rapidly as an unpronounceable version of the same word written with initial and final consonant clusters reversed, "skseabl." According to the idea of grapheme-phoneme correspondence, the consonant clusters *bl* (when it is in the initial position) and *sks* (in the final position) are treated as perceptual units. In the braille study it was shown that words like "bleasks" are read faster than their difficult-to-pronounce counterparts. These results suggest that in spite of the successive nature of haptic perception, units larger than single letters function in braille reading. The limits of size of units in braille reading have not been determined nor have the mechanisms by which these larger units are achieved.

In considering the encoding of information we must confront the question of meaning of patterns of stimulation. With stimuli like braille the meaning of each character is arbitrary, but there are representational patterns of stimulation which naturally reflect the meaning of the thing they are supposed to represent. Again there is not much knowledge of how to naturally represent things, but consideraton of such issues is of major importance when designing representational tactile stimuli. For example, it would be obviously incorrect to represent the size of cities on a braille map (or a visual map, for that matter) as an inverse function of the real size—the larger the city the smaller the symbol.

Let us consider a few examples of what may be natural ways of representing

5

information. Schiff, Kanfer, and Mosak (1966) found that spatial direction could be encoded effectively in the texture elements constituting a dotted line. Each element of texture in a line gradually increases to a peak height and then abruptly drops to the base of the paper. As in feeling along a sawtooth edge, movement in one direction feels like a "smooth bumpy line" while movement in the other direction feels like a "rough bumpy line." The smooth direction is arbitrarily specified as the direction of interest. Perception of direction represented in this way is faster for both blind and sighted subjects feeling the line than when direction is represented by more traditional arrow figures made of either dots or raised lines. Texture might also be used to represent distance or length in a natural way. If perception of amount of movement over a surface is partially determined by the number of transitions of high and low points of surface texture, traversed coarseness of texture may influence the perceived length of a surface or line. If the texture is very coarse, few transitions would be traversed and the distance might be perceived as short. If texture were finer there would be more transitions and perhaps perception of greater distance—until the texture became so fine that some of the transitions were missed. In studies of the relation between texture and perceived length, Baird (1971), and Corsini and Pick (1969) found evidence for the correctness of the above analysis. There was a curvilinear relation between roughness and perceived length. The length of coarse-textured stimuli was underestimated in comparison with the extreme smoothness of oak tag paper. It would be possible to use this fact on tactual maps or pictures to represent or accentuate distances and differences in distance.

A somewhat more abstract example of a possibly natural way of representing information was discovered by White, Saunders, Scadden, Bach-Y-Rita, and Collins (1970) in developing and testing a visual substitution device. The device consisted of a 20 x 20 matrix of tiny vibrators strapped to the skin surface of the back or front of a person's body. The vibrators are driven by the output of a TV camera so that areas of high luminance activate the vibrators; in a sense, painting a vibratory picture of the camera's view on the skin. Subjects being trained to use this device would explore objects by pointing the camera. It was observed that congenitally blind subjects would sometimes duck when the lens was unexpectedly "zoomed" in a magnification direction. The vibratory pattern on the skin (like the visual pattern on the retina) when something approaches is one of increasing area of stimulation. Apparently with very little experience such a skin pattern could provide a vivid impression of rapid change in distance of an external object. A possibly important component of the brief experience during which such sensitivity develops is the *self-produced* tactual stimulation which the subject receives as he explores with the camera. White (1973) suggests this may very well be important for the fact that subjects quickly perceive this stimulation on the skin surface as being something outside and in front even when the matrix is stimulating their back. In designing tactual representation systems it may be very important to capitalize on such natural correspondences between symbols and meaning.

Transformation of Information

What happens to tactual and haptic information after it is encoded? It is often the case in real life that we have to remember information or we have to transform information before it is useful. The problem of short-term memory or storage of information may be particularly important in haptic and tactual perception because of the successive nature of information input. This is particularly unfortunate because there is at least some evidence to suggest that proprioceptive memory decays relatively more than visual memory over a short delay (Posner,

1967). In this study, subjects were asked to remember a particular arm position or a distance they had moved their arm. When they performed without vision there was considerable increase in error when waiting 20 seconds. With vision there was no increase in error over that period if the subject was not required to engage in a distracting task. A similar increase in error in memory over 25 seconds for proprioceptive position was found by Smothergill (1973). These results would suggest trying to provide considerable opportunity for rehearsal and review when tactual and haptic explorations were taking considerable amounts of time.

Transformation of perceived information is going on all the time. In the case of verbal information, we can often not recall the exact words we have been reading but we know the meaning. That is so commonplace we hardly think of it as transformation of information. Indeed it can be shown that we go beyond the literal information and make inferences that are not in the text at all. But what about nonverbal perception? Do we, or can we, transform information about objects? The answer is yes. A recent dramatic example of this ability is provided by Marmor and Zaback (1976). They asked congenitally blind subjects to feel a shape and then to describe whether a second shape was identical to the first or a mirror image of the first shape. Across a number of repetitions of this procedure the second shape was rotated with respect to the first by varying amounts. Reaction time for responding was measured and the results indicated that the greater the rotation the longer was the reaction time to judge whether the second shape was a mirror image or not. The interpretation of the results was that subjects were "mentally rotating" the first shape in order to see whether the two were congruent. The farther the shape had to be rotated the longer it took. Except for isolated examples of transformation of information we know little about how this works for tactual and haptic information. One can imagine a number of practical tasks where such transformations would be useful for the visually impaired. Consider trying to tell which key will fit into a particular keyhole. Or what will be the composite shape when two shapes are put together? Are there procedures for training this capacity? The answers are yet to be found.

CONCLUSION

The attempt here was to describe the state of knowledge and general approaches in the basic study of tactual and haptic perception. Where possible, this basic information was made relevant to problems faced by the visually impaired. However, there is a considerable gap in most cases between the basic research and application to the world by the blind. An attempt was made to describe how haptic perception of objects proceeds and the strengths and weaknesses in research on it, followed by a consideration of the psychophysics of haptic perception. Psychophysical studies formed the basis of the classical research in perception and they still are fundamental in an analytic approach to perception. No discussion of haptic perception would be complete without a description of the underlying physiological and behavioral mechanisms. Again the purpose was to try to show how these mechanisms result in functional information. The cognitive side of tactual and haptic perception was treated in the final section on information processing. In some ways this topic is the most exciting perhaps because it is the one where our ignorance is greatest.

Bibliography

Ananev, B. G., Lomov, B. F., Vekker, L. M. & Yarmolenko, A. R. *Osyazanie v prostsessakh poznaniya i truda. (Touch in the processes of cognition and work.)* Moscow, USSR: RSFSR Academy of Pedagogical Sciences, 1959.

5

Baird, R. M. Effect of texture on tactually perceived size. Unpublished master's thesis, University of Louisville, 1971.

Berla, E. P., & Murr, M. J. Psychophysical functions for active tactual discrimination of line width by blind children. *Perception and Psychophysics*, 1975, **17**, 607-612.

Bliss, J. C. Summary of three Optacon-related cutaneous experiments. In F. Geldard (Ed.) *Cutaneous Communication Systems and Devices*. Psychonomic Society, 1973.

Blumenfeld, W. The relationship between the optical and haptic construction of space. *Acta Psychologica*. 1937, **2**, 125-174.

Boring, E. G. *Sensation and perception in the history of experimental psychology*. New York: Appleton-Century-Crofts, Inc., 1942.

Bower, T. G. R. Blind babies see with their ears. *New Scientist*, February 3, 1977.

Brumaghim, S. H., & Brown, D. R. Perceptual equivalence between visual and tactual pattern perception: An anchoring study. *Perception and Psychophysics*, 1968, **4**, 175-179.

Corsini, D. A., & Pick, H. L., Jr. Effect of texture on tactually perceived length. *Perception and Psychophysics*, 1969, **5**, 352-356.

Crewdson, J., & Zangwill, O. L. A note on tactual perception in a blind subject. *British Journal of Psychology*, 1940, **30**, 224-229.

Davidon, R. S., & Cheng, M. H. Apparent distance in a horizontal plane with tactile-kinesthetic stimuli. *Quarterly Journal of Experimental Psychology*, 1964, **16**(3), 277-281.

Duran, P., & Tufenkjian, S. Tactile-kinesthetic methods for measuring length used by congenitally blind children. *Perceptual and Motor Skills*, 1969, **28**, 395-400.

Ekman, G., Hosman, J., & Lindstrom, B. Roughness, smoothness, and preference: A study of quantitative relations in individual subjects. *Journal of Experimental Psychology*, 1965, **70**, 18-26.

Fischel, H. Transformationserscheinungen bei Gewichtshebungen. *Zeitschrift für Psychologie*, 1926, **98**, 342-365.

Fraiberg, S. Parallel and divergent patterns in blind and sighted infants. *Psychoanalytic Study of the Child*, 1968, **23**, 264-299.

Fraiberg, S., Siegel, B. L., & Gibson, R. The role of sound in a search behavior of a blind child. *Psychoanalytic Study of the Child*, 1966, **21**, 327-357.

Gaydos, H. F. Sensitivity in the judgment of size by finger span. *American Journal of Psychology*, 1958, **71**, 557-562.

Gibson, E. J., Gibson, J. J., Pick, A. D., & Osser, H. A developmental study of discrimination of letter-like forms. *Journal of Comparative and Physiological Psychology*, 1962, **55**(6), 897-906.

Gibson, J. J. The useful dimensions of sensitivity. *American Psychologist*, 1963, **18**, 1-15.

Gibson, J. J. *The senses considered as perceptual systems*. New York: Houghton Mifflin, 1966.

Gliner, C. R., Pick, A. D., Pick, H. L., Jr., & Hales, J. A developmental investigation of visual and haptic preferences for shape and texture. *Monographs of the Society for Research in Child Development*, 1969, **34**, (Serial No. 130), No. 6.

Harper, R. S., & Stevens, S. S. A psychological scale of weight and a formula for its derivation. *American Journal of Psychology*, 1948, **61**, 343-351.

Harper, R. S., & Stevens, S. S. Subjective hardness of compliant materials. *Quarterly Journal of Experimental Psychology*, 1964, **16**, 204-215.

Hatwell, Y. Etude de qualques illusions geometriques tactiles chez les aveugles. (A study of geometrical tactile illusions among the blind.) *Annae Psychologique*, 1960, No. 1, 11-27.

Howard, I., & Templeton, W. B. *Human spatial orientation*. New York: Wiley, 1966.

Hunter, I. M. L. Tactile-kinesthetic perception of straightness in blind and sighted humans. *Quarterly Journal of Experimental Psychology*, 1954, **6**, 149-154.

Jenkins, W. O. The tactual discrimination of shapes for coding aircraft-type controls. Chapter 14 (pp. 199-205) in P. M. Fitts (Ed.) *Psychological research in equipment design*. Washington: U.S. Government Printing Office, 1947.

Kederis, C. J. The legibility of braille characters. Unpublished master's dissertation, University of Louisville, 1963.

Kelvin, R. P. Discrimination of size by sight and touch. *Quarterly Journal of Experimental Psychology*, 1954, **6**, 23-24.

Lazlo, J. I. Role of visual and kinesthetic cues in learning a novel skill. *Australian Journal of Psychology*, 1968, **20**, 191-196.

Marmor, G. S., & Zaback, L. A. Mental rotation by the blind: Does mental rotation depend on visual imagery? *Journal of Experimental Psychology: Human Perception and Performance*, 1976, **2**, 515-521.

Merton, P. A. Human position sense and sense of effort. *Homeostasis and feedback mechanisms: The 18th Symposium of Society for Experimental Biology*. London: Cambridge University Press, 1964, **18**, 387-400.

Mountcastle, V. B. Physiology of sensory receptors: Introduction to sensory processes. In V. B. Mountcastle (Ed.) *Medical physiology, Volume II*. St. Louis: C. V. Mosby Company, 1968.

Mountcastle, V. B., & Darian-Smith, I. Neural mechanisms in somesthesia. In V. B. Mountcastle (Ed.) *Medical physiology, Volume II*. St. Louis: C. V. Mosby Company, 1968.

Over, R. A comparison of haptic and visual judgments of some illusions. *American Journal of Psychology*, 1966, **79**, 590-595.

Owen, D. H., & Brown, D. R. Visual and tactual form complexity: A psychophysical approach to perceptual equivalence. *Perception & Psychophysics*, 1970, **7**(4), 225-228.

Paillard, J., & Brochon, M. Active and passive movements in the calibration of position sense. In S. J. Freedman (Ed.) *The neuropsychology of spatially oriented behavior*. Homewood, Ill.: The Dorsey Press, 1968.

Pick, A. D. Improvement of visual and tactual form discrimination. *Journal of Experimental Psychology*, 1965, **69**, 331-339.

Pick, A. D., Thomas, M. L., & Pick, H. L., Jr. The role of grapheme-phoneme correspondences in the perception of braille. *Journal of Verbal Learning and Verbal Behavior*, 1966, **5**, 298-300.

Pick, A. D., & Pick, H. L., Jr. A developmental study of tactual discrimination in blind and sighted children and adults. *Psychonomic Science*, 1966, **6**, 367-368.

Pick, H. L., Jr., & Pick, A. D. A developmental and analytic study of the size-weight illusion. *Journal of Experimental Child Psychology*, 1967, **5**, 362-371.

Posner, M. I. Characteristics of visual and kinesthetic memory codes. *Journal of Experimental Psychology*, 1967, **75**, 103-107.

Reid, R. L. An illusion of movement complementary to the horizontal-vertical illusion. *Quarterly Journal of Experimental Psychology*, 1954, **6**, 107-111.

Renshaw, S., Wherry, R. J., & Newlin, J. C. Cutaneous localization on congenitally blind vs. seeing children and adults. *Journal of Genetic Psychology*, 1930, **38**, 239-248.

Ringel, R. L., Saxman, J. H., & Brookes, A. R. Oral perception: II mandibular kinesthesia. *Journal of Speech and Hearing Research*, 1967, **10**(3), 637-641.

Rubin, E. Haptische untersuchungen. *Acta Psychologica*, 1935, **1**(3), 18-380.

Schiff, W., Kanfer, L., & Mosak, S. Informative tactile stimuli in the perception of direction. *Perceptual and Motor Skills*, 1966, **23**, 1315-1355.

Skramlik, E. von Psychophysiologie der Tastisinne *Archiv fur Gesamte Psychologie*, 1937, vierter erganzungband Teil 1, 935.

Smothergill, D. W. Accuracy and variability in the localization of spatial targets at three age levels. *Developmental Psychology*, 1973, **8**, 62-66.

Stanley, G. Haptic and kinesthetic estimates of length. *Psychonomic Science*, 1966, **5**(10), 377-378.

Stevens, S. S., & Stone, G. Finger span: Ratio scale, category scale, and j.n.d. scale. *Journal of Experimental Psychology*, 1959, **57**, 91-95.

Stevens, S. S., & Harris, J. R. The scaling of subjective roughness and smoothness. *Journal of Experimental Psychology*, 1962, **64**(5), 489-494.

Stevens, S. S., & Guirao, M. Scaling of apparent viscosity. *Science*, 1964, **144**, 1157-1158.

Stone, L. A. Subjective roughness and smoothness for individual judges. *Psychonomic Science*, 1967, **9**(6), 347-348.

Taub, E., Ellman, S. J., & Berman, A. J. Deafferentation in monkeys: Effect on conditioned grasp response. *Science*, 1966, **151**, 593-594.

Teghtsoonian, M., & Teghtsoonian, R. Seen and felt length. *Psychonomic Science*, 1965, **3**, 465-466.

Torrey, C. C. *The distance-weight effect: An exploratory study in weight perception*. Unpublished Ph.D. dissertation. Cornell University, 1963.

Tsai, L. S. Müller-Lyer illusion by the blind. *Perceptual and Motor Skills*, 1967, **25**, 641-644.

White, B. W., Saunders, F. A., Scadden, L., Bach-Y-Rita, P., & Collins, C. C. Seeing with the skin. *Perception and Psychophysics*, 1970, **7**, 23-27.

White, B. W. What other senses can tell us about cutaneous communication. In F. Geldard (Ed.) *Cutaneous communication systems and devices*, Psychonomic Society, 1973.

Audition

William R. Wiener

Audition, or hearing, is one of man's most important senses, playing an important role in day-to-day functioning, and making it possible to communicate with others easily and effectively. The process starts when the child begins to associate specific sounds with the objects that emit them. As a direct result of auditory stimulation, the child later begins to acquire language, accumulating a storehouse of commonly shared sounds to form a network of symbols representing, at first, objects, and, later, abstract concepts that allow immediate exchange of ideas. As the child grows and acquires auditory symbols for more abstract ideas, higher conceptual functioning can begin. Hearing also allows one to participate in social activity. Auditory communication facilitates cooperative and interdependent relationships by sharing knowledge and feelings. Hearing also helps a person to experience pleasure from the environment. The sounds of nature add much to the enjoyment extracted from the other senses, as the sound of waves breaking on the beach greatly add to the visual pleasure of the ocean. One can appreciate a fine symphony orchestra or a well acted play through hearing, but hearing also serves as a warning system to avoid danger. The sound of a car approaching from the rear or around a corner, or sounds of yelling or a siren may alert one to danger or an emergency.

Audition is especially important to a visually impaired person. When vision is not functioning or not functioning well, hearing may provide some of the information about the environment usually received through vision. Hearing like sight is a long distance sense which can tell an individual what is farther out in the environment. It helps one to appreciate depth by identifying the existence of space and the distance through space to a reflecting surface or a sound emitting object. Hearing also enables comprehension of some of the characteristics of the environment. A person entering a room can learn to use reflected sound to determine whether the room is large or small and what type of furnishings are present. Outdoors, hearing may be used to determine the type of environment through which one is navigating. The sound of heavy traffic may identify a business area.

Hearing provides information that permits independent movement in complex environments. Indoors, reflected sound helps a person to avoid contact with obstacles or walls. Outdoors, hearing is used to determine when it is safe to cross the street. At a residential crossing, the absence of sound provides the necessary clue. In a business or downtown area, accelerating parallel traffic indicates that the light has changed and it is safe to cross.

Hearing also helps a visually impaired person to establish and maintain orientation in the environment. To ascertain one's position in the environment, an individual must be aware of his relationship to significant objects. Hearing facilitates this by providing information to help identify known landmarks and information points. In a public building, for example, a person may identify a sound from a ventilator fan that could signify his position within a particular hallway. Outdoors, one may verify a position in the environment perhaps by identifying the sounds of children playing in a playground. Sound localization may further help in orientation by allowing determination of the exact location of a sound source. Indoors, one can determine position in relation to an elevator door by localizing the sound of the opening door and determining the relationship to it. Outdoors, one can determine position at a street corner by localizing the sounds of the cars stopped behind the crosswalk. During a street crossing localization or tracking the sound of moving vehicles can determine whether one is in a position parallel to them to insure a straight crossing to the opposite side.

Fine sound discrimination is also helpful in orientation. The ability to differentiate between similar sounds may enable the traveler to determine his location more accurately by deciding that the sound he is hearing is, for example, the sound from the fan at the drug store and not the air conditioner at the restaurant next door. Visually impaired people can also learn to use reflected ambient sound to determine position. A wall in a person's path can be detected by the reflected sound of footsteps as one approaches it. It may also tell the individual that he is reaching the end of a corridor or a large object within a hall. Similarly walls and objects beside an individual can reflect sound that will make their presence known. Using this information, a visually impaired person can determine when he has reached a particular intersecting hallway by the absence of reflected sound at the junction.

In order to understand the auditory functioning of the visually impaired person, the mobility specialist must comprehend audition itself and the special uses of audition in independent travel. This chapter is, therefore, divided into two parts. The first examines the perceptual, physical, and biological bases for hearing; the second focuses upon the special auditory needs of the visually impaired.

Part I—The Basis of Sound

AUDITORY PERCEPTION

A complex picture emerges when one tries to determine what hearing is. Sound results from an energy source moving a medium such as air and causing waves to be transmitted to a more distant point. But does sound exist when there is no receiver present? If a disturbance of air was caused by a rock slide on a planet devoid of life, would a sound have been created? A physicist might answer that a sound would have been created in that situation since pressure waves in the air were generated. A psychologist might argue that a sound would not have been created because there was no organism present to receive it. The psychologist also might argue that sound is dependent upon an individual's perception. The same sound may be different to different individuals. While the age-old question may seem unanswerable, it points out that hearing can be considered from different perspectives. Sound can be thought of as a mechanical process that can be explained by the principles of physics and independent of reception by an organism. Sound can also be considered as part of the receptive process, the biological reaction to stimulation by pressure waves. In other words, the vibrations in the air cause corresponding vibrations within the ear. One must go beyond these basic explanations and consider sound from a perceptual viewpoint, which acknowledges that the reception of sound is not just a passive biological reaction, but an active cognitive one shaped by perception. Interpretation of sound is more than just mechanical generation and biological reaction but also is based upon the individual's past and present experiences.

Stimulus

Auditory functioning is built upon the same perceptual model that is the basis for other sensory functioning. The environment is classified or organized according to the commonalities received through the senses. Perceptual skills become a way of ordering or interpreting sensory information. In auditory perception, this process starts when the individual searches for sound clues and begins to attend to specific stimuli while rejecting others. Meaning is associated with the stimuli as a result of previous experience and groups of patterns of stimuli are integrated into an organizational framework or schemata that adds to the understanding of the environment. New information, when received, verifies and adds to existing conceptions, or changes the framework to allow for new perspectives. For example, a visually impaired person moving through a familiar indoor environment is continually searching out sensory information which may be useful. He decides to concentrate on one specific stimulus that is present among the various stimuli within the particular environment and begins to identify the stimulus based on previous experience with this particular sound. He goes through a period of checking the stimulus and rejecting or accepting it into his classification. If the sound is an elevator door opening or closing, he may accept this information realizing that his organizational framework of indoor environments indicates elevators as common within this setting. If the sound happens to be a motorized vehicle, he then must do more checking to classify this stimulus within his schemata, or framework. Eventually, he may decide that this particular stimulus does not fit or he may determine that a new schemata is necessary incorporating motorized vehicles in indoor settings. His understanding of the environment and movement through it will depend upon his perceptual process.

Identification

Auditory perception unfolds as the child begins to associate meaning with various auditory stimuli and starts to seek out and classify sound. As the child matures, various perceptual skills emerge that make such interpretation of information possible (Sanders, 1971; Gibson 1966). Auditory perception begins with an awareness of the existence of sound. The child is first aware of stimulation present in his environment. Later, he learns to discriminate between different stimuli and to recognize certain specific stimuli among several alternatives in the environment. This discrimination is based on acoustic qualities of the sound such as the frequency, intensity, phase, and duration of the signals. At first, the child learns to discriminate between sounds that are grossly different; later he acquires discrimination skills which allow him to differentiate between similar sounds. Maturation of discrimination occurs as the child is repeatedly exposed to sounds within the same context. He begins to associate sounds with specific environmental stimuli and to associate particular acoustic stimuli with other sensory stimuli; the sound of his mother's voice may be associated with her soft touch. A multisensory recognition of sound-producing objects develops and, finally, identification of a sound is possible solely on the basis of its acoustic properties. The child eventually identifies the sound of his mother's voice based on pitch, intensity, and other acoustic qualities.

While sound discrimination and identification are developing, figure-ground perception is also emerging. At first, the child may be aware of one sound from a background of sounds, without recognizing what it is. Later, as discrimination and identification emerge, figure-ground becomes more selective and meaningful sound stands out from a background of less significant sounds. The individual learns to shift from one figure to another at will, and selective listening becomes possible. Sound localization contributes to this ability. The individual begins to identify the source of the sound-emitting object and learns to focus upon it. This skill is very important for visually impaired people.

Closure

Closure is another important perceptual skill for auditory functioning. The individual begins to perceive an incomplete stimulus as representing the complete stimulus based on prior experience with the complete or whole stimulus. Groups or patterns of stimuli are recognized as an integrated whole even though the complete stimuli or pattern of stimuli are not present. An example of this is commonly seen when a person is able to understand speech even though the complete stimulus is not heard or is distorted. He experiences closure of the incomplete stimulus and can gain the complete meaning from the spoken word. The hearing impaired person learns to interpret auditory stimuli with missing parts or distorted frequency components by recognizing that these parts represent a more complete gestalt which was not present aurally.

Perceptual Constancy

Perceptual constancy also plays a role in auditory functioning. Surroundings can affect the quality of the sound stimuli while the object emitting the sound stimuli remains the same. Softer sounds are recognized as not necessarily coming from smaller objects, but instead, objects farther away in the environment. The visually impaired person who is listening to the sound of a car traveling parallel to the direction he is facing, may perceive its path incorrectly unless perceptual constancy comes into play. At first the car may seem to be traveling towards a point ahead which is in the center of the environment rather than parallel to the way he is facing. Auditory perspective, the same as its visual counterpart, makes objects seem to merge in the center off in the distance. Constancy helps the individual to adjust for this phenomenon and to assess more accurately the path of the sound-emitting object. In both of these examples constancy allows the person to perceive a reality that is different from the sensory impressions.

UNDERSTANDING AND MEASURING SOUND

Various terms and definitions are helpful for an understanding of the properties and transmission of sound. According to Newby (1964), sound is a form of energy consisting of molecular movements in a series of pressure waves through a medium. For example, if the medium is air, pressure waves are generated by a force which pushes the molecules against each other. This disturbance of the medium consists of a compression and a rarefaction. Compression is that part of the disturbance which is due to an external force causing a reduction of the distance between molecules. Rarefaction is the removal of the force and the return of the molecules past the resting position. Again using air as an example of a medium, one would find that compression takes place when a force starts a chain reaction that compresses one air molecule into its neighboring molecule. When the energy is expended, each air molecule returns beyond its original starting point in a settling motion. In nature, however, the molecules are usually set into motion again by a new stimulus before they come to a rest. The sound that is generated through the medium travels in all directions in concentric circles. As the waves travel from the energy source, they continually lose intensity.

The medium's characteristics are responsible for the transmission of the sound. First, the medium must be elastic so that it resists being twisted, stretched, or compressed. This resistance results in the molecules of the medium springing back after removal of the force. Second, the medium must possess mass or a quantity of matter such as molecules of air or some other material. The density of the medium's molecules determine the speed at which sound may pass through the medium. In a very dense material, the molecules are closer together and do not have to move far during compression and rarefaction. Therefore, in dense material sound travels faster than in material with more space between molecules. Because of this phenomenon, sound travels faster in solids than in liquids or gases, and can clearly be seen by comparing the speed of sound in steel, water, and air representing the three states of matter. In steel, sound travels at 15,000 ft-per-second (4500 m-per-second) in water, 4500 ft-per-second (1350 m-per-second), and in air, 1100 ft-per-second (330 m-per-second).

Intensity, Frequency, Phase

A sound's three most important characteristics are intensity, frequency, and phase (Martin, 1975). The intensity of a sound is related to the particle displacement or the distance the molecule in the medium travels from its resting position. The particle amplitude is the point of greatest particle displacement above its resting position and determines the intensity or loudness of the sound. When the particle amplitude is great, the intensity will also be great. Large particle-amplitude is achieved when the energy moving the molecules is great.

Frequency is the number of compressions and rarefactions which take place within one second. It can also be thought of as the rate of vibration. In the past, frequency has been labeled in cycles-per-second (cps). More recently, frequency is labeled as Hertz (Hz) after the German physicist Heinrich Hertz. If a tone is identified as vibrating at a frequency of 1000 Hz, it is completing 1000 compressions and rarefactions in one second. Any tone which is composed of one and only one frequency is called a pure tone. Pure tones are artificial and rarely exist in nature. Instead, complex tones are found resulting from a combination of many pure tones.

The phase of a sound refers to the position of the sound wave within the cycle. This is best explained through graphic representation of sound waves. First, a graphic representation of intensity and frequency serves to introduce the concept of phase. The representation known as a sine wave shows the backward and forward movement of molecules in the medium as they are compressed and then returned past the starting position. Time is represented by drawing the compressions and rarefactions over a distance. The compressions are represented by curves drawn upward while rarefactions are curves drawn downward (Fig. 1-6). The

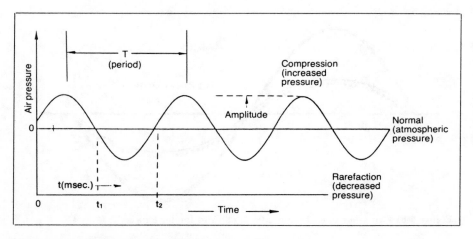

Figure 1-6. Compression and rarefaction in sound waves.

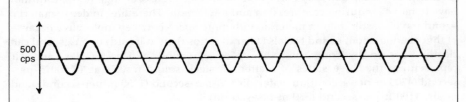

Figure 2-6. Higher frequency (500 cycles-per-second).

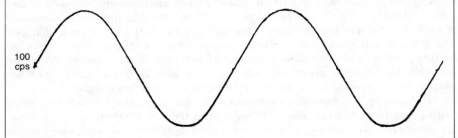

Figure 3-6. Low frequency (100 cycles-per-second).

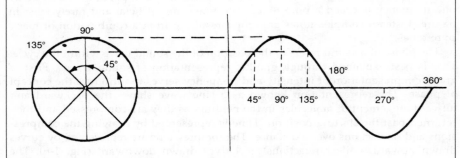

Figure 4-6. Points along the soundwave labeled in degrees.

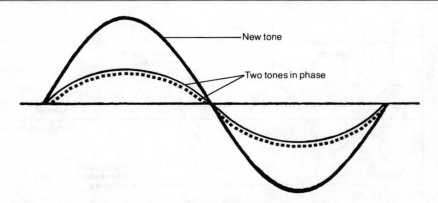

Figure 5-6. Two tones in a phase producing a third louder tone.

height of the curve from the starting point or base line represents the particle amplitude or intensity. The relative positioning of the peaks and valleys of the curves give information about the frequency. When they are closer together, more peaks and valleys can fit into the same space which represents a given amount of time. Since a compression and rarefaction represent one vibration, it is easy to see that a larger number of vibrations in a given area means a higher frequency while a lower number means a lower frequency (Fig. 2-6 and Fig. 3-6). To draw a complete sine wave, the actual number of compressions and rarefactions which occur in one second of time would have to be represented.

It is now possible to explain phase through a representation of position of the sine wave. If the sine wave is thought of as a circle which is disconnected and the lower half rotated, degrees of position can be assigned to the wave as depicted in Fig. 4-6. The start of the curve is designated as zero. The point where the upward slope or compression peaks is labeled as 90°. The point where the curve returns to the base line or resting point is identified as 180°. The point of greatest depression in the rarefaction curve is designated as 270°. Finally, the return from rarefaction to the resting position is 360°. The total circle represents one complete cycle of the tone. The portion of the wave above the base line is in a positive direction while that below the line is in a negative one. Phase is the relative position of the sound wave at a given time in the cycle. Two sounds are said to be in phase with each other when the comparative compressions and rarefactions occur at the same time in the positive and negative directions. In Fig. 5-6, two tones are in phase, and because they are the same frequency and amplitude, they combine to form a new wave which has an amplitude proportionately higher. In the next example, Fig. 6-6, the two tones are in phase, but are of slightly different frequencies. When this occurs, the two tones through a process of mathematical summation are merged into a complex tone by the addition and subtraction of the intensities of the two pure tones. When the compression of one tone occurs while a

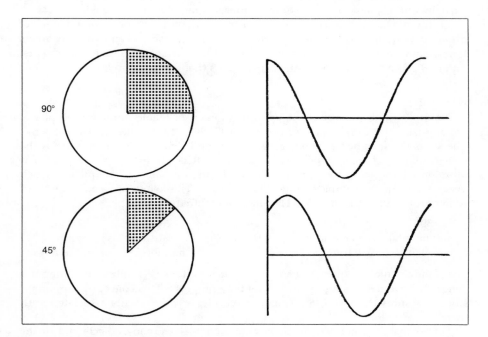

Figure 6-6. Two tones slightly out of phase.

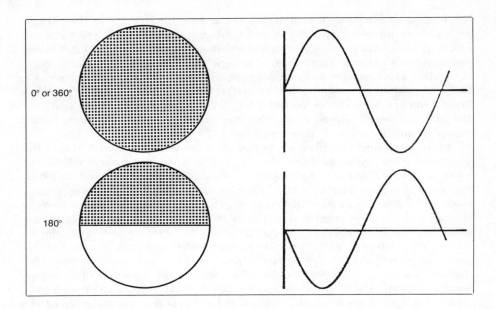

Figure 7-6. Two tones 180° out of phase.

second tone is undergoing rarefaction, the two tones are said to be out of phase. In Fig. 7-6 the two tones are 180° out of phase because they are exactly opposite. When two tones are out of phase and are of the same frequency and intensity, they cancel each other out leaving an absence of sound. If they were not 180° but only partially out of phase, sound would be present but altered in intensity.

Ordinarily sound consists of a combination of pure tone components of different frequencies, amplitudes, and phase relationships, known as complex tones. They are the result of the summation of the various pure tone components. Figure 8-6 is a series of pure tone components that form a complex tone.

Harmonics

Natural sounds are also made up of harmonics, or whole-number multiples of the fundamental frequency. According to Gerber (1974), the fundamental frequency is the specific frequency at which a sound producer is vibrating. It is the lowest frequency in the spectrum of sound that is produced by the particular vibrator. The vibrator generates multiples of the fundamental frequency which become part of the complex sound that is heard. The following is an example of harmonics resulting from a 500-Hz fundamental frequency:

500	1000	1500	2000	2500 etc.
fundamental	second	third	fourth	fifth
frequency	harmonic	harmonic	harmonic	harmonic

The fundamental frequency has the greatest intensity while the harmonics generally have decreasing intensities as they progress. This concept is important since it assures that even low sounds have higher components associated with them.

Sound that is generated in the environment strikes many objects and in the process may undergo reflection, defraction, refraction, or any combination of these processes. The resulting sound that returns to the environment may be changed in some way which will alter its quality. Sound that undergoes only reflection returns to the environment unchanged except for its direction. The angle of incidence equals the angle of reflection in these instances. This can best be illustrated by the example of a pool ball striking the bank of the table. The angle at which it strikes is equal to the angle at which it leaves. The defraction of sound can occur when sound breaks up in all directions as it passes through an object smaller than itself such as is the case when talking into a megaphone. A sound is refracted after striking an object when part of it is absorbed and changed or distorted. The distortion may take the form of frequency, phase, or amplitude change. The returning sound is different than the original sound and as a result helps one to determine the characteristics of the environment responsible for changing the sound. Indoors, the material in a room may alter sound by absorbing it or changing it as it is refracted. If the room has a great deal of carpeting, drapery or upholstery, much of the sound will be absorbed and changed, resulting in what is commonly called a dead room. A room without such soft absorbing material will reflect more of the sound-creating acoustic reverberation or the prolongation of the sound after the source has stopped vibration (Sanders, 1971), resulting in an acoustically live room. The sound quality resulting from either of these situations may help the visually impaired person to determine the furnishings of the room and its approximate size. A small room has less reflections than a larger room. Often distortion in the returning sound takes place because the materials in a room are frequency specific, absorbing some frequencies more than others. In general, the change in sound provides useful information for some one trained to notice the differences.

MEASUREMENT OF SOUND AND HEARING

To determine level of auditory functioning it is necessary to understand the individual's sensitivity to sound. The unit of physical measurement of intensity is the decibel (dB) (Martin, 1975), which is one tenth of a larger unit called a Bel, after Alexander Graham Bell. The decibel is a measurement on a logarithmic scale which involves a ratio between the intensity of a sound being heard with a standard

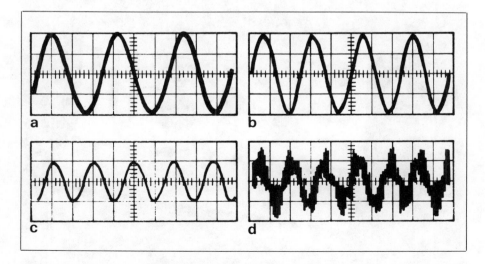

Figure 8-6. Pure tone components forming a complex tone.

reference intensity. The formula for the decibel is:

$$dB \ (SPL) = 10 \ Log_{10} \ \frac{Pressure \ 1^2}{Pressure \ 2^2}$$

SPL refers to sound pressure level, a way of stating that the measurements being taken and the resulting intensity level are based upon the actual pressure of the sound molecules of the medium. The Pressure 1 is that of the sound which is being measured while the Pressure 2 is the standard reference intensity of .0.0002 dynes-per-centimeter squared.

An audiologist uses an audiometer (Fig. 9-6) to attempt to determine a person's threshold of sensitivity to sound by measuring the intensity or dB level at which the subject hears a tone 50 percent of the time. (The tone is sounded four times and the subject should respond two or more times.) The instrument measures thresholds at specific frequencies. For the threshold measurements to have meaning, however, they must be interpreted in comparison to normative data. In 1935-36, the United States Public Health Service under Beasley conducted a survey that established data for average hearing thresholds (Martin, 1975). In 1951, these thresholds were accepted by the American Standards Association (ASA). At that point, American audiometers were standardized to the ASA values. It was later found that these standards were not sensitive enough because the studies were not performed under well-controlled conditions. Later, both European and American studies of average thresholds disclosed values that were closer to absolute audibility. These values were then averaged and accepted by the International Organization for Standardization (ISO) as the interim standard or norm. In 1964, United States accepted the ISO standards as an interim norm. The American National Standards Institute (ANSI) published a work in 1969 accepting the ISO standards and balancing them for use with the current headphones. New audiometers are calibrated to the ANSI 1969 standards which is very similar to the ISO standard. Some older audiometers may be calibrated to ASA 1951, and data from these instruments must be corrected to conform to the ANSI calibration.

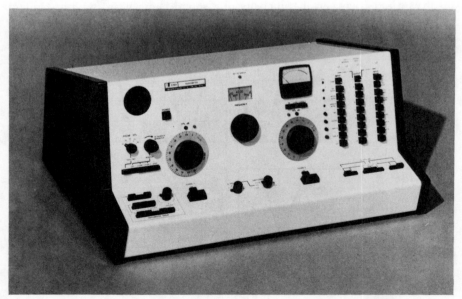

Figure 9-6. Diagnostic Audiometer (Courtesy Grason-Stadler, Inc., Littleton, Mass.)

Hearing Threshold Level

Audiometers are calibrated so that the actual dB (SPL) level needed for most normal people to hear a frequency is labeled 0 dB HTL. HTL stands for hearing threshold level (or HL, hearing level) and means in reality that at 0 dB on the audiometer dial, a specific decibel level is being generated for each frequency tested even though the dial reads 0 dB HTL. For example, under the ANSI standards, 11 dB of actual intensity or sound pressure level (SPL) are necessary for a 500-Hz tone to be heard by the person with normal hearing, and 6.5 dB SPL are necessary at 1000 Hz. In both above instances, however, the point of audibility is referred to as 0 dB HTL. In other words, the HTL level is a way of indicating that the decibel level needed for threshold is an adjusted level and not the actual level being generated by the audiometer. In testing hearing, an audiologist may indicate an individual's threshold for a 1000-Hz frequency to be, let us say, 10 dB HTL. In reality, however, the audiometer is putting out 16.5 dB SPL to achieve this level or 6.5 dB plus 10 dB.

To interpret audiological data, it is necessary to understand the dimensions of hearing sensitivity exhibited by the human hearing mechanism. The audible intensity range is generally between 0 dB HTL and 140 dB SPL. While the lower limit is usually designated by 0 dB HTL, some individuals can hear sounds at certain frequencies below this level at −5 dB HTL or −10 dB HTL. The upper limits for the normal individual of 140 dB SPL is considered the threshold of pain. At this intensity of sound, the individual begins experiencing pain in association with the sound. Just below the threshold of pain at 130 dB SPL is the threshold of tickle where vibrations are felt in the ear. Just below this threshold at 120 dB SPL is the threshold of discomfort. It is generally at this point where one begins to feel that sounds are too loud and are annoying. Some people who experience this discomfort at a lower level are suffering from an anomaly called recruitment which causes a disproportionate growth in perceived loudness as sound becomes slightly more intense. The audiometer is able to measure intensities in most cases beginning below 0 dB HTL and extending to 110 dB HTL.

In terms of frequency sensitivity, the human ear can perceive sound between the frequencies of 20 Hz to 20,000 Hz. Sounds below 20 Hz, termed infrasonic, are inaudible to most individuals. Sounds above 20,000 Hz are usually inaudible also and are termed ultrasonic. The normal frequencies tested by the audiologist are 125, 250, 500, 1000, 2000, 4000, and 8000 Hz. Each doubling of frequency is called an octave. On occasion, the audiologist may test the frequencies of 3000 and 6000 Hz when he is concerned about hearing sensitivities in the upper frequencies. Special importance is given to those frequencies of 500, 1000, and 2000 Hz, generally thought to be most important for the understanding of speech. It is these frequencies which are used to determine the severity of a hearing loss. Mobility specialists, however, must be concerned with *all* tested frequencies, not just the speech frequencies. Losses in lower or higher frequencies will certainly have an impact upon orientation and mobility.

ANATOMY AND FUNCTION OF THE EAR

An understanding of the anatomy of the ear will help the mobility specialist to understand the functioning of the hearing mechanism and the nature of hearing losses. The types of hearing losses correspond to disease processes found in the various portions of the ear. Diseases can affect the outer ear, middle ear, inner ear, and neural pathways beyond the inner ear. The portion of the ear affected will result in hearing losses characteristic to that specific part of the ear. Audiometric tests, in effect, assess the amount of hearing loss which may result from problems in the aforementioned portions of the ear. Some tests are designed to discover

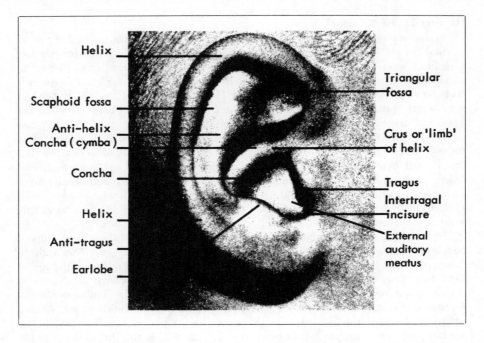

Figure 10a-6. The pinna. (From Willard R. Zemlin, *Speech and Hearing Science: Anatomy and Physiology*, © 1968, p. 365. Reprinted by permission of Prentice-Hall, Inc., Englewood Cliffs, N.J.)

overall loss. Others are used to differentiate loss occurring in the specific portions of the hearing system.

The Outer Ear

The outer ear consists of the pinna and the external auditory meatus, or ear canal (Zemlin, 1968). The pinna is a cartilaginous structure composed of grooves and depressions. The rim around the pinna is called the helix. The deepest depression is called the concha, an area that leads into the auditory canal. The tragus is a flap that partially blocks the opening into the canal. The external auditory meatus is an S-shaped canal 25 to 35 mm (0.8 to 1.4 in.) in length, and from 6 to 8 mm (0.24 to 0.32 in.) in diameter. The first third of the canal or meatus is cartilaginous while the remainder is osseous. The entire canal is covered with epidermis or skin. Within the first third of the canal are hair follicles called cilia and two types of glands. The sebaceous glands produce an odor that discourages penetration by insects and is also a possible antibacterial agent. The ceruminous glands produce wax to cleanse the canal and keep it from drying out (Figs. 10a-6 and 10b-6).

The outer ear conducts sound waves through the medium of air into the next section, the middle ear. The pinna in animals is movable and quite helpful in localizing sounds. In man, the pinna is immovable, but offers some assistance in localization. The auditory meatus is a pathway to direct sound waves to the end of the canal where the eardrum is found.

The Middle Ear

The middle ear, according to Zemlin (1968), consists of the eardrum or the tympanic membrane, the three ossicles, or the middle ear bones, and the

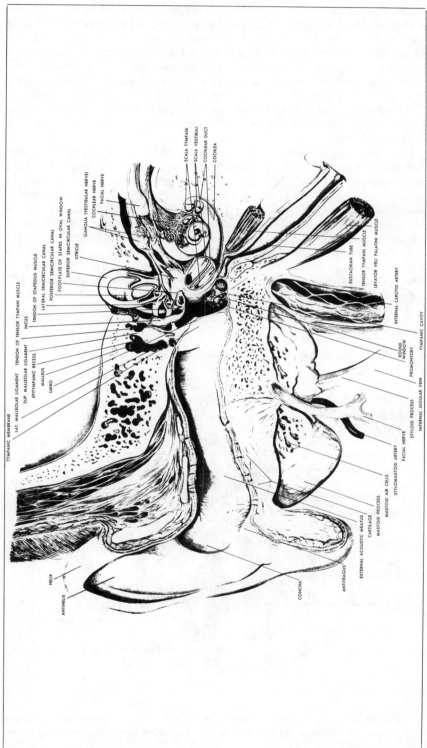

Figure 10b-6. The hearing mechanism. (Drawn by Ernest W. Beck, copyright 1957. Reprinted by permission of Zenetron Inc.—Manufacturer: Zenith/Zenetron Hearing Aids.)

eustachian tube, all housed in the middle ear cavity in the petreous portion of the temporal bone. The tympanic membrane is a circular tissue attached to the wall of the osseous portion of the meatus or ear canal. It has a fibrocartilaginous ring around the exterior which ends at the top. The top section is therefore weaker and is called the pars flaccida. The remainder of the membrane is tense and called the pars tensa. The tympanic membrane has three distinct layers. The outside layer which is continuous with the external auditory meatus is called the cutaneous layer. The middle layer called the fibrous layer provides the strength for the membrane. The internal layer is a mucous membrane continuous with the·middle ear cavity (Fig. 11-6).

The cavity between the tympanic membrane and the next section, the inner ear, is called the middle ear cavity or tympanic cavity. The cavity is lined with a mucous membrane and is about 15 mm (0.6 in.) high and 2 to 4 mm (0.08 to 0.16 in.) wide. The tympanic membrane on the lateral wall of the cavity is connected to the medial or inner wall of the cavity by three bones or ossicles. The first bone which connects with the eardrum is the malleus or hammer. It attaches to the drum at the middle, pulling it inward somewhat like a cone. The malleus has a head, a neck, and three extensions or processes. The posterior surface of the bone has a facet which attaches to the next ossicle called the incus or anvil. The junction of the two bones is called the incudomalleal joint. The incus has two processes, one which points posteriorly and one which points medially. At the end of the medial

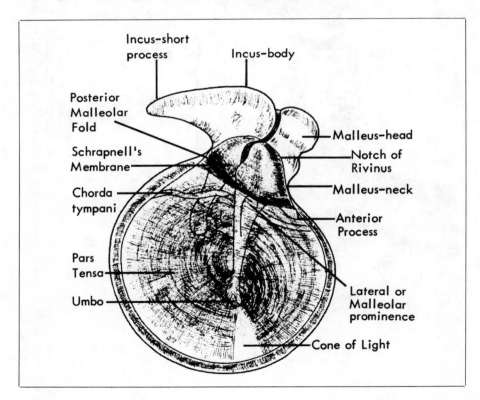

Figure 11-6. The tympanic membrane. (From Willard R. Zemlin, *Speech and Hearing Science: Anatomy and Physiology,* © 1968, p. 369. Reprinted by permission of Prentice-Hall, Inc., Englewood Cliffs, N.J.)

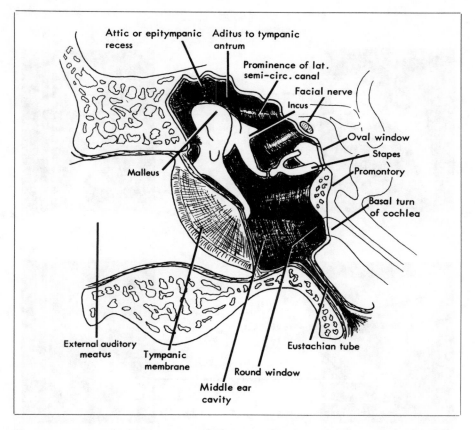

Figure 12a-6. Bones of the middle ear. (From Willard R. Zemlin, *Speech and Hearing Science: Anatomy and Physiology.* © 1968, p. 372. Reprinted by permission of Prentice-Hall, Inc., Englewood Cliffs, N.J.)

process, the incus joins with the next ossicle, the stapes or stirrup. At the incudostapedial joint, the stapes has a head, two arms called crura, and a footplate. The head of the stapes connects to the medial process of the incus, while the footplate attaches to the oval window, a structure marking the beginnings of the inner ear. Also located within the middle ear cavity is the eustachian tube, a structure which connects this cavity to the outside air. This permits changes in outside air pressure to influence or equalize air pressure within the middle ear cavity. In addition, it allows drainage to the throat of secretions that sometimes occur within the middle ear (Figs. 12a-6 and 12b-6).

The middle ear contains two muscles which are believed to protect the ear from excessively loud noise. The stapedius muscle innervated by the seventh facial nerve pulls the stapes posteriorly away from the oval window while the tensor tympani innervated by the fifth trigeminal nerve pulls the malleus anteriorly toward the inner ear increasing tension on the tympanic membrane. Together, the action of these two muscles changes the tension and the balance of the ossicles preventing transmission of intense sound.

The middle ear acts as a transformer of energy, the purpose of which is to change the airways of the outer ear to mechanical vibration that is passed to the inner ear through the rocking and sliding motion of the ossicles. During this

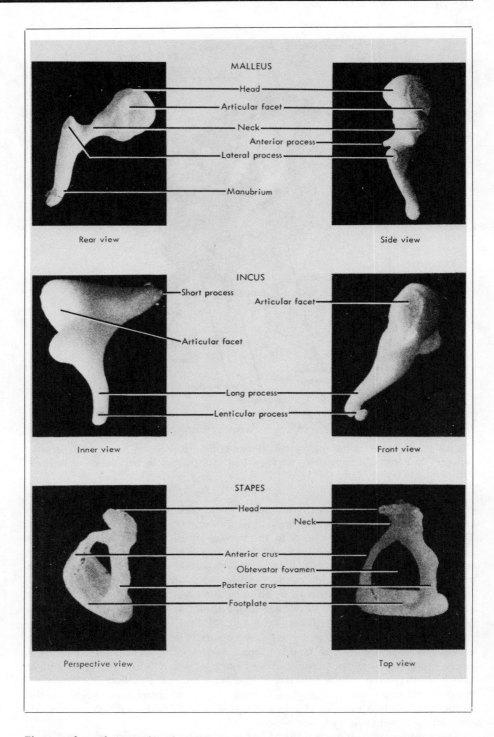

Figure 12b-6. Photographs of middle ear bones. (From Willard R. Zemlin, *Speech and Hearing Science: Anatomy and Physiology,* © 1968, p. 377. Reprinted by permission of Prentice-Hall, Inc., Englewood Cliffs, N.J.)

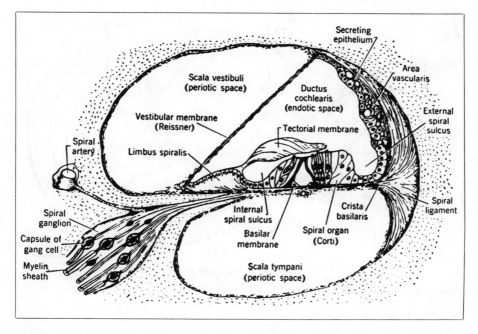

Figure 13a-6. The cochlea. (From S. S. Stevens, Ed., *Handbook of Experimental Psychology.* John Wiley & Sons, Inc., New York, 1951.)

transformation of energy, 30 to 35 dB of intensity are lost. It is theorized that 22.5 dB are regained due to the areo-ratio hypothesis which explains that the transference from the large drum of the tympanic membrane to the small drum of the oval window of the inner ear regains the lost intensity. Furthermore, another 2.5 dB are regained in the lever advantage of the ossicular chain. Together, this regained energy results in intensity almost equal to that initially entering the middle ear.

The Inner Ear

The final portion of the ear, the inner ear, consists of two systems—one concerned with hearing and the other with balance (Zemlin, 1968). This chapter is concerned only with the structures responsible for hearing. Refer to Chapter 4 for information about balance functions of the ear. The inner ear, located in the petreous portion of the temporal bone, is called the cochlea or labyrinth because of its winding construction. It is a snail-like chamber composed of 2¾ turns with the basal end closest to the middle ear and the apical end farthest away. It has a hard outer shell called the bony labyrinth and an inner membrane called the membranous labyrinth. The membranous labyrinth is a closed system or passage called the cochlear duct or scala media. This system contains a special fluid called endolymph.

The scala media divides the cochlea into an upper chamber and a lower chamber filled with a spinal-like fluid called perilymph (Figs. 13a-6 and 13b-6). The upper chamber is called the scala vestibuli and is in line with the entrance to the inner ear, the oval window. The lower section of the scala vestibuli is separated from the scala media by a tissue called Reissner's membrane. The lower chamber is called scala tympani and is in line with the round window, a structure leading out of the inner ear. This chamber is separated from the scala media by the basilar

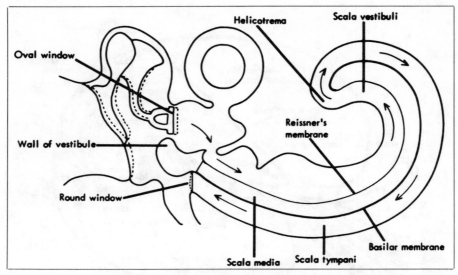

Figure 13b-6. Cross section of the inner ear. (From Willard R. Zemlin, *Speech and Hearing Science: Anatomy and Physiology,* © 1968, p. 417. Reprinted by permission of Prentice-Hall, Inc., Englewood Cliffs, N.J.)

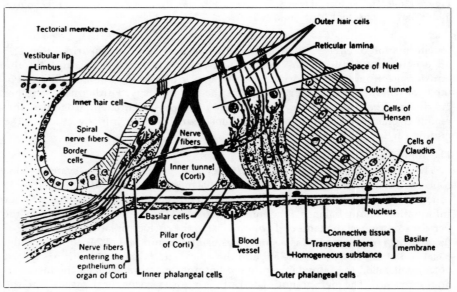

Figure 14a-6. The organ of Corti. (From S. S. Stevens, Ed., *Handbook of Experimental Psychology.* John Wiley & Sons, Inc., New York, 1951.)

membrane. The two chambers or scalae connect at a junction called the helicotrema. At this junction, the perilymph from both chambers is continuous. Within the endolymph of the scala media is located the organ of Corti, the nerve endings of the hearing mechanism (Fig. 14a-6). These endings are located on the basilar membrane and consist of four rows of hair cells, one inner row, and three

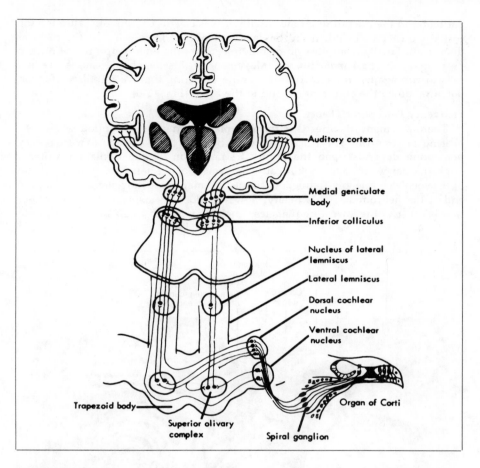

Figure 14b-6. The neural pathways. (From Willard R. Zemlin, *Speech and Hearing Science: Anatomy and Physiology,* © 1968, p. 414. Reprinted by permission of Prentice-Hall, Inc., Englewood Cliffs, N.J.)

outer rows. They are covered by the tectorial membrane. The hair cells run along the scala media and each attach to nerve fibers that join to form the acoustic branch of the eighth nerve. The eighth nerve in turn connects to the medula oblongata of the brain stem. The nerve pathway progresses up the brain stem to the auditory cortex of the brain (Fig. 14b-6).

The purpose of the inner ear is to transform one form of energy to another. The inner ear changes the mechanical energy of the middle ear to hydraulic and later electrical-chemical impulses which travel along the eighth nerve to the auditory lobe of the brain where they are interpreted as sounds. The inner ear receives the mechanical energy and eventually changes it to electrical impulses that the brain can interpret. This is accomplished through the vibration of the ossicles which eventually set in motion the oval window in the scala vestibuli. This in turn sets up pressure waves within the scala vestibuli which travel around the helicotrema and continue through the scala tympani, finally creating a reverse bulge of the round window at the end of the scala tympani. In addition, this compression is transmitted through the cochlear duct or scala media besides traveling along the path around the duct through the two outer scalae. This compression through the cochlear duct presses down on Reissner's membrane forcing it into the cochlear duct itself. Finally, compression or bulging causes the endolymph in the duct to press upon the basilar membrane. Movement of this membrane causes the hair cells to rub against the tectorial membrane initiating a nerve impulse or action potential down the eighth nerve and to the brain (Fig. 15-6).

Frequency Perception Theory

There are many theories that try to explain frequency perception within the hearing mechanism. The Place Theory by Békésy (1928) stresses that frequency perception depends upon the point of stimulation on the basilar membrane. High-frequency stimulation may cause movement of the hair cells in the basal end of the cochlea while low-frequency stimulation may cause movement in the apical end at the helicotrema. This theory, however, does not explain all pitch perception because at the lowest frequencies, this may not hold true. Another theory to

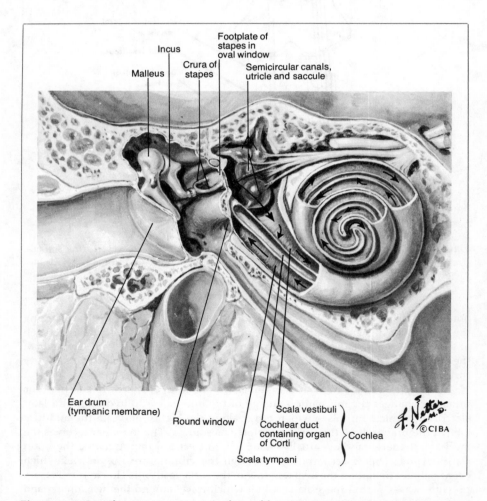

Figure 15-6. Soundwave transmission in the cochlea. (© 1962 CIBA Pharmaceutical Company, Division of CIBA-GEIGY Corporation. Reproduced with permission from *Clinical Symposia*, illustrated by Frank H. Netter, M.D. All rights reserved.)

explain frequency perception called the Telephone Frequency Theory (Rutherford, 1886) indicates that frequency is determined by the rate of firing of each hair cell. However, it has been shown that hair cells cannot be fired over 500 times-per-second. Therefore, frequencies above 500 Hz should not be possible. In still another frequency theory, called the Volley Theory, Weaver (1949) states that a number of neurons may fire together. For example, ten neurons firing 500 times-per-second will add up to 5000 Hz. Many audiologists currently feel that a combination of the various theories may account for frequency perception. At low frequencies up to 400 Hz, the Telephone Frequency Theory may be functioning. At frequencies from 400 to 5000 Hz, the Volley Theory may be responsible. Finally, between 5000 and 20,000 Hz, the Place Theory may account for pitch perception.

CLASSIFYING AND QUANTIFYING HEARING LOSS

Classification of hearing loss is based upon site of disease or breakdown in any of the sections within the hearing mechanism. For purposes of classification, losses are identified according to the anatomic areas affected. If the site of lesion or disease is located in the outer ear or in the middle ear, the loss is classified as *conductive*. If the dysfunctioning is within the inner ear or beyond, it is classified as a *sensori-neural* loss. The hyphenated word "sensori-neural" indicates a broad category which can be further broken down. A cochlear abnormality may be the cause of the sensori-neural hearing loss, or a retrocochlear or eighth nerve site of lesion may possibly be the cause of such a loss. Another explanation of loss may be a central or brain stem lesion. Finally, a dysfunction of the cortical area of the brain may be the cause. Each type of sensori-neural loss has its own distinctive characteristics which can be discovered through a battery of special tests.

The mobility specialist, however, need be concerned primarily with differentiating between the conductive and the general category of sensori-neural losses. An understanding of the differences between these categories will help the specialist to interpret basic audiometric test results and to understand the auditory functioning of his students. The audiologist, in order to determine whether the site of lesion is in the conductive domain or sensori-neural domain must first test the transmission system as a whole and then compare the results to a testing of the sensori-neural system in isolation. If the test of the system as a whole shows abnormality, the test of the sensori-neural system will help to disclose where the abnormality lies. When the sensori-neural system works adequately, then through the process of elimination, the fault must lie within the conductive system. If the sensori-neural system is dysfunctioning, then the loss must, at least in part, and possibly in total, be a result of sensori-neural problems. The distinction as to whether the loss is a pure sensori-neural loss or a mixed loss containing elements of both conductive and sensori-neural components can be made by carefully examining the differences between the total system measurement and the sensori-neural measurement.

The test used to measure the functioning of the total system is called *air conduction testing*, while the test for sensori-neural function is called *bone conduction testing*. In air conduction testing, the audiologist begins by placing headphones over the patient's ears and generating signals through the audiometer which pass through the outer ear, middle ear, and inner ear, finally up to the brain. The patient indicates when he is aware of hearing the signals by raising his hand or finger. Each ear is tested separately for the threshold measurements of the frequencies 125, 250, 500, 1000, 2000, 4000, and 8000 Hz. In contrast, bone conduction testing is accomplished by directly stimulating the inner ear while bypassing the outer and middle ear structures. This is typically done by placing a bone vibrator over the portion of the mastoid bone just behind the pinna. The

135

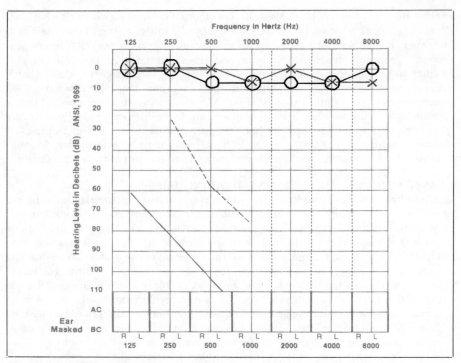

Figure 16a-6. Air conduction symbols, unmasked (right ear—circle, left ear—X).

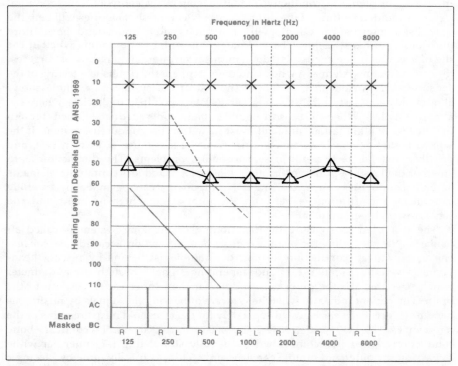

Figure 16b-6. Symbols for the right ear air conduction testing (triangle—left ear masked).

6

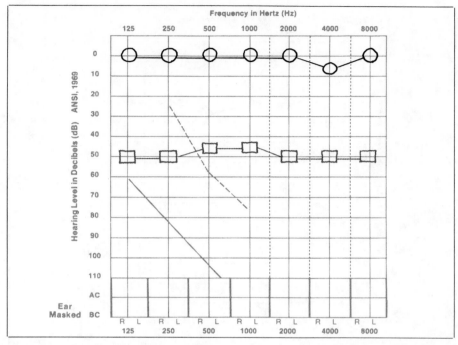

Figure 16c-6. Symbols for left ear air conduction testing (unmasked right ear and masked left ear).

vibrator oscillates and stimulates the inner ear through vibration of the bones of the skull. The vibration causes the fluid of the membranous labyrinth to become compressed due to the general compression of the skull while the inertial lag of the ossicles further stimulates the organ of Corti. Each ear is tested separately to establish threshold measurements for the frequencies of 250, 500, 1000, 2000, and 4000 Hz. The frequencies of 125 and 8000 Hz are not tested during bone conduction because the audiometer generating the high energy needed at these frequencies would distort the sound.

Audiogram

The severity of the hearing loss and the type of loss is computed by examining and comparing the values of the measurement as plotted on an audiogram, a chart which lists test frequencies along the top horizontal line and intensity level in dB HTL on the left vertical line beginning with 0 dB and progressing downward to 110 dB. Plottings are made at each frequency for each ear representing the dB-level necessary to reach the individual's threshold or 50 percent point of recognition for the frequency. These plottings are recorded for air-conduction testing by using a different symbol to represent each ear; the right ear by a circle, and left ear an X, (Fig. 16a-6). (In actual audiograms the circle is red and the X is blue.) On occasion, one of the two ears will be so much less sensitive than the other that the more sensitive ear will interfere with the tests of the poorer ear by actually hearing the high-intensity sound presented to the poorer ear. When this is the case, a masking sound may be used to keep the more sensitive ear busy, so that it cannot interfere. When the masking sound has been used it is indicated on the audiogram by a triangle (red) for the right threshold plotting (Fig. 16b-6), and a square (blue) for the left threshold plotting (Fig. 16c-6).

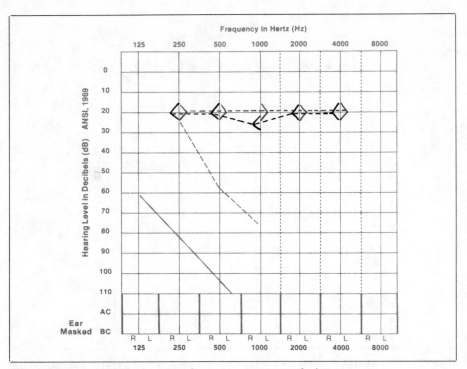

Figure 17a-6. Symbols for bone conduction testing, unmasked (caret).

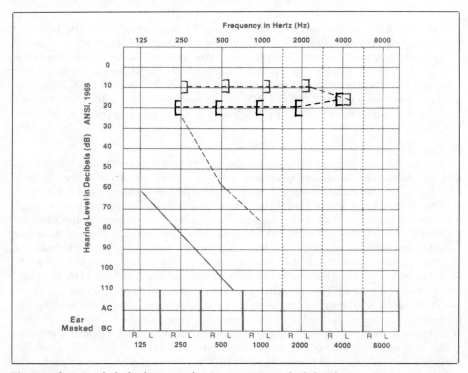

Figure 17b-6. Symbols for bone conduction testing, masked (bracket).

Plottings for bone-conduction testing use different symbols to represent each ear (Fig. 17a-6). Unmasked the right ear is indicated by a caret (red) pointing to the left and located to the left of the frequency line, as the ear would be if one were facing an individual. The left ear is indicated by a caret (blue) pointing in the opposite direction to the right side of the line (Fig. 17a-6). When it is used in masked bone-conduction testing, the symbol for the right ear is a bracket (red) pointing to the left, while the symbol for the left ear is a bracket (blue) pointing to the right (Fig. 17b-6).

Air conduction plottings enable one to determine if a hearing loss exists and its severity by averaging the threshold dB levels for the three frequencies of 500, 1000, 2000 Hz, (Fig. 18-6) and comparing the obtained pure tone average (PTA) with the categories in Goodman's (1965) classification system. If the hearing loss is much greater at one frequency than at the other two frequencies, 20 dB or more, the

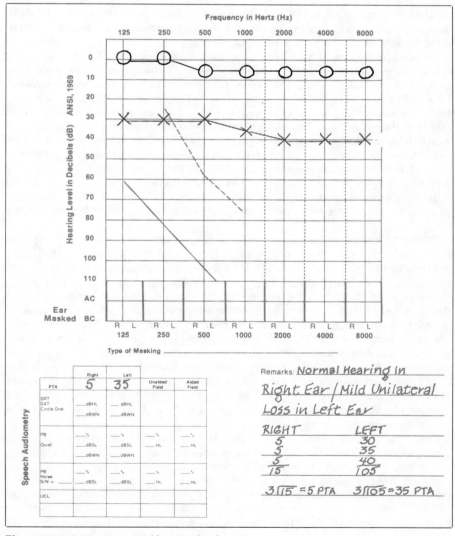

Figure 18-6. Determination of hearing loss severity.

frequency with the large loss should not be used in determining the average. This method of computation is known as the Fletcherian two-frequency method of averaging.

Goodman's categories of hearing-loss severity provide a way to classify auditory functioning. The figures in each category are based upon audiometers calibrated to the 1964 ISO standards or the 1969 ANSI standards. Category one, – 10 dB to 26 dB HTL, indicates normal limits or normal hearing. Category two, 27 to 40 dB HTL, indicates mild hearing loss. Category three, 41 to 55 dB HTL, indicates a moderate hearing loss. Category four, 56 to 70 dB HTL, indicates moderately severe hearing loss. Category five, 71 to 90 dB HTL, indicates a severe hearing loss. The final category, 91+ dB HTL, indicates a profound hearing loss. Goodman warned that it is not helpful to interpret the table too strictly because different types of hearing loss may impose different degrees of handicap and the dB loss in and of itself can be only one source of information used to determine handicap. With this qualification, it is possible to use the classifications for cautious determination of the probable handicap and the needs of the individual. Someone with a mild hearing loss may have some difficulty hearing faint or far-away speech. A person with a moderate hearing loss may be able to understand conversational speech only in close proximity of approximately 3 to 5 ft (90 to 150 cm) and have great difficulty in group discussion. An individual with a moderately severe hearing loss may find that conversation must be very loud for comprehension and that he cannot generally participate in group communication. Someone with a severe hearing loss may be able to hear a loud voice approximately 1 ft (30 cm) from the ear and may be able to identify environmental sounds. A person with a profound hearing loss may hear various loud sounds, but cannot rely upon them consistently as a primary channel for communication. Deafness is commonly defined in a functional manner. According to the Conference of Executives of American Schools for the Deaf, a person is deaf when hearing is nonfunctional for ordinary purposes of life. Such an individual may be aware of loud or random sounds, but may not be able to comprehend speech even with the use of hearing aids.

When a hearing loss exists, the audiologist compares air-conduction and bone-conduction thresholds to determine the type of loss (Newby, 1964; Martin, 1975). When looking at the relationship between the air-conduction plottings and the bone-conduction plottings, he looks to see if a gap exists between the two at the frequencies tested by both methods. If it is found that normal bone-conduction thresholds exist, but air-conduction testing shows a gap of 15 dB or more at all the tested frequencies, a pure conductive hearing loss has been identified and a medical referral to an ear, nose and throat specialist (otolaryngologist) is essential. The inner ear and neural pathways register as normal by bone conduction while the depressed air conduction thresholds indicate that the problem, by process of elimination, must lie in the remaining part of the system, the outer or middle ear. Figure 19-6 is a plotting of a typical bilateral conductive hearing loss with normal bone conduction and an air conduction gap of 15 dB or more in the same ear at all tested frequencies.

If it is found that a gap does not exist between air and bone conduction, or if a gap is less than 15 dB at each and every frequency, a sensori-neural hearing loss is identified. When there is a hearing loss with bone-conduction and air-conduction thresholds nearly the same, the loss must be due to dysfunction in the inner ear mechanism since hearing can be no better than the neural functioning. Figure 20-6 is plotting of such a sensori-neural hearing loss with nearly identical air and bone conduction thresholds (less than 15-dB difference between air and bone in the same ear).

At times a mixed loss may be found consisting of a combination of conductive and sensori-neural loss. This occurs when there is a hearing loss by bone conduction with a more severe loss by air conduction. Figure 21-6 is an example of such a loss (worse by 15 dB or more in the same ear). A further example of a mixed loss (Fig. 22-6) may be found when bone-conduction thresholds are within normal limits but an air-bone gap of 15 dB or more at one or more frequencies exists (conductive component) while less of a gap is found at one or more frequencies (sensori-neural component).

Conductive and sensori-neural hearing losses present hearing characteristics which are generally different from each other. People with conductive hearing losses generally have flat-line trajectories on the audiogram with somewhat poorer hearing in the low frequencies. The amount of loss is fairly consistent at all frequencies which means that sound will not be distorted but will just be softer.

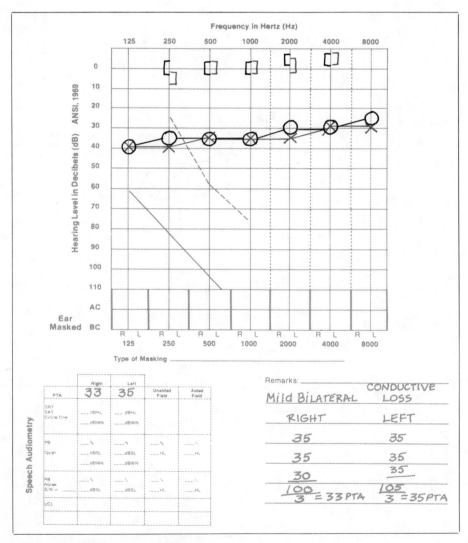

Figure 19-6. Bilateral conductive hearing loss.

People with conductive hearing losses generally benefit from increased volume. Hearing aid amplification is helpful but surgery and medication, however, are usually the preferred remedy. People with unremediated conductive losses tend to talk either softer than usual or with normal intensity because they can hear their own voices through bone conduction but do not hear competing noise. They may hear better in loud, noisy environments than they do in quieter environments.

The audiograms of people with sensori-neural losses generally have sloping curves. The amount of hearing loss may be more severe at the upper frequencies, meaning that sound will not only be softer but distorted as well. At present, surgery has not been developed which can remediate this type of loss, nor will increased volume alone entirely make up the deficit. Hearing aids which amplify sounds and augment upper frequencies are helpful but do not return perfect hearing. Before obtaining hearing aids, people with sensori-neural losses often

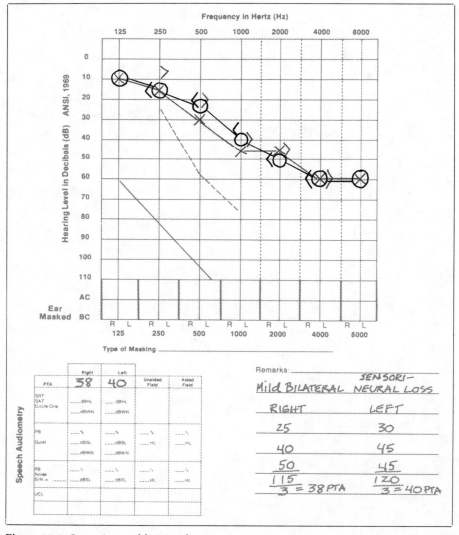

Figure 20-6. Sensori-neural hearing loss.

talk louder than normal since they may not be able to hear their own voice as loudly through bone conduction as they talk. To compensate, they speak up. People with this type of loss tend to hear more poorly in noisy environments than in quiet environments. Communicating with such an individual is facilitated by speaking distinctly, as much of normal speech is received as though it had been mumbled or muffled. In general it is helpful for a hearing impaired person to position himself so as to use any vision to see the speaker's face and lips.

Speech Audiometry

The second major category of tests audiologists perform is speech audiometry (Hopkinson, 1972) to provide information about a person's functional ability to hear and understand speech. While the pure tone audiogram provides information about threshold responses to pure tone signals, speech audiometry procedures test the individual's ability to receive speech signals that consist of complex tones.

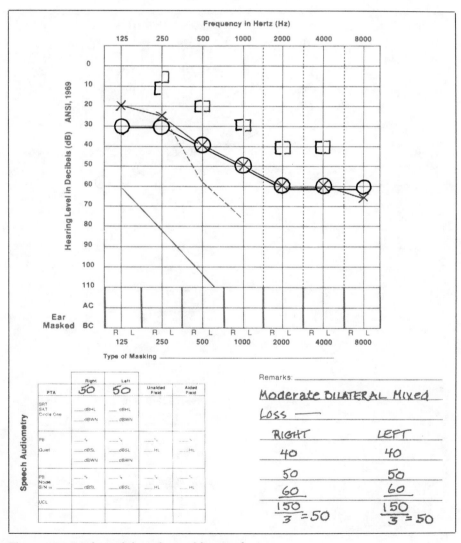

Figure 21-6. Moderate bilateral mixed hearing loss.

The *speech reception threshold* or SRT is commonly the first test given in the speech audiometry battery. It is a measure of threshold for the reception and understanding of speech, determined by presenting to the individual through headphones, in decreasing intensity, simple two-syllable words called spondees. When the individual can repeat only 50 percent of the words correctly, the SRT has been established. This particular test is used for two purposes. First, it is used as a way of checking the reliability of the pure tone average of the speech frequencies 500, 1000, and 2000 Hz as obtained on the audiogram. The SRT measurement should be no further than ±7 dB away from the pure tone average. If it is greater than this, one might suspect that the subject is malingering or may be exhibiting pathologies associated with brain dysfunction. Second, the SRT is used as a base for the determination of the next measure, speech discrimination.

Speech discrimination testing provides the audiologist with an evaluation of

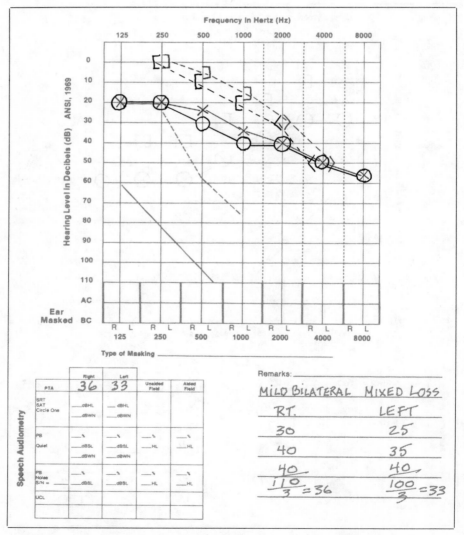

Figure 22-6. Mixed hearing loss with bone conduction within normal limits.

the functional ability of subject to hear and understand speech when it is presented at a volume loud enough to be heard comfortably. The test provides functional information regarding one's ability to receive communication auditorily. The audiologist presents through headphones a standardized list of 50 monosyllabic words at an intensity level usually between 20 and 40 dB above the SRT, loud enough to be easily heard. The percentage of words repeated correctly by the subject is called the speech discrimination score (DISCRIM) which gives useful information about one's ability to understand speech. When based on common word lists such as the Northwestern University Word List #6, Central Institute for the Deaf CID22 form, the computed score can be interpreted according to the following standards. A score of between 90 and 100 percent indicates understanding ability within normal limits. A score between 75 and 90 percent indicates slight difficulty comparable to listening over a telephone. A score between 60 and 75 percent indicates moderate difficulty. A score of between 50 and 60 percent may indicate poor speech discrimination with marked difficulty in following a conversation. Finally, a score of below 50 percent indicates very poor speech discrimination with probable inability to follow running speech. Figure 23-6 is an example of the way information is recorded for both an SRT and a speech discrimination test.

When a person has a pure conductive hearing loss, expect that the speech discrimination score will be 90 percent or better because speech is tested at a level loud enough to overcome the loss and the signal is relatively undistorted. When someone has a sensori-neural loss, it will usually be found that he has a lower speech discrimination score because the signal is distorted and for which loudness alone cannot compensate. Speech discrimination tests are also useful as an aid in fitting a hearing aid. The audiologist looks for improved scores as he tests the individual with different hearing aids in the sound field (through speakers in a sound treated room). He also bases his judgment on the client's subjective evaluation of differences between hearing aids.

In performing the various tests of the audiometric battery, the audiologist has as

Speech Audiometry		Right	Left	Unaided Field	Aided Field
	PTA				
	SRT SAT Circle One	___dBHL ___dBWN	___ dBHL ___dBWN		
	PB Quiet	_70_% _35_dBSL ___dBWN	_50_% _35_dBSL ___dBWN	___% ___HL	___% ___HL
	PB Noise S/N = ___	___% ___dBSL	___% ___dBSL	___% ___HL	___% ___HL
	UCL				

Figure 23-6. Record of speech audiometry testing.

his prime goal the evaluation of ability to receive and understand speech. The audiogram and the speech tests are used to determine what difficulty, if any, the individual will have in following conversation. In many cases the tests are used to recommend hearing aids that will help to make up the deficits in hearing and improve the reception of verbal communication. The mobility specialist must be able to understand the audiometric testing so that he can understand the student's ability to follow speech. This understanding is important so that the mobility specialist can be prepared for communication problems that might arise. The specialist armed with such information will be better able to communicate with his student. In some cases, he might have to use manual communication skills or an interpreter. Equally important is the specialist's sensitivity to communication problems which the student may have with the sighted public. Audiometric data can also be used to help the mobility specialist to evaluate the use of sound for independent travel.

PATHOLOGIES OF THE EAR

The mobility specialist must, from time to time, turn to medical history to gain more complete information on the ear pathology exhibited by an individual. To help the mobility specialist to understand the particular pathology indicated in the report and the functional expectations associated with it, this section presents an overview of the more commonly found diseases of the ear (Martin, 1975; Davis & Silverman, 1970; Newby, 1964).

Outer Ear

The external ear can exhibit a variety of pathologies that may lead to hearing loss of up to 50 or 60 dB HTL. A common cause of such a hearing loss, usually in the lower frequencies, is the accumulation of cerumin (ear wax) in the ear canal. If the cerumin presses against the ear drum, a tinnatus or a ringing sound may occur. Ear drops are often needed before removal of hardened cerumin. Otitis externa is an infection of the skin in the external canal which, in most cases, does not cause hearing loss. It is usually treated by antiseptics, but if not treated, bacteria can work inward and cause more serious problems. Serous externa occurs when a clear fluid accumulates under the skin lining in the canal and it swells. Again, no hearing loss occurs unless the canal becomes completely occluded. Antiseptics are usually an effective treatment. Hematoma, another outer ear problem, is caused by external injury to the ear resulting in the breakage of blood vessels and the accumulation of blood under the skin. It generally must be severe for any kind of a hearing loss to be sustained. One of the more common outer ear problems in children occurs when a foreign body is pushed into the ear canal. Usually no hearing loss occurs unless the canal is totally occluded. The audiologist must be concerned with perforation of the tympanic membrane when a foreign body is present in the canal. Such perforation could introduce bacteria into the middle ear causing more severe pathology.

Middle Ear

Middle ear pathologies may lead to a hearing loss of up to 50 or 60 dB HTL. The most common is an inflammation or infection known as otitis media. There are several different varieties of this disease. Acute serous otitis media, one of the least damaging, is a noninfectious build up of fluid which occurs when the eustachian tube becomes blocked as is sometimes the case with a head cold. Negative pressure is sustained in the middle ear cavity when the oxygen within the blocked cavity becomes used up. As a result, fluid begins to build as the negative pressure draws such material from the surrounding tissues. The tympanic membrane becomes distended or pushed out from the pressure. Usually there is considerable pain. Antibiotics and decongestants are usually successful in opening the eustachian tube. Chronic serous otitis media is a stage of recurring noninfectious acute serous which has progressed to a chronic condition. Acute supporative otitis media is associated with the buildup of infectious pus. The bacteria infection if left unchecked will erode the ossicles of the middle ear cavity and put pressure upon the tympanic membrane. Antibiotics usually clear it up, but in some instances an incision in the drum is needed to drain the pus. A further stage, chronic supporative otitis media, occurs when the tympanic membrane becomes ruptured in the center due to pressure buildup of the infectious material. After the rupture, the pressure is relieved and the pain disappears. If this is allowed to continue without proper treatment, the pus continues to accumulate and can lead to more serious pathology. Finally, cholesteotoma may result from otitis media. This is a smooth gray or pearl white growth that often results when chronic supporative otitis media remains untreated, allowing the pus to accumulate and erode the ossicles in the middle ear cavity. It then continues to eat away the mastoid bone and finally the brain meninges. If untreated, death can occur.

Hemotympanum, another ear disease, is the result of injury to the ear and the accumulation of blood in the middle ear behind the tympanic membrane. Generally this condition clears up by itself. This particular problem is sometimes seen after surgery.

Another middle ear problem often found is simple tympanic membrane perforation generally occurring from the introduction of foreign bodies and will heal itself quickly unless bacteria has also been introduced into the middle ear cavity. There are three types of such perforations: solid perforations, fluid perforations, and air perforations (changes in air pressure from explosions).

Systemic diseases also cause middle ear problems. Such diseases as mumps, scarlet fever, measles, and whooping cough are sometimes responsible for hearing loss. The amount of loss resulting may depend upon such factors as the severity of the disease and at what age it is incurred.

Otosclerosis is the most common cause of hearing loss in adults. An inherited disease of the middle ear often associated with middle age, it is a formation of spongy tissue around the head of the stapes which eventually immobilizes it. This material invades the cavity and in some situations can even go farther into the inner ear causing labyrinthine otosclerosis. The disease is usually insidious, taking years to develop. One out of ten individuals in the general population has it but only 5 percent sustain a hearing loss as a result. It is twice as common in females as in males, and during pregnancy it is reported that a 25- to 63-percent increase in its growth can take place. This disease is usually bilateral and has the associated symptoms: tinnatus or ringing in the ears in 80 percent of the cases; vertigo in 25 percent of the cases; and a red hue on the tympanic membrane. Individuals with this disease often hear better in noisy environments than in quiet areas, a situation termed paracusia willisiana. Otosclerosis can be surgically corrected by removing the stapes and creating a prosthetic link between the incus and the oval window. This procedure, called a stapedectomy, results in normal or near normal hearing in approximately 90 percent of the cases.

Inner Ear

There are many commonly found inner ear or sensori-neural losses. Generally speaking, there are no surgical remedies for sensori-neural pathology. Hearing loss can be anywhere from mild to profound in severity. Presbycusis, a very common sensori-neural pathology, is generally believed to be caused by advancing age and is found in the sixth or seventh decade of life, although many times it can be found earlier. It may be associated with heredity, but may also be due to noise exposure and dietary deficiencies, resulting in a loss of sensitivity to high frequencies. Pathology is due to atrophy of the blood supply to the organ of Corti and degeneration of the eighth nerve and associated structures. Usually the loss never becomes complete.

Another pathology of the inner ear is damage to the head, usually caused by a fracture of the petrous portion of the temporal bone. During the fracture, part of the inner ear may be damaged. This type of injury is usually not bilateral.

Meniere's disease or endolymphatic hydrops is usually unilateral and results from a buildup of the endolymph fluid causing undue pressure and possibly rupturing Reissner's membrane. Symptoms are at first fluctuating loss of hearing, dizziness, tinnatus, and fullness in the affected ear. The dizziness at times can become severe and on rare occasions the inner ear may have to be surgically altered to relieve severe symptoms. A 2000-Hz peak may be present on the audiogram in this type of disease.

Acoustic trauma is a result of excessive noise exposure. There is a great deal of individual susceptibility associated with this disease. Strong noise attacks the supporting structures in the organ of Corti and then attacks the nerve cells themselves. Initially exposure to such noise results in temporary threshold shift or TTS. Following the shift of threshold sensitivities, hearing usually works itself back to normal, but if exposure continues daily, the loss may eventually become a permanent threshold shift or PTS. Generally a 4000-Hz depression or notch is present on the audiogram with this disease entity. With continued exposure the sensitivities of the bordering frequencies are also reduced.

Neuritis, another cause of inner ear pathology, is due to viral infections such as scarlet fever, mumps, or measles. These diseases may attack the cochlea along with other parts of the system. Within this category rubella or German measles is of particular significance because it also may impair vision and produce defects of the heart and nervous system.

Vascular occlusion and lack of oxygen may cause damage to the inner ear. In both cases, oxygen is denied to the cochlea, resulting in damage to the organ.

Finally, syphilis can be devastating to the inner ear and can completely destroy hearing. Congenital syphilis affects hearing in children or teenagers.

Retrocochlear Pathology. Dysfunction along the eighth nerve is known as retrocochlear pathology. It occurs beyond the cochlea up to the brain stem. Retrocochlear tumors are a major form of disease that affect this part of the hearing mechanism. They are usually benign in nature and are located at the site of the internal auditory meatus, applying pressure on the eighth nerve in that vicinity and cutting out the function in the nerve. They can result in partial to complete hearing loss. A battery of audiometric tests given early can usually identify the tumor. Surgery can be performed but part of the affected nerve must be removed.

Central Pathology. Pathology along the central auditory nerve-fiber system of the brain is classified as central pathology. This can be further broken down into brain stem and cortical involvement. One form of brain stem pathology, erythro-blastosis fetalis, is due to RH factor incompatibility occurring when the mother has RH negative, the father has RH positive, and the developing fetus has RH positive blood type. With the RH incompatibility, antibodies may attack the ganglion within the brain stem forming fibroid material within the ganglia. There can be a partial or complete hearing loss. Other brain stem pathologies include tumors that affect tone thresholds and speech discrimination.

Another central pathology occurs within the cortex of the brain. Audiological tests cannot always locate such tumors. Symptoms may include tinnatus, imbalance, and a difficulty in understanding speech even though pure tone thresholds may be normal. These tumors often may be removed surgically.

Functional Pathologies. A special case of auditory dysfunction is known as nonorganic or functional hearing loss. This type of auditory impairment does not appear to have any organic basis or only limited organic involvement with a functional overlay. It is thought to be due to psychological factors that affect attention, motivation and understanding.

Part II—The Special Auditory Needs of the Visually Impaired

Part II examines: those functions of hearing that are used specifically by the visually impaired for independent travel, approaches that have been used to improve the use of these auditory skills, and correction of hearing loss through hearing aid amplification.

PRINCIPLES OF BINAURAL HEARING

The visually impaired traveler benefits greatly from the reception of binaural sound receiving information through both ears—each of which is a complete and independent system for the reception of auditory stimuli. However, the response must be to one signal, not two independent ones. Cherry and Bowles (1960) emphasize that binaural summation forces the integration of signals received through the two ears. Sayers and Cherry (1957) explain that the invariants of two stimuli, or those properties that they have in common, are detected in the brain by a cross-correlation analysis that results in fusion, or at least partial fusion, when the two stimuli are related. A combination of two systems attending to the same stimuli provides advantages for the traveler.

Differences in the signal characteristics reaching each ear make it possible to localize the sound source. It is important to understand fully the principles of sound localization. To a visually impaired traveler, sound localization emerges as a perceptual skill of paramount importance going beyond the usual selective listening skills of a sighted person. It takes on the added function of helping to locate objects within the environment and to travel safely through that environment.

Signal Differences

According to Carhart (1958) the listener uses his ears to obtain an auditory triangulation on every sound source, which results in signal differences. Carhart (1958), Bergman (1957), and Sayers and Cherry (1957) all report four characteristic differences between signals reaching the ears. The first difference between incoming signals is the time of arrival. Since the ears are separated by the head and are approximately 8 in. (20.3 cm) apart, the ear closest to the sound source may receive the signal just before the opposite ear. The second difference in signal reception between the two ears is signal intensity. The ear closest to the sound source will receive a more intense signal because of the separation of the ears and the defraction effect of the head, which tends to reduce the intensity to the far ear. The third difference is found in the phase relationship of the signals reaching the ears. Again because of the distance between the ears, the phase position of the sound wave reaching the farthest ear will be different from the phase of the signal reaching the first ear. The final difference between signals is the spectral composition. According to Wiener (1947), and Perrott and Elfner (1968), the head acts as a filter, reducing high-frequency sound as the signal moves around the head. Low-frequency sounds, with wide-phase amplitude tend to bend around the head while the shorter wavelength of the high-frequency sound prevents the same from occurring as easily. As a result, the ear away from the sound source will receive a sound of lower-frequency components. Furthermore, Sayers and Cherry (1957) state that additional spectral differences may be perceived due to the reflective properties of the environment and different angles-of-incidence of sound waves as they hit the ear orifices.

Pinna Shadow

When a signal comes from the side, one of the ears receives the signal earlier and with more intensity than the other ear. Phase and spectral differences are also present. All these differences permit the individual to localize the position of the sound source accurately. If the sound comes from directly in front of or behind the individual, the signals to the two ears will be very similar and will complicate determination of source position. In this situation, a person may turn the head slightly to create a difference between the signals that enables localization. According to Noble (1975), spectral components may also help one to localize sound where the source is directly ahead of or behind the person. According to the "pinna-shadow hypothesis," the pinna acts to shadow the ear canal when the signal approaches from the rear and as such allows passage of low frequencies more easily than high frequencies. Therefore, a complex sound will provide different spectral components to the inner ear depending upon whether it is emanating from in front of or behind the individual. Furthermore, Hirsh (1950) explains that the pinna may also serve to reduce the intensity of a sound approaching from the rear while not interfering with sounds entering from the front. A similar intensity reduction theory is postulated by Stevens and Newman (1936). These theories state that the pinna by altering spectrum and intensity helps a person to determine whether a sound is coming from the front or the rear.

Frequency

Focusing even more sharply on the mechanism for sound localization, Harris (1974) has indicated that certain signal differences become more important at specific frequency ranges. At lower frequencies, time of arrival and phase clues are most important. According to Harris, this holds true only until the frequency reaches 1500 Hz. The sensitivity to both time of arrival and phase is better in the low frequencies and diminishes as the frequency rises. At the upper frequencies, intensity clues are most important for localization. Mills (1960) reported a minimum intensity difference perceivable between the two ears to be as small as 0.5 dB at 1500 Hz and above. Harris concludes that for the low frequencies, phase/time is all that is necessary to determine direction, while intensity is sufficient at the higher frequencies. He further states that while phase differences diminish to zero about 1500 Hz, the time cue remains for high-frequency tones and transients. He concludes that time is, therefore, the prepotent cue. Moushegian and Jeffress, as reported in Harris (1974), have found a trading relationship in responsibility for lateralization between phase/time and intensity which is dependent upon frequency, sensation level, and individual differences.

In discussing localization, Harris explains that it is necessary to have approximately an 11-millisecond (msec) difference in time of arrival at each ear to perceive each degree of azimuth change between 1° and 60° from the midline. This correlates with the minimum interaural time difference of 10 msecs reported above, and means that an individual should be able to localize differences as small as 1° at least to 60° off the midline. Mills (1958) confirms this minimum detectable difference for localization as being between 1° and 2° at all frequencies. In actual field testing, however, it is not uncommon to find a 15° error in localization.

According to Stevens and Newman (1936), the accuracy of localization is relatively constant at low frequencies and becomes less accurate as the frequency approaches 3000 Hz. Above 4000 Hz, the ability to localize again becomes better and by 10,000 Hz is as accurate as it was at 1000 Hz. Localization of tones between 2000 and 4000 Hz is not exact because of the properties of the clues of phase and intensity. They state that since phase is most effective in localizing low tones and intensity with high tones, we find the middle region of 3000 Hz has neither phase nor intensity as an effective cue. They further report that localization is most accurate at the median plane and poorest at the extreme lateral positions such as 90° to either side. This information is supported by Wiener (1947) indicating that sound is most easily localized at a 0° or 180° position. Therefore, the individual often turns his head to place the sound at those positions when localizing.

Head Movement

Movement of the head plays an important role in localization of sound, Hirsh (1950) indicates that localization effects are the greatest when the individual moves his head to use both ears. According to Briskey in Katz (1972) sounds of long duration may require head movements to maximize localization by utilizing the head-shadow effect to identify sound-intensity differences. According to Koenig (1950) our directional perception is in part related to our ability to analyze the way binaural sounds are affected by head movements. He noted that in an experiment using a binaural telephone system, localization to the right and left were possible but the listener seemed to identify all sounds as emanating from a semicircle behind his head. Similar experiments using binaural tapes with blind subjects by Norton (1960) resulted in the same confusion when head movements did not make changes in the signals reaching the two ears. Sayers and Cherry (1957) explained that physical acoustic clues may be correlated with kinesthetic neck-muscle clues to further process direction. The brain may analyze the sound and correlate it with these other clues as it attempts to fuse the signals from the two ears.

While much study of localization has been conducted, very little research has been conducted on the ability to judge the distance of a sound. According to Whetnall (1964) estimation of distance of a sound is determined by the ratio of reflected sound to direct sound reaching the ears. When the sound source is near, a greater proportion of the sound comes directly from the source. When the sound source is farther away in the environment, more of the sound comes from reflection.

Intensity

Often when there is unilateral hearing loss or when the ears have different thresholds, there are implications for sound localization. Bergman (1957) indicates that when individuals have markedly different thresholds between the two ears, localization ability depends primarily upon the level of intensity of the sound. He performed a study in which he tested localization of hearing impaired individuals by continually raising the sound stimulation in steps of 5 dB beginning 10 dB above speech-detection threshold for spondee words in a free-field presentation. His results showed that the ability to localize in a person with a significantly better ear occurred when the level of sound was sufficient to stimulate the poorer ear as well. It was found that at low sensation levels the subjects tended to judge the sounds to be emanating from the side near the better ear or from in front of them. Only when the sounds reached the level above auditory threshold of the poorer ear, was the subject able to localize more accurately.

Monaural Localization

Accurate localization is not generally possible without binaural hearing. Perrott and Elfner (1968) agreed that sound localization is primarily a binaural process, but further explained, however, that monaural localization is possible with persistent sounds and by head movements. This can be accomplished if a unilaterally deaf person moves his head to seek out the area of maximum intensity. They further reported that some subjects were able to show monaural localization without head movements. Their performance was poorer than normal, but still significantly better than chance alone could predict, and for some subjects performance was nearly as good as the performance of normal-hearing individuals. Wright and Carhart (1960) further confirmed that some individuals were able to localize monaurally. Perrott and Elfner suggested that binaural clues were essential for localization of pure tones but that complex sounds could be localized monaurally. They explained that the pinna may be the central ingredient in such localization because its many surfaces might act to change the spectral components of the sound.

In order to test Perrott and Elfner's theory, six subjects were given localization tests under three conditions: normal binaural localization, normal monaural, and modified monaural. During normal binaural localization, the subjects were asked to identify which of two speakers a sound was coming from when head movements were not possible. In the normal monaural condition, one ear was occluded so that a 35-dB loss was experienced. The sounds in both speakers were presented 10 dB above threshold of the occluded ear. The modified condition equally matched sounds from the two speakers so that the speaker near the occluded ear presented a sound 10 dB above the threshold of that ear while the other speaker presented a sound 10 dB above the threshold of the better ear. This procedure eliminated loudness as a factor that could be used to localize sound, forcing the individual to rely upon spectral differences. The results of the experiment showed that the first condition produced no errors. The normal monaural produced errors during the early trials, but results improved after practice. The modified monaural condition produced performance no better than chance. The preliminary data, therefore, indicated that monaural localization was possible with practice based upon distinguishing intensity differences. A further experiment was run with two subjects under the modified condition. Both subjects were given additional trial combined with immediate feedback. Subject 1 was given the correct feedback while Subject 2 was given incorrect feedback. The result was that Subject 1 learned to localize sound accurately based only upon spectral differences. Training coupled with immediate feedback allowed the subject to learn how to use frequency changes of the sound bending around the head in order to identify the direction of the sound source.

Implications for the hearing and visually impaired traveler suggest that monaural localization is possible when training is provided with feedback. Such localization can be based upon intensity changes and spectral changes. Furthermore, since monaural localization with one ear is most effective with sound sources of long duration, mobility specialists may find that individuals with such a hearing handicap may be able to learn to localize traffic sounds to some degree. Traffic sounds, of course, consist of long continuous complex noise that allows the individual time enough for head movements to permit loudness judgments to enable determination of the direction of the sound. In addition, those with a large discrepancy between threshold sensitivities in each ear may also be able to learn to localize with some degree of accuracy using these principles. Hearing aid amplification, however, can be used to improve sound localization where certain hearing impairments exist.

There are further advantages to binaural hearing which seem, in most cases, to be subjective and, in others, clinically founded. Koenig (1950) found that very loud sounds were easier to tolerate when heard binaurally. He felt that a "squelch" effect was functioning that suppressed reverberation and background noise. He cited an experiment using a binaural telephone system which was switched back and forth from a monaural to a binaural system. When the system was switched to binaural, the blind subject reported that background noises gradually faded away to a low level. Schubert and Schultz in Dirks and Wilson (1969) reported that while the advantage of listening to a voice binaurally in competing noise resulted in a threshold improvement of only 3 dB, subjectively, the experience was described as a dramatic improvement in hearing. Bergman (1957) indicated that less effort was required for comfortable listening with binaural hearing. Finally, there were various studies by Decroix and Dehaussy (1964), Jerger, Carhart and Dirks (1961), and Chappell, Kavanagh, and Zerlin (1963) which showed that people with binaural hearing have 10 to 20 percent better word discrimination than individuals with monaural hearing.

Binaural hearing, for a visually impaired person, has the further advantage of providing space perception by facilitating the separation of two sounds in space. The differences in signals reaching the two ears allow for figure-ground comparisons. Cherry and Bowles (1960) stated that two simultaneous voices were easier to distinguish if they were spatially separated and that this principle of image-separation enhancement served to give an individual his impression of "subjective space." Bergman (1957) indicated that separation of speech signals from a competing signal of noise is closely related to localization and that this process allows the separation of the signals in space without the conscious awareness of the listener. Blind persons similarly learn to separate environmental sounds to gain an appreciation of space. This perceptual skill is greatly hampered when one ear is noticeably less sensitive than the other. When this is the case, the differences in the reception of signals between the two ears are complicated by the introduction of unequal hearing.

Finally, it must be remembered that even if unequal hearing or unilateral hearing greatly disrupts localization, mobility may still be possible. A person traveling from corner to corner along the block will not be greatly hampered by poor localization skills. Crossings in a residential area can be attempted on a go, no-go basis. If one can discriminate between traffic sounds being present and not present, he may cross when he is sure that traffic is not around. The following section on the interpretation of audiograms for travel purposes examines the hearing sensitivity which may be needed for an individual to hear traffic early enough to make this go, no-go determination. Crossings at traffic-light controlled intersections do require localization ability and, therefore, should be made only with sighted assistance when accurate localization of traffic cannot be made.

INTERPRETATION OF AUDIOMETRIC DATA FOR USE OF TRAFFIC SOUNDS

The mobility specialist should go beyond using audiometric data solely as a means to understand the student's communication ability. He must also be able to use audiogram data to gain understanding of a student's ability to process auditory information for independent travel.

One of the main concerns of the mobility specialist is how the visually impaired person will be able to interpret traffic sounds. The ability to use such sounds will in part determine how successful a traveler can become. It is, therefore, important to understand the measurement and composition of traffic sounds.

Traffic Sounds

The intensity of traffic sounds can be measured with a sound level meter, an instrument capable of measuring the intensity of sound at various frequencies. Spectrum analysis is accomplished by using a system of filters attached to the sound level meter, each of which allows passage of a certain band of frequencies. Usually the analysis is made at each octave such as 125, 250, 500, 1000, 2000, 4000, 8000 Hz, etc. However, for more detailed analysis, third octave filters can be used to analyze the intensities at even more frequent intervals. In addition to measuring intensity at the various frequencies, the sound level meter is able to provide an average reading of the various frequencies as they would be heard through the audible range of human hearing. It is a weighted measurement and is designated by the suffix dBA, which reports only those frequencies audible to man.

According to Bugliarello, Alexandre, Barnes, and Wakstein (1976), the sound of a car is primarily caused by the tires against the pavement because of compression and decompression of air trapped between the tire treads as the tire rolls on the road. Additional sound can be recorded from mechanical components such as the motor. Measurements with the sound level meter indicate that tire noise generates sound which covers the entire audible frequency range from 20 to 20,000 Hz. Rough pavement can increase the sound intensity by about 12 dBA in the frequency range from 100 to 1000 Hz. Weather conditions also affect the sound. A car riding in the rain can produce a sound 10 dBA louder than the normal intensity. Snow tends to reduce intensity but studded snow tires on dry pavement increase intensity in the high frequencies. The average sound intensity of traffic becomes greater when the number of vehicles increases. The sound level is increased when there are heavy trucks present because the average heavy truck is 10 dB louder than the average car. The loudest traffic is that which is continuous at high speeds. Speed in general tends to influence intensity level. Acceleration of vehicles can increase intensity 10 to 20 dB beyond that of normal driving. Motorcycles can produce extremely intense sound that can easily mask other traffic.

Traffic Intensity

Wiener and Goldstein (1977) conducted a study to measure approximate traffic intensities in various settings for the purpose of examining the relationship between auditory thresholds at various frequencies and the ability to use traffic sounds for independent travel. A sound level meter B+K type 2209 was used with a 1/3-octave band filter B+K type 1616. Measurements of traffic sounds were made at the frequencies of 125, 160, 200, 250, 315, 400, 500, 630, 800, 1000, 1250, 1600, 2000, 2500, 3150, 4000, 5000, 6300, 8000, 10,000, and 12,500 Hz, in a quiet residential area, a residential area with intermittent traffic, a residential area with continuous traffic, a small business area, and downtown Cleveland. All measurements were taken at a corner in a position comparable to where someone would stand before crossing. In a quiet residential area, measurements were taken when no traffic was passing the intersection. The overall intensity was 52 dBA SPL reflecting ambient sound from wind, pedestrians, etc. A spectral analysis of the sound found the most intense sounds in the lower frequencies, with intensities beginning at 54 dB SPL at 125 Hz and decreasing to 13 dB SPL at 12,500 Hz. In a residential area with intermittent traffic, measurements were taken with one car passing the intersection. This measurement resulted in an overall rating of 72 dBA SPL, with intensities highest in lowest frequencies decreasing from 69 dB SPL at 125 Hz to 36 dB SPL at 12,500 Hz. In a residential area with continuous traffic, measurements were taken as cars passed by in several lanes. The measurements resulted in an overall rating of 71 dB SPL. The greatest intensity was in the lowest frequencies starting at 74 dB SPL at 125 Hz and decreasing to 38 dB SPL at 12,500 Hz. In a small business area, measurements were taken with more than one lane of cars passing, however measurements were not taken when heavy trucks passed by. The overall rating was 76 dB SPL. The most intense sound was in the lowest frequencies starting at 73 dB SPL at 125 Hz and decreasing to 42 dB SPL at 12,500 Hz. Finally, measurements were taken in the downtown area and included both trucks and buses. The overall rating was 84 dB SPL with the most intense sounds in the lowest frequencies starting at 78 dB SPL at 125 Hz and decreasing to 45 dB SPL at 12,500 Hz.

Since the human ear is not equally sensitive to all frequencies, the intensity needed to stimulate the ear at each frequency must be examined. According to Davis and Silverman (1970), the human hearing mechanism is much more sensitive to middle frequencies than low or very high frequencies. Therefore, it requires much more intensity to hear a very low and very high sound than mid-frequency sounds of 1000-4000 Hz. Davis and Silverman indicated that it requires 20 dB SPL of intensity in a sound field for a sound to reach threshold level of 125 Hz. This amount decreases to 11 dB SPL at 250, 7 dB SPL at 500, and 4 dB SPL at 1000 Hz. It continues declining until it reaches 6000 Hz where it begins ascending once again to 10 dB SPL and 13 dB SPL at 8000 Hz. Applying this information to traffic sounds, it can be seen that while traffic sounds produce more intensity in the low frequencies, the loudness is offset by the fact that it requires even more intensity to hear such sounds because the ear is less sensitive to these frequencies. For example, in the residential area with one car passing, intensity in the frequency of 125 Hz was found to be 69 dB SPL. Because it requires 20 dB SPL for a normal hearing person to begin to hear a sound at that frequency, the sound will actually be perceived as only 49 dB SPL loud. On the other hand, it takes only 4 dB SPL to begin to hear the intensity of the car at 1000 Hz. If the intensity at that frequency is 60 dB SPL, there is a remainder of 56 dB SPL that is audible to the normal listener. Therefore, the human ear has the most sensitivity for interpreting traffic sounds between 500 and 4000 Hz. However, those frequencies below 500 also provide a good deal of useful auditory information, but with slightly less audible intensity.

It can be clearly seen from the data that in all settings the most intense traffic sounds were present in the lowest frequencies and decreased in intensity as higher frequencies were measured. It appears that the fundamental frequency for traffic is low, creating harmonics in the higher frequencies. It is possible, therefore, to conclude that hearing sensitivity in the low to mid frequencies is most important for use of traffic sounds. This is contrary to what is needed for communication purposes. For speech reception and discrimination, sensitivity in the mid to upper frequencies is most important. The implications of this finding are that persons classified as having communication problems based upon the pure tone averages of speech frequencies and lowered speech discimination scores, may not necessarily have the same degree of difficulty with traffic sounds. If someone has a hearing loss in the upper frequencies with a less severe loss in the mid to low frequencies, travel or use of traffic sounds may not be impaired as much as would be expected.

Sensitivity

To gain further information regarding the sensitivity that may be necessary for one to identify the presence of traffic sounds, the Wiener-Goldstein study was continued. Measurements of intensity were again taken in a residential area as traffic approached while a subject was waiting to make a crossing. A residential area was chosen because the previous data indicated that traffic sounds were least intense in that setting. Therefore, if someone had the sensitivity necessary to travel in that area, travel in areas with louder traffic sounds should be possible if localization was intact. Measurements were taken as cars approached within 78 ft (23.4 m) of the instrument. This distance was chosen because a study by the American Automobile Association (1957) indicated that a car traveling 30 mph (48 kph) would require 78 ft (23 m) to stop including 33 ft (9.9 m) reaction time and 45 ft (13.5 m) braking time, under clear conditions. A pedestrian making a crossing in a residential area, therefore, must be able to detect an approaching car at least 78 ft (23.4 m) away. The measurements of the study found that the most intense sound recorded at 78 ft (23.4 m) was 56 dB SPL at 125 Hz. As in the other measurements, this decreased as the frequency rose. More specifically, the decibel figures were in the low 50's through 400 Hz and then down through the 40's until 4000 Hz. Again, considering the sensitivity of the human hearing mechanism, it should follow that an individual having sound-field thresholds lower than 36 dB

HL in low frequencies or 45 dB HL in the mid frequencies should be able to detect the presence or absence of vehicles for a crossing. In practice, however, this should be used only as an approximate indicator. Other factors may intervene such as the fact that some individuals make better use of the same amount of hearing than others. Actual evaluation of the person's hearing ability on the street must be conducted. Also, some people with a hearing loss may be able to achieve adequate thresholds with hearing aid amplification.

USE OF REFLECTED SOUND

Visually impaired persons gain much useful information for orientation and mobility by using the presence or absence of reflected sound. The traveler who is able to make good use of this source of stimuli, learns to travel in a more sophisticated, more graceful manner than those unable to do so. Use of reflected sound enables a person to avoid large obstacles before making contact, to locate alleyways and recesses for purposes of orientation, to detect corners by the absence of reflected sound from buildings, and to make turns within a complicated building without having physical contact with the walls. Originally, the ability to use reflected sound was not understood by the public, and misconceptions persist to this day. A survey of the development of research into use of reflected sound will help in understanding present knowledge of the subject.

Early History—Bat Studies

The first investigation into the use of reflected sound centered on the ability of bats to avoid bumping into obstacles (Griffin, 1958). In 1793, natural scientist, Lazzaro Spallanzani noticed that an owl, which flew into his room, accidentally extinguished a candle and became disoriented in the dark room. The owl crashed into the walls and other obstacles. Later, Spallanzani experimented with bats and discovered that these animals did not lose their orientation in the dark, but instead flew quite well. To decide whether the bats were using vision to accomplish this, he blinded them. The bats were able to remain oriented and avoided obstacles, and he concluded that the ability to avoid obstacles was not a function of sight, but of a sense we knew nothing about. In 1794, Charles Jurine demonstrated that when the ears of a bat were tightly plugged with wax or other material, it crashed helplessly. Spallanzani continued his experiments by using various hoods and bags to cover different portions of the bats' heads, demonstrating that the bat would crash with its ears or mouth covered. He felt that the wings or body made a sound which was reflected back from the obstacles to the bat. His contemporaries, however, did not accept his conclusions. He varnished the bodies of bats to cut down tactual sensitivity and repeated his experiments. The bats were still able to avoid obstacles, even with deadened tactual sensitivity, but his theories were still not accepted by fellow scientists.

Roughly 100 years later, Hahn (1908) verified Spallanzani's experiments concluding that the bat lost orientation with only his ears plugged. Maxim (1912) reported that bats detect obstacles by feeling reflections of low-frequency sound caused by their wingbeats. Hartridge (1920), who was familiar with acoustics, said that bats might emit sounds of high frequency and short wavelength. Griffin (1958) later used G. W. Pierce's sonic detector to listen to the sounds of bats. He found that bats produced ultrasonic frequency as they approached objects, with maximum use of reflected sound obtained at 50,000 Hz. The sound was in the form of pulses originating from the mouth. In an experiment, he tied the jaws of the bat closed, sealed the lips, and found that it lost orientation and crashed. Later, investigation found that the frequency of orientation sounds of bats are as high as 50,000 to 70,000 Hz in the vicinity of an object, and 30,000 Hz when flying freely in the air. Using reflected ultrasonic sound, bats are able to perceive an object 1 mm in diameter. Whales, porpoises, sea lions, and some nocturnal birds also use ultrasonic echoes in similar ways.

Facial Vision

Unfortunately, investigators studying the use of reflected sound for blind persons were not familiar with Spallanzani's or Jurine's experiments with bats and had to build a base of knowledge without the benefit of the bat experiments. As early as 1749, Diderot (1916), reported that a blind friend had the ability to perceive the presence of objects and to determine their distance accurately. His explanation of this phenomenon, was that the objects were perceived because they compressed a column of air against the individual's face as he walked towards the object. He felt that the blind might have increased sensitivity of facial nerves and end organs, and his explanation was accepted by contemporaries. According to a summary by Bürklen (1924), Zeune in 1808 and Knie in 1821 said that the blind used their cheeks and foreheads as feelers with air pressure being the stimulus. Levy (1872) named this ability "perceptio facialis" or facial perception or vision, and described the performance of remarkable feats.

Investigators began experimenting to find a more accurate explanation for the ability to perceive obstacles. Heller (1904) stated that obstacle detection was a twofold process. He believed that the traveler used changes in the sound of his own footsteps in order to alert himself to sensations of pressure against his forehead. He believed the sound of the footsteps served to inhibit other processes which could interfere with full attention. At the same time, William James (1890) suggested that awareness of obstacles might result from pressure sensations against the tympanic membrane, but independently of hearing. Dressler (1893) tested James' idea and found that the amount of pressure needed to stimulate the tympanic membrane far exceeded the amount actually present from the air-wave pressure caused by approach to an object. Dressler did further research by covering the face of his subjects as they approached obstacles. He concluded that perception of obstacles was due to differences in sound. Javal (1905) introduced the term "the sixth sense of the blind." He believed that this sense was similar to touch but was aroused by ether waves. Truschel (1906) believed that detection resulted from a rising pitch in the sound of footsteps as a person approached an obstacle. He also concluded that localization of stationary objects outside of the path of the individual was due to reflected sounds. In 1918 Villey (1930) concluded that the ears were responsible for avoidance of obstacles by the blind. He stated that sounds are present around us all the time and that when there is some change in these sounds, they are interpreted as an object present between the traveler and the sound source. He explained the feelings of pressure upon the face as an auditory illusion.

In a dramatic step backward, Romains (1924) said that blind people detected obstacles through what he called vestigial ranvier corpuscles, or little eyes located in the forehead of an individual which were brought into function by the blind. He did not present his method of experiment. Dolanski (1931) experimented by covering subjects' faces and later their ears in an attempt to discover the source of obstacle perception. He concluded with a physiological theory that any clues from any sense cause contraction of small muscles in the skin. Mouchet (1938) determined that an auditory process, subliminal auditory stimuli, was involved in obstacle perception.

THE CORNELL EXPERIMENTS

In the 1940s, a series of modern scientific experiments called the Cornell experiments investigated the obstacle perception phenomenon. In "Facial vision: The perception of obstacles by the blind," Supa, Cotzin, and Dallenbach (1944) designed an experiment to determine if sound was the explanation for the phenomenon. They used a long hallway over 60 ft (18 m) in length and conducted experiments asking blind or blindfolded subjects to detect a masonite board ¼ in. (6 mm) thick, 4 ft (120 cm) wide and 4 ft 10 in. (145 cm) high. They had each subject walk on a hard floor with hard soled shoes, and stopping when an object was perceived. The subjects were then to walk as close as possible to the object without touching it. At first, the sighted subjects wearing the blindfold could not detect the board well, but began having some success after the ninth trial. The blind subjects picked up the presence of the board much sooner, but did not get closer without touching. When the same experiment was tried on soft carpet with bare feet the performances of all subjects were poorer, but they could still locate the board. Next, the facial areas were covered and the subjects could still detect the board, suggesting that air waves or pressure against the skin were not necessary for this detection. Next, the subjects had their ears plugged and it was found that none could detect the board. In fact, they began veering into the walls.

The experiment was repeated using a 1000-Hz masking sound. Again the subjects were unable to detect the board. Next, any possible air or pressure waves against the skin were eliminated by isolating the subjects in soundproof rooms while having them wear headphones and listening to the sounds another individual made as he walked down the hallway towards the board carrying a microphone. The microphone had a dynamic range of between 70 and 9000 Hz. The subjects in the soundproof room could detect the board by listening to the changes in sound as perceived over the headphones. This experiment more credibly ruled out air pressure as the source of obstacle detection. Later, the subject walked down the hall in a monaural experiment to determine if a blocked ear would interfere with detection of the object. It was found not to interfere. A final experiment using pseudophones to switch the sound from one side of the head to the other by rerouting the stimulus before it could affect the ears, did not affect obstacle detection.

Dr. Ivo Kohler (1964) carried on further experiments to determine whether the facial area had any role in obstacle perception. He used novocaine to anesthetize the facial area, and found that in spite of the anesthetic his subjects still reported skin perception when approaching an object. He later used pseudophones and found that the subjects experienced skin sensations on the sides opposite from what would normally be expected. Therefore, the sound was responsible for detection but was *perceived* as facial pressure.

Facial Vision and the Deaf-Blind

In another Cornell experiment, Worchel and Dallenbach (1947) conducted a study for the purpose of determining further whether stimulation of the cutaneous surfaces of the external ear, the external auditory meatus, and the tympanic membrane were, as James had theorized earlier, responsible for obstacle perception. A group of subjects were selected for their ability to travel well. They were put through the same experiences as the previous Cornell experiment subjects and were expected to locate the masonite board. All the deaf-blind subjects with the exception of one ran into the board many times and did not improve with practice. The subject who did consistently detect objects was found later to be using vision. In the dark, this individual was unable to detect the board. They concluded that the inability of the deaf-blind to detect obstacles ruled out the possibility that pressure on the surfaces of the ear canal, or tympanic membrane, was responsible for obstacle detection.

Pitch and Loudness

Cotzin and Dallenbach (1950) investigated the role of pitch and loudness in perception of obstacles by the blind. The purpose of the study was to determine what frequencies were involved in obstacle perception. The subjects were placed in soundproof rooms and fitted with earphones that were connected to a microphone with an upper frequency limit of 12,000 Hz. A sound stimulus was moved toward the test object on a trolley suspended from the ceiling and was controlled by the subject so that it could be accelerated, decelerated, or stopped. A 10,000- to 12,000-Hz hissing sound was generated as the trolley and microphone approached the test object. All subjects did well in locating the board. Each noted a rise in pitch as the noise approached the object. The noise worked better than the footsteps had. Next, 125-, 250-, 500-, 1000-, 2000-, 4000-, 8000-, and 10,000-Hz pure tones were used separately for each trial. Collisions were numerous during the trials when stimulus tones of 8000 Hz and less were presented. Between 65 and 75 percent of the trials resulted in collisions and no improvement was evident. At 10,000 Hz, the results changed and the subjects did much better. The loudness of the sounds were found not to affect the perception of obstacles, but frequencies of 10,000 Hz and higher were needed for effective obstacle perception. The authors in conclusion stated that the high frequencies allowed for a rise in pitch as the object was approached, a phenomenon known as the *Doppler effect*. In the Doppler effect, a sound appears to have a slightly higher frequency if heard by a listener who is moving toward its source. Conversely, a listener who is receding will hear the sound at a distinctly lower pitch. The magnitude of the Doppler effect depends upon the ratio between the velocity of the individual and that of the sound wave. Higher frequencies are necessary because the sound at such frequencies travels fast enough to reflect off the object and return to the listener soon enough for the Doppler effect to be perceived while walking at normal speeds.

Environment

Ammons, Worchel, and Dallenbach (1953) conducted a study to determine whether the results of the Cornell experiments held true outdoors. They also wanted to learn whether everyone with normal hearing could acquire object perception. They found that the subjects learned more slowly outdoors than under more ideal conditions found indoors. Wind, shade, and olfactory stimulation interfered with the trials. At night, the subjects did better because there was less noise masking out important sounds. They concluded that all normal hearing individuals could learn the skills outdoors. Those, however, with hearing losses performed poorly.

Practice

Worchel and Mauney (1950) conducted a study to determine the effect of practice on the perception of obstacles. They selected 7 of 34 students who had failed to develop obstacle perception in a study conducted at the Texas State School for the Blind, to determine whether those who had failed could develop this ability with proper training. Training and testing of the seven subjects took place outdoors on a concrete walk 65 ft (19.5 m) long and 8 ft (2.4 m) wide. The subjects were taught to detect the standard masonite board. Each subject was given 7 series of 30 trials for a total of 210 trials. The results of the study showed that all subjects improved considerably, and all showed striking improvements within the first 30 to 60 training trials. They concluded that systematic training made the difference. The trial and error procedures to which the blind naturally resort are not always efficient.

The results of the Texas experiment were similar to the data on the amount of practice necessary to acquire object perception in two other studies. Supa, Cotzin, and Dallenbach (1944), while working with two sighted persons, found that they were able to achieve 25 successes in 44 trials. In another study with 10 sighted subjects, Worchel and Ammons (1953) found that 30 to 90 trials were needed to obtain success in 25 out of 30 cases. Implications for training based on these studies indicates that mobility specialists should not give up prematurely in training efforts and should make more systematic efforts at teaching object perception.

DISCRIMINATION ABILITY

Kellogg (1962) investigated the size, distance, and material of objects that could be perceived aurally. He stationed his subjects in a soundproof room with small plywood discs capable of holding targets. The discs would move noiselessly toward or away from the subjects. The subjects were allowed to make any noise they wanted to help them to detect the object. Seven distances were measured between 30 cm (12 in.) and 120 cm. (48 in.). Sighted subjects with blindfolds did poorly while the blind subjects did much better. In comparing the size of test objects, the blind revealed discrimination ability at 30 cm (12 in.) but became poorer with distance. Objects between 15 cm (6 in.) and 30 cm (12 in.) in diameter were used for this phase of the experiment. Later in material discrimination, discs measuring 30 cm (12 in.) in diameter made of six different materials were compared. Subjects were able to distinguish metals from the other materials except glass. Glass was confused with both metal and wood. Plain wood and wood that was painted were indistinguishable. Cloth was distinguishable from the four materials above. Surprisingly, blind subjects could even differentiate between velvet and denim. Comparisons between hard and soft materials were made with 99 percent accuracy. When evaluating the above results, one must remember that the subjects were allowed to generate artificial sounds to help them with the differentiations. Ambient sound may not allow for such fine discrimination.

Rice (1967a) investigated the influence that the shape of the target has on detectability. The only significant information was found to be related to dimension ratios. He found that there were significantly less detections of the objects as the ratio of the rectangle's width-to-length dimensions increased. For example, a 2 in. by 8 in. (5 cm by 20 cm) target was perceived less often than a 4 in. by 4 in. (10 cm by 10 cm) target, or a 1 in. by 16 in. (2.5 cm by 40.6 cm) target less often than a 2 in. by 8 in. (5 cm by 20 cm) target. No increase in detections was noted when the long dimensions were changed to either a horizontal or vertical plane. The practical application of this study should alert mobility specialists to the fact that very thin objects, such as the edge of a door left ajar, a pole, or a thin shelf may go undetected. When the shape of the targets was changed, it was found that concave targets bounced back more sound and could be detected more easily, while convex objects bounced back less sound and were the hardest to detect. Round objects, therefore, may be harder to perceive.

Myers and Jones (1958) in England presented different sized objects at different distances to gather data about object perception. When the subject was silent, he was poor in detecting the object, but did much better when generating artificial noise. Clicking was an excellent sound source. They concluded that most blind people while stationary could detect an object 2 ft (60 cm) wide at 6 ft (180 cm). Some could even detect an object 2 in. (5 cm) wide at 6 ft (1.8 m). Young blind children can develop this ability by four years of age. From various studies, it seems that artificially generated noise increases chances of perception. This may be the reason that young blind children click or snap their fingers when not sure of their orientation.

J. Juurmaa (1965) in a study at the Institute of Occupational Health in Helsinki revealed that object perception was demonstrably present in about 85 percent of the blind. Obstacle perception correlated with early onset and long duration of blindness, and was independent of intelligence. Juurmaa also gives an explanation for the subjective facial pressure that has been associated with obstacle perception. He feels that because the head is likely to be injured first, the person unconsciously detecting a wall due to reflected sound will also experience a tenseness in his face due to an associated rise in the tension in his facial muscles.

CONCLUSIONS—USE OF REFLECTED SOUND

Various studies have shown that obstacle perception is a process of determining the presence of an object in one's path by hearing reflected sound returning from the object. On approaching an object, one may become aware of a rising pitch that is a result of the Doppler effect. For some individuals object perception is experienced as a facial pressure even though it is a function of hearing in the upper frequencies. Echo detection or echo location is a related phenomenon that refers to detecting the presence or absence of a surface or object outside of one's path by utilizing reflected sound. There are two possible ways of using obstacle perception and echo detection. Obstacles and surfaces can be detected by the artificial generation of sounds. Tongue snapping, finger clicking, heel clicking, whistling, and others, have been used to generate sounds to create usable echoes for orientation. This, however, draws undue attention to the blind traveler. Observation of this type of behavior to gain orientation may be a clue that the traveler is uneasy in a particular area or is gathering additional information. Reflected ambient sound can be used to give the traveler the necessary sound information. Indoors, the sounds of people, footsteps, and the natural noise level create enough sound to generate reflecting echoes. Outdoors, traffic and other existing ambient sounds can be utilized for the detection of objects and surfaces. The use of ambient sound is superior in that it is a natural way of traveling that does not focus unnatural attention on the traveler. As mentioned earlier, the use of reflected sound by blind persons allows a high degree of sophistication in travel. The traveler can make less contact with objects and building lines, and can walk through a building in the middle of the hall without needing to trail the walls except to locate specific objectives. Outdoors, the traveler is more easily able to locate objectives by using recessed areas such as alleys and store entrances as landmarks.

This research indicates that useful reflected sound is found primarily in the frequencies between 10,000 and 12,000 Hz. Audiologists generally do not consider such high frequencies important because they do not directly influence speech reception. Therefore, relatively few audiometers test above 8000 Hz, and those that do, test only to 10,000 Hz. Researchers interested in comparing upper-frequency threshold sensitivity with obstacle detection performance, have therefore been limited in their investigation by the use of frequencies only up to 8000 Hz.

Kohler (1964) conducted a study to determine the correlation between auditory thresholds of frequencies up to 8000 Hz and ability to detect obstacles. He found a low correlation between the thresholds and performance in obstacle detection which ranged from .20 for the low to mid frequencies to .40 at 8000 Hz. He also investigated age of subjects and obstacle detection performance to see if good performance would correlate strongly with youth, since younger people usually have better thresholds in the upper frequencies. He found poor correlation between the age of the subjects and obstacle-detection performance resulting in a −.30 value. Furthermore, Kohler found that those with equally good hearing who participated in training courses for obstacle detection developed very different levels of performance in the skill. Kohler concluded, therefore, that while hearing capacity is crucial to the ability to detect obstacles, hearing capacity may cover two different, separate faculties.

He hypothesized that obstacle-detection performance may be more directly related to the ability to detect small differences in sound than to the actual hearing threshold of the individual. In order to prove his hypotheses, Kohler constructed a sound modifier which emitted a constant hissing noise at an intensity of about 30 dB. The device produced fluctuation of sound intensity that increased or decreased in response to a button pressed by subjects. The subjects were asked each time the fluctuations became less obvious to press the button to increase the differentiation. When they felt they could detect the fluctuations again, they pressed the button again, decreasing the differentiation. A recording device automatically recorded the subjects' sensitivity to small differences in sound. Results obtained from 48 subjects led to a correlation of +.74 between sensitivity to fluctuations and obstacle-detection performance. Kohler concluded that an individual's ability to detect variations in sound is more important than absolute threshold.

De l'Aune, Scheel, Needham, and Kevorkian (1974) investigated the relationship between seven variables and echo-detection performance. They formulated a forced-choice detection task in an intersecting "T" hallway which required the subject to determine whether he was at the intersection or the closed-in area after being led by a sighted guide. A total of 50 trials per subject were given after which the percent correct score was correlated with each of the following variables: auditory thresholds for frequencies between 250 and 8000 Hz, age, educational level, extent of visual impairment, Wechsler Adult Intelligence Scale (WAIS) Verbal IQ score, and personality trait scores from the Minnesota Multiphasic Personality Inventory (MMPI) and the California Psychological Inventory (CPI). The data showed no significant correlations between echo detection-performance and any of the investigated variables with the exception of the psychological variables. The performance scores were significantly correlated with the CPI Scales of Well Being .59, Achievement via Conformance .60, and Intellectual Efficiency .71. They concluded that auditory discrimination in mobility situations was significantly related to personal adjustment.

These two studies make it clear that variables other than just auditory thresholds are related to echo-detection or object-perception performance. If auditory thresholds were the sole determinant of this skill, we would find a high correlation between the two. However, auditory thresholds do play an important role in use of reflected sound. Worchel and Dallenbach (1947) in their study of obstacle perception by the deaf-blind pointed out that adequate hearing is necessary for success at this task as did the 1953 study by Ammons, Worchel, and Dallenbach. The mobility specialist can gain information regarding auditory thresholds in the upper frequencies by reviewing the audiometric data. The curve of the audiogram can be used as a basis from which to draw inferences regarding the higher frequencies. If it becomes apparent that a person's hearing is progressively worse in the upper frequencies, it might be suspected that there will be a similar loss in the frequencies beyond 8000 Hz. It must be remembered, however, that impaired thresholds at these frequencies may not greatly affect use of reflected sound until they make it impossible to detect the presence of the returning sound. As long as sound can be detected and one has the capacity for detecting fine changes in the sound, obstacle perception or echo detection should be possible. At present, threshold sensitivity necessary for this task has not been identified. Furthermore, other variables may modify this level for each individual. For example, the research of De l'Aune, Scheel, Needham, and Kevorkian seems to indicate that personal adjustment affects auditory functioning. Those most comfortable with themselves and the task at hand may be less hampered by anxiety and better able to attend to the auditory stimuli.

AUDITORY TRAINING

Effective use of sound is essential for the visually impaired individual to become a well-oriented successful traveler. Mobility specialists concerned with helping their students to develop auditory skills have provided auditory training for them. An audiologist defines auditory training as a systematic procedure to improve communication that includes lip reading, use of auditory training equipment, speech and language therapy, counseling, and hearing aid fitting and orientation. The mobility specialist, however, should provide a kind of auditory training that focuses on the auditory skills necessary for independent movement.

The first and most widely used approach to auditory training is done in natural settings. It is generally recognized that actual experience coupled with immediate feedback is most effective for improving auditory functioning. Mobility specialists, therefore, have developed training procedures that use real environments and actual sounds. Two approaches to this type of training have evolved. The mobility specialist may provide auditory training on a one-to-one student-teacher ratio as an integrated part of the travel lesson, or may provide such training removed from the travel lesson as a separate sensory training class. Both approaches have advantages and disadvantages. In the first approach, the mobility specialist using the sighted guide technique helps the student to sort useful auditory information from that which is not useful. As training progresses, exercises are given to teach the student to use specific auditory skills that relate directly to travel situations. Often the use of auditory skill and the actual travel procedure are taught together, which has the advantage of illustrating to the student, in the most direct way, the actual use to which auditory skills are put. Motivation is thus increased by this procedure. In addition, working on a one-to-one ratio, the instructor is able to individualize such training, taking into consideration the abilities and needs of each student.

Separating auditory training from the actual travel lesson also has advantages. In such an approach, the student is free to concentrate fully upon the sounds without worrying about related navigation skills or being inhibited by fear of dangerous situations. Another advantage is that auditory training can precede formal travel lessons and prepare the individual for travel before actually taking part in such a program. This allows building of essential skills in young children before teaching navigation. More than one student can be taught in such a class, permitting interaction between students to share problems, frustrations, and successes. Each student benefits from the experience of others.

Perceptual Skills

Whether auditory training is taught as part of the travel lesson or separated from it, there are many important skills that must be learned. The following is an outline of possible methods for teaching many of these skills. It is not meant to be an exhaustive list of procedures to be followed, but suggested activities upon which practitioners can expand. The tasks are based upon the perceptual skills necessary for effective interpretation of auditory information, and may be taught as part of travel instruction or separately. They can be used with totally blind students or when appropriate with low vision students. The question always arises as to whether or not it would be beneficial to blindfold those with low vision to help them to learn to use their hearing more effectively. Experience shows that it is better not to blindfold, but instead to teach the student how to use hearing to interact with vision. Only in certain unusual situations is it helpful to blindfold.

I. Use of direct sound coming straight from a sound source to the listener.
   A. Training in sound localization
      1. In a large room
         a. Have trainee stand in center of room.
         b. Instructor move around trainee and clap at different positions.
         c. Trainee turn and point to the instructor each time instructor claps.
         d. Trainee walk to instructor each time instructor claps hands.

e. Repeat Steps c. and d. without instructor clapping; trainee must localize point at which instructor's footsteps stopped.

f. Using self-protective techniques, have trainee find way out of room by localizing sound coming through doorway.

g. Repeat Step f. in different rooms.

2. With audible ball
   a. Have trainee stand in center of larger open area.
   b. Trainee must localize audiball rolled to him by instructor.
   c. Trainee must turn, judge when the ball is close to him, bend, and pick it up.

3. Coin localization. (Can be taught in conjunction with the basic skills used in picking up dropped objects.)
   a. Instructor throws a coin into the air.
   b. Have trainee localize sound as coin hits floor.
   c. Have trainee point to coin and walk toward it.
   d. Have trainee pick up the coin, using proper techniques.
   e. Repeat above procedure many times with up to as many as three coins dropped at the same time.

4. Continued practice in sound localization can be incorporated into training sound identification in next section.

B. Training in sound identification
   1. In a building
      a. Take trainee through building, and have him identify and localize varying sounds as he passes through halls and into some rooms. The following sounds should be included: people typing, phones ringing, doors opening, people walking, people writing, elevator doors opening, etc.

   2. Sound maneuvers, (sounds made by instructor). Tell trainee that by listening to maneuvers he can discover much about what a person is doing and about what is in the room.
      a. Seat trainee, and have him listen to what the instructor does from the time he enters room until he leaves.
      b. Have trainee later tell instructor what he did on his maneuvers.
      c. The instructor should go to different parts of the room on different maneuvers and use different equipment. The instructor may enter room, pull out a chair, sit at a desk, open a drawer, take out paper, write a few sentences, stand up, walk to a filing box, and file paper.

   3. In a residential neighborhood
      a. Using sighted guide technique, take trainee through a residential neighborhood to identify and localize sounds. Emphasis should be on determining width of street, number of pedestrians in a group, and identifying car sounds, lawnmowers, etc.

   4. In a semi-business area
      a. Take trainee through a semi-business area to identify and localize sounds of buses, trucks, cars, motorcycles, people entering cars, cars pulling away from traffic lights, cars slowing down, etc.
      b. Have trainee estimate distance from corner by listening to cars going to traffic.
      c. Have trainee identify type of street by listening to traffic.
      d. Have trainee estimate distance from corner by listening by cars going by on street in front of him.
      e. Take trainee into different stores to identify type of store by sounds made.

5. Sound identification with cane. (Many common objects that the cane will strike have identifiable sounds. Learning to identify these sounds will aid in orientation.)
   a. Have trainee strike a long aluminum cane against common objects outdoors to teach identification of objects by the sounds.
   b. Include following objects: automobile fenders, automobile bumpers, mail boxes, wooden poles, etc.

C. Training in discrimination between varying sounds
   1. Teach trainee to distinguish between different sound producing objects such as bells or rattles with different pitches, and pair or match those which sound alike.
   2. Coin sounds
      a. Drop a penny, nickel, dime, and quarter on the floor and ask trainee to memorize sound of each coin.
      b. Drop each coin and have trainee identify order in which they were dropped.
   3. Environment sounds
      a. Plan routes through environments that expose trainee to similar sounds, and have him differentiate between those sounds.
   4. Automobile sounds
      a. At intersection with traffic light, teach trainee to differentiate between cars pulling away and cars idling in accordance with changing traffic light.
      b. Go to different intersections and have trainee tell instructor when to cross street by listening to traffic sounds.

D. Teaching use of sound shadow. (A visual shadow is created when an object is between a light source and an observer. The object blocks out light that would ordinarily fall upon the observer. A sound shadow is similar to a visual shadow except that sound is substituted for light. An object between a sound source and an observer will block or muffle sound. The sound bending around the object and reaching the observer's ears will be softer and will lack the higher frequency components.)
   1. Purpose—sound shadow enables trainee to become aware of an object between him and sound source. A trainee can use sound shadow to identify poles and parked cars along a street or at a corner.
   2. Methods
      a. Take the trainee outdoors in a semi-business area, and place him facing street in front of a large object such as a truck or car.
      b. Teach trainee to listen for blocking out of sound as other motor vehicles pass the truck or car.
      c. Place trainee in front of a space where a large object may be present, and have him indicate if something is present by listening to passing vehicles.
      d. Repeat until trainee is able to hear the sound shadow.
      e. Repeat above procedures, first using wide poles and then thinner poles.
   3. Reinforcement
      a. Take trainee to different intersections, and have him indicate if poles or parked cars are present.
      b. Have trainee walk along street with instructor, telling instructor when he passes poles and parked cars.

165

E. Teaching use of sound tracking or taking direction from a sound. (Sound tracking is the process of listening and mentally tracing the paths of moving vehicles as they pass by.)

1. Purpose

   This technique may be used to place oneself parallel to the traffic before crossing a street, enabling one to walk straight across the street rather than walking near moving traffic on one side or into automobiles behind crosswalk on the other side. It is also useful in determining one's position while walking along a sidewalk.

2. Review possible paths of moving vehicles with trainee, using a model intersection.

3. Track instructor.

   a. Place trainee in center of large room.

   b. Instructor stands to the right in front of the trainee and explains that he will walk parallel to the side of the trainee's body to represent an automobile moving toward, alongside, and past him. (A path parallel to the trainee means that a passing object be the same distance away when it starts moving, when it is alongside, and when it has passed. In other words, the path of the trainee and object will never meet.)

   c. Have trainee listen to instructor as he claps his hands and walks alongside him.

   d. This time, as the instructor walks the same route, clapping hands, have trainee trace instructor's path mentally and at the same time point to him as he walks along the route.

   e. The instructor should walk several routes, some parallel and some not parallel to trainee. After each walk, have trainee tell whether the route was parallel or not.

   f. Have trainee demonstrate whether the next route is parallel to him. If it is not, have trainee turn and make *his* projected path parallel to the instructor's path. Repeat until trainee performs satisfactorily.

   g. Repeat Steps a. through f. with instructor on right side of trainee, but starting behind him and walking to a position ahead of him.

   h. Repeat Steps a. through f. with instructor on left side of trainee, starting in front of him, and walking to a position behind him.

   i. Repeat Steps a. through f. with instructor on left side of trainee but starting behind him and walking to a position in front of him.

   j. Repeat Steps a. through f. with trainee trying to stand perpendicular to the path the instructor walks.

4. Intersections

   a. At an intersection have trainee track traffic and line up to it.

   b. Take trainee across street the way he is facing. This provides immediate feedback and should help to improve sound tracking.

   c. Repeat above two steps until performance is satisfactory.

II. Use of reflected sound coming to a listener after bouncing off another object.

A. Training to use object perception

1. Use of large board with trainee in stationary position

   a. Seat trainee and stand in front of him with a large board.

   b. Move the board towards trainee until he is aware of it by utilizing ambient reflected sound. Then move the board back until he can no longer perceive it.

   c. Repeat above until trainee is able to detect the board effectively.

   d. Hold board parallel to front of the trainee's face. Tilt the board to right or to left, and have trainee identify direction in which the board was tilted.

2. Object perception combined with movement
   a. Hold a board eye level to trainee at other end of a hall. Have trainee walk and try to stop before touching board.
   b. Repeat above until trainee can stop in time.
   c. When trainee can identify presence of the board, have him continue walking until he walks as close as possible without touching it.
   d. Next, have trainee walk toward a wall, using self-protective techniques, and stop within 1 ft (30 cm) of the wall by listening to the echo created by his footsteps as he approaches it.
   e. Repeat above until trainee is able to stop very close to the wall.
   f. Repeat above two steps with shoes off. Instead of relying on the echo of his footsteps, trainee should now rely on sound from natural noise in hall.
   g. Stand between trainee and the end of a long hall. Instruct trainee to walk through hall and use the upper hand and forearm technique when he feels that an object is in front of him.
   h. Repeat above until trainee begins using upper hand and forearm technique early enough to protect himself.

B. Training to use echo detection
   1. Indoors
      a. Using sighted guide, walk student down a hall toward an intersecting corridor.
      b. Walk him at brisk speed close to wall.
      c. Have student, using echo detection, identify point at which wall ends at intersecting corridor.
      d. Repeat above until trainee locates opening consistently.
      e. Next, walk trainee and sighted guide past several open doorways with trainee close to the wall.
      f. Have trainee identify openings as they are passed.
      g. Have trainee travel down the hall independently, listening for the intersecting corridor.
      h. After this is done with confidence, have trainee travel down hall and count all open doorways.
      i. Using self-protective techniques, have trainee practice making turns in halls without touching walls.
   2. Outdoors
      a. Walk trainee along a street with many buildings that are close to sidewalk and an occasional alley between buildings. Start at corner and have trainee determine when building line begins. Have trainee indicate presence of alleys.
      b. After mastering the above, have trainee locate recesses or open doorways while walking along other streets.
   3. Determining room characteristics by use of dampened sound. (Dampened sound is the muted or distorted quality of sound heard when a sound is absorbed by draperies or carpeting. It reveals information about room furnishings.)
      a. Take trainee into rooms containing sound absorbing objects, and acquaint him with the sound quality present.
      b. Take trainee into rooms with varying furnishings and have him

identify those rooms that contain soft objects, such as drapes, soft chairs, or thick carpets.

Recorded Sounds

The second and less widely used approach to auditory training involves improving auditory skills by the use of recorded sounds. It may be done with binaural training tapes using headphones, and/or monaural training tapes played free field through speakers. The procedure used for binaural training is to record environmental sounds on a two-track tape recorder with each track recording the sound received at ear level of the respective ear. The recording microphones are placed in positions which correspond to each ear. They may either be implanted in an artificial head at ear position or may be worn at ear level by a person. The separation of the microphones coupled with the head-shadow effect combines to create authentic recordings of reproduced localization of sounds. With high quality equipment having a wide-frequency response, fidelity approaches realistic levels. Reproduction is accomplished by amplifying the sounds and playing them back over headphones.

There are many advantages to such a system. Tapes provide sounds of the environment without presenting the fear usually associated with traffic and other hazardous situations. Tapes also allow better control of environmental sounds for training situations. Instead of random experiences which are often encountered in on-the-spot training procedures, tapes permit planned sequencing, to present principles in an order that will facilitate learning of the skills. Tapes can also be played over and over for repeated study, and can be used as a supplement to the actual travel training on the street.

There are also disadvantages to such a system. When used as a substitute for practice with actual environmental sounds, the student is deprived of the necessary experience of combining the use of sounds with actual travel. Another drawback concerns problems with front-rear localization, which seems to be inherent in such pre-recorded tapes. Many students undergoing such training have reported that while they could easily distinguish between sounds coming from the left versus the right, they had difficulty determining whether some sounds originated from the front or the rear. This problem occurs often enough to be considered a serious drawback, and is inherent in binaural recording. Because localization is due to differences in the time of arrival, phase, intensity, and spectral components between the two ears, in an authentic listening situation, sounds coming directly from either the front or the rear are easily confused until the head is moved slightly. The movement changes these differences between the ears enough to permit accurate localization. In a taped situation, the turning of the head does not resolve localization difficulties because the turning does not change the signals of the two ears. Instead, the auditory environment turns with the head via the headphones. Some individuals rely more heavily upon head movements to localize sound than others. Those more dependent on such movement find difficulty in localization with tapes. They report hearing all sounds as coming either from the front or from the rear.

In 1959, an auditory training method using binaural tapes was begun at the Shilling Auditory Research Center (Harris, Dupress, Wright, Curtis, Winer, Gropper, & Kelsey, 1963). A program of binaural taping was designed to be incorporated into existing mobility training programs to provide well presented auditory training to a large number of people in a consistent way. Its goals were to develop auditory skills and to teach a person how to orient himself to an environment by utilizing taped sounds of that environment. Head-position identification and street-crossing decisions were stressed as two important auditory skills.

In head-position identification, an artificial head with microphones was positioned at the side of the road in one of five positions with respect to traffic flow: 0°, 45° right, 45° left, 90° right, 90° left. Traffic sounds were recorded for 15 seconds with 5 seconds of silence between each recording. At the conclusion of each 15-second playback exposure, the subject was asked to indicate which way the head was turned, and whether he was sure or unsure of his decision. The results were surprisingly poor in that the best scores were only 80 percent correct.

In street-crossing decisions, a judge stood by and decided when it was time to cross and when it was too late. The period in between was called the safe crossing interval and was indicated for each recording. A blind subject listened to the tapes and had 13 trials in determining when to cross.

The tapes were also used to teach the student to coordinate environmental sounds with the travel area by using them in combination with a miniaturized relief map of the particular area. The maps indicated important terrain, and man-made objects such as buildings, hydrants, or poles. The subject would listen to the tape and trace the corresponding section of the relief map by wheeling a miniature cart along the route. The attempt was unsuccessful, in part, because the tapes were not of high enough auditory quality to allow for accurate judgments regarding the placement of the head in the environment. It was necessary to move the artificial head to within 1 ft (30.5 cm) of the building line to record the reflected sound from the building, and even this did not work well when a high level of traffic noise was present.

In conclusion, this taping effort met with many difficulties. The positioning of the artificial head at the curb during the recording was critical. When the head was too close to the curb the tape sounded like the car was running through the listener's head. It was also found that moving the artificial head along a route was disadvantageous until a more advanced stage of training had evolved. The first tapes should develop an awareness of sound while later tapes should concentrate on skills. A lack of success with the tapes may have been due to the complexity of the map and the area used. However, ideas for future projects sprang from this initial project.

Binaural Auditory Training

Binaural auditory training was attempted at the Cleveland Society for the Blind in 1960 (Norton, 1960). With support from the Office of Vocational Rehabilitation, a program was developed for the purpose of compiling a manual complete with recordings and exercises that would enhance orientation either in travel or in the home. The program concentrated on basic hearing skills of localization and identification followed by "you are there" recordings. The application of the skills were for travel or for general orientation, but it was recognized that the recordings did not provide sufficient experience for immediate travel ability. Norton developed a series of tapes that were played in sequential order progressing from basic hearing skills to a more sophisticated programming. Tape 1 consisted of a calibrated pure tone; Tape 2 described the importance of hearing and accustomed the individual to headphone listening; Tape 3 taught a clock face reference system for localization, and gave a pretest in sound localization; Tape 4 provided practice in localization along with a self test; Tapes 5 through 7 provided further sound localization training such as seating a client in a chair and asking him to point to positions on a giant clock face from which sounds were emanating; Tape 8 was sounds heard in a kitchen; Tape 9 was sounds heard in a living room; Tape 10 asked the client to locate sounds in a strange kitchen and encouraged future listening for typical sounds to learn the interior of rooms. The recordings were made with microphones embedded in an artificial head made of latex over balsa wood, and recorded on a reel-to-reel machine at a speed of 15 inches-per-second (ips), (38 cmps) for optimum fidelity. In addition to the recordings, specific auditory exercises in natural settings were suggested.

In evaluating his work with the original ten tapes, Norton indicated that client response had been very positive. They stated that the training had made them more conscious of the use of hearing or had emphasized it. Upon being asked to make a comparative rating of the training, they indicated that it would be useful to most blind people. Norton recommended an audiological examination before starting binaural training in order to reveal any hearing loss. However, there was no research to ascertain whether an individual with an imbalance in hearing thresholds could benefit from the training procedure. He reported that some people had difficulty separating sounds originating in front from sounds originating from the rear. In experiments, he reported that clients had less trouble with the separation when told that the sound would be coming from the front or the back, but some individuals still tended to imagine the situation as all from the front or all from the back. After 90 people had received this training his conclusions were that he could report localization and identification of sounds in real situations to be significantly improved with binaural recordings.

Another attempt at auditory training through binaural taping was more recently instituted at the Michigan Rehabilitation Center in Kalamazoo. The program focused sharply upon auditory skills essential for orientation and mobility, with recordings made by mobility specialists for this purpose. Sounds were recorded on a reel-to-reel machine at a speed of 15 ips (38 cmps). Microphones were worn by a person at ear level on a headphone band. Five tapes were developed, beginning with elementary skills and progressing to harder tasks. Tape 1 was concerned primarily with the identification of various sounds and their localization. Tape 2 attempted to record echolocation as a person walked parallel to a wall. Also included were recordings of ambient sounds in various rooms while asking for identification of those rooms. Tape 3 introduced the student to traffic sounds recorded in the middle of a block on a one-way street and later on a two-way street. Tape 4 consisted of traffic sounds recorded at different kinds of intersections. Tape 5 consisted of auditory discrimination tasks such as distinguishing between cars, trucks, buses, and identification of sounds in an enclosed shopping mall. Of all the tapes, Tape 2 was the least successful in simulating echo detection through the system. Only when sounds in the environment were generated for the recording was it possible to perceive the presence of absence of the parallel wall in the recorded situation.

Tapes with Auditory Maps

Wiener and McLaughlin (1973) developed a comprehensive binaural taping program at the Syracuse Association of Workers for the Blind which included auditory maps with authentic sounds from the mapped areas. Sounds were recorded on a portable reel-to-reel machine at a speed of 7½ ips (19 cmps). Microphones were imbedded into a styrofoam head complete with pinna to augment sound localization. The program consisted of a graduated sequence of tapes which began with basic auditory skills and led to more sophisticated auditory judgements.

The beginning tapes focused upon sound localization instruction and practice. Later, practice in sound identification was given. Then the student listened to an "auditory" map of a training area in a form similar to that suggested by Blasch, Welsh, and Davidson (1973). In addition to the usual description afforded by such auditory maps, the tape incorporated actual sound characteristics of the specific area. Sound localization practice was also given. Another tape showed the difference between parallel and perpendicular traffic by taped examples. Other advanced tapes helped the student to trace the paths of moving vehicles. One tape was devoted to identifying objects by the sound that is made when a cane contacts them. Various tapes provided practice in determining when to cross different types of residential streets, and streets with traffic-light control. Tests were provided on these tapes followed by immediate feedback. Interspersed within the various tapes were additional auditory maps explaining street patterns of the training areas. When auditory landmarks were present in an area, they were recorded on the tape. Traffic patterns on the described streets were also recorded. The program was designed not to replace travel lessons with auditory tapes, but to supplement them by providing additional practice. They were intended to help a blind person to build confidence in the ability to interpret auditory information correctly. It is interesting to note that this program like others had been relatively unsuccessful in developing tapes that might help to train for object perception or echo location. The Syracuse program reported that the same localization problems existed that Norton reported earlier—sound coming from the front can be confused with sounds coming from the rear, with some people experiencing this problem more than others.

Echolocation

A study was conducted at the Eastern Blind Rehabilitation Center in West Haven, Connecticut to determine whether binaural taping could be useful in developing echolocation skills (De l'Aune, Scheel, Needham, & Kevorkian, 1974). Using microphones implanted in an artificial head, sound was recorded in closed-in areas and in open areas. Two groups of subjects who had previously done poorly in echo detection tasks were given two different types of binaural training programs. The first group listened to tapes which contained sound experiences in open areas and closed areas. The total exposure amounted to 300 seconds of training. The second group received tapes of all closed areas. The subjects were then given a posttest that consisted of identifying presence or absence of an opening in an actual corridor. The results indicated that the first group at posttest performed significantly better than the second group. From these results, De l'Aune concluded that binaural taping may be a valuable part of auditory training for orientation and mobility.

Conclusions

Based on experience with taping programs, several conclusions can be drawn. Auditory binaural taping has several strong points. Programmed exposure can be given to environmental clues to allow for sequencing. This facilitates efficient teaching by reducing the uncontrolled random exposure ordinarily found on the street. Listening to auditory tapes reduces anxiety while helping the individual to gain auditory skills. In addition, much practice is possible in a short period of time. Auditory maps can also be made with actual sounds of an environment to prepare individuals for travel in a new area. Finally, confidence in auditory functioning can be facilitated through feedback provided by a taping program. Weak points in binaural taping programs are that localization difficulty is a significant problem for some people; the system is ineffective if it becomes a substitute for actual environmental experience, instead of adding to it; and special equipment, and sophistication in its use, are necessary for binaural programs.

If an auditory binaural taping program is initiated, candidates should be screened to eliminate those who have difficulty with localization. They can be given alternative auditory training. Actual experiences should be integrated with taped training in the mobility program. The tapes should be of a graduated complexity, beginning with stationary tasks and proceeding to movement. Binaural taping has good potential for training that it has not been able to reach, and more research is needed.

While the most authentic sounding recordings are made with binaural tapes, some instructors have provided auditory training using monaural systems. Such systems are less complex, less expensive, and more easily available. The disadvantages are that the sounds are not as authentic and do not have directionality. Monaural tapes are best suited to teaching such skills as sound identification, sound discrimination, and figure ground relationships. With well-prepared tapes, students can become familiar with various sounds, can learn to distinguish between them, and pick out important sounds from unimportant background information. Tapes or records presenting useful auditory information can be prepared by the mobility specialists or can be purchased commercially.

HEARING AIDS

So far this chapter has dealt with auditory training for people with normal hearing. For many people who do not have normal hearing, a hearing aid may improve their ability to process auditory information. An appropriate hearing aid, instruction in its use, and auditory communication training are prerequisites for auditory training for independent travel. A mobility specialist should be knowledgeable about hearing aid amplification and its uses for the blind-hearing impaired traveler.

Hearing aids amplify the sound reaching the inner ear by adding energy to the existing signal using four major components and an earmold (Berger, 1974).

The microphone acts as a transducer to change air molecule vibration, generated by a sound producing force, into electrical energy. It can be omnidirectional or directional. The omni-directional microphone emphasizes all sounds equally regardless of incoming direction. The directional microphone emphasizes sounds emanating from the front and from positions 45° to the right and left of forward. It has two inlets that allow the back opening to delay noisy environment. At present, there seems to be no evidence of negative effect on sound localization using this type of microphone.

The battery, or the energy cell, supplies the electrical energy that is added to the original sound signal. Battery cells are of four general types: mercury, silver oxide, alkaline, and rechargeable nickel cadmium. They provide power of between 1.35 to 1.5 volts.

The amplifier uses the power of the battery to amplify the incoming signal through a series of transistors, resistors, capacitors, switches, and wires.

The receiver is basically a transducer that changes the electrical energy back into air molecule vibration. It may take the form of a bone conduction vibrator or, more commonly, an earphone receiver. The receiver connects with the ear canal through a plastic earmold individually fitted to the contours of the pinna and ear canal. Earmolds of various types can completely occlude the canal or leave an opening for ambient sound to enter. Special venting can also be introduced to allow reception of unamplified sound.

There are four electroacoustic characteristics which must be considered in hearing aid amplification (Pollack, 1975). First, and most important, is the maximum *power output* of the aid. The output is tailored for the individual user based upon level of tolerance for loud sounds. The maximum output is set to protect the user from discomfort that could result from intense amplification. The output is also limited so as not to reach a level that will overload the receiver and cause sound distortion.

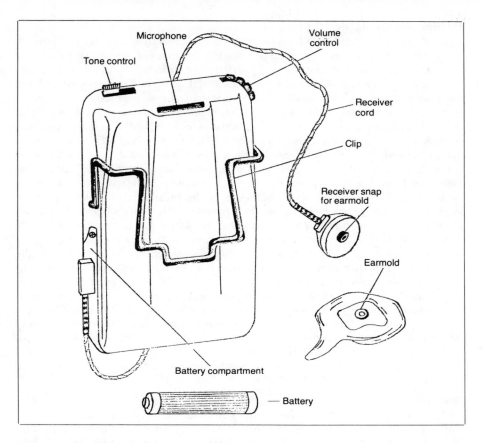

Figure 24-6. Body hearing aid components.

The second characteristic is *frequency response*. There is a specific curve on a person's audiogram to indicate threshold sensitivity at varying frequencies. A hearing aid must augment or enhance those frequencies to correspond to hearing loss. It has been shown that lower frequencies between 62 Hz and 500 Hz supply 60 percent of the intensity for speech, but supply only 5 percent of the information for intelligibility. Conversely, the frequencies between 500 Hz and 8000 Hz supply only 40 percent of the intensity for speech but supply over 95 percent of the information for intelligibility (Gerber, 1974). For this reason, the upper frequencies are more meaningful to the audiologist than the lower frequencies. They provide intelligibility information for communication, while the lower frequencies provide intensity that often transmits noise in the environment. Therefore, each individual is usually fitted with a hearing aid designed to augment specific hearing losses in the upper frequencies, more so than in the lower frequencies.

A third characteristic of a hearing aid is *gain*, the difference between the level of signal input and the level of output. Gain is also prescribed individually to correspond to severity of hearing loss.

Distortion, the fourth characteristic, is an unplanned difference in the intensity of the frequency components between the original input signal and the amplified output. Some research indicates that distortion has a negative effect on interpretation and must be kept at a minimum.

173

Hearing Aid Candidates

Traditionally, a candidate for a hearing aid has a threshold average of 25 dB HL or poorer in the better ear, or when hearing in the worst ear is no lower than 85 dB HL. In the past, audiologists have classified users into the following categories: those with thresholds of between 0 and 25 dB HL were not generally considered candidates, between 25 to 40 dB HL were considered part time users, between 45 to 80 dB HL were considered full time users who obtained the most benefit from the aid, and someone with a hearing threshold of 85 dB HL or greater was considered a full time user who would benefit only partially. Today, audiologists are much more functionally oriented to their selection of candidates for hearing aid use. More frequently, audiologists are recommending aids based upon the communication problem rather than upon the degree of hearing loss. They are basing their judgments on the total needs of the individual, not just upon the degree and slope of the hearing loss. Someone with thresholds better than 25 dB HL may be recommended for a hearing aid if the audiologist and candidate believe it will be beneficial. At the other end of the spectrum, an audiologist generally recommends a hearing aid for someone with a loss greater than 85 dB HL, especially a child. Amplification may even be prescribed as an aid in gathering information to supplement speech reading (lip reading) even if improvement in speech discrimination cannot be documented. Of all hearing aid users, only 10 percent have a conductive hearing loss which they are aiding with amplification, because conductive hearing losses for the most part can be remediated by surgery. Ninety percent of all hearing aid users suffer from sensori-neural pathology. At present, cochlear surgery is not an alternative solution.

There are four basic types of hearing aids in use today, some of which can be modified for specific problem fittings.

Body Aid

The microphone and amplifier of the body aid are worn clipped to the user's clothing or worn on the torso, and the receiver is snapped to the ear mold (Fig. 24-6). They are large and, because of their size, have been able to deliver the best frequency response along with highest gain and output. They also have more control modifications and thus more flexibility. However, the body aid reduces necessary auditory information because of its location. The body acts as a baffle, reflecting sound into the microphone. The reflected sound is augmented 2 to 6 dB in the low frequencies and reduced in the mid-frequencies by 5 to 15 dB (Erber, 1973). This is the opposite of what is needed for increased intelligibility of speech. In addition, clothing noise is often picked up by the microphone. Furthermore, the body aid is used as a monaural aid unless two aids are used and placed far apart on the body. However, this does not result in true binaural amplification because the microphones are not at ear level. Today, such aids are being used less often, but are still recommended for very young children with severe hearing losses where highest gain and output are needed. Traditionally, someone having a loss of between 85 to 100 dB with an equal loss across the frequencies would be considered a candidate for such an aid.

Behind-the-Ear Aid (BTE)

The second type is the post aural or behind-the-ear aid (BTE), contoured to fit behind the ear (Fig. 25a-6). All components are either contained within the unit behind the ear or they can be separate. It is becoming common to use an external receiver when extreme output is needed (Fig. 25b-6). The BTE does away with the problems of body baffle and clothing noise because of the ear level microphone location, and it is much less conspicuous. There are many advantages in positioning the microphone at ear level. First of all, defraction of the sound around the head increases

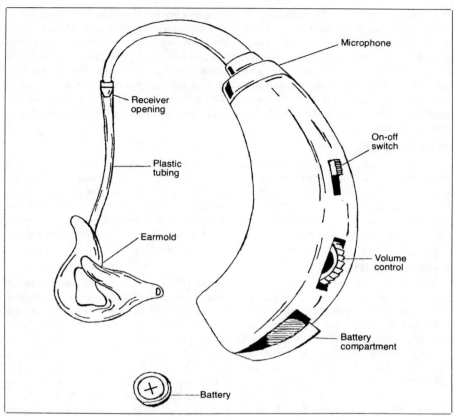

Figure 25a-6. Components of a behind-the-ear aid with internal receiver.

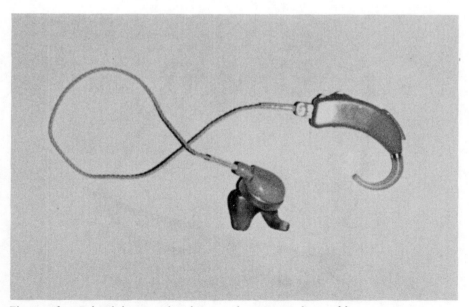

Figure 25b-6. Behind-the-ear aid with external receiver and earmold.

amplification by 2 to 5 dB, therefore requiring less power from the aid. Also, when two aids are used together for symmetrical losses, true binaural amplification can be attained, permitting accurate localization in many instances. Recent advances in technology have put the frequency response of this aid on a par with the body aid and have greatly improved its gain and output characteristics. Previously this aid was recommended for individuals who had hearing no better than 25 dB HL and no worse than 70 dB HL. Now with the technological advances, there are no limitations. A person with thresholds of between 15 to 110 dB HL can be fitted with variations of such an aid.

Eyeglass Aid (EG)

The third type, the eyeglass aid (EG), is similar in design to the BTE. The components of the EG are enclosed within the temple of the glasses, and can be installed in any pair of glasses with a 5-or 7-barrel bridge. All the advantages of the BTE aid are also valid for the EG. They can also be more comfortable for the visually impaired individual who must wear glasses and who may be uncomfortable wearing in addition a BTE. The owner of an EG should have an extra pair of optical glasses for the times when the aid is in repair (Fig. 26-6).

In-the-Ear Aid (ITE)

The fourth type is the in-the-ear hearing aid (ITE), a fairly recent advancement that allows the aid to be worn inconspicuously entirely within the ear canal and pinna. At first, there was controversy about the aid because size limitations restricted its gain and frequency response, but some of this has now been overcome. It has many advantages. The microphone is housed within the concha of the pinna in a natural position (Griffing and Preves, 1976). In this position, the aid can take advantage of the pinna effect. The pinna cups the sound giving a rise of from 10 to 15 dB in intensity at middle and high frequencies. The aid also takes advantage of the peak resonance of the ear canal, supplying up to 15 dB of gain at 3000 Hz. With both of these advantages, the aid requires less output and gain. Head defraction also helps to amplify the sounds. Since one aid can be worn

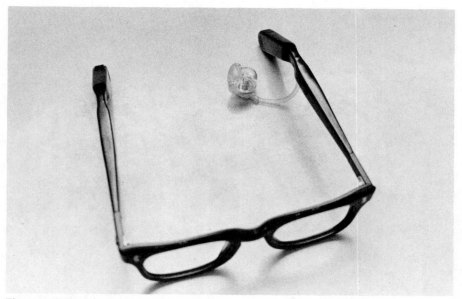

Figure 26-6. Eyeglass aid.

on each ear, true binaural amplification is also possible, and with it better directionality and localization. Originally, because of gain restrictions, the aid was recommended for mild to moderate losses, but recent technological advances have made it possible to be used for losses from mild to severe (Fig. 27-6).

Modification CROS

One of the modifications available for problem fittings is the contra-lateral routing of signal (CROS), a recent development to provide information and directionality for someone who has one normal or near normal ear and one totally deaf ear. To accomplish this, a microphone is mounted behind the ear that is totally deaf. The receiver and amplifier are located on the other side of the head. The microphone picks up sounds on the deaf side and transfers them around the head to the good ear where they are transformed into sound energy giving an awareness of sound from the deaf side (Fig. 28-6). Sounds coming from the side near the good ear are received without amplification and are able to enter the ear through an open earmold. That same earmold, however, is responsible for delivering the amplified sound from the opposite side to the good ear. The amplified sound from the deaf side can easily be distinguished from the normal sound because of the different frequency characteristics of the amplified sound. In other words, the sound that is amplified will have a tinny characteristic, much different from the normal sound. Once the separation is identified, a degree of sound localization is possible. The aid can be fitted on a person who has total hearing loss in one ear and one normal ear or with a loss of up to 45 dB HL. It is difficult to fit, however, if the better ear has thresholds of better than 20 dB HL. CROS can be fitted, as a behind-the-ear aid, an eyeglass aid, or an in-the-ear aid. Usually wiring around the head is necessary, but can be camouflaged when connected through eyeglasses. An eyeglass wireless CROS is a new development that requires no wiring around the head because it has a radio transmitter and receiver to send and receive the message. Many types and adaptations of CROS are now on the market and may be beneficial in special applications.

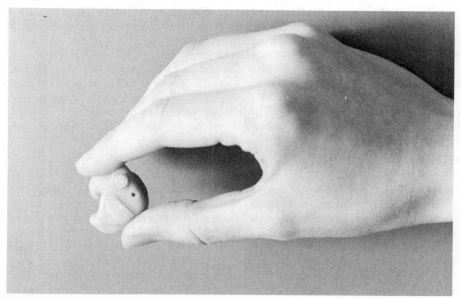

Figure 27-6. In-the-ear aid.

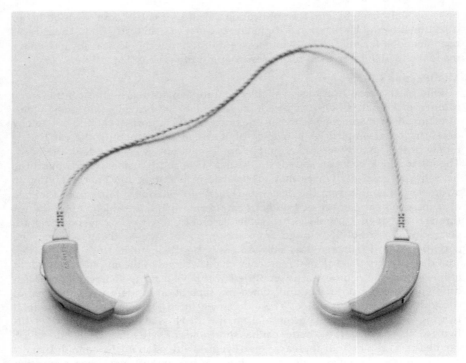

Figure 28-6. CROS aid.

BiCROS

A second modification available for complex fitting problems is the CROS with bilateral routing of signal (Bi-CROS). This aid is used in cases where the better ear has a 50-dB HL loss or greater and needs amplification while the opposite ear is totally deaf or unaidable. A microphone is mounted on the side of the deaf ear and a complete aid (microphone, amplifier, and receiver) is mounted on the side of the hearing ear. The signals from the two microphones are mixed together in the one amplifier, giving the wearer reception of sound on both sides of the head. In this situation, directionality both aided and unaided is totally absent because there is no way of separating sounds as to their origin at one side of the head or the other. The aid is helpful, however, for those who want to receive information generated from either side of the head, even though the aided condition cannot restore directionality.

Potential

Hearing aids have a great potential as a rehabilitation tool for the hearing-impaired blind traveler. At present, however, they fall short of providing the assistance of which they are capable. Most aids are built to function within a limited frequency range of 400 to 4000 Hz, and fitting trends today support major amplification between 1000 to 4000 Hz. The frequencies within this range provide 85 percent of the intelligibility for speech, and the audiologist or hearing aid dealer, in fitting an aid, is most concerned with solving speech reception and discrimination problems and not with providing an instrument of wider frequency response that would facilitate reception even within this limited frequency range. The lower frequencies are generally not amplified as much as the upper frequencies because they are the major carriers of noise, and enhancing them generally makes communication more difficult.

Traffic Sounds

A spectral analysis of traffic sounds (Wiener & Goldstein, 1977) showed that the greatest absolute intensity of traffic sounds was found within the lower frequencies. After considering the threshold sensitivity of the human ear, it became evident that the greatest amount of actual traffic-sound intensity available to the individual was between 500 and 2000 Hz. The audiologist, in emphasizing the upper frequencies, is disregarding some useful information for interpretation of traffic sounds. This may be especially true for someone who has a "typical" sensori-neural loss with only a small amount of loss in the lower frequencies but a much greater loss in the mid and upper frequencies. This person is unable to hear traffic sounds easily in the mid to upper frequencies and therefore has to rely more on the lower frequencies. The lower frequencies play an important role in enabling him to benefit from the use of traffic sounds to improve mobility. To improve the ability to process traffic information, the hearing aid should allow for the amplification of low-frequency sounds by a user-operated tone control capable of augmenting the lower-frequency range and the upper frequencies as the situation calls for it. With such an aid, the user could switch to an augmentation of high frequencies for communication purposes, or an augmentation of low and high frequencies for travel purposes. This would be helpful not only in use of traffic sounds but also other low-frequency ambient sounds present in the environment.

Frequency Discrimination

In addition to de-emphasizing the low frequencies, most modern day hearing aids limit the reception of high frequencies above 4000 Hz. Successful use of audition for independent travel, however, requires use of frequencies well beyond 4000 Hz; especially true in situations where spectral components of sound are needed for localization, for judgment of distance, and for use of echo information. Research has demonstrated that frequencies of 10,000 Hz and above are needed to make the best use of reflected sound. Hearing aids which amplify only to 4000 Hz will not assist the blind traveler in this instance. At present, even the hearing aids with extended range receivers can not reach much beyond 7000 Hz in their upper frequency of amplification. Because high-frequency sounds can not readily bend around the head (or around the pinna), the traveler learns to identify the direction of the sound, in part, by recognizing the direction from which the higher freqeuncy sounds are originating. The hearing aid wearer may not be able to detect higher frequencies if the ear is blocked with an earmold, and if the aid is not capable of processing higher frequencies.

Sound localization has been shown to be more accurate in both the lower and higher frequencies than in the middle frequencies that are emphasized most in hearing aids. This ability to localize sound is critical for acquisition of good mobility skills. If a hearing impaired individual is capable of frequency discrimination, it is important to have higher frequency capabilities in their hearing aids.

According to De l'Aune (1976), the ability to judge the distance of a sound-emitting object may be impaired by some hearing aids. He explains that sounds in the environment that are closer to the individual have higher frequency spectral components than sounds farther away. The more distant sounds lose high frequencies as they travel through the air. Hearing aids which do not have a sufficient frequency response at the upper end may not allow the individual to receive the high frequency necessary for distance and judgment. De l'Aune further states that hearing aids used by the severely hearing impaired, which are designed to limit greatly the intensity of their output in response to loud sounds, may also make distance judgment difficult. The use of an automatic volume control (AVC) in a hearing aid can prohibit sounds from becoming loud enough to cause discomfort, but may reduce the intensity differences between the near and far sounds. Ordinarily this form of output limitation does not suppress loud sounds enough to cause problems in judging distance. However, in the case of those needing large amounts of amplification and suffering from recruitment (an abnormal sensitivity to small increases in loudness), hearing aids may be specifically designed to limit output greatly as sounds begin to get louder. Therefore, sounds of loud objects close by are kept softer and are judged to be farther away than they really are. In the case of a fast moving automobile, this can be a dangerous situation. De l'Aune recommends hearing aids for these users with an AVC switch that would permit output limitation circuitry to be turned off during travel times. However, user-operated output controls are not commonly manufactured at present.

Unilateral vs. Bilateral Loss

Theoretically, hearing aids should be able to help the hearing impaired person to improve sound localization skills. When there is unilateral hearing loss, localization is distorted because the better sensitivity of one ear forces the perception of sound as coming from the direction closer to that ear. As reported earlier (Bergman, 1957), when the level of the sound stimulus reaches the threshold of the poorer ear, ability to determine the direction of the sound is greatly improved. The closer the sensitivity of the two ears, the better the localization will be. Therefore, a hearing aid that provides more intensity to stimulate the poorer ear should help to improve localization.

Binaural hearing aids for the visually impaired who have bilateral hearing loss should be used whenever appropriate to achieve more equal hearing sensitivity. In reality, it has been reported that amplification does help to determine if a sound is coming from the right side of the environment, the left side or somewhere in between, but often results in front-rear reversals. This is not a severe problem for sighted people because vision is used to verify sound origin. The blind traveler who experiences these reversals has no other sensory information to help localize the sound.

At present, there seems to be no proven reason for the reversal phenomenon or an explanation as to why some individuals are affected more than others. A theory by Keane (1965) attempts to explain the reversals. In most head-level hearing aids, the microphone is behind or above the pinna of the ear and is not shadowed from the rear by that structure. The hypothesis is that the location of the microphone outside of the ear canal is responsible for the reversals. Research is needed to determine whether placing the microphone in the canal would solve the problem. In-the-ear hearing aids with a concha microphone might provide the answer, but they occlude the ear entirely and would prevent any unamplified sound from entering.

Because of sound localizing difficulties with hearing aids, De l'Aune (1976) suggested those visually impaired individuals with mild hearing losses who experience this might do better to remove their hearing aids for travel purposes. He cautions, however, that such a decision be made only in collaboration with an audiologist. Those with more severe losses will have to depend upon hearing aids.

When hearing aids are worn for localization, every attempt should be made to provide localization training coupled with immediate feedback to improve accuracy. Often, when inaccuracies are found in pinpointing position of right from left, the difficulty can be overcome by adjusting the gain control of the hearing aid. A simple "fusion test" can help a person to adjust the gain control or controls to equalize the sensitivity of both ears more closely and thus improve localization (Keane, 1965). The mobility specialist should stand directly in front of the trainee and instruct him to adjust the gain control on the aid or aids until the specialist's voice sounds as though it is coming from directly ahead. Noting the control position at this point will facilitate return to it when necessary.

A person with one near-normal ear and one totally-deaf ear may have trouble localizing sound accurately. With a CROS aid, localization can be greatly improved. Successful use of the aid for independent travel has been documented (Rintelmann, 1970), but unfortunately, some audiologists are unaware of the auditory needs of blind people. If they are concerned only with helping someone to understand speech, they may not consider use of the CROS worth the effort. Interpreting information with it takes practice. The necessity for a blind person to be able to localize traffic and other environmental sounds makes the extra time needed to learn to interpret the CROS well worthwhile.

MOBILITY SPECIALIST'S ROLE IN AUDITORY REHABILITATION

In order to prepare students for independent travel, the mobility specialist must have a realistic understanding of the auditory functioning of each one. Along with a battery of social, medical, and ophthalmological information available on each student, there should be appropriate audiometric evaluation. The specialist should be skilled in the interpretation of audiograms to evaluate general auditory function as a starting point in communication with the student. Audiograms are useful, but must be combined with observed auditory functioning in natural environments because people with very similar audiograms can function very differently. It is a known fact that some learn to use hearing more effectively than others, therefore actual observation is necessary. Speech discrimination scores can be a useful supplementary tool for functional measure of speech comprehension. Pathology and type of hearing loss may give a mobility specialist some expectation of functional problems. For example, it should be remembered that conductive losses are generally free from distortion. Sensori-neural losses, on the other hand, are prone to distortion even with hearing aids. The mobility specialist should be constantly alert to the possibility of hearing problems. If a hearing loss is suspected, the mobility specialist should refer the client to an audiologist or otolaryngologist. When such referral leads to the discovery of a hearing loss, the mobility specialist is in a position to work with the audiologist to describe functional difficulties and acquaint the audiologist with the special auditory needs of blind people. When hearing aids are prescribed, the mobility specialist should work closely with the audiologist and follow up the fitting with an appraisal of the individual's functioning with the aid, both in communication and orientation. Together the mobility specialist and the audiologist can help the visually and aurally impaired person to achieve a higher level of rehabilitation.

The mobility specialist is responsible for development of a training program to teach the necessary auditory skills for independent travel. As indicated earlier, this may be accomplished before formal travel techniques training, along with it, or integrated into it. The training may be provided in natural settings or in a combination of natural settings and taping. The mobility specialist is often in a position to consult with parents and teachers on auditory training activities. Explaining to parents the necessity for stimulating the child with auditory toys and games to initiate exploration and auditory development is most helpful. Providing curricular suggestions to the classroom teacher is also beneficial. All in all, the mobility specialist should function as a member of the auditory rehabilitation team working alongside the otolaryngologist, the audiologist, and the parent or family.

Bibliography

American Automobile Association. *How to drive*. Washington, D.C.: AAA, 1957, 58.

American Automobile Association. *Sportsmanlike driving*. New York: McGraw-Hill, 1965, 94.

Angell, J. R. & Fite, W. Monaural localization of sound. *Psychology Review*, 1901, **8**, 225-245.

Ammons, C. H., Worchel, P., & Dallenbach, K. Facial vision: The perception of obstacles out of doors by blindfolded and blindfolded deafened subjects. *American Journal of Psychology*, 1953, **40**, 519-553.

Apps, D. C., Recent developments in traffic noise control. *Noise Control*, September, 1957.

Bauer, R. W., Matuzsa, J. L., Blackmer, R. F., & Glucksberg, S. Noise localization after unilateral attenuation. *The Journal of the Acoustical Society of America*, 1966, **40**, 441-444.

Bekesy, G. von. Zur Theorie des Horens. Die Schwingungsform der Basilarmembran. *Physik. Zeitschrift*, XXIX, 1928, 793-810.

Berger, K. W. *The hearing aid: Its operation and development*. Detroit: National Hearing Aid Society, 1974, Chapters 2-5.

Bergman, M. Binaural hearing. *Archives of Otolaryngology*, 1957, **66**, 572-578.

Bergman, M., Rusalem, H., Malles, I., Schiller, V., Cohan, H., & McKay, E. Auditory rehabilitation for hearing-impaired blind persons. *ASHA Monographs*, March, 1965. No. 12.

Blasch, B., Welsh, R., & Davidson, T. Auditory maps: An orientation aid for visually handicapped persons. *New Outlook for the Blind*, April, 1973, 145-158.

Briskey, R. J. Binaural hearing aids and new innovations. In J. Katz (Ed.), *Handbook of clinical audiology*. Baltimore, Maryland: Williams & Wilkins Co., 1972, 572-578, 590-601.

Bugliarello, G., Alexandre, A., Barnes, J., & Wakstein, C. *The impact of noise pollution — A socio-technological introduction*. New York: Pergamon Press Inc., 1976, 81-92.

Bürklen, K. *Blinden-psychologie*. Leipzig, Germany: Johann Ambrosius Barth, 1924, BF 233.

Calearo, C., & Antonelli, A. R. Audiometric findings in brain stem lesions. *Acta Oto-Laryngologica*, 1968, **66**, 305-318.

Carhart, R. The usefulness of the binaural hearing aid. *Journal of Speech and Hearing Disorders*, 1958, **23**, 42-51.

Chappell, R. G., Kavanagh, J. F., & Zerlin, S. Monaural versus binaural discrimination for normal listeners. *Journal of Speech and Hearing Research*, 1963, **6**, 263-269.

Cherry, C., & Bowles, J. A. Contribution to a study of the "Cocktail Party Problem." *The Journal of the Acoustical Society of America*, 1960, **32**, 884.

Conkey, H. The effect of contralateral routing of sound on auditory localization and mobility of a blind person. *Exceptional Children*, 1968, **34**, 705-706.

Corso, J. F. Aging and auditory thresholds in men and women. *Archives of Environmental Health*, 1963, **6**, 330-356.

Cotzin, M., & Dallenbach, K. Facial vision: The role of pitch and loudness in the perception of obstacles by the blind. *American Journal of Psychology*, 1950, **63**, 485-515.

Curtis, J., & Wener, D. M. The auditory abilities of the blind as compared with the sighted. *Journal of Auditory Research*, 1969, **9**, 57-59.

Daugherty, K. M. Listening skills: A review of the literature. *The New Outlook for the Blind*, 1974, **68**, 363-369, 415-421, 460-469.

Davis, H., & Silverman, S. R. *Hearing and deafness*. Holt, Rinehart, & Winston, Inc., 1970, 83-176.

Deatherage, B., & Evans, T. Binaural masking: Backward, forward, and simultaneous effects. *The Journal of the Acoustical Society of America*, 1969, **46**, 362-371.

Decroix, G., & Dehaussy, J. Binaural hearing and intelligibility. *The Journal of Auditory Research*, 1964, **4**, 115-134.

De l'Aune, W., Scheel, P., Needham, W., & Kevorkian, G. Evaluation of a methodology for training indoor acoustic environmental analysis in blinded veterans. Proceedings of the Conference on Engineering Devices in Rehabilitation, Tufts University: New England School of Medicine, 1974.

De l'Aune, W., Lewis, C., Dolan, M., Grimmelsman, T., & Needham, W. Two sensory aids having profound effects on the blind. *IEE International Conference on Acoustics*, April, 1976.

Di Dea, A. Detection of obstacles by blindfolded persons. *Biological Review*, C.C.N.Y., 1947, **9**, 9-15.

Diderot, D. Letter on the Blind in *Early Philosophical Works* (trans. M. Jourdian). Chicago and London: The Open Court Publishing Company, 1916, 68-141.

Dirks, D. D., & Wilson, R. A. Binaural hearing of speech for aided and unaided conditions. *Journal of Speech and Hearing Research*, 1969, **12**, 650-664.

Djupesland, D., & Zwislocki, J. Sound pressure distribution in the outer ear. *Acta Oto-Laryngologica*, 1973, **75**, 350-352.

182

Dolanski, V. Do the Blind Sense Obstacles? *And There Was Light,* 1931, **1,** 8-12.

Dressler, F. B. On the pressure sense of the drum of the ear and facial vision. *American Journal of Psychology,* 1893, **5,** 344-350.

Dupress, J. K., & Wright, H. N. Identifying and teaching auditory cues for traveling by the blind. *AFB Research Bulletin,* 1962, **1,** 3-9.

Duttman, D., & von Bergeryk, K. On the mechanism of binaural fusion. *The Journal of the Acoustical Society of America,* 1969, **46,** 362-371.

Erber, N. Body baffle and rear ear effects in the selection of hearing aids for deaf children. *Journal of Speech and Hearing Research,* **38,** 1973, 224-231.

Fisher, G. H. Spatial localization by the blind. *AFB Research Bulletin,* 1968, **15,** 147-158.

Freedman, S. J. *The neuropsychological of spatially oriented behavior.* Homewook, Illinois: Dorsey Press, 1968.

Gerber, S. *Introductory learning science.* Philadelphia: W. B. Saunders Co., 1974.

Gibson, J. *The senses considered as perceptual systems.* Boston: Houghton Mifflin Co., 1966.

Goodman, A. Reference zero level for pure tone audiometry. ASHA, **7,** 1965, 262-263.

Griffin, D. R. *Listening in the dark.* New Haven, Connecticut: Yale University Press, 1958.

Griffin, D. R. *Echoes of bats and men.* Garden City, New York: Doubleday and Co., 1959.

Griffing, T., & Preves, D. In-the-ear: Part 1. *Hearing Instruments,* 1976, **27,** 22-24.

Hahn, W. L. Some habits and sensory adaptations of cave-inhabiting bats. *Biology Bulletin.* 1908, **15,** 135-193.

Hare, B., Hammill, D., & Crandell, J. M. Auditory discrimination ability of visually limited children. *The New Outlook for the Blind,* 1970, **64,** 287-292.

Harris, J., Dupress, J., Wright, H., Curtis, J., Winer, D., Gropper, F. K., & Kelsey, P. *Identification and teaching of auditory cues for traveling in the blind.* Groton, Connecticut: C. W. Shilling Auditory Research Center, 1963.

Harris, J. D. *Psychoacoustics.* Indianapolis: The Bobbs-Merrill Company, Inc., 1974, 66-79.

Hartridge, H. The avoidance of objects by bats in their flight. *Journal Physiology* 1920, **54,** 54-57.

Hauptvogel, R. Das Ferngefuhl der Blinden. *d. Blindenfreund,* 1906, **26,** 23-25.

Heller, T. *Studien zur blinden Psychologie.* Leipzig: Wilhelm Englemann, 1904.

Hirsh, I. J. Binaural hearing aids: A review of some experiments. *Journal of Speech and Hearing Disorders,* 1950(a), **15,** 114-123.

Hirsh, I. J. The relation between localization and intelligibility. *The Journal of the Acoustical Society of America.* 1950(b), **22,** 196-199.

Hopkinson, N. T. in Katz, J. (Ed.) *Handbook of clinical audiology.* Baltimore: Williams and Wilkins Co., 1972, 143-180.

Howard, L. P., & Templeton, W. B. *Human spatial orientation.* New York: John Wiley and Sons, 1966, 139-174.

Huss, M. F., & McShane, W. R. Noise in transit systems. *Traffic Quarterly,* April 1973.

James, W. *Principles of psychology,* Vol. 2. New York: Henry Holt and Co., 1890.

Javal, E. *On becoming blind.* New York and London: The Macmillan Co., 1905.

Jerger, J. (Ed.) *Handbook of clinical impedance audiometry.* New York: American Electronedics Corporation, 1975.

Jerger, J., Carhart, R., Dirk, D. Binaural hearing aids and speech intelligibility. *Journal of Speech and Hearing,* RES, 4, 1961, 137-148.

Juurmaa, J. An analysis of the components of orientation mobility and mental manipulation of spatial relationships. *Report Institute Occupational Health,* August, 1965, No. 28.

Juurmaa, J. The effects of training on the perception of obstacles without vision. *The New Outlook for the Blind,* 1970, Part I, **64,** 65-72, Part II, **64,** 104-118.

Kabelek, A. K., & Pickett, J. M. Monaural speech perception through hearing aids under noise and reverberation with normal and hearing-impaired listeners. *Journal of Speech and Hearing Research,* 1974, **17,** 724-739.

Kasten, R. N., Lotterman, S. H., & Hinchman, M. J. Head shadow and head baffle effects in ear level aids. *Acoustica,* 1967, **19,** 154-160.

Keane, G. *Auditory rehabilitation for hearing-impaired blind persons.* ASHA Monograph #12, 1965, 31-51.

Kellog, W. N. *Porpoises and sonar.* Chicago: University of Chicago Press, 1961.

Kellog, W. N. Sonar systems of the blind. *Science,* 1962, **137** (3528), 399-404.

Knie, J. *Versuch uber den Unterricht der Blinden,* Breslau, 1821, quoted in K. Burklen, *Blindenpsychologie.* Leipzig: Verlag Von Johann Ambrosius Barth, 1924, 325.

Koenig, W. Subjective effects in binaural hearing. *The Journal of the Acoustical Society of America,* 1950, **22,** 61-62.

Kohler, I. Orientation by oral clues. *AFB Research Bulletin,* 1964, **4.**

Ladefoged, P. *Elements of acoustic phonetics.* Chicago: University of Chicago Press, 1962, 34-39.

Lax, B. The effects of environmental conditions on blind and sighted children as measured by structured sound situations. *Dissertation Abstracts International*, 1971, **31**, (11A), 5851.

Levy, W. H. *Blindness and the blind*. London: Chapman and Hall, 1872.

Liddle, D. The effect of signal strength on reaction times to auditory signals in noise. *AFB Research Bulletin*, 1969, **19**, 129-190.

Ling, D. Implications of hearing aid amplification below 300 CPS. *Volta Review*, **66**(12), 723-729.

Martin, F. *Introduction to audiology*. New Jersey: Prentice-Hall, 1975.

Maxim, H. The sixth sense of the bat. *Scientific American*, Suppl., Sept. 7, 1912, 148-150.

McCarty, B., & Worchel, P. Rate of motion and object perception in the blind, *The New Outlook for the Blind*, 1954, **48**, 316-322.

Mills, A. W. *The Journal of the Acoustical Society of America*, 1958, **30**, 237-246.

Mills A. W. Lateralization of high-frequency tones. *The Journal of the Acoustical Society of America*, 1960, **32**, 132-134.

Mills, A. W. Auditory perception of spatial relations. *Proceedings of the International Congress on Technology and Blindness*. New York: American Foundation for the Blind, 1963, **2**, 111-139.

Moncur, J. P., & Dirks, D. Binaural and monaural speech intelligibility in reverberation. *Journal of Speech and Hearing Research*, 1967, **10**, 186-195.

Mouchet, E. Un Nuevo Capitaula de Psicofisiologia; el Tacto a Distanci o Sentibo de les Obstaclos en los Ciegos. *An. Inst. Piscol., Univ. Buenos Aires*, 1938, **2**, 419-441.

Myers, S. O., & Jones, C.G.E.F. Obstacle experiments: Second report. *Teacher Blind*, 1958, **46**, 47-62.

Newby, A. H. *Audiology*. New York: Appleton-Century-Crofts, 1964.

Noble, W. G. Auditory localization and its impairment. *Maico Audiological Library Series*, 1975, **14**, (Report One).

Northern, J., & Downs, M. P. *Hearing in children*. Baltimore, Maryland: Williams & Wilkins Co., 1974.

Norton, F. T. Training normal hearing to greater usefulness: A progress report. *The New Outlook for the Blind*, 1960, **54**, 199-205.

Organization for Economic Co-operation and Development (OECD). *Motor vehicle noise*. Paris: November, 1971.

Perrott, D. R., & Elfner, L. F. Monaural localization. *The Journal of Auditory Research*, 1968, **8**, 185-193.

Perrott, D. Limits of the detection of binaural beats. *The Journal of the Acoustical Society of America*, 1969, **46**, 1477-1488.

Perrott, D., Elfner, L. F., & Homick, J. L. Auditory spatial organization. *Perception and Psychophysics*, 1969, **5**, 189-192.

Pollack, I., & Mitchell, R. Effects of head movement on the localization of sounds in the equatorial plane. *Perception and Psychophysics*, 1967, **2**, (12, Part A), 591-596.

Pollack, M. C. Special applications of amplification. In M. C. Pollack (Ed.), *Amplification for the hearing impaired*. N.Y.: Grune & Stratton, 1975, 243-256.

Rice, C. E., & Feinstein, S. H. Echo detection ability of the blind: Size and distance factors. *Journal of Experimental Psychology*, 1965(a), **70**, 246-251.

Rice, C. E., & Feinstein, S. H. The influence of target parameters on human echo-detection tasks. *Proceedings of the American Psychological Association*, 1965(b).

Rice, C. E., & Feinstein, S. H. Sonar systems of the blind: Size discrimination. *Science*, 1965(c), **148**, 1107-1108.

Rice, C. E. Human echo perception. *Science*, 1967(a), **155**, 656-664.

Rice, C. E. Quantitative measures of unaided echo detection in the blind: Auditory echo localization. In R. Dufton (Ed.), *Proceedings of the International Conference on Sensory Devices for the Blind*, London: St. Dunstan's, 1967(b), 89-102.

Riley, L. H., Luterman, D. M., & Cohen, M. The relationship between hearing ability and mobility in a blinded adult population. *The New Outlook for the Blind*, 1964, **58**, 139-141.

Rintelmann, W., Harford, E., & Burchfield, S. CROS for blind persons with unilateral hearing loss. *Archives of Otolaryngology*, 1970, **91**, 284-288.

Road Research Laboratory (RRL). *A review of traffic noise*. Report LR 347 (U.K.), 1970.

Romains, J. *Eyeless sight*, (trans. by G. K. Ogden). New York and London: G. P. Putnam and Sons, 1924.

Rosenweig, M. R. Auditory localization. *Scientific American*, 1961, **205**, 132-142.

Rutherford, W. A new theory of hearing. *Journal of Anatomy and Physiology*, 1886, XXI, 166-168.

Sanders, D. *Aural rehabilitation*. New Jersey: Prentice-Hall, 1971.

Sayers, B. M., & Cherry, E. C. Mechanism of binaural fusion in the hearing of speech. *The Journal of the Acoustical Society of America*, 1957, **29**, 973-987.

Sivian, L. J., & White, S. D. Minimal audible sound fields. *The Journal of Acoustical Society of America*, 1933, **4,** 288-321.

Stevens, S. S., & New man, E. B. The localization of actual sources of sound. *American Journal of Psychology*, 1936, **48,** 297-306.

Supa, M., Cotzin, M., & Dallenbach, K. M. "Facial vision": The perception of obstacles by the blind. *American Journal of Psychology*, 1944, **57,** 133-183.

Tillman, T. W., Kasten, R. N., & Horner, J. S. Effect of head shadow on reception of speech. Paper for the 1963 Convention of ASHA, Abstract in *ASHA*, 1963, **5,** 778-779.

Tobias, J. V. Binaural recordings for training the newly blind. *Perceptual and Motor Skills*, 1965, **20,** 385-391.

Truschel, L. Der sechste Sinn der Blinden, *Z.f. Exp. Padagogik*, 1906, **3,** 109-142; 1907, **4,** 129-155; 1907, **5,** 66-77.

Twersky, V. An obstacle detecting device for the blind. *Biological Review*, C.C.N.Y., 1947, **9,** 16-21.

Twersky, V. Obstacle detector vs. guidance device. *Biological Review*, C.C.N.Y., 1949, **2,** 14-19.

Twersky, V. On the physical basis of the perception of obstacles by the blind. *American Journal of Psychology*, 1951, **64,** 409-416.

United States Environmental Protection Agency. Report to the President and Congress on noise. Washington, D.C.: December, 1971.

United States Environmental Protection Agency. Proposed emission standards for interstate rail carrier noise. The Bureau of National Affairs, Washington, D.C.: July, 1974.

Villey, P. *The world of the blind: A psychological study.* London: Duckworth, 1930, 101-131.

Welch, J. A psychoacoustic study of factors affecting human echo location. *AFB Research Bulletin*, 1964, **3,** 1-15.

Wever, E. G. *Theory of hearing.* New York: John Wiley and Sons Inc., 1949.

Whetnall, E. Binaural hearing. *Journal of Laryngology and Otology*, 1964, **78,** 1079-1089.

Wiener, F. M. On the diffraction of a progressive sound wave by the human head. *The Journal of the Acoustical Society of America*, 1947, **19,** 143-146.

Wiener, F. M. Experimental study of the airborne noise generated by passenger automobile tires. *Noise Control*, July/August 1960, 13-16.

Wiener, W., & Goldstein, B. A spectral analysis of traffic sounds in residential, small business, and downtown areas, 1977, in progress.

Wiener, W., & McLaughlin, D. Description of Auditory Training Program, unpublished, 1973.

Worchel, P., & Ammons, C. The course of learning in the perception of obstacles. *American Journal of Psychology*, 1953.

Worchel, P., & Dallenbach, K. Facial vision: Perception of obstacles by the deaf-blind. *American Journal of Psychology*, 1947, **60,** 502-553.

Worchel, P., & Mauney, J. The effect of practice on the perception of obstacles by the blind. *Journal of Experimental Psychology*, 1950, **41,** 170-176.

Wright, H. N., & Carhart, R. The efficiency of binaural listening among the hearing-impaired. *Archives of Otolaryngology*, 1960, **72,** 789-797.

Yates, J. L., Johnson, R. M., & Starz, W. J. Loudness perception of the blind. *Audiology*, 1972, **2,** 368-376.

Zelnick, E. The importance of inter-aural phase differences in binaural hearing aid fittings. *Paper presented at Oticongress 4, Copenhagen*, 1974, 66-74.

Zelmin W. R. *Speech and hearing science*, New Jersey: Prentice-Hall, 1968.

Zeune, A. *Belisar: Uber den Unterricht der Blinden*, Berlin, 1808, quoted in K. Burklen, *Blindenpsychologie.* Leipzig: Verlag Von Johann Ambrosius Barth, 1924, 329.

Low Vision

Marianne M. Apple, Loyal E. Apple, and Donald Blasch

At one time, severely visually impaired but not totally blind persons were either educated, trained, or rehabilitated as though they had no useful vision or were not considered in need of any special services at all. In residential schools for the blind, children with useful vision were usually taught to read braille and in general to learn through senses other than vision. Most low vision adults were taught mobility techniques developed for the totally blind with few adaptations that took into account their ability to see.

There were several reasons for this approach:

1. Until the early 1950s, use of very limited vision was thought to cause it to deteriorate, and terms such as sight conservation and sight-saving classes were used to describe the educational philosophy.

2. Techniques and materials developed for the education and rehabilitation of the visually impaired were based on experience with the totally blind and the need to rely completely on other senses.

3. The problems of the totally blind were, perhaps, considered more serious.

4. There was a lack of knowledge about the unique aspects of seeing with very limited vision which would allow for the development or adaptation of techniques and training methods.

RECOGNITION AND DEVELOPMENT

Fortunately, this situation has been changing rapidly since the mid 1960s. Interest in providing education and rehabilitation services tailored to the specific needs and problems of persons with low vision is growing. Research in areas such as visual perception and optics has reached the point where implications for the low vision population are becoming apparent. This chapter will familiarize the reader with the historical and theoretical basis of low vision orientation and mobility and discuss the practical aspects of training. Table 1-7 is a chronological sampling of important events in the area of low vision.

Research that would later have important implications for increasing the low vision person's ability to use that vision began in the 1920s. Important work in mapping of the acuity of visual fields and of color vision appeared throughout the 1920s and 1930s (Ferree, Rand, & Hardy, 1931; Kleitman & Blier, 1928). During World War II much work on visual phenomena, visual learning, visual search, and adaptation to darkness was produced by perceptual psychologists and advanced by later military science studies (Low, 1946; Mandelbaum & Sloan, 1947; Morris & Horne, 1960). During this period the work of Renshaw provided the basic research which became the foundation for the systematic training of vision to improve

TABLE 1-7.
Low Vision—Historical Development

1918	Bates course of eye training
1928	Kleitman and Blier, color and form discrimination; American Optometric Association (AOA)
1930	Ferree, Rand, and Hardy, visibility factors testing; refraction for peripheral field
1939	Renshaw, psychological optics
1940	Research in visual search, adaptation to darkness
1942	AOA Department of Visual Adaptation and Rehabilitation
1944	Luckiesch, lighting; M. Bender, perception in perimetrically blind fields
1946	F. Low, peripheral vision studies
1947	American Printing House for the Blind (APH) begins regular publication of large print books
1949	D. Hebb, *Organization of behavior*
1950	J. J. Gibson, *Perception of the visual world;* Gesell, vision development in infants
1953	E.J. Gibson, effects of training on perceptual judgments; Industrial Home for the Blind Low Vision Clinic; Megascope developed by AFB
1954	First exhibit of low vision aids organized by Ritter for International Congress of Ophthalmologists
1955	F. Allport, *Theories of perception and the concept of structure*
1957	Hoover's functional definition of blindness; optical aids clinics win federal approval as component of vocational rehabilitation program
1958	AOA—Department of Vision Care of the Aging
1959	AOA—Committee on Aid to the Partially Blind
1960	M. von Senden translated; first graduate mobility program at Boston College
1961-2	Kohler, Riesen studies on goggles and sensory deprivation; Fonda evaluates telescopic spectacles for mobility
1964	AAWB Mobility Interest Group IV "informally" formed at annual convention in New York, Rod Kossick, Chairman; Barraga study on increased visual functioning; Frostig, *The Frostig program for development of visual perception; Teacher's guide*
1965	Replication of Barraga's work begun; AAWB annual convention, Denver, Group IX "formally" formed, Loyal E. Apple elected first chairman
1966	J. J. Gibson's *Senses considered as perceptual systems;* R. L. Gregory; *Eye and brain*
1967	Low vision clinic established in Western Michigan University program; "two visual systems" theory developed
1970	San Francisco Low Vision Mobility Conference; *Visual efficiency scale and teachers' guide* published by APH; CCTV commercially available; L. Apple and M. May, *Distance vision and perceptual training*
1971	*Low Vision Abstracts* begins publication; A. Valvo, *Sight restoration after long-term blindness*
1972	First required low vision course in mobility curriculum, Western Michigan University; mobility application of night viewing goggles; Low Vision Clinical Society founded; Low Vision Diplomate Program established, American Academy of Optometry, Edwin Mehr, Chairman
1974	Vision stimulation for mobility purposes documented by A. Smith at Western Pennsylvania School for the Blind.
1975	Low Vision Mobility Workshop at Kalamazoo; AAWB Low Vision Interest Group formed; Goodrich and Quillman, eccentric viewing training; Fresnel lenses used for mobility; low vision section formed, American Academy of Ophthalmology
1976	Academy of Ophthalmology *ad hoc* low vision committee formed
1977	National Eye Institute conference on low vision usage; revision of Barraga/APH material begun; AFB survey of low vision clinics services

academic achievement. Other perceptual psychologists and developmental vision optometrists followed this applied research trail (Getman & Kephart, 1950-1960; Kephart, 1958).

Research into visual phenomena as they relate to brain damage resulted in increased understanding of perceptual anomalies frequently associated with severe sight loss (Bender & Teuber, 1948; Bender & Teuber, 1946; Bender & Krieger, 1951). Williams and Gassel (1962, 1963) and Teuber, Battersby, and Bender (1960) did some of the first work to interpret the patient's subjective report f visual field.

The Literature

During the 1950s the number of disciplines interested in vision expanded considerably and there was a rapid growth in the literature (May, 1978). The work of Eleanor and James Gibson began and spanned the next 25 years. James Gibson developed theories which account for the use of vision in human behavior. His papers can be easily understood because of their relevance in mobility (*The Senses considered as perceptual systems*, 1966; Gibson, J., 1954). E. Gibson's work on the effects of practice on perceptual judgments is summed up in *Principles of perceptual learning and development* (1969).

The 1960s produced some work of great value to low vision, including the first significant broad scale application of the state of the art of perceptual psychology to low vision services.

The limited literature on the effects of sight restoration in persons who have never seen, offers some clues to the stages of visual learning and organization that take place before visual functioning is possible (von Senden, 1960; Valvo, 1968). This literature (Gregory, 1966; Gregory & Wallace, 1963) raises questions regarding the psychological effects of maladaptation to restored vision. This area still remains relatively unexplored by current research.

Several crucial studies were done which indicated the great flexibility of human beings in adapting to highly restricted, displaced, or distorted vision (Kohler, 1962, 1975; Riesen, 1961). The technical developments which allowed Kohler and Riesen to conduct their studies opened the subject of artificially reducing or degrading visual acuity and fields in order to develop low vision training techniques.

Without doubt, the strongest impetus to application of this knowledge to persons with low vision was Barraga's (1964) research on increasing the visual efficiency of children who had very limited amounts of vision through the use of specialized materials and instruction. Barraga's study of children who had previously been educated as though totally blind provided the evidence that sequential visual stimulation training was highly effective as a way to improve near visual functioning even without significant changes in near vision acuity. Several replications of Barraga's study (Holmes, 1967; Tobin, 1973) have shown similar rates of success. Use of vision stimulation techniques with low vision children not previously educated as though totally blind also proved successful (Montgomery County Board of Education, 1969). Similar work was taking place and similar techniques were also being applied to children with developmental disabilities (Frostig & Horne, 1964).

Another early effort that directed attention to and stimulated interest in the unique problems and attributes of persons with low vision was Hoover's (1957) attempt to propound a more functional definition of blindness.

Mobility Techniques

Following the establishment of the first university programs to train mobility specialists in 1961, the numbers of agencies and schools that provided mobility training to clients and students grew quickly (Chapter 19). Mobility specialists began to encounter clients who obviously had useful vision which with training could be used for travel. As early as mid-decade (Richterman, 1966), it was apparent that mobility techniques developed for the totally blind were not entirely appropriate for the low vision person. Hughes (1967) identified several problems that low vision children attending a residential school for the blind had with orientation and mobility and called for better methods of training and the use of optical aids. Concurrently, the relationship of distance vision to mobility began to be examined (Blasch, D., & Apple, L., 1967).

Distance Vision

Because mobility does depend mostly on distance vision, the early visual efficiency and stimulation studies, which stressed near vision tasks, did not provide the answers mobility specialists working with low vision clients needed. They did, however, provide a model that could be used to begin investigating the development of distance vision training techniques.

The first national conference on low vision and mobility was held in 1970 in San Francisco under the sponsorship of the U.S. Office of Education. Entitled "Visual Abilities—Their Behavioral Assessment and Possible Methods for Their Improvement in the Individual with Severe Visual Impairment," the conference was multi-disciplinary in nature and was the first concerted effort to deal with the distance use of small amounts of vision (Apple, L. & May, M., 1970). The primary purpose of the conference was to lay a sound basis for the use of techniques and knowledge developed by perceptual psychologists, ophthalmologists, optometrists who dealt with visual training and perceptual problems, educators of low vision children, educators of the perceptually handicapped, and mobility specialists who had worked with low vision clients. Major areas covered by the conference were: characteristics of eye conditions related to low vision, measurement of visual effectiveness, effects of severe visual impairment on psycho-social behavior, functional assessment of low vision visual perception as it relates to low vision, and training methods for increasing visual effectiveness. This conference greatly stimulated interest in providing mobility training for low vision clients. It firmly established the need for information from a variety of disciplines and the concept of the multi-disciplinary team approach to the rehabilitation of the low vision client.

GROWTH AND DEVELOPMENT

Considerable progress was made during the years immediately following the 1970 conference. Apple and May (1970) formulated a program model based on application of perceptual and educational psychology, physiological optics, neurology, human engineering, and mobility literature. The program model was based on sequential learning in several core areas involving actual mobility: depth perception, perception of motion, light adaptation, and perception and memory for distinctive features and form. In 1972, Western Michigan University, Kalamazoo, became the first university blind rehabilitation professional training program to offer a required course on low vision. *Low Vision Abstracts* was established in 1971 to deal with the literature that had implications for mobility training of low vision persons.

In 1975, the Veterans Administration sponsored a second national conference on low vision and mobility. This conference, held at Western Michigan University, was designed to synthesize the state of the art in orientation and mobility for low vision persons, in visual science and in ophthalmological and optometric work in distance vision, and to devise an integrated plan of action for the future (Apple, L. & Blasch, B., 1976).

At this second conference, which like the first was multi-disciplinary, participants came with a good understanding of the body of knowledge, of the various disciplines involved in low vision rehabilitation, and considerable direct experience working with low vision persons. The topics discussed at the second conference clearly reveal the growing sophistication. The discussion of evaluation of visual functioning centered around peripheral stimulation, processing of visual information, vestibular-optical reflexes, and perceptual learning. The section on visual training without aids dealt with perceptual problems, processing of information, early intervention, and training of the adventitiously low vision person. In the section on optical aids, their use was considered in terms of life conditions and problems resulting from diminished visual perception, the team approach to services, the complex nature of evaluation for aids, an in-depth look at distance aids themselves. Finally, the section on psycho-social aspects of persons with low vision dealt with their marginal status in society, definitions, common characteristics, and the role of the rehabilitation specialist.

Professionalism

Today, most university programs for the training of professional rehabilitation personnel for the visually impaired emphasize low vision along with total blindness either in special courses or integrated into all other courses. Administrators of low vision clinics have begun to recognize the value of providing mobility training to clients who need it (Jose, Cummings, & McAdams, 1975; Faye & Hood, 1975b; Sprague, 1977).

There is, in addition, much more awareness on the national level of the needs of persons with low vision. Three professional organizations, and one consumer organization have emerged to provide forums in which low vision treatment can be discussed: the Clinical Society for Low Vision, which is a part of the American Medical Association; the Low Vision Diplomate Section, which is a part of the American Optometric Association; and the Low Vision Interest Group, which is a part of the American Association of Workers for the Blind and the Council of Citizens with Low Vision, an affiliate of the American Council of the Blind. The American Foundation for the Blind offers national consultative services on low vision and has a Low Vision Advisory Committee. Professional publications such as the *Journal of Visual Impairment and Blindness**, *Education of the Visually Handicapped*, *Long Cane News*, *Optometric Monthly***, *Optometric Review*, and *Sensory Disabilities* regularly report on low vision research and practice and, as mentioned previously, *Low Vision Abstracts* covers literature pertinent to training of near and distant vision.

Nevertheless, knowledge of both the theoretical and practical aspects of training of low vision is still in the very early stages. There are a number of unanswered questions and gaps in methodology and services that need serious attention in terms of research, training of professionals, program development, and delivery of services. While many of these problems are, strictly speaking, outside the purview of this chapter, the mobility specialist does need to be aware of them and how they might relate to mobility training of a low vision client.

Providing mobility services to low vision persons is a complex undertaking that ideally involves a number of disciplines and a number of skills, and possibly several settings (Apple, L. & Blasch, B., 1976). Low vision services are most effective when they are integrated and inter-disciplinary. The following flow chart provides a suggested model for an integrated approach to providing these services:

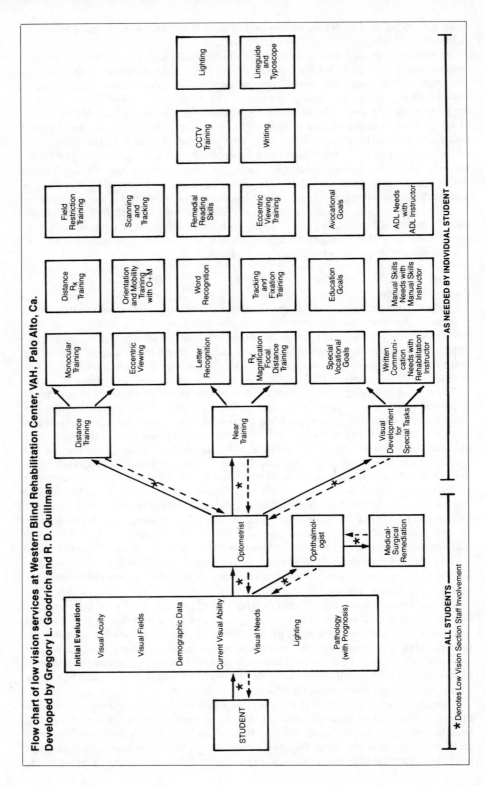

Flow chart of low vision services at Western Blind Rehabilitation Center, VAH, Palo Alto, Ca. Developed by Gregory L. Goodrich and R. D. Quillman

Ideally, the mobility specialist will provide travel training to a low vision client as a member of a multi-disciplinary rehabilitation team that includes clinical vision specialists, social workers, educators, etc. While such situations do exist (Faye & Hood, 1975b; Jose, Cummings, & McAdams, 1975; Friedman, Kayne, Tallman, & Asarkof, 1975), low vision services are not easily available in all parts of the country nor are they all comprehensive and multi-disciplinary in nature (American Foundation for the Blind, 1978). For some years to come, it is likely that many mobility specialists will find themselves working with low vision clients in setting where professionals from other disciplines are not readily available (Carter, & Carter, 1975).

LOW VISION DEFINED

Mobility specialists will also have to contend with the confusion surrounding the definition of low vision and the profusion of terms used to describe the condition itself and the people who have it. Hoover (1957) first proposed the term severe visual impairment which has since come to be accepted as the general term describing serious visual problems from inability to read newsprint with ordinary glasses and would include total blindness. Low vision has come to be accepted as the term that best describes the condition that has been called in the past, partial sight, cecutiency, residual or remaining vision, near blind, purblind.

Definitions of what constitutes low vision also vary widely although there is considerable agreement on the importance of not limiting the term and services available to persons who fall within the "legal" definition of blindness. Four recent definitions reflect this understanding.

Mehr and Freid (1975) say that, "Low Vision may be defined as reduced central acuity or visual field loss which even with the best optical correction provided by regular lenses results in visual impairment from a performance standpoint."

Colenbrander on behalf of the International Society for the Prevention of Blindness, the World Health Organization (1977), defines a low vision person as "having a significant visual handicap but also having significant usable residual vision."

Faye and Hood (1975a) define a person with low vision as having "visual acuity that falls below a norm, that the acuity cannot be corrected with conventional spectacle refraction, and that the person has many problems in daily existence related directly to reduced visual acuity or a field defect."

Genensky (1970, 1978) has developed a functional classification for blindness and severe visual impairment. A person is *functionally blind* if he is either totally blind, or has at most light perception or light projection. A person is *partially sighted and legally blind* if he is legally blind but not functionally blind. A person is *partially sighted* if the acuity in his better eye even with ordinary corrective lenses does not exceed 20/70 *or* if the maximum diameter of his visual field does not exceed 20° *and* if he is not functionally blind.

While these definitions are not exactly the same, they do have several points in common that make them useful to mobility specialists and other education and rehabilitation professionals: None attempt to categorize a person with low vision in terms of specific acuity and field defect levels; by implication, all four suggest the presence of *useful* vision; they suggest that the person with low vision encounters problems in daily functioning that stem from the visual deficit.

Partly because of the uncertainty about the definition of low vision, partly because of the way in which statistics on visual impairment have been collected, estimates of the size of the low vision population in the U.S. are difficult to make.

There are two primary sources of statistical data that have been used to describe the characteristics and size of the population with visual loss:

1. The Model Reporting Area for Statistics on Blindness (MRA)—a roster of legally blind persons registered with 16 states, which observed standardized procedures in collecting information. The data were compiled and analyzed annually from 1962 to 1970. In 1970, there were 99,347 persons on the MRA registers (Kahn, & Moorhead, 1973).

2. The Health Interview Survey of the National Center for Health Statistics (NCHS-HIS)—an annual national household interview sample survey from which an estimate of the number of persons with severe visual impairments is derived. Severe visual impairment is defined by NCHS-HIS as the inability to read ordinary newspaper print, even with the aid of glasses.

In 1970, 10.6 percent of the registered legally blind MRA population had "absolute blindness" and 11.4 percent had "light perception" only, making a total of 22 percent who had no useful vision, and 78 percent who had useful vision (Table 25b, Kahn & Moorhead, 1973).

Since 1957, NCHS-HIS has made national estimates of the number of persons with severe visual impairments. However, it was only in the 1963-64 Health Interview Survey that persons were asked whether or not they could "see light." Among persons reported to have severe visual impairment, 6.1 percent were unable to see light (Table D, National Council for Health Statistics, 1968). In the absence of evidence to the contrary, and since neither the methodology nor definition have changed since the 1963-64 survey, it can be assumed that the same proportion of severely visually impaired persons is unable to perceive light at the present time. The unpublished, provisional NCHS-HIS estimated number of severely visually impaired persons in the U.S. in 1977 is 1,391,000. Assuming approximately 94 percent of these can perceive light, it can be estimated that more than 1,300,000 persons could probably benefit from low vision aids and training.

The mobility specialist must also appreciate the newness of training persons to use small amounts of vision, the resulting lack of an accepted best practice, and especially how this relates to difficulties in understanding the extraordinarily diverse low vision population. There are people born with low vision. There are persons whose vision becomes severely impaired later in life. Some low vision persons are identified (and treated) by themselves and others as blind. Some are identified by others and identify themselves as sighted. There are a wide variety of physical reasons for low vision. Even when the physical visual problem is identical, the functional problems it creates can vary widely from person to person (Margach, 1968). A wide variety of psychological characteristics, differing in kind from those experienced by the totally blind, also affect the functioning of persons with low vision.

Thus while the remainder of this chapter deals separately with the specific aspects of mobility training of low vision clients, vision assessment, visual functioning, training techniques and psychosocial aspects, the mobility specialist must continually keep in mind that in actual training situations, these factors cannot be so neatly separated.

ASSESSMENT OF VISUAL FUNCTIONING

An appropriate mobility training program for a low vision person must be preceded by assessment of the client's visual functioning. This is particularly true in view of the wide range of visual conditions represented within the group labeled as low vision persons. Table 2-7, adapted from similar charts, identifies and keys eye diseases by category, functional characteristics, and physical needs (Table 2-7).

There are three major ways to assess visual functioning: clinical assessments, self-reports of visual functioning, and functional vision assessments. All of these methods must be used for every low vision client. Special attention must be given to the interaction between the information obtained through each method and any discrepancies that result from the various methods.

TABLE 2-7.
Characteristics of Eye Diseases

Disease	Category	Functional	Physical
Achromatopsia	Cnp	d, g	h, i
Albinism	Cnp	f, g	h, i
Amblyopia ex anopsia	Ap	b, f	h, i, m
Aniridia	Cs	f, g	i, m
Aphakia, surgical	Anp, s	f, g	h, i, l, m
Cataract	Cnp, p	f, g	i, m
	Anp, p	f, g	h, i, j, m
Chorioretinitis	Anp	a or b, e, f, g	i, m
Coloboma of iris, choroid or disc	Cnp	a, e, f	i, j
Corneal dystrophy	Cnp, p	e, f	i
Corneal graft, uveitis or scarring	Anp, s	f, g, e	h, i, l, m, j
Detachment of retina surgically treated	Anp, p	a or b, c, e, f	h, i, l, m
Diabetic retinopathy	Ap, s	b, c, e, f	h, i, j, l, m
Glaucoma	Cp	a, c, e, f	i, j, m
Hypertensive retinopathy	Ap	b, e, f	i, j, l, m
Keratoconus	Ap, s	a, e, f	h, i, k
Macular degeneration juvenile	Cnp	b, d, f, g	h, i, l
senile	Anp, p	b, d, e, f, g	i, j
Myopia, degenerative axial	Cnp, s	a or b, c d, e, f	h, k, l, m
Primary optic atrophy	Anp	f, g	h, i, k
congenital	Cnp	b, e, d	h, i, j
neurological	Anp, p	a, c, d, e, f	i, j, l, m
Retinitis pigmentosa	Ap	a, c, e, d	h, i, j
Retrobulbar neuritis	Anp, p	a, b, d, f, g	i, j, m
Retrolental fibroplasia	Anp, s	a or b, e, f	h, i, k, l

Key:

Category

Congenital or Hereditary	C
Non-progressive	np
Progressive	p
Secondary Complications	s
Adventitial	A
Non-progressive	np
Progressive	p
Secondary Complications	s

Functional Characteristics
a. Peripheral field loss
b. Central field loss
c. Defective night vision
d. Defective color vision
e. Bright light preferred
f. Average light preferred
g. Dim light preferred

Physical Needs
h. Distance glass or aid
i. High-plus reading spectacle
j. Hand-held lens preferable
k. Can read without glasses
l. Physical activity may be restricted
m. May be on eye treatment or medication

Clinical Assessment

Clinical assessments are formal procedures used by ophthalmologists, optometrists, and other vision specialists under somewhat controlled conditions. This term is used to refer to those assessments which are performed in specially designated "low vision clinics" as well as those which are performed by any vision specialist in his own office or other service setting.

Clinical assessments should yield information that is essential to understanding the needs of an individual low vision client. It is important to understand certain medical conditions and other health-related information that would lead to a specific approach for a client with certain characteristics. For example, eye-health conditions, such as retinal detachment or a susceptibility toward a detachment, mitigate against rigorous physical activity. Other eye conditions, medications that a client takes, or fatigue combined with certain conditions, can result in fluctuating visual functioning and should be noted (Green & Spencer, 1969). A clinical assessment should also reveal other health and medical conditions which would affect the person's vision and his treatment.

The strength of the clinical assessment should be to yield detailed acuity and field and color measurements under a variety of lighting conditions, and, most appropriate, refractions for both near and distance tasks. Visual acuity, which is a measure of the resolving power of the eye or the ability of the eye to discriminate between two visible points, is usually measured through the use of the system developed by Snellen. The Snellen measurement system involves the concept of visual angle. In the normal eye, the ability to discriminate between two distant points, such as distinguishing that there are two stars rather than one, is considered to represent the ability of the eye to resolve a visual angle of one minute of arc, which is equivalent to 20/20 vision in Snellen terminology. A Snellen measurement of 20/200 indicates that the eye has the power to resolve a visual angle of ten minutes of arc or greater, which means that two objects must be farther apart to be distinguished as two separate objects by the eye.

A Snellen chart is designed in such a way as to distinguish in a standardized manner an individual's ability to resolve visual angles of increasing magnitude when the chart is viewed from standard distances. These distances are such that the Snellen system measures only distance visual acuity.

Near visual acuity is measured using symbol charts such as the Feinbloom Subnormal Vision Reading Card, the New York Lighthouse Near Vision Test for Children, and Sloan reading cards which are viewed at distances of 16 in. (40 cm), the normal distance for reading.

For clients with very low levels of vision, their abilities are sometimes reported as the ability to detect hand movements or to count fingers at distances less than 60 in. (152 cm). Counts fingers at 12 in. (30.5 cm) is equivalent to 1/200; counts fingers at 24 in. (61 cm) is equivalent to 2/200, etc. While this is reported by the clinician, it is a less standardized and less reliable measure than other clinical reports.

A clinical assessment will also provide a standardized measure of the amount of area which the client can see. This is called the visual field. The various methods devised for estimating visual fields should be preceded by visual acuity measurements so that an appropriate sized test object can be selected.

One gross, qualitative procedure of field testing is the confrontation test. The examiner faces the client on the same level at a distance of 24 in. (61 cm). Each with an eye occluded, the client and the examiner fixate the exposed opposite eye of the other. The examiner should be in front of a uniform dark background with the source of illumination behind the client. The examiner then moves a test object (white disc on wand, flashlight, toy, large sheet of white paper) in from the periphery and notes when it comes into the client's field of view. This procedure is then repeated with the object being moved in from each of the eight cardinal meridians of the field. Two test objects can be used on opposite sides of fixation to elicit visual extinction (Berman, 1978).

The confrontation method of visual field testing can be done anywhere; it is not restricted to use in the clinic. While it is sometimes used there, a more standardized approach is testing done with a tangent screen and/or perimeter. A tangent screen, primarily used to test the central 30° of the visual fields, is a black screen with a fixation target in the center that is customarily fixated by the client at a distance of 1 or 2 yds (1 or 2 m). A test object or an illuminated target is moved in from the periphery and the field plotted with markers on the screen. The standard illumination for testing is 7 footcandles.

Other methods, such as amsler grids, may be used to test the central field. Peripheral fields are usually tested with arc or bowl perimeters. The client sits with his head and chin resting on the instrument at the proper testing distance 13 in. (330 mm) as he fixates a center point. A test object is moved in from the periphery and the point at which it becomes visible, when it disappears, and when it flickers or grays out is noted (Stein & Slatt, 1968). A person's visual fields can be reported graphically as in Fig. 1-7. Isopters (a line circumscribing an area in which a given size and color test object is seen) are usually written on the visual field chart as a fraction:

$$\frac{\text{size of target} \quad \text{(color)}}{\text{testing distance}}$$

Ideally a clinical examination should also indicate the client's color discrimination abilities. Generally, the Farnsworth Color Test adapted for low vision

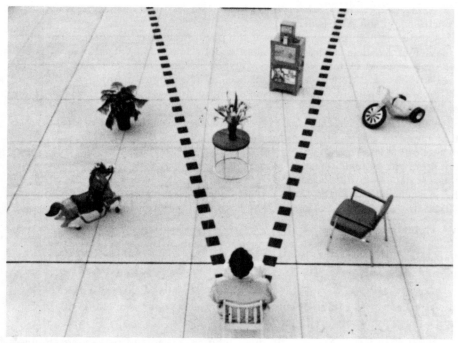

Figure 1-7. Field of vision.

persons and the Primary Colors Test provide suitable information on color discrimination (Wood, 1975; Mehr & Freid, 1975).

Other components of visual functioning which are assessed through a clinical examination include the optical power of the eye, accommodation, convergence and divergence ability, light and dark adaptation, aligning ability, and binocularity.

Self-Report

A second general method of learning how a person sees is the client's self-report of visual functioning (Apple, M., 1973; Apple, L., & May, 1970). A subjective report provides information about what the low vision person expects from and experiences with his vision. Visual anomalies, such as phosphenes, floaters, and photophobia should be discussed and documented on the client's record. The low vision person should be helped to document his visual functioning by sketching how he sees or understands his visual field defects (Apple, M., 1973).

In a self-report, the client should be helped to discuss what he is able to see using his distance vision, such as road signs, billboards, television, movies, etc. He should share his reactions to various illumination levels and how they affect his visual functioning. Does he see better when it is bright and sunny or when it is dark and/or cloudy? Do certain levels of illumination cause him discomfort? Which colors can he see most easily and recognize most consistently? Such a report should also consider the person's near vision. Can he read print? What type of print can he read comfortably? What kind of lighting is needed? At what distance away from himself does he hold the text? What other kind(s) of activities does he perform which require near vision, such as hobbies, recreation, etc.

The self-report should also pay attention to other characteristics of the client which may help to explain his visual functioning. It should consider the client's literacy, his attitude toward seeing, his level of expectation for the return of vision, and his role in the family.

Functional Vision Assessment

A third method of determining what a person sees is to do a functional vision assessment. While a clinical assessment is done in a standardized manner which attempts to hold extraneous factors constant so as to achieve the most reliable measure of visual deficit, a functional vision assessment attempts to achieve an observational measure of the person's ability to use the vision he has under ordinary conditions.

A functional vision assessment systematically places the client in a representative range of travel situations under a variety of conditions. The role of the evaluator is to assess how the client uses his vision to travel through the various environments or to do the other tasks required. The person's visual performance in these situations is affected, of course, by variables such as anxiety or the challenge he might experience, the skills he has developed for anticipating or analyzing situations, and the past experience he has had in similar situations.

VA Guidelines

The guidelines for a functional vision evaluation that were developed at the Veterans Administration's Western Blind Rehabilitation Center in Palo Alto were presented by Hennessey (1975). The major elements considered are:

Line of travel.   An erratic or poor line of travel may indicate weaknesses in such areas as scanning techniques, contrast awareness, or a preoccupation with the very immediate environment.

Object avoidance.   Many individuals who are capable of perceiving an object under ideal conditions, fail to detect it in travel situations. Persons with restricted field may see the smallest of obstacles, but lose perspective and fail to avoid them.

Drop-offs.   Does the client have the ability to detect irregular surface conditions; the depth perception to detect stairs, curbs, etc.?

Street crossings.   Typical performance factors are the individual's ability to locate and interpret traffic signals in varying conditions, and the ability to judge speed and direction of traffic which may be dependent on either auditory or visual information.

Adaptation.   Changes in lighting involve behavioral adaptation to them such as travel on the sunny (rather than the shady) side of the street; travel with the sun to one's back; shadow and glare areas; need for sunshades; and need for cane.

Visual identification of landmarks.   It is essential to identify the characteristics of landmarks which the client can consistently locate.

Travel in crowded areas (indoors and outdoors).   Differences between stated and actual travel ability are resolved through exposure to those travel environments in which the client expresses a proficiency. The evaluation environment should become more complex or more simple until a realistic evaluation has been achieved.

Night travel.   Evaluation of travel under night conditions should place special emphasis on factors involving ability to remain on the sidewalk, judge depth, avoid obstacles, detect landmarks, react to headlights of on-coming traffic, and use street lights as a means of establishing direction.

Orientation skills.   The client should be evaluated on knowledge of cardinal directions, spatial concepts and mapping, accuracy of directional sense, and ability to use vision to place onself in the environment.

Considerations

The procedures developed for functional vision assessments should systematically determine whether the client can see a wide range of objects under a variety of illumination levels such as daylight, nighttime, and twilight; on cloudy days and sunny days; with indoor lighting where appropriate, when a light source is in front of, behind, or beside the object; when facing oncoming headlights from cars; and when there is glare (Ensor, 1976; Welsh & Wiener, 1976). In assessing visual field restrictions, the evaluation should also consider how well the client sees objects that are above, below, and to either side of his area of central vision, and to what extent the client uses extensive head scanning to see objects in these various positions.

Although functional vision assessments cannot be as standardized as clinical procedures, there should be, and has been, an effort to standardize procedures and the visual stimuli in those particular settings where assessments are done. To whatever extent such an effort would be successful, the information generated by standard procedures may be a more consistent predictor of the most appropriate type of intervention for particular clients.

Some early efforts to develop checklists to standardize assessment procedures were published in *Low Vision Abstracts* (Fall, 1972 pp. 15-20).

The three methods of assessing visual functioning of the person with low vision should not be perceived as alternative methods of accomplishing the same thing, but rather they should be regarded as complementary methods each of which should be included in the ideal effort to determine visual functioning. Traditional clinical measures are designed to preclude existing compensatory mechanisms on the part of the individual, and, therefore, measure visual deficiency and not the ability to overcome the deficit. The mobility specialist as well as the special educator or other rehabilitation specialists are oriented toward assisting the person to compensate for the visual loss and therefore they must focus not only on the loss but also on the person's ability to compensate for the loss.

Recently mobility specialists and special educators of the visually impaired have become more and more concerned about children whose clinical assessments indicate "vision nil" or "no vision, should be taught braille" but who in the course of their education or training are discovered to have usable sight. Many of these children are able to read and to travel using sight after a special training program involving the development of visual functioning (Barraga, 1964; Smith, 1974). Some educators feel that medically oriented vision specialists have made little progress in diagnosing the presence of impaired but essentially useful vision in babies. To the extent that this is the case, it speaks to the need for improved communication between those who assess visual functioning so that the most accurate assessment results lead to the most appropriate educational or training intervention for the child.

IMPROVING VISUAL FUNCTIONING

Once the assessments have been completed, the mobility specialist and other members of the multi-disciplinary low vision rehabilitation team should be well into the planning and administration of a program to improve the individual's ability to use the vision. There are two basic methods of enhancing an individual's ability to see, vision training and the prescription and use of optical aids. For some low vision persons, a combination of vision training and the use of optical aids will be necessary; and rarely are optical aids of any value without vision training. For others, vision training alone will suffice.

Vision Training

Training of the visual skills of individuals in order to increase overall performance is currently being practiced in the military services, sports, optometry, and in special education. The military trains spotters, ground observers, and pilots in visual search procedures that have implications for low vision mobility (Morris & Horne, 1960). These procedures include scanning techniques, search logic, figure-ground discrimination, use of distinctive features, and transformation.

Because outstanding peripheral vision has been identified as a characteristic of superior athletes, programs to increase this ability have also been instituted. Some optometrists trained in developmental vision have demonstrated changes in performance through vision training. Most of the literature in this area is available from the Optometric Extension Foundation, Duncan, Oklahoma.

Barraga (1964) pioneered the use of vision stimulation training techniques to increase the near vision efficiency of low vision children. Once the implications of vision stimulation programs for young "blind" children were clear, several mobility specialists extended this practice to orientation and mobility programs (Hennessey, 1975; Jose & Shane, 1978). An especially interesting effort of this sort, dealing with 42 youngsters at the Western Pennsylvania School for the Blind, was documented on videotape (Smith, 1974).

LOW VISION PROGRAM PLANNING

Mobility specialists familiar with the fundamentals of orientation and mobility training for the totally blind will find that they are making differential decisions in four basic areas, length of training, use of the blindfold, and development of lesson plans, when they begin planning special programs for low vision persons.

Length of Training

Increases in age, health problems, psychological problems, and learning rate will, in large measure, determine need and length of training time. If the functional evaluation reveals minimal difficulties, it appears that approximately 20 hours should be the minimum of training to insure efficiency and safety of any low vision person.

Training is lengthened to allow for learning but is again shortened for severely impaired individuals because of diminished capacity. When the client is hearing as well as visually impaired, decreases in hearing plotted against training time result in a curved line with mild and profound hearing losses requiring somewhat less training time than moderate losses. Use of blindfold will tend to increase training time. Knowledgeability of the mobility specialist in low vision will tend to increase training time. It appears that the more basic content knowledge the mobility instructor has, the less likely he is to cut the training program short. He is able to recognize the client's needs based on depth of understanding.

Use of Blindfold

The blindfold has distinctive advantages and disadvantages when used in the training of low vision persons. Use of the blindfold permits low vision persons to be trained to use the same techniques as persons who are totally blind. This deprives the low vision person of instruction in use of vision in orientation and mobility. Use of the blindfold permits low vision persons to be trained for night travel using the blindfold as a simulator. It is not a true simulation because it deprives the person of use of visual cues at night. The blindfold permits training of persons when vision is fluctuating with greater comfort and certainty for the low vision person. The blindfold permits the person to better appreciate and perhaps rely on other sensory stimuli.

Non-use of the blindfold allows for the organized presentation and solution of low vision problems experienced by low vision persons. The "two-way" lesson is used to allow both visual and blindfold instruction for better integration of training. The blindfold is used to reach the objective and removed for the return over the same route. Another method involves the use of the blindfold until the mobility specialist is certain the low vision person is making optimum use of other sensory stimuli. Empirical evidence seems to indicate that judicious use of the blindfold may result in the client feeling that his vision is improved (Hines, 1961). In reality, he is making optimum use of other sensory stimuli.

The mobility specialist should have very concrete reasons for use of the blindfold. It must be a reason that relates to the student. It should enable the student to integrate other sensory stimuli with his residual vision to enable him to function better and this should be part of the lesson plan. It should not be based on the instructor's need to instruct.

Use of Cane.

The cane has several uses in the mobility training of low vision persons (Blasch, B.G., 1975). Functional vision evaluation should be designed to illustrate need for the use of the cane in ordinary travel situations to both the instructor and the student. Night lessons are frequently the most important deciding factor of need for cane travel skills. There will be a tendency for persons with lower acuity to utilize the cane for both day and night travel. Persons with peripheral field losses will use the cane somewhat more for night travel than day travel. Persons with central field losses tend to be those who do not require the cane for travel either day or night. The collapsible cane is frequently utilized as a ready explanation to the public that the user cannot see normally, and is for occasional use. There will be certain situations and environmental conditions, for example, under poor lighting conditions, unfamiliar areas, or unusual terrain when it will be advisable for the client to make use of his cane technique even though he is capable of traveling without it in most ordinary circumstances.

Development of Lesson Plans

Lesson plans for low vision programs have four distinguishing features. They will have a section devoted to instruction in the use of telescopes and other optical aids. They will provide for night lessons. In addition to tactual and auditory cues, they will provide the use of visual cues and landmarks. Routes of travel will be selected for their visual content, as well as to meet skill-building requirements.

There are a large number of concepts having to do with visual performance and visual learning which must find their place in a training program for low vision persons.

In training low vision persons to perform mobility tasks, the mobility specialist should consider: ability to learn to attend to stimulus dimensions, selecting the right dimensions, and that dimensions in the task might change as the learner becomes more proficient. (Initially he may need quite a bit of visual information for identification purposes, but as he becomes more proficient, he will require less visual information.) The mobility specialist must teach the low vision person to concentrate on what to look for and what features are important for his particular task; begin with exaggerated differences in the critical stimulus dimensions and reduce these differences as training proceeds.

Four critical stimulus dimensions may be used to determine the "seeability" of the environment (Apple & May, 1970). The brightness level, or actual amount of light available, makes it possible to see the environment, but too much light will tend to degrade visibility of the environment. The brightness contrast or extent to which things can be distinguished from their background by their color or shade is the most important dimension, if enough light is present for the low vision person to see. The size of objects becomes critical with lowered acuity but is more easily managed by the student because, by halving the distance between himself and the object, he can double the size of its image on his retina. Unless the low vision person has sufficient time for viewing, objects will not be visible to him: the required time for viewing decreases with experience.

A program of training for the adventitious low vision person should focus on the effects of his particular visual problem and the strategies to maximize information. The loci of the visual disorder, whether central or peripheral, or both, makes a considerable difference in the type of vision available to the client for training. Literature on vision tends to focus on the fovea and its function, despite the fact that this comprises a very small portion of the visual field. The periphery, on the other hand, accounts for more than 98 percent of the retina (Goodrich & Quillman, 1977). The fovea and periphery complement each other, but their function and physiology are different (Johnson, 1976). Many studies have demonstrated that visual training improves response to visual stimuli, particularly through use of peripheral vision. Studies by Low (1946a, 1946b, 1951) indicate a marked improvement in peripheral vision with practice. Similar results were produced by Johnson and Leibowitz (1974).

The "two visual systems" model suggested during the late 1960s (Ingle, 1967; Schneider, 1969; Trevarthen, 1968; Held, 1968, 1970; Humphrey, 1974) has become a particularly useful concept in regard to the functional properties of the visual system and problems associated with visually-guided behavior. The "two visual systems" model basically states that there are two modes of processing visual information. One visual system, a predominantly peripheral localization system, maintains a marginal awareness or a vague diffuse awareness over a large portion of the visual fields and provides a monitoring and selection mechanism. In effect, this visual system answers the question of the "where" of visual stimulation. The second visual system, predominantly involving the fovea, includes central fixation, gives full attention to analysis of form and contour, and answers the question, "what." It should be noted that this dichotomy is relative rather than absolute (Johnson, 1976); Apple, L. & Blasch, B., 1976 . In normal visual information processing, the "where" system or the motor response of turning the head provides information as to where the eye should fixate to provide the "what" information or verbal response.

The predominantly peripheral "where" system or the ability to monitor and localize stimuli such as cars, pedestrians, etc., assumes a significant role in independent travel. The "two visual systems" theory has been a useful tool in understanding the visually-guided behavior of persons during adaptation to prisms, visual rearrangement, and other visual-motor skills (Held, 1970). It is suggested that visual-vestibular and other cross-modal visual interactions should be considered, with regard to the "two visual systems" model and also in relation to perceptual learning and visual training (Johnson, 1976).

There is a functional difference for the central "what" versus peripheral "where" functions. With respect to the visual stimulus, luminance or brightness level is generally considered the most important stimulus variable for the visual system (Apple, L. & Blasch, B., 1976). For example, by increasing luminance, visual resolution, intensity discrimination, and depth perception are improved, and color discrimination is possible only at the higher luminance levels (Apple, L. & Blasch, B., 1976). However, when considering the functions of peripheral vision, the ability to discriminate detail becomes essentially independent of luminance as discussed by Kerr (1971). In a study by Leibowitz, Meyers, and Grant (1955a, 1955b), subjects were asked to localize the stimulus in space. Results indicated that luminance had no effect as long as the stimulus was visible. Therefore, in training, the variable of luminance is important for the "what" function but not particularly important for the "where" function.

Based on the results of previous research and the importance of peripheral vision for certain tasks, it is also important to consider refractive errors of peripheral vision.

The optical quality and clarity of the retinal image is critical for foveal vision. For this reason and because it is important to see clearly, clinical refraction tends to concentrate on central vision without paying due attention to peripheral vision. Yet it has been demonstrated (Ferree, Rand, & Hardy, 1931; Lotmar & Lotmar, 1974) that peripheral refractive characteristics may differ from those in the fovea. Leibowitz, Johnson, and Isabelle (1972) found that with respect to perception of motion, a marked improvement in motion threshold resulted from correction of the peripheral refractive error. It must also be kept in mind that specific visual tasks are related to particular aspects of vision. For example, loss of foveal vision is a greater problem for those whose work requires heavy reading or discrimination of detail. A person with reduced vision in the peripheral area would have greater difficulty with mobility tasks such as driving or anticipating a collision path with other pedestrians. This implies that the results of impairment to the visual system are specific in terms of limitations rather than general.

A person who experiences a sudden loss of central vision often experiences various apparent distortions of space. The neurological resolution capability of the peripheral retina produces a non-optical "blur" of the image whereby low vision persons interpret location as farther away, therefore contact is made sooner than expected; conversely, if fitted with a distance magnification aid, location appears nearer so that contact is expected sooner than it occurs. If a central defect covers a

203

large retinal area, it may cause sudden disappearance and/or reappearance of objects as the observer or object moves. Low vision as a result of brain injury brings about unique distortions in vision not found in other eye conditions. Bender and Teuber (1948) describe some of these perceptual disturbances involving motion:

1. Drifting of images

2. Distortions in the perceived path of moving objects within the impaired visual field

3. Changes in apparent speed of moving objects within the impaired visual field

4. Apparent multiplication of single moving objects

5. Visual perception of true motion varies with the speed of the viewed moving object; slow motion produces an impression of a single stationary object; more rapid motion produces an apparent elongation or duplication of image; fast motion causes object to appear as multiple image.

Certain strategies flow from the "two visual systems" model. Johnson (1976) reports that for both absolute thresholds (Abernathy & Leibowitz, 1971) and motion detection (Johnson & Leibowitz, 1974) in the periphery, a small amount of practice and feedback of results (4 to 5 one-hour sessions) will result in marked improvement in performance in the periphery. This improvement can be maintained for relatively long periods of time (Johnson & Leibowitz, 1974). Improvements, with practice on specific tasks in the periphery, appear to generalize to some extent to other performance characteristics of peripheral vision (Johnson, 1976). Visual performance is better if attention is focused on a known specific part of the visual field rather than spread over the entire visual field. It follows, therefore, that depending upon the visual environment and tasks to be performed, and the demands upon the low vision person, training procedures that allow the person to concentrate attention to a specific portion of the visual field may be very helpful (Johnson, 1976).

This type of training for low vision persons is generally referred to as eccentric viewing training (Goodrich & Quillman, 1977; Quillman & Goodrich 1977; Mehr & Freid, 1975; Holcomb & Goodrich, 1976). Eccentric viewing training teaches the use of the peripheral vision system to obtain information in cases where there is decreased central vision functioning. The low vision person is trained to use that remaining portion of the vision field which is closest to the center of the fovea. Several techniques have been developed for training eccentric fixation, but all such training is naturally based on accurate data on the client's visual fields and acuity, and follows an easy-to-difficult progression (Goodrich & Quillman, 1977; Holcomb & Goodrich, 1976). A consistent relationship between the new eccentric fixation and eye-hand, eye-foot coordination must be established.

Scanning activities can be taught to partially compensate for the loss of visual field. A blind spot on the right would be the basis for teaching the client to make head and eye movements to the right sufficient to maintain information needed for safe mobility. In this as well as in instances where there is a constriction of the visual field, it is important that the client establish a system for scanning the visual environment. The mobility specialist can give the guidance to the client which will lead him to establish a compensatory system of scanning. Although it appears that the cadence and flow of scanning is highly individualized (Held, 1974) it is important that the client have a system.

Persons with vision in only one eye can be taught the cues which will allow them to estimate distance and depth. Some of these are relative size, linear and textural perspective, brightness and shadowing, placement of one object in front of another, and the relative motion of the object within the visual field.

Perception can improve, and such improvements occur with practice. *Training is a systematic exposure to learning activities, which results in more improvement in visual functioning than random experience for most low vision clients.* Random experience can organize in a negative way. Where training tasks differ from the actual real-life performance, attention should be given to how to transfer learning from the training situation to the real world. The low vision person can be taught to use specific information available in the visual environment by learning to attend to available but previously unused visual and nonvisual information. The role of reinforcement in visual training is self-regulatory: conscious improvement "rings a bell" and external reinforcement becomes less central to progress. "Looking harder," straining neck and facial muscles, and general tension make visual perception less effective, and relaxation should be encouraged. The straining to see which occurs early in training is acceptable because it may be an indication of motivation.

Verbalization during the development of perceptual awareness helps the low vision person to organize and retain visual stimulation and to assist the instructor in assessment and clarification. The following hierarchy for visual performance may be of value to mobility specialists in their communication with low vision persons as it presents a model for use in obtaining information about the way the low vision person understands his environment: Questions about what he sees can follow this outline:

1. A vague awareness of difference in the visual field

2. A generic object in the visual field (the "like" stage)

3. A specific object in the visual field (the "unlike" stage)

4. Object reorganization (combining and ordering like and unlike)

5. Search for meaning (what it is, what is it for, etc.)

6. Naming stage (identification)

7. Elaboration and expansion through visualization (beginning of concept).

It is possible to increase visual efficiency through the type of training described in this section but often it may be necessary and/or advantageous to use optical aids as well.

OPTICAL AIDS

Despite the interest in the mobility problems of low vision persons, skills in prescribing optical aids for distance vision in general, and for mobility in particular, lag well behind the prescription of such aids for reading and other close work. Most low vision clinics report that between 10 and 15 percent of their patients are prescribed telescopes and that frequently patients receive corrective spectacles or contact lenses for distance use.

Optical aids for distance vision fall into the following categories: spectacles or contact lenses, hand-held telescopes, head-mounted telescopes (bioptics or clip-ons), contact lens telescopes, "field expanders" (Fresnel, reverse telescopes, fisheye lenses), image intensifiers (nightscopes or goggles), and illumination control devices.

Spectacles and contact lenses. Because of their convenience and general acceptability, spectacles and contact lenses are the preferred form of distance vision aid if a good correction can be obtained. It is very desirable to have the correction improve the acuity in the peripheral field.

Hand-held telescopes. The small Galilean-type telescope of high magnification is used basically for orientation purposes and observation from a stationary position.

Head-mounted telescopes. Bioptics are prescription telescopes mounted on the corrective spectacle lens. The telescope is placed on either the upper or lower portion of the spectacle lens and the head is tilted to use the telescope for spotting. This kind of telescope has been used by low vision persons for driving automobiles (Kelleher, 1976; Keller & Eskridge, 1976). Clip-ons are clipped on to the spectacle frame, are easily removed, and are useful for spotting.

Contact lens telescopes. This system utilizes a minus lens in the contact lens in combination with a plus lens in a spectacle which is usually on an extended frame. One of the characteristics of this system is a ring scotoma. This system has also been used successfully for mobility purposes including driving.

Field expanders. The Fresnel paste-on, prism-type lenses have been used for field "expansion" (Gadbow, Finn, Dolan, & De l'Aune, 1976; Jose & Smith, 1976). They are strips of Fresnel prisms pasted on corrective distance lenses, just outside the field of view of persons with very narrow fields. Looking through the Fresnel prism allows the person to see a distorted view of objects to either side.

Generally, patients with fields of 10° or less will use Fresnel prisms most successfully and experience greater optical enhancement. Students with greater than 10° field generally benefit more from training in scanning techniques. In like manner, the sharper the acuity (20/200 or better), the better the chance for success (Jose & Smith, 1976; Gadbaw, *et al.*, 1976). Some of the advantages of Fresnel prisms (Apple, L., & Blasch, B., 1976) include reduction of nystagmus and gross head turns due to eccentric viewing. However, instruction should include the training in judgment of apparent and actual location of objects.

The use of reverse telescopes is sometimes called minification in that by reversing the telescope, the user can have a miniature image of a larger field of view than the client might be able to obtain with his own restricted field (DeBruin, 1977; Ricker, 1978; Drasdo, 1976; Holm, 1970). These require good central acuity.

Fisheye lenses can be mounted in spectacle frames and give a wider but highly distorted view for persons with narrow fields. They are infrequently prescribed because of the distortion and unusual appearance.

Nightscopes. The growth of "image intensifier" technology has allowed development of night goggles and night telescopes particularly useful to persons with impaired night vision (Coursey, McGowan, & Apple, 1972; Berson, Mehaffey, & Rabin, 1973; Davidson & Echols, 1976). Previous "nightscope" technology involved use of rather large infrared light source. Image intensifiers developed in the early 1960s photomultiply ambient light. Currently, most of the uses of the nightscope are in military and police surveillance work.

International Telephone and Telegraph (ITT) has produced applications of the image intensifiers: Pocketscope and Medical Pocketscope. The Medical is 5 in. (13 cm) long and weighs 12 oz (336 g). It can be adjusted in brightness gain up to about 600 times, depending on the requirements of the user. It is available only by ophthalmologist's prescription.

In the present state of the art, the nightscope and night-viewing goggles are used mostly in rural or other poorly lighted areas, and are not now in a form convenient for general nighttime mobility use. It is expected that further research will produce a more acceptable version.

Illumination Control Systems (sunglasses). The illumination needs of individuals vary as well as the sensitivity to light (photophobia). The specific aid should be selected depending on degree of problems the individual has with lighting and glare. Examples of such illumination control systems include AOlite True Tone absorption lenses, NoIRs plastic glasses, Visorettes, and Filterwell lenses.

TELESCOPES

Training in the use of the Galilean telescope most often falls to the mobility specialist. This fact merits some discussion of the characteristics of this type of telescopic system. The Galilean telescope is made up of relatively low power plus lens at the objective (lens closest to the object being viewed) and a relatively high power minus lens at the ocular (lens closest to the eye). A plus lens is a convex lens so that the objective lens brings the light rays from the object being viewed to a focus at a point somewhere between the lens and eye. The minus lens, which is really a concave lens, is separated from the ocular lens by a distance that is equal to the sum of the focal lengths of both lenses. Concave lenses spread the light rays wider apart and since the concave lens is of a higher power than the convex lens the result is that the light rays are spread over a larger area. The function of such optics is to enlarge the image received by the retina with the effect of making the image look both larger and closer.

Both the prescribing specialist and the mobility specialist will probably take an active part in the final selection of an appropriate telescope(s) following some general guidelines which have been found to suit client needs. It should be expected that the client will change telescopes during the course of training from one with low magnification and wide field to one with high magnification and narrower field. A wide field is needed at first in order to develop a system and skill in searching for useful information. The ability to find the information must precede the ability to acquire the information. Magnification is increased to the point which will insure that the low vision person can read needed information. Magnification beyond the minimum is a luxury at the cost of visual field, as given in the following example: the Selsi 7X to 12X focusable zoom prism monocular has a field of 5° to 6°; whereas; the Selsi 2.5X focusable has a field of 10°.

Apparent field of view is a concept which the mobility specialist should understand and be able to apply in the selection of the most effective low vision aid. As one looks at the magnified scene in the eyepiece, the eye itself covers a much greater field in moving from one extreme edge of the scene to the other. For example, 10X monoculars with 8° real field-of-view will have an apparent field angle of 80°. The apparent field is determined by multiplying the real field, which is usually listed in the aids catalogue, by the power of the instrument. Therefore, if you have a choice between using a 4X monocular with 8° field-of-view and a 6X monocular with an 8° field-of-view, the latter would be a better choice in terms of apparent field, since the former would have an apparent angle of 32° while the latter has an apparent angle of 48°.

The relative light efficiency (RLE) or relative brightness (RB) should also be taken into account. These terms are intended as a means of comparing how efficiently the aid transmits the light that is collected at the objective lens. RLE is generally 50 percent higher than RB. For the low vision person who is very sensitive to light it would be better to choose an aid with a lower value. For an individual with a very small pupil, a higher value might be more suitable. This is generally determined by the prescribing specialist.

It is also important to consider whether the optical aid is primarily for orientation, spotting and locating information, or for mobility purposes. Hand-held aids such as Selsi Monoculars, Miniscopes, and Miniatures, and the Zeiss and Walters' pocket monocular telescope (Fig. 2-7) are used primarily for orientation purposes as it is difficult to hold the hand steady while moving. Head-mounted telescope lenses such as the bioptic wide-angle lenses, (Fig. 3-7), Selsi Sportscopes, Vision Bioptic spectacle inserts, and Bioptic Keppler Telescope may be useful for both orientation and mobility.

The convenience and cosmetic appearance of telescopes are important too. Users tend to prefer telescopes that are small, lightweight, and as convenient as possible. Head-mounted telescopes of the sportglass type involve a cosmetic "obstacle" which can be overcome through practice, desensitization, and the basic rewards of the telescope. Bioptic telescopes are probably the most convenient telescope with a minimum of cosmetic problems. It appears, however, that the bioptic is being underprescribed and its great value and flexibility not adequately explored.

Genensky (1973) reports the use of binoculars for a variety of tasks including: determining the status of a traffic light, taking notes on or copying from a chalkboard, determining the number and destination of a bus, ascertaining a street address, locating an article that has become misplaced, watching a ball game, determining what friends and family really look like. Under some circumstances, a large powerful telescope may be quite helpful, for example, to a farmer looking for stock or a movie projectionist focusing the projector. These advantages plus the obvious advantages for orientation, spotting, and identification in mobility serve to reinforce the use and prescription of such aids.

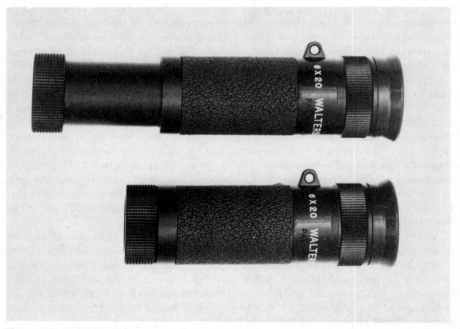

Figure 2-7. Walters' pocket monocular.

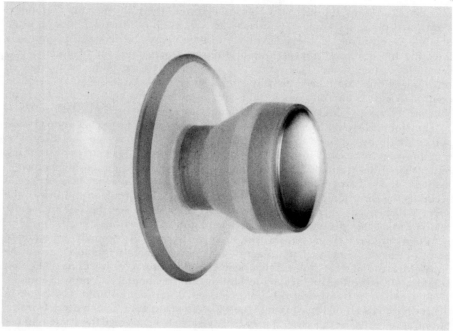

Figure 3-7. Head-mounted telescopic lens.

Training with Telescopes

The optics which make telescopes possible mandate some principles and guidelines for training which differ from those for persons using ordinary spectacles or unaided vision.

Initially three to five minutes of work with the telescopic system should be followed by a rest period. The time can be gradually increased when the student experiences no "complications" from shorter training periods.

Initial learning experiences should take place in controlled, visually simple environments with the client and target stationary. The basic learning task is to focus the aid and to locate selected object targets. Subsequent learning tasks involve development of horizontal and vertical scanning patterns.

Once the student can effectively locate stationary object targets, tasks involving tracking of moving objects can be introduced. It is helpful if the first tracking exercises involve a person who begins to walk slowly from a standing position. The client, sitting or standing, is bypassed by such a person moving parallel, perpendicular, and then diagonally to him. Verbal and tactual clues are used to help the client interpret the true position. These sequences lead naturally into adaptation to the distance distortion inherent in telescopic systems.

Once the client can visually relate to moving objects from a stationary position, positions can be reversed and the client moves up to, about, parallel, diagonally, etc. to stationary objects. Initial travel experiences utilizing head-mounted aids can be guided by an instructor; subsequently the low vision person may want to use a cane. A slight side-to-side scanning of the head may be used while walking in order to provide a larger field for side clearance. When making any turn, the head is kept in a low position (i.e., gaze directed near the feet) after turning the body, then lifted slightly. By lifting the head, the intended line of travel is cleared for obstacles. Dropping the head before beginning the turn prevents discomfort from "sweeping" telescope gaze in a 90° arc. If a curb, an irregular surface, or an obstacle is observed in the field of view, then it can be fixated by gradually lowering the head and approaching at a reduced pace until the obstacle can be satisfactorily negotiated (Davidson, 1972). As the client develops proficiency in traveling within controlled, visually simple environments, lessons can begin in controlled indoor and outdoor settings free of pedestrians and motor congestion (Burton, 1975; Cory & Prince, 1975; Quillman, 1977; Wiener, *1976; Staley, 1978).

The mobility specialist should make a list of the types of objects the low vision person might be expected to locate and then list the logical search and identification questions for each. This will help to develop an organized pattern of scanning rather than indiscriminate scanning. For example, bus stop sign, barbershop pole, mailbox. If the barbershop pole is the visual landmark, at what height does it occur? Is the direction of approach going to place the landmark on the side of the client which needs search training? Is the client able to see the red and white colors? From what distance and under what lighting conditions?

When outdoor training advances to street crossings it is extremely important to point out to the student that a magnifying optical system tends to decrease the apparent speed of a car approaching head-on; therefore, a car traveling at 40 mph would appear through binoculars to be traveling at about 11-12 mph (Thouless, 1968). Caution in training at this point is needed in order to build confidence in the individual's ability on judging when to cross a street on which there is traffic but no stop lights. In this case, it may be advisable to encourage the student to use auditory as well as visual cues (Burton, 1975).

Cory and Prince (1975), Quillman (1977), Burton (1975), and Staley (1978) have suggested lesson plans for most types of mobility situations or environments using optical aids: room familiarization; residential travel, including street crossings and numbering systems; traffic lights; business travel; store familiarization; and bus travel.

One final note about optical aids is their vulnerability to effects of weather. Wind may affect the low vision person's tolerance by causing excessive tearing. Some forms of precipitation may interfere to the extent that the aid is useless (Burton, 1975).

VISION REDUCTION EQUIPMENT

Vision reduction simulation is suggested here as a means for mobility specialists to better understand the learning experiences possible with severely reduced or distorted visual information (Apple, L., Apple, M., & Blasch, D., 1976; Blasch, B., 1972; Morris, 1976). Such simulation puts the instructor in the position of working through the same decision-making process that the student is likely to go through in interpreting the visual environment.

Increased familarization with severe visual impairment created via artificially reduced visual information should allow the mobility specialist to select appropriate environmental stimuli. Also, use of the vision reduction equipment can help the family to understand what is a "friendly" yet challenging environment for the client. Practicum with vision reduction equipment will call attention to problem areas in the environment or to visually guided behavior which must be further developed for adequate coping with reduced or distorted visual information.

Sessions using the vision reduction equipment should be of sufficient length or allow for repeated sessions. Persons using vision reduction equipment will

---

*Distance Vision Training with Optical Aids, a videotape available for sale or rental from the Social Service Department of Cleveland State University, 1983 E 24th Street, Cleveland, Ohio 44115.

observe a gradual accommodation to the reduced visual cues. It has been observed that there is a certain shock value associated with "instant" sensory deprivation, and persons are tempted to believe that they are experiencing what a visually impaired person is feeling. This reaction is typical of both the experience with the blindfold and with the equipment which artificially reduces visual information. Pastalan (1974) noted in his studies of the use of simulation to develop an empathic model for sensory problems associated with aging, that it is how one begins to perceive the environment after overcoming the preoccupation with the deficit that allows one to begin to concentrate on evaluation of the degraded visual information.

At present there are certain caveats and technical limitations concerning the construction of vision reduction equipment (Apple, L., Apple, M., & Blasch, D., 1976). Vision reduction equipment can only reproduce loss of visual acuity as measured by the Snellen chart and loss of peripheral field. The equipment should not be thought to reproduce or simulate any known eye condition. There is a real temptation during practicum with such equipment to want to compare the equipment with a particular client's eye condition, i.e., macular degeneration, congenital cataract, or retinitis pigmentosa. The equipment does not have the ability to reproduce some of the more subtle but functionally limiting characteristics of severe visual impairment such as visual fatigue, eye discomfort, phosphenes, and photophobia. Most of the equipment, in fact, does not reduce the wearer's visual acuity, but rather degrades visual stimulus so that it is equivalent to loss of visual acuity.

There are many ways to construct vision reduction equipment. Some are more crude than others and may not provide a satisfactory learning experience. There are several desirable characteristics for vision reduction equipment. The carrier frame should allow for as complete a field as possible. The user should be able to wear his own glasses comfortably under the equipment. The equipment should permit ventilation without allowing light through the carrier frame and should be lightweight. The lenses or templates should be easily changeable to allow for a variety of acuity of field restrictions or any combination of the two. Frosted lenses should have the frosting on the inside to prevent the smudging and soiling that results from handling.

Vision reduction equipment is made up of three basic components: the carrier or frame, acuity reduction panel or lens, and the field reduction panel. Suggested materials, include welding, safety, or ski goggles; plano, Fresnel, or high magnification lenses; mylar, wax paper, opaque templates, and small funnels (Apple, L., Apple, M., & Blasch, D., 1976).

There are a number of activities which should be used for practicum with vision reduction equipment. Two or more sessions are necessary in order to develop strategies for accomplishing a given task, as well as for development of skill. Suggested tasks include activities of daily living such as eating, dressing, and cooking; throwing and kicking games with balls of different colors; and standard orientation and mobility "runs" (National Mobility Centre, 1976). Observations made during this type of practicum should aid in the analysis and development of some effective ways of managing the situation under conditions of reduced vision. The kinds of questions raised by this experience are: Will the low vision person have to rely on color cues? Will he try to control the distance to obtain his preferred viewing distance? Will he scan, manipulate the lighting, etc.?

After the mobility specialist has gained experience viewing the environment using vision reduction equipment, he might wish to use the equipment on occasion in developing lesson plans, analyzing a particular route, or illustrating something to a sighted family member.

Up to this point, the chapter has dealt with methods and techniques and aids and equipment that may help the low vision person to increase his visual efficiency. Another, and equally important, facet of adjustment and training requires an understanding of the psychological effects of low vision.

PSYCHOSOCIAL ASPECTS

Psychosocial factors seriously affect attempts to rehabilitate low vision persons (Mehr, H., Mehr, E., & Ault, 1970). The mobility specialist providing training to such a client must have a good understanding of how the individual feels about the attitudes of the public, the family's role in the individual's life, the client's perception of his own vision, his ability to handle the stress created by poor vision and/or sight loss, and his motivation.

Despite statistics estimating that up to 94 percent of the severely visually impaired population has some useful vision, the general public tends to think in terms of the two extremes (blind or sighted). Lukoff and Whiteman (1970) studied the extent to which low vision persons identify with the blind, the sighted, or both populations, in terms of their willingness to accept offers of assistance. They found that the greater the amount of residual vision, the less willingness to accept offers of assistance. However, the amount of vision did not necessarily determine which population the low vision person identified with. Independence (unwillingness to accept assistance) was highest among persons who identified with both the blind and the sighted population, next highest among those who identified with the sighted population, and least among those who identified with the blind.

On the other hand, many low vision people are perceived as having no useful vision, as being blind. Many have never been taught or encouraged to use their remaining vision and some, for economic reasons, are reluctant to admit to the sight they do have.

It is extremely important for the mobility specialist at the outset of training to gain a good understanding of how the low vision person feels about himself and his situation. His attitudes will tend to reflect the attitudes of those around him toward visual difficulties. The low vision person who has been labeled "blind" may need considerable encouragement to begin to use his vision.

There are several strong motivating factors for the use of vision. The desire to cope with life with minimal assistance from others is a strong motivator as is the desire to work and support oneself and family. Use of his vision enables the low vision person to regain some measure of privacy by allowing him to take care of his own affairs (Mehr, E., Freid, A., & Mehr, H., 1975).

Even well-meaning people unwittingly betray misguided attitudes. While they realize that a totally blind person uses his other senses as a result of his visual loss, they do not understand that the low vision person often finds it necessary and productive to combine the use of the remaining vision with use of the other senses.

Many low vision people, especially those who have experienced visual loss in adulthood, identify strongly with the general public's attitudes toward blindness, especially during the early stages of visual loss. The mobility specialist must be very sensitive to the fear of blindness, or the hope for return of sight (Mehr, E., Freid, A., & Mehr, H., 1975). During the initial stages of adjustment to loss of sight, the nearer the training and equipment come to being defined as specifically for the blind, the more resistant the low vision person will be to training (Thackeray, 1975; Ault, 1976). No matter what the prognosis for vision is, it is impossible, impractical, and possibly deleterious to educate a person for eventual total loss of sight (Blasch, D., & Apple, L., 1967; Genensky, 1978). This applies even to low vision persons with progressive disorders such as diabetic retinopathy

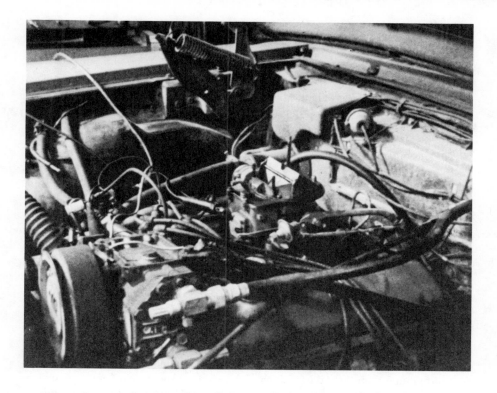

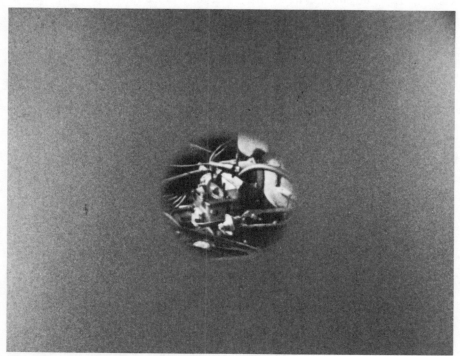

Figure 4-7. Normal vision—tunnel vision.

that can lead to total blindness. Diabetes and other progressive conditions result in a continuous series of adjustments to sight loss and an uncertain future. This contributes to the low vision person's feelings of insecurity and anxiety (Mehr, Mehr, & Ault, 1970).

The mobility specialist should concentrate on the technical and social skills that will allow the low vision person to function more independently and productively with his present level of impaired vision. While the specialist should not encourage the client to dwell on the possibility of return of vision, neither should he attempt to train for further loss of vision without strong clinical evidence.

The mobility specialist must also recognize the low vision child's special problems. Unlike the low vision adult who went through childhood, adolescence, and a considerable part, perhaps, of adulthood as a normally sighted person, the low vision child may have developed as a "blind" child not encouraged or trained to use his vision. He may be experientially deprived. Sophisticated guidance is needed to keep this child from assuming an inappropriate role and identity. Marshal (1969) suggests that because vision is learned, how well a child learns to see may affect his development and personality.

Closely related to the attitudes of the general public and authorities are the attitudes of the client's family and friends. It is strongly recommended that the client's family and friends be assisted to understand the low vision person's ability to function. Family members and friends not only may share the general public's attitudes but may have also developed specific understandable fears, doubts, embarrassments, false perceptions, and negative attitudes (Glass, 1970). These can be diminished considerably when the family and friends go through a sequence of systematic observation, guided discussion, and didactic experience.

A program for family and friends should include observation of one or more low vision persons functioning in a variety of social and mobility situations, under a variety of lighting conditions, and the viewing of films* and reading of print materials followed by discussion of them (Veterans Administration, 1974). The film, *Not without sight*, discusses several common eye conditions. It shows the types of vision experienced as a result of these eye conditions and something about the kinds of techniques and aids considered helpful. Examples of normal vision and the visual impairment are shown in Fig. 4-7, tunnel vision; Fig. 5-7, macular degeneration; and Fig. 6-7, cataract.

Positive attitudes and appropriate methods of dealing with problems are acquired via active didactic participation in the rehabilitation process including some experience under the blindfold or using vision reduction equipment.

The family should also be involved in realistic planning for the future along with the low vision person and the total rehabilitation team. One of the rehabilitation team's main functions is to educate and encourage the total family to handle problems by using their own ingenuity and resources available to them in their community.

There are several other psychosocial factors that the mobility specialist will encounter. The low vision person's understanding and/or ability to articulate what he sees frequently poses communications difficulties with the mobility specialist and others. Low vision persons tend to find it easier and more profitable to explain the limitations arising from their poor vision to only those people with whom they work every day or meet frequently socially, rather than to persons with whom they come into contact on a more casual basis (Herkes, 1978).

Because many persons with low vision claim less vision than they are theoreti-

---

Not without sight, 35 mm, color, American Foundation for the Blind, 1973; *What to do when you meet a blind person*, 35 mm, color, American Foundation for the Blind, 1971.

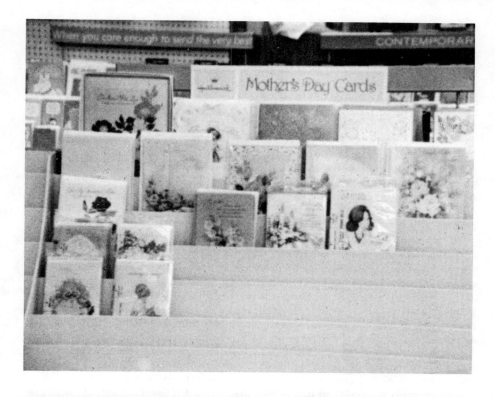

Figure 5-7. Normal vision—macular degeneration.

cally supposed to have, several factors must be examined before proceeding. First, as mentioned previously, the possible reasons why the low vision person is claiming less vision than he has—fear of losing economic benefits, having been labeled blind, never having received training in use of vision, lack of motivation, fear of stress and failure, etc. The mobility specialist must also be aware of his own feelings toward low vision and blindness. If the client is sensitive about his visual loss or deficit, fostering and maintaining a meaningful relationship should be uppermost, not pursuit of discussions on visual loss.

Frequent questioning of the low vision person about his vision during the initial stages of adjustment may lead to resistance or rejection of the total rehabilitation program. For example, the low vision person whose income depends on being labeled legally blind may become suspicious that training represents an attempt to remove him from that category. Conversely, extensive questioning may reinforce denial of the impairment—and the training that will ease it—if the person is using that defense mechanism.

Proper timing, reassurance and the appropriate approach when discussing level of vision with the client may help to save the low vision person from months or years of frustrating attempts to feign excessive loss of vision. Conversely, some students try to act as though they see more than they actually do usually out of fear of losing or jeopardizing status, friendship, or employment possibilities (Herkes, 1978). Premature confrontation regarding visual status may force a low vision person into physically hazardous activities, keep him from attempting positive activities, and/or destroy whatever personal relationship has been developed. Any inference on the mobility specialist's part that the client has an "intent to deceive" based on superficial evidence will be more destructive to rehabilitation than the client's own trial and error method of coming to terms with his visual loss.

The mobility specialist should not be discouraged if several meetings with the client are necessary before motivation for training appears. An initial contact might give the mobility specialist the impression that motivation is lacking and attitudes are negative while further meetings and exploration may reveal capabilities and goals in the client that had not appeared earlier. The mobility specialist must constantly evaluate and frequently revise his expectations of the client to correlate with training, counseling, visual equipment, feedback, adaptations, and learning.

If capability increases as the client becomes familiar with places and situations, further development of mobility skills should be encouraged. Amount of vision should still not be raised or questioned. Many low vision persons see better at some times and under some conditions than at others. In these situations, again do not question vision but repeatedly tell such persons that it is normal to experience such differences.

Motivation to use remaining vision often plays an important role in a client's willingness to communicate how much vision he has and to receive training.

Negative reactions and behaviors are common indicators of stress in low vision persons. "For a partially sighted person a face-to-face situation may demand constant alertness or even bluff in order that an aspiration to be treated as 'sighted' is confirmed. Unless the parties are well known to one another, there is plenty of opportunity on both sides for impatience, body tension, anxiety, withdrawal, fatigue, and frustration" (Thackeray, 1975, p. 103). The person who has recently experienced loss of vision is usually preoccupied with a multiplicity of problems. Problems concerning employment or schooling, with the family and friends, with daily living, with coping with the environment in general, and gathering and assimilating information, particularly about training. Statements and responses of persons in this stage of adjustment often seem to indicate memory loss, loss of the

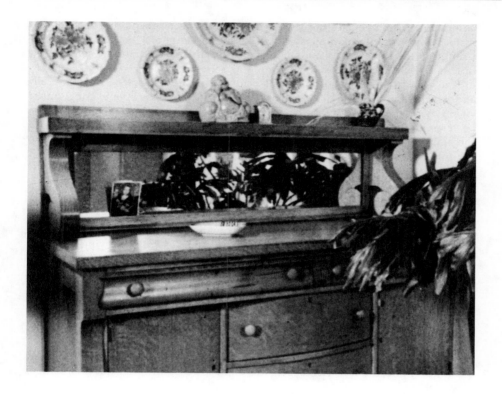

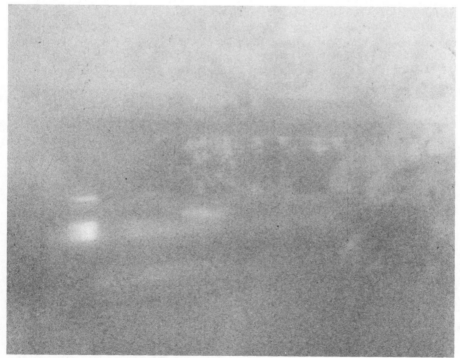

Figure 6-7. Normal vision—cataract.

ability to reason, negativity. Most of these behaviors are normal reactions to distorted visual information and may lead to frustrations that cause extreme irritability, fatigue, loss of judgment, and uncooperative or nonresponsive attitudes (Thackeray, 1975; Ault, 1976).

The very act of seeing with residual vision can create stress. It can be physically and psychologically tiring (Thackeray, 1975). Yet its efficiency and range make vision by far our most effective sensory modality. Even when restricted it still can be very effective in enabling a person to gather needed information. The better we can aid a person in understanding its limitations and finding the best methods to use this remaining vision, the more effectively he will be able to function.

CONCLUSION

Knowledge about the special services needed by persons with low vision and the ways in which these services are best provided is growing. Rehabilitation professionals, including mobility specialists, will find that the percentage of their clients who have some useful vision keeps expanding. Because they are trained to help a client make use of all sensory cues for the purpose of improving functioning and importance, mobility specialists can play a pivotal role in the development of low vision services. As techniques and practice evolve and experience is gained, mobility specialists will undoubtedly learn to work as successfully with visual cues as with aural and tactile ones.

The interdisciplinary approach to the treatment of low vision clients should address itself to two highly significant issues which were identified and developed by a committee of low vision persons themselves: The low vision person's right to make full use of vision through the provision of all necessary aids, services, and techniques; and the low vision person's right to recognition of his capabilities, potential, and needs.

One factor that has often confused or complicated the provision of treatment and services to low vision persons is that the disability is invisible to most people. While it certainly does not have the visibility of total blindness or paraplegia and other major crippling diseases and disorders, it can be just as devastating in many areas of life such as mobility, work, daily living, and reading.

Some of the concepts which must be considered when addressing the major aspects of this functional disability are:

1. Aids, services, and techniques should "pay their own way" in terms of increased function

2. Low vision is a *separate* disability and low vision persons should not be encouraged to "pass" for either sighted or blind

3. Discrimination against low vision persons takes place both when they use aids and when they do not use aids

4. Training and other methods of facilitating personal adjustment are crucial in the areas where there are functioning problems.

The possibilities for successful rehabilitation of low vision persons when the appropriate interdisciplinary approach is used are clear. There is no other disability group in which such great improvements in functioning can be obtained by a majority of the population. Using prescribed techniques, the cost of rehabilitating a low vision person is usually far less than the cost of leaving him with his disability. Measured in terms of return of function, comprehensive low vision services are highly cost-effective.

Finally, as recognition of the need for increased services to the low vision population increases, several critical issues have emerged which must be faced by mobility specialists and other vision rehabilitation professionals:

1. Funding for low vision services must have a broader base than it does at present. This low-cost, highly-effective service is not covered by most federal programs and private insurance policies. Consequently, a substantial number of low vision persons who could benefit from services either cannot afford them or have no access to them

2. The need for expansion and proliferation of the kinds of services already available and a clearer concept of comprehensive low vision service

3. The need for uniform reporting and data collection systems that cover the effectiveness of various techniques, aids, and comprehensive care programs

4. The need for growth in strength and vitality of the professional organizations in the area of low vision

5. The need for expansion of high-quality low vision training programs in disciplines in which practitioners are likely to be responsible for the care of the low vision persons

6. The absolute necessity, if an interdisciplinary approach is going to work, that the various disciplines involved learn to work effectively together for the development of these services.

Bibliography

Abernathy, C., & Leibowitz H. The effect of feedback on luminance thresholds for peripherally presented stimuli. *Perception & Psychophysics*, 1971, **10**(3), 172-174.

Allen, D. Orientation and mobility for persons with low vision. *Journal of Visual Impairment and Blindness*, January 1977, **71**(1), 13-15.

Allport, F. H. *Theories of perception and the concept of structure*. New York: Wiley & Sons, 1955.

American Foundation for the Blind. *Directory of Agencies Serving the Visually Handicapped in the U.S.* 20th Edition. New York: Author, 1978.

Apple, L., Apple, M., & Blasch, D. The artificial reduction of visual cues as a means of preparing training programs for low vision clients. *Low Vision Abstracts*, Fall 1976 **II**(4) [4-6].

Apple, L., & Blasch, B. (Co-directors) *Report of the Workshop on Low Vision Mobility, Western Michigan University, Kalamazoo, Mich., Nov. 3-5 1975*. Washington, D.C.: Veterans Administration, Department of Medicine & Surgery, 1976.

Apple, L., & May, M. *Distance vision and perceptual training: A concept for use in mobility training of low vision clients*. New York: American Foundation for the Blind, 1970.

Apple, M. Subjective field examination, *Low Vision Abstracts*, Fall 1973, **1**(5), 8-13.

Ault, C. The marginal man. (Unpublished manuscript.) Western Blind Rehabilitation Center. Palo Alto, Ca.: Veterans Administration Hospital, 1976.

Barraga, N. *Increased visual behavior in low vision children*. New York: American Foundation for the Blind, 1964.

Barraga, N., Collins, M., & Hollis, J. Development of efficiency in visual functioning: A literature analysis. *Journal of Visual Impairment and Blindness*, Nov. 1977, 387-391.

Bender, M., & Krieger, H. Visual functions in perimetrically blind fields. *Archives of Neurology and Psychiatry*, January 1951, **65**, 72-79.

Bender, M., & Teuber, H. Disorders in the visual perception of motion. *Transactions of the American Neurological Association*, 1948, 191-193.

Bender, M., & Teuber, H. Phenomena of fluctuation, extinction, and completion in visual perception. *Archives of Neurology and Psychiatry*, January 1946, **55**(29-33), 627-658.

Berman, R. Fundamentals of the visual fields. *Review of Optometry*, Sept. 1978, **115**(9), 53-64.

Berson, E., Mehaffey, L., & Rabin, A. A night vision device as an aid for patients with retinitis pigmentosa. *Archives of Ophthalmology*, August 1973, **90**(2), 112-116.

Blasch, B. The use of the long cane by clients with visual acuity of 10/200 as an aid or an identification device. (Unpublished.) Abstracted *Low Vision Abstracts*, 1975, **2**(2), 8.

Blasch, B. B. Simulation: An approach to low vision research. *Low Vision Abstracts*, Spring 1972, **1**(2) 1)2.

Blasch, D., & Apple, L. Severe Visual Impairment, Pt. I. *Long Cane News*, **II**(1), 1967, 1-4.

Brandt, T., Dichgans, J., & Konig, E. Differential effects of central vs. peripheral vision on egocentric and exocentric motion perception. *Experimental Brain Research*, 1973, **16**, 476-491.

Burg, A. Lateral visual field as related to age and sex. *Journal of Applied Psychology*, 1968, **51**(1), 10-15.

Burton, R. A guide for training clients to utilize low vision distance aids for mobility. (Unpublished paper.) Orientation and Mobility Program, Western Michigan University, Fall 1975. Abstracted *Low Vision Abstracts*, 1976, **2**(4) 10.

Carroll, H., & Hibbert, F. The perceptual ability of a class of partially sighted children. *The Visually Handicapped International Archives for Research*, 1973, **3**, 106-118.

Carter, K., & Carter, C. Itinerant low vision services. *New Outlook for the Blind*, June 1975, **69**(6), 255-260, 265.

Colenbrander, A. Dimensions of visual performance. *Ophthalmology Transactions, American Academy of Ophthalmology and Otolaryngology*, 1977, **83**, 332-337.

Cory, D., & Prince, J. A report on the incorporation of low vision aids into the orientation and mobility program of low vision clients. (Unpublished paper) Orientation and Mobility Program, Western Michigan University, Fall 1975, abstracted *Low Vision Abstracts*, 1976, **2**(4)8.

Coursey, T. Telescopes as low vision aids, unpublished manuscript, Denver, Colorado, 1976.

Coursey, T., McGowan, D., & Apple, L. Night viewing goggles for night-blind travelers. *Bulletin of Prosthetic Research*, Spring 1972, 191-194.

Davidson, T. Disaster or not? Telescopics for distance vision in mobility. *Low Vision Abstracts*, **1**(2), Spring 1972, 3-8.

Davidson, W., & Echols, C. The development of the Generation II as an aid for patients with retinitis pigmentosa and night blindness. *Optometric Weekly*, Sept. 16, 1976, **67**(38), 47-56.

DeBruin, D. A detailed look at expanding the visual field with a reversed monocular. (Unpublished paper) Orientation and Mobility Program, Western Michigan University, Kalamazoo, Mich., 1977, abstracted *Low Vision Abstracts*, Fall 1977, **3**(2), 8.

Dichgans, J., & Brandt, T. The psychophysics of visually induced perception of self-motion and tilt. In F. O. Schmitt & F. G. Worden (Eds.) *The Neurosciences* III. Cambridge, Mass.: MIT Press, 1974, 123-129.

Drasdo, N. Techniques, instruments, cases: Visual field expanders. *American Journal of Optometry and Physiological Optics*, 1976, Pt. 1, 464-467.

Ensor, S. L. Orientation and mobility project: A low vision orientation and mobility evaluation. (Unpublished paper.) Orientation and Mobility Program, University of Northern Colorado, Dec. 1976. Abstracted *Low Vision Abstracts*, Fall 1977, **3**(2), 7.

Faye, E. & Hood, C. (Eds.) *Low vision*. Springfield, Illinois: Charles C Thomas, 1975a.

Faye, E., & Hood, C. Low vision services in an agency: Structure and philosophy. *New Outlook for the Blind*, June 1975b, **69**(6), 241-148.

Ferree, C., Rand, G. & Hardy, C. Refraction for the peripheral field of vision. *A.M.A. Archives of Ophthalmology*, 1931, **5**, 717-731.

Friedman, D., Kayne, H., Tallman, C., & Asarkof, J. Comprehensive low vision care: Pt. II. *New Outlook for the Blind*, May 1975, **69**(5), 207-211.

Frostig, M., & Horne, D. *The Frostig program for development of visual perception; Teacher's guide*. Chicago: Follet Publishing Co., 1964.

Gadbaw, P., Finn, W., Dolan, M., & De l'Aune, W. Parameters of success in the use of Fresnel prism lenses. *Optical Journal & Review of Optometry*, Dec. 1976. **113**(12) 41-43.

Genensky, S. *Binoculars: A long-ignored aid for the partially sighted*. R-1402-HEW, Nov. 1973, Rand Corp.

Genensky, S. Data concerning the partially sighted and the functionally blind. *Journal of Visual Impairment and Blindness*, May 1978, **72**(5), 177-180.

Genensky, S. Functional classification system of visually impaired to replace the legal definition of blindness. Memorandum RM-6246-RC, Santa Monica, Calif.: Rand Corp., 1970.

Getman, G., & Kephart, N. *Developmental vision*. A series of papers released by the Optometric Extension Program to its membership. Dec. 1950-Sept. 1951, G. N. Getman; Oct. 1957-Sept. 1959, G. N. Getman and N. C. Kephart; Oct. 1959-Sept. 1960, G. N. Getman. Duncan, Okla.: Optometric Extension Program.

Gibson, E. *Principles of perceptual learning and development*. New York: Appleton-Century-Crofts, 1969.

Gibson, J. *The perception of the visual world.* Boston: Houghton Mifflin, 1950.

Gibson, J. The visual perception of objective motion and subjective motion. *Psychological Review,* 1954, **61,** 304-314.

Gibson, J. The senses considered as a perceptual system. Boston: Houghton Mifflin, 1966.

Glass, E. The social psychological adjustment to low residual vision. In Apple, L., & Apple, M. (Eds.) *Proceedings of the low vision conference—visual abilities—their behavioral assessment and possible methods for their improvement in the individual with severe visual impairment.* U.S. Office of Ed. Grant #0-8-071112-2995(607), Nov. 29-Dec. 1, 1970.

Goodrich, G. L., & Quillman, R. D. Training eccentric viewing. *Journal of Visual Impairment and Blindness,* 1977, **71**(9), 377-381.

Graybiel, A., Jokl, E., & Traff, C. Russian studies in vision in relation to physical activity and sports. *Research Quarterly,* 1955, **26,** 212-223.

Green, H., & Spencer, J. Drugs with possible ocular side effects. London: Barrie & Rockliff, 1969.

Gregory, R. *Eye and brain.* New York: McGraw-Hill, 1966.

Gregory, R. & Wallace, J. Recovery from early blindness: A case study. *Experimental Psychology Society Monograph No. 2.* Cambridge, 1963.

Hebb, D. O. Organization of behavior. New York: Wiley & Sons, 1949.

Held, R. Dissociation of visual functions by deprivation and rearrangement. *Psychologische Forshung,* 1968, **31,** 338-348.

Held, R. (Ed.) *Image, object and illusion.* San Francisco: W. H. Freeman & Co., 1974.

Held, R. Two modes of processing spatially distributed visual stimulation. In F. O. Schmitt, (Ed.) *The Neurosciences: Second Study Program.* New York: Rockefeller University Press, 1970.

Hennessey, J. A pragmatic approach to the orientation and mobility needs of a low vision client. *Blindness Annual,* AAWB 1974-75, 80-88.

Herkes, J. Partial sight: Some psycho-social aspects. *The New Beacon,* March 1978, **62**(731), 57-59.

Holcomb, J. & Goodrich, G. Eccentric viewing training. *Journal of the American Optometric Association,* 1976, **47**(11), 1438-1443.

Holm, C. A simple method for widening restricted visual fields. *Archives of Ophthalmology,* 1970, **84,** 611-612.

Holmes, R. *Training residual vision in adolescents educated previously as non-visual.* Unpublished master's thesis, Illinois State University, 1967.

Hoover, R. A new look at the definition of blindness. In *Proceedings of the Thirty-first Convention of the American Association of Workers for the Blind.* Washington, D.C.: 1957.

Hughes, R. K. Orientation and mobility for the partially sighted. *International Journal for the Education of the Blind,* May 1967, 119-120.

Humphrey, N. Vision in a monkey without striate cortex. *Perception,* 1974, **3**(3), 241-255.

Ingle, D. Two visual mechanisms underlying the behavior of fish. *Psychologische Forschung,* 1967, **31,** 44-51.

Johnson, C. Some physiological considerations for visual training. *Low Vision Abstracts,* 1976, **2**(4), 1-3.

Johnson, C., & Leibowitz, H. Practice, refractive error, and feedback as factors affecting peripheral movement thresholds. *Perception and Psychophysics,* 1974, **15,** 276-280.

Johnson, C., Millodot, M., & Lamont, A. Peripheral vision acuity and refractive error: Evidence for "two visual systems"? *Perception and Psychophysics,* 1976, **20**(6), 460-462.

Jose, R., Cummings, J., & McAdams, L. The model low vision clinical service: An interdisciplinary vision rehabilitation program. *New Outlook for the Blind,* June 1975, **69**(6) 249-254.

Jose, R., & Shane, *Help me become everything I can be.* N.Y.: American Foundation for the Blind In Press.

Jose, R. & Smith, A. Increasing peripheral field awareness with Fresnel prisms. *Optical Journal and Review of Optometry,* 1976, **113**(12), 33-37.

Kahn, H. & Moorhead, H. *Statistics on blindness in the model reporting area, 1969-1970.* DHEW Pub. No. 73-427. Washington, D.C.: Government Printing Office, 1973.

Kelleher, D. Driving with low vision, from the patient's perspective. *American Journal of Optometry and Physiological Optics,* Aug. 1976, **53**(8), 440-441.

Keller, J., & Eskridge, J. Telescopic lenses and driving. *American Journal of Optometry and Physiological Optics,* Nov. 1976, **53**(11), 756-759.

Kephart, N. C. Visual behavior of the retarded child. *American Journal of Optometry,* 1958, **35,** 125-133.

Kerr, J. Visual resolution in the periphery. *Perception and Psychophysics,* 1971, **9,** 375-378.

Kleitman, N., & Blier, Z. Color and from discrimination in the periphery of the retina. *American Journal of Physiology.* 1928, **85,** 178-190.

Koestler, F. *The unseen minority.* New York: David McKay Co., Inc., 1976.

Kohler, I. Experiments with goggles. *Scientific American,* 1962, **206,** 62-72.

Kohler, I. Past, present, and future of the recombination procedures. *AFB Research Bulletin,* No. 29, June 1975, New York: American Foundation for the Blind, 118-120.

Leibowitz, H., Johnson, C., & Isabelle, E. Peripheral motion detection and refractive error. *Science,* 1972, **177,** 1207-1208.

Leibowitz, H., Johnson, C., & Isabelle, E. Peripheral motion detection and refractive error. *Science,* **189,** 1975, 1207-1208.

Leibowitz, H., Meyers, N., & Grant, D. Radial localization of a single stimulus as a function of luminance and duration of exposure. *Journal of the Optical Society of America,* 1955a, **45**(2), 76-78.

Leibowitz, H., Meyers, N., & Grant, D. Frequency of seeing and radical localization of single and multiple visual stimuli. *Journal of Experimental Psychology,*1955b, **50**(6), 369-373.

Lotmar, W., & Lotmar, T. Peripheral astigmatism in the human eye: Experimental data and theoretical model predictions. *Journal of the Optical Society of America,* 1974, **64,** 510-513.

Low, F. N. *Effect of training on acuity of peripheral vision.* Report No. 68, Civil Aeronautics Admin., Division of Research, 1946a.

Low, F. Some characteristics of peripheral visual performance. *American Journal of Physiology,* 1946b, **146,** 573-584.

Low, F. Peripheral visual acuity. *AMA Archives of Ophthalmology,* 1951, **45,** 80-99.

Lukoff, I., & Whiteman, M. *The social sources of adjustment to blindness.* New York: American Foundation for the Blind, 1970.

Mandelbaum, J., & Sloan, L. Peripheral visual acuity with special reference to scotopic illumination. *American Journal of Ophthalmology,* 1947, **30,** 581-588.

Margach, C. Pacific University, College of Optometry, "Spatial perceptions in low-visioned persons." Presentation at 1968 Biennial Conference of AEVH, Toronto, Canada, June 1968.

Marshall, G.H. Detecting visual dysfunction. *Special Education,* Sept. 1969, **58**(3), 21-22.

May, M. *Low vision literature pertaining to education and rehabilitation: A keyword index.* New York: American Foundation for the Blind, 1978.

Mehr, E., & Freid, A. *Low vision care.* Chicago, Ill.: Professional Press, Inc., 1975.

Mehr, E., Freid, A., & Mehr, H. Psychological and sociological factors. In E. Mehr and A. Freid *Low Vision Care.* Chicago, Ill.: Professional Press, inc., 1975.

Mehr, H., Mehr, E. & Ault, C. Psychological aspects of low vision rehabilitation. *American Journal Optometry & Archives American Academy Optometry,* August 1970, **47**(8), 605-612.

Minor, J. (personal correspondence with Loyal E. Apple) May 19, 1976, Northeastern Rehabilitation Center, 301 Washington Ave., Albany, N.Y. 12206.

Montgomery County Board of Education. *Vision stimulation.* Bulletin No. 227, Rockville, Maryland, 1969.

Moore, L. The Moore contact lens-spectacle system. *Nearpoint,* Spring 1976, **1**(5).

Morris, A., & Horne, E. (Eds.) *Visual search techniques.* Washington, D.C.: National Academy of Sciences, National Research Council, Publication 712, 1960.

Morris, O. Simulation of visual impairments as a training technique. *New Outlook for the Blind,* Dec. 1976, **70**(10), 417-419.

National Center for Health Statistics. *Characteristics of visually impaired persons: United States-July 1963-June 1964.* Visual and Health Statistics Series 10, No. 6. DHEW Pub. No. 1000. Washington, D.C.: Government Printing Office, 1968.

National Mobility Centre. Low vision practicum. *Report of the Annual Course/Conference, 6-7 May, 1976, Birmingham, England,* 5-8.

Oppel, D., Pascuzzi, D., Pikovsky, R., Williams, J.A., & Moore, M.W. Utilization of visual information functional signs. *Low Vision Abstracts,* Spring 1977, **3**(1), 4-13.

Orientation and Mobility Section. *Orientation and Mobility Indoor Functional Vision Evaluation.* Palo Alto, Ca.: Western Blind Rehabilitation Center, Veterans Administration Hospital, May 1970.

Pastalan, L. The simulation of age-related sensory losses: A new approach to the study of environmental barriers. *New Outlook for the Blind,* Oct. 1974, **68**(8), 356-362.

Quillman, R. D. Utilization of telescopic lenses in low vision mobility. *Long Cane News,* November 1977, **10**(2), 3-9.

Quillman, R. D. & Goodrich, G. L. Eccentric viewing training: A case report. *Long Cane News,* Nov. 1977, **10**(2) 9-14.

Richterman, H. Mobility instruction for the partially seeing. Ad Hoc Committee Meeting, Washington, D.C. April 18, 1966.

222

Ricker, K. Visual field wideners: A personal report. *Journal of Visual Impairment and Blindness*, Jan. 1978, **72**(1), 28-29.

Riesen, A. Studying perceptual development using the technique of sensory deprivation. *Journal Nervous & Mental Diseases*, 1961, **132**(1), 21-25.

Schneider, G. Two visual systems. *Science*, 1969, **163**, 895-902.

Smith, A. (Narrator). "Consider Me Seeing" (Videotape). Documentary of low vision stimulation program for mobility purposes at Western Pennsylvania School for Blind. (1974) A/V Dept., Hillman Library, University of Pittsburgh, Pittsburgh, Pa.

Sprague, W. Low vision: Its impact on an agency. *Journal of Visual Impairment and Blindness*, **71**, 1977, 197-202.

Staley, K. Low vision lesson plans for Illinois Visually Handicapped Institute Unpublished paper. Orientation and Mobility Program, Western Michigan University, Kalamazoo, Mich., April 1978, abstracted *Low Vision Abstracts* Fall 1978 **4**(2).

Stein, H., & Slatt, B. *The ophthalmic assistant: Fundamentals and clinical practice*. St. Louis: C. W. Mosby Co., 1968.

Teuber, H., Battersby, W., & Bender, M. *Visual field defects after penetrating missile wounds of the brain*. Cambridge, Mass.: Harvard University Press, 1960.

Thackeray, D. People with limited residual vision. In V. Carver, Gill, J., Reid, F. (Eds.) *The handicapped person in the community. Unit 6*. London: The Open University Press, 1975.

Thouless, R. Apparent size and distance in vision through a magnifying system. *British Journal of Psychology*, 1968, **59**(2), 111-118.

Tobin, M. *A study in the improvement of visual efficiency in children registered as blind*. Birmingham, England: University of Birmingham Research Centre for the Education of the Visually Handicapped, 1973.

Trevarthen, C. Two mechanisms of vision in primates. *Psychologische Forschung*, 1968, **31**, 338-348.

Valvo, A. Behavior patterns and visual rehabilitation after early and long-lasting blindness. *American Journal of Ophthalmology*, January 1968, **65**(1), 19-24.

Valvo, A. *Sight restoration after long-term blindness: The problems and behavior patterns of visual rehabilitation*. New York: American Foundation for the Blind, 1971.

Veterans Administration. *Program Guide Social Work Service* (G-3, M-2, Part XI). Washington, D.C.: Author July 25, 1974.

von Senden, M. *Space and sight: The perception of space and shape in the congenitally blind before and after operation*. (trans. Peter Heath). Glencoe, Ill.: Free Press, 1960.

Welsh, R., & Wiener, W. *Travel in adverse weather*. New York: American Foundation for the Blind, 1976.

Wiener, W. *Distance vision training with optical aids*. (Videotape) Cleveland, Ohio: Social Service Department, Cleveland State University, 1976.

Williams, D., & Gassel, M. Visual function in patients with homonymous hemianopia. Pt. I. The visual fields. Pt. III. The completion phenomenon: Insight and attitude to the defect, and visual functional efficiency. *Brain*, 1962, 85; and 1963, 86.

Wilson, J. McVeigh, V. McMahon, J., Bauer, A., & Richardson, P.C. Early intervention: The right to sight. *Education of the Visually Handicapped*, Fall 1976, **7**(3), 83-90.

Wood, A. (Ed.) *Instructional manual for visual skills*. Palo Alto, Ca.: Western Blind Rehabilitation Center, Veterans Administration Hospital, 1975.

Psychosocial Dimensions

Richard L. Welsh

The impact of psychological and social variables on the physical and cognitive behaviors of people is well known and readily accepted. People generally believe that nervousness or a strong desire to win can affect the success of the athlete's performance. Fear of failure or firm confidence can influence a student's performance on an examination. Similarly, the presence of others who support one's efforts can influence success, just as the attention of those who threaten can detract from performance.

The interaction of the emotions, the mind, and the body has been demonstrated in the research of a number of disciplines. The reality of psychosomatic disorders has been established in medicine. The decisions of others have been shown to influence the judgments of subjects in studies of perception. Studies of experimentally induced fear have demonstrated the impact of that psychological variable on a wide range of physical and cognitive behaviors. The influence of personality factors on the academic performance of culturally disadvantaged students has been documented.

Psychological and social variables play an important role in understanding the cognitive and physical behaviors that result in orientation and mobility. A common sense understanding of these variables seems quite prevalent among mobility specialists, yet relatively little formal research has been done to explicate them. This lack of systematic study may reflect the complexity of these variables and the highly individualized nature of human experiences in this area. It may also reflect the lack of sophistication in our current ability to study and understand the psychosocial dimensions of our human conditions.

While psychological and social variables are distinct and can be considered separately for the sake of certain types of analysis, efforts to understand their impact in applied situations must consider their interaction. Ekehammer (1975) reviewed the interactionist position on the study of personality and contrasted it with two other theoretical positions which emphasized either the "psychic structures" of the individual or environmental and situational factors as the primary determinants of behavior. According to Ekehammer, neither the person *per se* nor the situation *per se* can be emphasized, but the interaction of these two factors is the main source of variations in behavior.

Similarly, social psychology has grown as a result of the importance attached to understanding the impact of social stimuli on the behavior of the individual. The reactions of others to an individual's visual impairment seem to have a significant effect on the feelings, thoughts, and actions of that person. Support for this position is reviewed in Delafield's (1976) discussion of the concept of adjustment to blindness.

An underlying assumption of this discussion is that many if not all of the

225

psychological and social variables which appear to have an effect on the visually impaired person's ability to move through the environment in a purposeful way can best be understood through a dual and integrated focus. Insight into reactions of an individual will come only through an analysis of the interaction of a person possessing certain characteristics in a specific situation with its own characteristics, especially social ones.

A second basic assumption underlying the material presented in this chapter is that the impact and the importance of each variable on each visually impaired person is likely to be highly individualized. There has been little, if any, research which supports the concept of a special psychology of blindness. On the contrary, visual impairment occurs in all types of people. Research does seem to suggest that the basic personality of the visually impaired person has a greater impact on the subsequent behavior than does the blindness (Lokshin, 1957; Hallenback, 1967).

The goal of the chapter is to bring into focus certain characteristic reactions to disability that may be of assistance in understanding the particular experience of individuals who suffer visual loss. It will be evident from the discussion that focusing on one factor at a time can distort the reality to the extent that each factor is closely related to the others discussed.

The process of learning to move independently through the environment is integral to every phase of personal and social development. The personality of the individual emerges along with the ability to move independently as the one very much affects the other.

MOBILITY & ADJUSTMENT

A number of writers such as Wilson (1967) have suggested that immobility can create psychosocial problems. It may lead to "feelings of hopelessness, hostility, and dread of the outside world" (Wilson, 1967, p. 287). It can also create social problems since the person must be more dependent on others, which has the effect of increasing the sense of burden that others feel and further diminishing their expectations of the visually impaired person.

Studies of the adjustment of visually impaired persons done by Bauman and Yoder (1966) and Graham (1965) have indicated that success in mobility is associated with good adjustment to visual disability. It is impossible to say which comes first, whether good adjustment to a visual loss results in good mobility or whether the reverse is true. An interactive effect is likely to be closer to the truth which is also true for the other psychosocial variables that we will consider. The interaction between successful orientation and mobility and the self-concept, feelings of independence, motivation for rehabilitation, the attitude of the family, and the ability to cope with people on the street is complex and reciprocal. A positive self-concept can be both a cause and an effect of success in mobility. On the other hand, a negative self-concept can result from lack of independent mobility or can make progress toward independent functioning more difficult. Similarly, a sense of independence can contribute greatly to a person's success in learning to travel or can result from success in a particular mobility task. Excessive dependency, however, can hinder improvement in mobility or can be a by-product of the person's inability to move successfully. Such is the nature of psychosocial variables.

To reflect this complexity and reciprocity between orientation and mobility and psychosocial variables, seven such variables that seem to be particularly relevant will be considered. The discussion of each variable encompasses both positive and negative dimensions of the variable that seem to contribute to and/or result from orientation and mobility.

Before discussing the seven variables, some understanding concerning two components of the mobility training process that will be mentioned frequently in relation to several of the variables must be established. These components, the dimensions of mobility training which are most helpful in transforming negative psychosocial experiences into positive ones, are the lesson plan sequence and the relationship between the student and the mobility specialist.

LESSON PLAN SEQUENCE

An essential element of a good mobility training program is the use of a carefully structured and written sequence of lessons designed to accomplish several purposes. The lesson plans present the skills and techniques that must be learned in a developmental sequence that begins with the most basic skills and proceeds to the more difficult skills which frequently presuppose the skills of the previous section. This use of the sequence promotes more effective learning, and to that extent, it is characteristic of any good training methodology.

The developmental sequence of lessons also relates to many of the psychosocial variables. The sequence is structured to assist clients who may be struggling to develop a sense of their independence. When the lessons begin the client may depend a great deal on the mobility specialist, even to the point of using him as a sighted guide during the early stages. During this phase, however, the mobility specialist begins to expect the client to perform certain functions which make safe movement together possible. While walking with a guide, the client does not have to be oriented, but the lessons are structured so that concepts of orientation are introduced very early and the expectation is clear that the client must learn to remain oriented as he moves.

The mobility specialist has to make judgments at crucial stages in the sequence about the client's readiness for the next level of independence. As the client begins moving by himself in the indoor area where he has been traveling with a guide, the mobility specialist usually structures tasks that reflect the client's current level of proficiency and gradually increases the level of difficulty as the client is ready for new challenges. Similarly, the mobility specialist manipulates his proximity and accessibility to the client. This pattern of increasing the amount of the client's responsibility while decreasing the amount of interaction between the client and the mobility specialist is characteristic of each new area where successive lessons are implemented. As each new area presents demands for certain new skills, the mobility specialist is available to the client until the client is ready for independence. As the mobility specialist removes himself and interacts less, the amount of independent functioning that is required of the client increases. As the client moves through this sequence, he frequently also experiences positive change in his self-concept. This is particularly important for those clients who lack confidence in themselves.

The lesson plan sequence also exposes the client gradually to contact with the public. The initial lessons are usually conducted in a relatively controlled indoor area where any passersby are knowledgeable about the training. The presence of the mobility specialist during the early lessons discourages contact with other people. Successive lessons, however, take place in areas that are characterized by increasing numbers of people who are not familiar with the training. This fact, combined with the mobility specialist's plan to be farther removed from the client, results in gradually increased amounts of contact with the public. Of course, the mobility specialist must remain sensitive to how well the client is able to cope with the increased contact and adjust this component when necessary.

Still another dimension of the lesson plan sequence is the gradual exposure to more and more challenging problem-solving. The mobility specialist structures the lessons in a way that corresponds to the individual client's abilities to solve orientation problems. The mobility specialist's judgment in this area determines when he will allow a client to re-orient himself when confused as opposed to stepping in and assisting. This component also involves having the client plan reverse routes and alternate return routes from objectives that have been reached.

A significant problem that the client may be asked to solve at this point is the "drop-off." The drop-off lesson can be used as a part of indoor or outdoor lessons. On the outdoor drop-off lesson, the mobility specialist drives the client to a familiar neighborhood where previous lessons had been held, but drives there in such a way that the client will not know where within that neighborhood the lesson is beginning. The client is instructed that he is within a particular area and is given a destination to reach. In effect, the client is lost, and must establish his location using available clues in the environment and usually without depending on help from sighted pedestrians. This type of lesson provides the client with practice in realistic problem-solving. Success in this lesson, however, often also has a dramatic effect on the client's self-concept and sense of independence.

The lesson plan sequence is one of the most important methodologies that the mobility specialist uses to accomplish the goal of helping the client learn to travel more independently. It is important, however, that the methodology not take on more importance than the client. Concepts related to motivation that will be discussed later make it clear that successful instruction has to consider the client's current level of achievement as well as his level of aspiration in order to represent an appropriate challenge. In addition, all of the techniques and methodologies have to be used in a way that reflects the right of the client to participate in the planning of his own learning experiences.

RELATIONSHIP WITH CLIENT

The second essential element of mobility training as it is usually offered is the relationship between the client and the mobility specialist. It is likely, and frequently necessary, that this relationship become an important and positive experience for the client. It is likely because mobility instruction is offered in a one-to-one teaching mode. It is also likely for certain clients because the mobility training experience may generate fear and anxiety. The intensity of these emotions has a definite impact on the learning situation and on the relationship between the client and the mobility specialist.

For certain clients it is necessary that the relationship be strong and positive since it can become the vehicle through which the client learns to cope with some of the negative psychosocial variables that might be experienced. It may be through trust in the mobility specialist that the client is able to overcome some of the fear and anxiety that he experiences. It may be through discussion with the instructor about travel experiences that the client comes to really believe in his own abilities and to trust his own growing sense of independence. It may be the client's willingness to try again because of the relationship with the instructor that helps him to overcome the frustrating aspects of the training when he would rather not continue.

The importance of this relationship, particularly during the initial approaches to the previously immobile client, was stressed by Wilson (1967). Some of the problems that arise in the relationship between clients and mobility specialists were presented by Schulz (1972). It is clear from Schulz's discussion that for all the benefits that the relationship makes possible, it is not without cost in terms of the risks that such a close association presents.

The type of helping relationship that is most appropriate for mobility training situations was proposed for counselors and applied to the needs of teachers, rehabilitation specialists, and other helpers by Carkhuff (1972). According to

Carkhuff's theories, the mobility specialist must be honest and genuine with the client. At some point it may be necessary for the client to place his trust in the specialist at a time of great anxiety. When that happens, the client should have no reason to doubt that the mobility specialist is trustworthy. The specialist should share openly with the client where he will be during the lesson and whether or not he will be in a position to save the client from injury or embarrassment. The client should know when he is being observed and when he is functioning totally on his own. It is not uncommon for a mobility specialist to want to observe how his client functions when he is outside of the context of a lesson. To do this, he may tell the client that he is on a solo trip and then follow along to observe. Such a practice carries the risk that the instructor's presence will inadvertently be revealed through a remark of a passerby or when the client gets into trouble and the instructor feels obliged to intervene. When this happens, the basis of trust is destroyed and the relationship suffers.

The instructor must also communicate to the client a positive acceptance of him regardless of his success or failure during the lessons, and a respect for his right to be involved in planning and decision-making about his own program of instruction. In addition to being his right, the client's involvement in planning can have an important impact on his motivation to participate in the training.

Helper's Responses to Client

Carkhuff (1972) has presented types of responses which his research has shown to be of benefit to counselors, teachers, and other categories of helpers. Carkhuff has differentiated two types of responses, facilitative and action-oriented. A facilitative response acknowledges the feelings of the client, communicates that the helper understands what the client is experiencing, and enables the client to understand himself. The action-oriented response is one that enables the client to do something about the situation that is being discussed, to change in some way. Carkhuff has demonstrated that most helpers initially tend to respond in a way that communicates one or the other of these two dimensions but not both. The research further demonstrates that help is more likely to emerge from a relationship in which the helper is able to consistently give responses that encompass both dimensions. This suggests that for the mobility specialist the types of responses that will be of the most assistance to clients are those that acknowledge the emotional content of the client's statement and then go on to help him discover appropriate actions to take.

For example, when the client talks about his fear, some specialists may be inclined to minimize or pass over the fear quickly and prefer to talk about ways to handle the situation that would make the fear unnecessary. Other specialists may choose to interrupt the lesson and talk at length about the fear and encourage the client to understand his feelings completely. The more helpful approach, however, may be for the specialist to acknowledge and accept the fear as a genuine emotion in the client and to communicate his empathy with the client's experience. However, this alone is not sufficient. An empathic response is useful if it precedes a discussion about how the client might effectively overcome his fear. It is only when the specialist is sensitive to, respects and accepts the client's feelings and experiences that he will be able to help the client through some of the difficulties that he is experiencing and move on to solutions.

While the effectiveness of this approach has only recently been established empirically by Carkhuff and others, such an approach was characteristic of some of the early practitioners in mobility whom Bledsoe discussed in Chapter 18. In describing the teaching techniques of Richard Hoover, Bledsoe stresses the need to accept the client and his feelings and to communicate genuine caring for the client. He also stresses the need for an honest sharing with the client, especially in regard to his actual ability for independent travel.

MOTIVATION

Motivation is one of the most frequently discussed psychosocial variables in rehabilitation in general and in orientation and mobility in particular. Its importance reflects the central position it has held in most theories of human behavior. The centrality of this concept in psychology is perhaps responsible for the overwhelming collection of confounding literature on the topic. Its centrality in rehabilitation is manifested by the frequency with which it is cited as the explanation for why a client is more or less successful in his rehabilitation activity.

Like so many psychosocial variables, motivation is not unrelated to others that we will consider. What some might regard as a problem with motivation could be seen by others as an expression of dependency, and still others as a manifestation of a poor self-concept. It is less important to resolve this confusion than it is to elaborate certain reactions that seem characteristic of some visually impaired persons, even though they may be labeled differently by different theorists.

In this section on motivation, the focus will be on why persons with visual impairments participate or fail to participate in mobility training and/or independent travel. One explanation for a person's reluctance to begin traveling independently after experiencing a visual impairment or to begin mobility training may relate to his total adjustment to the disability itself. Psychoanalytically oriented writers such as Cholden (1958) and Blank (1957) have suggested the existence of a shock stage and a period of mourning following the news that blindness is permanent and irreversible. The purpose of these stages is to enable the ego to deal with this radical change and to integrate this information into its identity at a pace it can handle. The implications are that until the ego has assimilated this new identity the person cannot become motivated to participate in the activities related to rehabilitation. Instead, the person's attention is drawn more to thoughts of having vision restored and to efforts to find an ophthalmologist who would offer a different diagnosis.

While it seems likely that some people will not engage in rehabilitation training until they have accepted the reality and permanence of the visual disability, it is also possible that learning how to function successfully without vision may contribute to the person's ability to accept the reality of the visual loss and the possibility for a meaningful existence. This interpretation of the process suggests the value of early intervention in the event of vision loss and the use of a motivating relationship to encourage the person to participate in the training and to develop a more accurate view of the disability. It is too easy for the practitioner to "write-off" as unmotivated the client who merely does not understand what is involved in the training or who is reluctant to risk possible failure. Through a relationship that starts by acknowledging and accepting the reality of these early fears the person may be helped to take the action necessary to learn how to function.

Building Motivation

Any consideration of a client's motivation must focus on the question of "motivated for what?" It is necessary to understand how the client views the activity under consideration. Learning theory generally dismisses the concept of an internal motivating force. It considers that all behavior can be explained by an analysis of the reinforcers available in the environment. However, other aspects of learning theory contribute to the discussion at this point as a result of their emphasis on the arrangement of learning tasks in stages of difficulty and complexity. In attempting to motivate a client to begin mobility training, it is important to clearly delimit the task. Many clients have difficulty thinking of themselves as progressing from a point where they are totally dependent on others for travel to the point where they are crossing busy streets independently. For clients who are having this difficulty it is important to present the task in stages emphasizing the client's role in deciding how far the training will go and at what rate.

It is more likely that a client will be motivated first to learn how to travel more efficiently in a controlled area with a sighted guide than to consider traveling in public with the stigmatizing symbol of the cane. The success experienced at each stage contributes to the building of motivation for the next stage.

While the type of procedure discussed above resembles the concept of shaping developed by Skinner (1953), it also has antecedents in cognitive theory. Barker and Wright (1952) describe the operation and the importance of the "level of aspiration" in influencing the experience of success and the motivation to continue in an activity. Level of aspiration represents the goals that the person feels are attainable in his own situation. For most people, level of aspiration operates as a protective mechanism which serves to enhance the likelihood of their experiencing success regardless of their objective level of ability. People usually set their level of aspiration near the top of their ability level based on what they have accomplished in the past. The level tends to increase after success and decrease after failure. Because of the variable functioning of the level of aspiration, most people seem to experience relative success most of the time.

Client's Level of Aspiration

Difficulties arise, however, when the level of aspiration is placed inappropriately high or low. If placed too low, the person never really has the experience of success, even though the goals are accomplished. If placed too high the person frequently experiences frustration or failure and the loss of self-esteem. Setting the level of aspiration either too high or too low is characteristic of persons who have a high degree of fear of failure. The impact of failure seems to be greatest when the level of aspiration has been set at an appropriate level of difficulty.

The development and continuation of motivation usually depends on the experience of success. In view of the influence of the level of aspiration, the mobility specialist should take this variable into consideration when planning learning experiences for a client whose motivation is questionable. Accomplishing a task may not provide the experience of success that leads to motivation if the task is not perceived by the client as being of sufficient difficulty.

Another variable relevant to a visually impaired person's motivation for rehabilitation is the *"locus of control."* A thorough review of the theories and empirical findings related to this variable has been presented by Phares (1976). A growing base of empirical findings has given support to the validity of an enduring personality characteristic which reflects a tendency toward either internal or external locus of control. The person who tends toward external control typically perceives reinforcements that follow some actions of his own as a result of luck, chance, fate, as under the control of powerful others, or as unpredictable because of the complexity of the forces surrounding him. The person who has a belief in internal control tends to perceive that reinforcing events are contingent upon his own behavior or his own personality characteristics.

Much of the research done on this variable has applicability for understanding some of the motivation of persons who are entering rehabilitation (MacDonald, 1971; MacDonald & Hall, 1969; 1971). In addition, knowing the tendency of a person on this variable may also relate to how best to motivate the person. For example, the internally controlled person may be better motivated through appealing to his desire for competence or mastery; while the externally controlled person may be motivated more by praise from persons in authority or by peer support. The internal person also is more likely to engage in rehabilitation activities for his own purposes, but external people may be more susceptible to influence and persuasion when initially hesitant about entering training.

Recent research in physical medicine appears to be tapping into this same type of variable even though it does not use the concept of locus of control. Diamond, Weiss, and Grynbaum (1968) discovered that resigned attitudes concerning the disability and excessive guilt feelings were for the most part responsible where clients could not be influenced to participate in the rehabilitation program. Hyman (1972) found that attributing illness to supernatural causes was one of several factors that impaired motivation of persons entering a stroke rehabilitation program.

Locus of control research as well as that of Hyman (1972) and Diamond, Weiss, & Grynbaum (1968), cited above, tends to appear fatalistic unless it is examined in proximity to the motivational theory of Maslow (1954), which suggests that motivation is a multidimensional construct. There is not one type of motivation, but rather a hierarchy of motives that encompasses both lower deficit needs and higher self-actualizing needs. The hope that accompanies this theory lies in the notion that self-actualizing needs may not appear while the individual is preoccupied with gratification of the more basic deficit needs. Once the lower needs are at least partially gratified, then the self-actualizing needs may appear.

Client's Needs and Motivation

The five levels of needs described by Maslow include: 1) physiological needs, which include the basic survival needs such as for food and warmth; 2) safety needs, which encompass the need for security, stability, order, protection, and dependency; 3) belonging and love needs, such as the belonging to a family or a neighborhood group, or the need for an intimate relationship with another person; 4) esteem needs, including both the need for self-esteem as well as the need for respect and recognition from others; and 5) self-actualizing needs, such as the need to develop one's potential or to fulfill personal capacities.

While this categorization of needs is presented as a hierarchy, it is important to note that certain persons may be characterized by different needs at different times in a manner that does not reflect the hierarchy. The value of this concept for rehabilitation is in its suggestion for understanding the apparent lack of motivation exhibited by some clients. It may be difficult for an individual to engage in efforts to master the environment and to function independently when basic safety needs are unmet. This particularly applies to the mobility training situation as described by Murphy (1965). It is unlikely that a person will be motivated to learn how to function on his own if he feels threatened and unsafe. The safety of the person is assured initially by the presence and the attention of the mobility specialist until the client develops confidence in his ability to assure his own safety. Similarly, the instructor's respect or the family's support may have to be perceived by the client as fulfilling basic needs of belonging and esteem before he can become strongly committed to independent functioning for its own sake.

Similar to Maslow's discussion of the self-actualizing motives is the concept of competence or mastery as an important human motive. Trends in this direction were recognized and organized by White (1959) and applied to the rehabilitation situation by Smith (1974). While Maslow's hierarchy suggests the emergence of self-actualizing motives later in adult life after the basic needs have been gratified, White summarized studies that demonstrated the influence of the competence motive throughout life, even in the activities of children. Among those cited by

White were Hendrick (1942), who proposed the existence of an "instinct to master" which led to pleasure in exercising functions and which was responsible for the infant learning to suck, to manipulate, to walk, to speak, to comprehend, and to reason. A similar concept was proposed by Mittlemann (1954) who described motility as an urge in its own right that manifests itself in skilled motor activities such as posture, locomotion, and manipulation.

The concept of competence or mastery has been suggested as an explanation of curiosity and exploratory behavior, as well as of risk-taking and problem-solving. White (1959) summarized these concepts into an observable tendency on the part of people to want to use their capacities to produce effects on the environment, a tendency which appears most clearly when deficit drives have been at least partially gratified. Smith (1974) has pointed out some of the applications of this concept to rehabilitation. He suggests that certain qualities of the rehabilitation worker's approach to the client can support and reinforce the client's sense of competence. These include what Smith has characterized as "respectful, close attention" and a "toughminded faith" by the worker in the client's potential. In addition, the worker's careful selection and pacing of developmental tasks, selected in terms of the client's capacities and interests pose an appropriate challenge that can lead to success and increased motivation to take on the next level of challenge.

Increasing Feelings of Competence

The growth of evidence confirming the validity of the concept of competence as a source of motivation for human behavior is encouraging for the mobility specialist who can try to tap into this drive to support activities leading to increased competence in spite of a disability. It is important to note, however, that this drive can be suppressed by a history of failure which is frequently the early experience of persons with disabilities. This notion was addressed in a review of studies by MacMillan (1971), dealing with the problem of motivation in the education of mentally retarded children. He showed how early academic experiences of retarded children led to three motivational tendencies that he described as an expectancy for failure, positive and negative reaction tendencies toward interactions with adults, and an outer-directedness in seeking solutions to problems. MacMillan suggested that special education programs be modified to meet the motivational as well as the educational needs of these children. Among the solutions which he suggests are the use of a warm and accepting relationship between the teacher and student to help the student satisfy basic emotional needs before problem-solving motivations can be effective. MacMillan also pointed out the need for learning programs designed to eliminate failures and to create success experiences through the use of appropriate tasks that reflect the child's level of competence and level of aspiration, and meaningful rewards.

The major trend identified in the literature reviewed has been the growth of interest in and attention to the concept of competence and mastery as a powerful motivating force in human behavior. However, it has been established that this force can be suppressed or not highly active as a result of other needs or previous failure experiences. Based on some of the theories that have been reported, it seems likely that this powerful motivating force can be activated or facilitated by the use of developmental learning sequences and through a genuine, accepting relationship with the rehabilitation worker, the teacher, the mobility specialist, or some other significant person involved with the client in the rehabilitation process.

FEAR AND ANXIETY

Two psychosocial variables frequently associated with orientation and mobility are fear and anxiety. Uninitiated laypersons are particularly quick to project these attributes onto visually impaired persons who attempt to move independently.

While fear and anxiety can be distinguished and discussed separately, they are treated here together for two reasons. First, they are both experiences of threat and, as such, require similar methods of intervention. Second, they are frequently undifferentiated by theorists or differentiated in ways that are not in agreement from one theorist to another.

Fear seems to be considered most generally as a reaction to a clearly perceived threat or danger which most frequently results in flight from the danger or some other type of avoidance behavior. Anxiety seems to be a more diffuse reaction to a less specific or less clearly perceived threat. Frequently, anxiety seems to be the reaction to a general threat to the self and to the functioning of the ego. Anxiety seems to represent a less intense threat in which the reason for the discomfort is less well understood. It does not generally result in flight or avoidance, but rather occurs in situations where the person cannot escape, but must deal with the threat.

As with the other psychosocial variables, fear and anxiety can develop through interaction with other people. Many of the threats which the visually impaired person feels related to independent travel arise initially from the reactions of parents, family, and others who do not understand how safe movement can be accomplished without vision. Some fears are learned as a result of actual travel experience, especially when travel begins before orientation and mobility instruction.

Early empirical research on anxiety led to the classification of individuals according to high or low levels of anxiety as manifested by performance on measures such as the Manifest Anxiety Scale (Taylor, 1953). More recently, Speilberger (1966; 1972) differentiated between *state* and *trait* anxieties. Speilberger (1972) conceptualized state anxiety as a transitory experience of unpleasant, consciously-perceived feelings of tension and apprehension, associated with the arousal of the autonomic nervous system. This is an experience that affects all people at certain times to a greater or lesser degree and which varies from moment to moment and from day to day. On the other hand, trait anxiety has been described by Speilberger (1966) as the individual differences in the extent to which different people are characterized by anxiety states and by prominent defenses against such states. Certain people are more prone to experience anxiety more frequently and/or more intensely in response to a wider range of situations. The differentiation between these two types of anxiety carries implications for interventions related to them.

Limitation in the state-trait theory led Endler and Hunt (1966; 1968; 1969) to propose a person-by-situation interaction model for understanding anxiety. This model emerged from empirical research that indicated that the appropriate assessment of the trait of anxiety must consider both the responses that characterize anxiousness and the situations which are likely to arouse them. Further research with this model led Shedletsky and Endler (1974) to propose that the concept of trait anxiety as a characteristic level of anxiety response in individuals is a valid concept, but that it is better conceived as a multidimensional characteristic. The three dimensions that have been proposed as evoking differing amounts of anxiety are interactions with others, physical danger, and new or strange situations.

Fear and anxiety first enter the mobility situation as a deterrent to the visually impaired person entering the training and beginning to travel. The person's motivation to travel must be strong enough to enable him to overcome these avoidance tendencies. The individualized nature of mobility instruction may provide a sufficient guarantee of safety to encourage some fearful clients to begin. For others, the anxiety may be overcome by certain other motivational influences discussed previously, such as the drive to master a particular skill.

Positive Aspects of Anxiety

Once instruction has begun, fear and anxiety affect its success in other ways. Reactions to perceived threat can contribute to success in a positive way. There are certain real dangers for a person who attempts to travel without vision. The world has been constructed for people who can see. Obstacles, curbs, stairways, and moving vehicles present real threats to pedestrians, both blind and sighted. A normal fear of these dangers if followed by appropriate cautions can result in safe movement. Fear can also trigger the release of adrenalin and help the individual to deal with real threats.

Similarly, anxiety can contribute positively to successful mobility functioning. Mandler and Sarason (1952) indicated that some of the responses aroused by anxiety are directly related to the completion of the task at hand and reduce anxiety by leading to the completion of the task. Ryan (1962) indicated that minimal amounts of anxiety may be important in the learning situation and may serve as a motivator.

Fear and anxiety occupy the attention of the mobility specialist to whatever extent they prevent learning in the visually impaired person. While a number of studies have demonstrated that high anxiety may contribute in a positive way to the learning of simple tasks (Palermo, 1961; Sassenrath & Knight, 1965), the indications are in the opposite direction for complex tasks. The findings of a number of studies of these variables originally cited by Bauman and Yoder (1966) have been related to the mobility situation by Fluharty, McHugh, McHugh, Willits, and Wood (1976). It was noted that for highly anxious subjects learning was slower and the retention of what was learned was less (Diethelm & Jones, 1947), judgments of time and distance were distorted (Langer, Wapner, & Werner, 1961), and the efficiency in the performances of complex motor tasks was negatively affected (Ryan, 1962).

Negative Aspects of Anxiety

The dynamics by which anxiety lessens learning have been described by Mandler and Sarason (1952). They described how anxiety produces certain responses which may relate to the completion of the task at hand; however, other responses not directly related to the task might be produced. These other responses include: feelings of inadequacy, hopelessness, helplessness, heightened somatic reactions, anticipation of punishment or loss of status or self-esteem, and implicit attempts at leaving the situation. Campeau (1968) demonstrated that high anxiety subjects in a testing situation produced more task-irrelevant responses that served to disrupt their performance. When the threat was removed, the number of task-irrelevant responses was reduced and the performance of the high anxiety subjects was improved.

Easterbrook (1959) explained the effect of anxiety on learning and performance in terms of the reduction in the use of cues. The greater the anxiety the person experiences, the fewer the cues he uses to solve problems and make judgments. Bauman and Yoder (1966) extended this theory to explain how anxiety in moderate amounts may assist learning. They proposed that the reduction in cues tends to weed out those that are less relevant and makes the person more efficient by allowing him to focus on the more relevant aspects of the situation. Under conditions of serious threat or extreme anxiety, the person is focused more and more on the preservation of the integrity of the self and less on the task.

Another way of looking at highly anxious people has been suggested by Mandler (1968). Reflecting some of the early work by Lewin (1936), Mandler indicated that any organized activity is helpful in warding off a state of distress. A state of anxiety exists whenever a person is unable to draw upon some behavior or act to control his environment, whenever he is in a condition of helplessness and unable to control the stimulation and input from the environment. Highly anxious individuals are those who have very few mechanisms available for coping with helplessness and threat. They are faced with a world in which no behaviors are available for them to inhibit or avoid the threat.

The concept of *new psychological situations* was developed by Lewin (1936) and applied to the situation of disabled people by Barker, Wright, Meyerson, and Gonick (1953) was elaborated by Meyerson (1963). In discussing this concept Meyerson described a new psychological situation as one in which the goal and the path to reaching the goal is unknown. Entering the region where the goal exists both attracts and repels, and both the region and location of the goal will appear to change as the person's position changes. Many situations are new for a disabled person because he has never experienced them, because he lacks a culturally required tool for behavior in this situation, and/or because the social stimulus value of the disabled person makes usual situations new because the reactions of others are less predictable. This description of a "new psychological situation" closely relates to the description of anxiety as that stress that comes from the inability of the organism to cope with a situation that threatens to overwhelm him, or the absence of adequate behaviors to deal with environmental or intra-psychic events (Mandler, 1968).

It is not unusual, therefore, that a visually impaired person experiences anxiety. Since severe visual impairment is a low incidence disability, there are not many examples of independent functioning without vision available to the average person. The person who experiences visual loss has had very few examples of other persons within his own experience who have coped with this disability and continued to function normally. Even if the person has some awareness of the possibility of continued functioning, he has not usually been close enough to a visually impaired person to understand how that functioning is possible. This lack of knowledge comes at a time when the person is undergoing serious changes in his self-concept as a result of the visual loss and the different treatment he is beginning to receive from those around him. The reconstruction of his self-concept comes to be associated with his ability to learn how to function in his daily life, which has now become a new psychological situation both because it is a new experience and because he lacks the tools for coping with it. The possibility of not succeeding in this reorganization of the self overwhelms the person and leads to anxiety. This sequence of events is even more likely for those persons who are high in trait anxiety in any or all of the dimensions suggested earlier.

The congenitally visually impaired person's situation is different but similar. While they do not experience a reorganization of the self as do those who are adventitiously impaired, they do have a similar lack of awareness about how functioning will be possible. Much of their questioning in this regard is stimulated by the concern, lack of information, and the fears of their parents and those around them. While they can readily identify with the general goals of the culture as expressed in the value of employment and independent functioning, they do not have confidence of understanding how they will accomplish these tasks. This threat to the development and functioning of the self is not usually as clearly per-ceived as suggested here, but is experienced as a more diffuse threat and nervous-ness, which we call anxiety.

Strategies for Dealing with Anxiety

This conceptualization of anxiety as a reaction to new psychological situations, in which the person does not have the necessary tools to cope with the challenge or threat of living, is helpful in that it suggests a strategy for dealing with anxiety. The first stage in dealing with anxiety may be the recognition that it exists. Fear and anxiety frequently manifest themselves quite directly through avoidance behavior and attempted flight or through somatic symptoms such as dizziness, tachycardia, nervousness, sweating, and the inability to sleep. Often there are vague feelings of uneasiness and apprehension or diffuse fears and worry. The person may know what is behind such symptoms, but sometimes the cause is not readily apparent. Recognizing anxiety when it manifests itself through seemingly unrelated responses such as aggressive behavior, reduced activity, bragging or illness is particularly difficult.

It is important for the mobility specialist to recognize that a person is experiencing an increase in anxiety. This necessitates knowing each person well enough to recognize that person's unique way of revealing the sense of the self under threat. During times when fear and anxiety are particularly expected or suspected, it is important to relate to the client with empathy (Carkhuff, 1972) in an effort to help him be able to get in touch with the anxious feelings that are behind the symptoms and to be able to verbalize them.

In some cases, the fear may be so strong that it cannot be eliminated through ordinary learning activities. In this event, the client may need formal counseling or psychotherapy to assist in coping with the perceived threat. Perhaps the process of systematic desensitization as developed by Wolpe (1958) can be used. In this case, the mobility specialist will have to rely on the assistance of other professionals or members of the rehabilitation team.

In most cases, however, the client's anxiety and fears related to the mobility situation can be overcome or significantly reduced through a careful use of the relationship between the mobility specialist and the client and through the skillful use of the lesson plan sequence. As already indicated, the relationship between the mobility specialist and the client is quite important even in the initial phase of recognizing and identifying the influence of anxiety. It is also important that the mobility specialist establish a trust relationship with the client. Such a relationship enables the client to attempt behaviors he perceives as threatening as long as he can trust that the mobility specialist will guarantee his safety. At other points in the instruction, it is trust in the specialist's opinion that he can perform that will motivate the client to try new activities independently.

Schulz (1972) has stressed the importance of the emotional interaction between the mobility specialist and the client in the successful reduction of anxiety throughout mobility training. In a similar way, Fluharty, et al. (1976) have suggested that the mobility specialist communicate to the client that mistakes during training are expected and inevitable and that they will not result in rejection.

The developmental nature of the lesson plan sequence is the mobility specialist's other tool for combating the effects of anxiety. The sequence attempts to expose students to danger and anxiety-provoking situations only after he has had the opportunity to develop the skills to cope with that situation. This represents a direct effort to combat the new psychological situation by defining and training the client in the skills that are necessary for dealing with the challenge.

Use of Real Environments

It is also significant that mobility instruction takes place in real environments rather than simulated or artificial areas. In real environments the client will experience the actual fears and anxieties. It is only by experiencing these anxieties that the feeling of success that comes with the use of the proper techniques will have the effect of reducing the anxiety.

The unexpected nature of events that occur in real environments is also essential for the person to overcome his anxieties, especially those related to interacting with others. As the lessons progress, the mobility specialist retreats farther and farther from the client, increasing the chances that others will approach him and offer help or otherwise interact. As the client gets experience by dealing with people as well as evaluative feedback from the specialist about these interactions, some of these anxieties can be overcome.

While the ability to deal with the unexpected is a function of the lesson plans in real environments, the mobility specialist has an overriding responsibility to try to systematically expose the client to all possible contingencies that might occur while traveling independently. The importance of this procedure for dealing with emotional stress was presented by Haggard (1949) and applied to the mobility situation by Fluharty et al. (1976). While it is impossible to present all possible occurrences, the client should be exposed to a sufficiently wide variety of situations so that he will less likely experience anxiety as a result of not having tools to cope with new situations that come up.

Other methods of dealing with anxiety that have been presented by Heathers (1955) were applied to mobility by Fluharty, et al. (1976). These include the "distraction method" whereby the instructor relieves the client's feelings of anxiety during instruction by engaging him in conversation while at the same time providing instruction and practice in skills. In the "crutch method" the instructor supplies modes of dependence during the learning of a new technique which are gradually removed as the client becomes accustomed to the threatening situation. The example provided was beginning crossings at traffic lights by having the client use the instructor as a sighted guide and then progressing to more independent functioning. A third method of dealing with anxiety is by reassuring the client of the instructor's presence during particularly threatening experiences. This can be done verbally, but is particularly effective for some clients when done through a reassuring touch.

For clients who will continue to experience anxiety in mobility situations beyond the training period, Fluharty, et al. (1976) recommended that skills be overlearned through repetition and practice. Since anxiety interferes with the client's ability to cope with threatening situations, the more ingrained the behavioral pattern has become, the more likely it is that the person will be able to cope with the threats.

In summary, it seems the best way to help a client overcome the fear and anxiety related to traveling with reduced vision is by providing structured learning experiences which systematically expose the client to the real and imagined threatening situations in such a way that the client can develop techniques for coping with and reducing these threats.

INDEPENDENCE AND DEPENDENCE

The position of the visually impaired person on a scale of dependence/independence can relate to psychosocial problems in his adjustment to living. As with other psychosocial variables, the dependence/independence attribute is not unidimensional. The amount of dependence and independence can be assessed or analyzed in regard to several dimensions including financial, social, emotional, and others. For this discussion the focus will be on dependence/independence related to travel through the environment. It should be obvious, however, that there will be inevitable overlap among the various dimensions.

As Wright (1960) pointed out, a high value is placed on independence in western societies. This was demonstrated in a cross-cultural study of child-rearing practices by Whiting and Child (1953) and further verified by Sears, Macoby, and Levin (1957). Independence is associated with strength and leadership, while dependence has come to be associated with weakness, indecision, and helplessness. In reality, people are closely interdependent and becoming more so as society becomes more influenced by technology and specialization. As people must learn to rely more on each other and those with special skills, the inevitability of dependence becomes more apparent. Reliance upon others and the warmth and satisfaction of human interaction are important experiences for most people.

"Undesirable dependence" has been described by Havens (1967) as that which is concentrated on too few people or that which is unilateral instead of a reciprocal interdependence. Havens has also suggested that dependence is problematic to the extent that observing the highly dependent person threatens us by reminding us of our own inclinations toward dependency which we have struggled to reject.

Carroll (1961) has acknowledged the dual tendency within visually impaired individuals to desire both independence with its freedom and dependence with its protection, and has drawn attention to the need for both characteristics to maintain survival. Yet, Carroll has also pointed out some of the problems associated with the extremes of the dependence/independence scale. Both extremes, held zealously, can prevent an individual from fully realizing his potential. The person who resists dependence on others and interactions with others to achieve goals will be as handicapped as the person who must depend entirely on others without being able to contribute to mutual endeavors.

Problems in this area are associated with an individual's dissatisfaction with his position in the scale between the two extremes of dependency, or with the dissatisfaction of significant others in his environment. The position of greatest comfort is described by Carroll as an "inner independence" which he describes as the feeling of a person who has no difficulty accepting the occasional situations in which all of us have to be dependent.

A person's characteristic level of independence or dependence is not an innate psychological trait but rather a learned response that develops from the individual's past experiences. Bandura and Walters (1963) have defined dependency as a class of responses that are capable of eliciting positive attending and ministering responses from others. A number of empirical studies have indicated that the levels of dependency in children are determined to a large extent by the interactions between the children and their parents. Sears, Macoby, and Levin (1957), Bandura and Walters (1959), Rheingold (1956), and Levy (1943) have all presented evidence that suggests that parental demonstrativeness and warmth in response to dependent behaviors in children serves to reward these behaviors and leads to an increase in dependency.

In a similar way, independent functioning has been shown to be a learned response. Rosen and D'Andrade (1959) showed that the mothers of boys who displayed a great deal of self-reliance and effort at mastering tasks set higher performance standards for their sons, more readily gave approval when their sons' performance was good, and were more critical when their sons' performance failed to reach the standards than did the mothers of boys who showed less achievement-oriented behavior. Also, Crandall, Preston, and Rabson (1960) found that mothers who spontaneously rewarded and praised their children's efforts to achieve had children who displayed strong and frequent achievement efforts outside the home.

Vision loss, as well as other disabilities, is likely to cause disturbances in the individual's sense of dependence and independence. In some people, the problems that arise are quite natural and temporary, while in others the problems are more pathological and troublesome. Obviously, until the person learns techniques for functioning without vision, he will have to depend to a greater degree on others to assist him in performing many tasks of daily living, and especially for help in travel. This can, however, lead to a more serious problem if the individual has had dependency conflicts throughout his life. The loss of vision can be the "excuse" that a person uses to move into a socially acceptable dependent role that he has been reluctant to or unable to assume previously. The person may be getting additional benefits from his dependency relative to his role in his family or his interaction with significant others. Other individuals who have similar conflicts about independence may be threatened by even the necessary and natural dependency that accompanies visual loss. This person's response may be to strongly resist any assistance and to insist that he needs neither help nor any rehabilitation service.

Significant Others and Dependence

Some of the problems associated with dependency may come from people who are significant in the life of the impaired person or from the society at large. People around the visually impaired person may actively discourage any efforts or thoughts about learning to function independently again and they may reward and reinforce dependent functioning on the part of the visually impaired person. His dependence may also be satisfying the needs of other family members to dominate the impaired person. The role of family members in the development of dependency in the visually impaired person is especially significant in the experience of congenitally visually impaired persons. However, just as the family and friends can be forces that encourage and support dependency, so too, they can motivate and assist the person toward independent functioning when they are properly educated to the possibilities and how to proceed.

The problem associated with finding an acceptable balance between independence and dependence is a problem that all people face. However, the problem is more serious for the disabled person. He finds himself in a society that encourages independence generally but discourages it for disabled people in subtle ways, while the rehabilitation system of services focuses quite clearly on independence. He may also find himself between his family, who discourage independence and reward dependence, and his own feeling of freedom. It is also possible that the person's family and friends are burdened by the individual's dependence, while the individual himself is reluctant to learn to function on his own.

The person who is reluctant to learn to function more independently may eventually be motivated to do so for a number of reasons which were discussed earlier in the section on motivation. For example, the person may experience "dependency dissatisfaction." This occurs as the person discovers that the process of depending on others for certain tasks leads to results that are dissatisfying. Examples related to mobility include the person having to adjust his schedule for going and coming to meet the schedule of the person on whom he depends, or the person who is supposed to provide the guide service or automobile transportation forgetting and leaving the visually impaired person stranded or late for an appointment. A sufficient number of such experiences may eventually convince the person to learn to function more independently.

Once the person has entered training, excessive dependency may interfere with success and with the eventual transfer of the skills learned to new areas following training. The training experience itself can contribute to the lessening of the dependency needs and to the finding of a workable balance between independence and dependence. Carroll (1961), and Havens (1967) agree that one of the first important steps in helping a person overcome excessive dependence is to develop a new relationship between the client and the rehabilitation worker which is in effect a dependent one. Involved in the establishment of this relationship is the type of close and empathic communication in which the client and worker are together able to recognize and acknowledge that the dependency does exist. Once this first step is taken the worker should be able eventually to help the client wean himself from the need for the relationship to have this form, and to learn to depend on himself.

Through the developmental sequence of the lesson plans, the mobility specialist can manipulate the amount of independent functioning required of the client and thus reinforce that dependence on self. Research has shown that persons who have developed strong dependency habits are more influenced by social reinforcers than are persons in whom dependency responses have been only weakly reinforced (Baer, 1962; Cairns & Lewis, 1962). The specialist's skill must be to use his attention to reward independent effort and not to reinforce dependence. This requires that the specialist extend warm and accepting support while demanding more and more independence. The mobility specialist also uses his physical proximity to the client to assist in this effort. As the specialist withdraws farther and farther from the client, he communicates this to him and the client realizes that he must depend more and more on his own abilities. It is important that the client understand clearly the conditions under which the mobility specialist will re-enter the situation and assist, whether such re-entry is for the sake of assuring the client's safety, to control the level of difficulty of the situations that the client encounters, or for the sake of a more efficient and appropriate learning experience for that particular lesson. If the client does not understand why the instructor has intervened in a lesson that he was expecting to handle independently, he may perceive this as a contradictory message that will retard the growth toward independence.

The relationship described above is not without its hazards. There is a good possibility that members of the client's family will not understand this need to make demands on the client or that passersby will misinterpret the specialist's refusal to step into a situation when a client is disoriented. There are also dangers within the relationship itself which have been discussed by Schulz (1972). The close relationship that is necessary for the client to be able to put his trust in the mobility specialist could easily develop into one of excessive dependency. The specialist must be careful not to allow it to develop to the point where he becomes overprotective of his clients and does not have reasonable expectations of them. In addition, some clients may have difficulty severing strong attachments.

Absolute Independence Undesirable

A standard of absolute independence for a visually impaired traveler is neither feasible nor desirable. Inevitably he will encounter situations in which he will have to seek and obtain assistance from others on the street. It is ironic that the task of getting help from others requires quite a bit of skill if it is to be done efficiently. The average person on the street does not know how best to give directions to a visually impaired person. Thus, the person with the visual loss must take charge of the interchange and ask the right kind of questions that will bring the kind of information that he needs to achieve his objective. This is another skill that the mobility specialist must address in his lesson plans. Feedback from the specialist on how the client does on this task can help him learn how to manipulate interaction with sighted helpers so that the situation works to his advantage. The visually impaired person should also be helped to realize that the judicious use of help is not a threat to his independence. The truly independent person does not feel that he has to constantly prove himself to others. Therefore, reliance on others when necessary or chosen is quite acceptable.

In summary, it should be apparent that the variable of independence/ dependence provides a good example of the concept discussed at the beginning of the chapter related to psychosocial variables in general. It is difficult, if not impossible, to separate cause and effect when considering the interaction between independence/dependence and mobility. On one hand, immobility certainly leads to increased dependence, while success in learning to move through the environment diminishes the need to depend on others. On the other hand, a tendency to prefer dependence would discourage a person from engaging in mobility training, while a lack of success at early attempts to travel would seem to result in an increased desire to be dependent. The only way out of the circle seems to be through sequenced training in the context of an understanding and accepting relationship.

THE SELF-CONCEPT

Self-concept is another variable intertwined with the disabled person's ability to move through the environment. This central and complex variable has occupied the attention of psychologists and especially social psychologists since the treatment of the self by William James in his *Principles of Psychology* in 1918. It has occupied a prominent place in the theories of Mead (1934), Fromm (1941), Horney (1945), Sullivan (1953), Adler (1924) and Rogers (1951). In spite of this extensive treatment, or perhaps because of it, it still remains a complicated topic to understand and apply.

In this review, the self-concept is defined as that set of perceptions and feelings that an individual holds about himself. It also includes self-esteem, which implies an evaluative rating of the self with all of its parts considered as a whole. Many theorists have considered the self-concept to have various dimensions such as the physical self, the social self, the intellectual self, and the moral self. Other theories have proposed various levels of the self and various levels of self-awareness.

Some theorists, especially Rogers (1951), have suggested that the difference between the real self and the ideal self is responsible for many of the anxieties and conflicts that individuals experience. Therapy consists in helping the person to bring these two perceptions closer together. Horney (1950) proposed that an individual forms an ideal self-image to serve as a defense against anxiety and threat and to support a more favorable self-concept.

The distinctions made by Rogers and Horney suggest the various ways in which the self-concept is important to adjustment and interacts with behavior. Favorable self-esteem is regarded as an indicator of good adjustment. Another indicator of good adjustment in the theories of some is a minimal discrepancy between the ideal self and the real self. A person's self-esteem also has been demonstrated to alter his perceptions of other aspects of his world. It has been shown to affect his motivation for certain behaviors, particularly in the area of interpersonal activities and seems to be able to influence an individual's experience of success and failure and his level of aspiration. A good review of research related to these areas is contained in Stotland and Canon (1972).

Some of the concepts that have the most relevance to the topic of orientation and mobility for visually impaired persons are those related to the origin and development of the self-concept. Most theories stress the role of significant others in the formation of the individual's self-concept. Mead (1934) stated that an individual internalizes the ideas and attitudes expressed by significant others in one's life. An individual values himself as significant others value him and thinks less of himself to the extent that these others reject or ignore him. Adler (1924) attributed poor self-concepts to infirmities and weaknesses such as organ inferiorities and impairments. He proposed, however, that favorable outcomes can result in those situations as a result of encouragement, support, and acceptance of close associates.

Stotland and Canon (1972) identified a range of factors which they feel influence a person's sense of competence, which they see as equivalent to self-esteem. These factors were: 1) the person's perceptions of the effectiveness of his own actions, 2) her perceived freedom to select from a number of possible actions, 3) the number and specificity of the schemas, rules for understanding the regularities among events he has about a given situation, 4) his sense of similarity to other people, 5) his comparison of himself with relevant others, and 6) communication from others about his sense of competence.

In view of the importance of interactions with others in the formation and development of the self-concept, it is helpful to review how visual impairment is considered and evaluated by others in the environment of the person who has the visual loss. Some understanding of this may help in understanding how the self-concepts of visually impaired persons develop and how they might be improved when necessary.

Attitudes Toward Blindness

Most of the literature on the attitudes of people in general toward blind people is confusing. There are many indications of negative reactions to blindness and blind people. These were summarized recently by Monbeck (1973). Monbeck draws attention to the reports that blindness elicits pity, sympathy, and fear responses from people; some people seek to avoid contact with visually impaired persons; some project misery and unhappiness on blind people; while others feel that blind people are helpless. According to Monbeck, some people associate blindness with punishment for sin and with venereal disease; while others feel that blindness also results in intellectual deficits and other losses. There are few examples, although some do exist, in the literature, of positive attitudes toward blindness and of the association of special abilities with visual impairment along with the desire to help and be associated with persons so impaired.

Empirical efforts to establish exactly how people regard blindness have been confounded by a variety of measuring instruments, by different eliciting stimuli, and by basic confusion concerning whether they were measuring attitudes toward blindness or toward blind people (Lukoff, 1972). Much of the confusion can be explained by the more recent discovery that attitudes toward visually impaired persons as well as toward persons with other disabilities are not unidimensional as the early assessment instruments seemed to assume, but rather multidimensional.

A series of studies by Whiteman and Lukoff (1964a; 1964b; 1965) identified five factors or dimensions of attitudes toward blindness. These were 1) *personal attributes,* which differentiate respondents according to the degree to which they have a negative view of the emotional life and general competence of blind people; 2) *social attributes,* which relate to the readiness of sighted persons for interaction with the blind and to feelings about the interpersonal competence of blind people; 3) *evaluation of blindness,* which deals with the degree to which blindness is perceived as potentially threatening and as uniquely frustrating to one's self and others; 4) *non-protectiveness,* which relates to a lack of protectiveness and sympathy, and 5) *interpersonal acceptance,* which refers to an emotional acceptance of blind people in interpersonal situations.

The validity of this approach was supported by the work of Siller, Ferguson, Vann, and Holland (1967) who developed the Disability Factor Scale related to blindness that tapped seven different factors of attitudes toward blind people. These factors were: 1) *interaction strain,* which is associated with a distinct uneasiness in the presence of a blind person and an uncertainty in how to deal with him; 2) *rejection of intimacy,* which consists of a desire to avoid close, particularly familial, contact with a blind person; 3) *generalized rejection,* which reflects distinct anti-blindness reactions, negative descriptions of blind persons, and segregation of the blind person from others; 4) *authoritarian virtuousness,* which involves a double-edged type of endowing blind persons with exceptional qualities while pleading for tolerance and special treatment for their shortcomings; 5) *inferred emotional consequences*, which contains statements that refer negatively to the blind person's character and emotionality; 6) *distressed identification*, which involves highly personalized reactions to disability with the blind person named as a stimulus which activates anxiety about the person's own vulnerability; and 7) *imputed functional limitations*, which focuses on whether the blind person can function adequately in a number of typical and crucial situations.

While the appearance of multidimensional approaches to measuring and understanding attitudes toward blind people seems to complicate the issue and remove the facile ability to say whether the attitudes of a person are good or bad, this approach also helps in understanding how the self concepts of visually impaired persons might be affected negatively by interactions with persons who exhibit some or all of the attitude dimensions described above. In interactions with people who experience many of the above dimensions, the blind person is likely to perceive the strain or the imputations of lessened functioning that the other person is communicating. The visually impaired person is likely to sense the rejection or the personal distress and frustration that the other person feels. These attitudes develop from or are further affected by the relative lack of guiding norms for situations where blind and sighted persons first encounter each other (Lukoff, 1972). These strained interactions are disrupted by the blind person's lack of visual contact, different gestures and facial expressions, and lack of similar conversational cues (Monbeck, 1973).

Stress in Sighted-Blind Interactions

Because of the low incidence of blindness in the population, most people do not have an opportunity to develop comfort and skill in interacting with blind persons. People generally do not know what to expect of blind persons, and different people communicate varying expectations. This adds additional stress to the interactions between sighted and blind people. This situation is even more difficult for some low vision people. The expectations that people have for low vision people are even more varied since the range of actual conditions is wider. It seems that frequently the expectations for the low vision person that are held by others are not consistent with what the person can actually accomplish. These misperceptions negatively affect the interactions between people. The person with enough vision to move along the sidewalk without the use of a mobility device is expected to be able to read the sign on the bus and is answered rudely when he asks someone else to identify the bus that is approaching. Or the low vision person who uses a cane to ease those situations when he must ask for assistance may be helped onto the bus and into a seat when he could actually accomplish those activities without assistance.

The effect of these strained interactions on the self-concept of visually impaired persons was discussed by Scott (1969). Both Scott and Lukoff (1972) have pointed out, however, that the greatest effect on the self-concept does not result from the fact that these attitudes exist in the general population, but rather that they also often exist in those with whom the visually impaired interact the most, that is the family, friends, and those who provide services. According to the theories of self-concept formation, it is the significant other who will have the greatest impact on the self-concept of another person. These theories are helpful in that they also suggest a more feasible method of improving the self-concept of a visually impaired person.

Many writers about blindness have spoken of the devastating impact of visual loss on the self-concept. Cutsforth (1950) contended that an individual's self-regarding attitudes may be a greater incapacitation to him than the physical restrictions imposed by blindness. Carroll (1961) talked about blindness as a "destructive blow to the self-image which an individual has constructed throughout his lifetime."

Davis (1964) has suggested that the difficulties that visually impaired persons have in developing an accurate and realistic self-concept are related to their difficulty in developing an accurate image of their body structures. While this is particularly true for congenitally blind persons, Davis also implied that those blinded later in life must restructure a new body image and self-concept. These conclusions seem to relate to the research of Secord and Jourard (1953) and that of Weinberg (1960) who demonstrated that feelings about the body are very much related to feelings about the self.

Meighan (1971) discovered that visually impaired adolescents scored relatively low on the dimension of the Tennessee Self-Concept Scale which measured attitudes toward the physical self. They measured lower, however, on the dimension measuring basic identity and feelings about self. Meighan also reported that the self-concept scores of the visually impaired adolescents in the study were deviant in a negative direction from the normative scores for the Tennessee Self-Concept Scale.

The latter finding was contradictory to the earlier findings of Cowen, Underberg, Verrillo, and Benham (1961) and Jervis (1959) both of whom found no significant differences between the self-concepts of visually impaired and sighted adolescents. Jervis (1959) did report that the blind subjects in his study tended to perceive themselves as either very positive or very negative. He felt that blind persons are either forced into having a very poor self-concept, or if they are "fortunate enough to find positive attributes," they tend to exaggerate them. Jervis felt that this indicated that visually impaired persons have difficulty in making a normal adjustment.

In related research dealing with other disabilities, Bice, (1954), Grayson (1951), and Krider (1959) have studied the effect of disability on the self-concept of young children. In rehabilitation research, Barry, Dunteman, and Webb (1968) and MacGuffie, Janzen, Samuelson, and McPhee (1969) have demonstrated that high self-esteem is conducive to good motivation during rehabilitation. While Hyman (1972) found that patients entering a stroke rehabilitation program with extremely low self-esteem may succeed as a result of the fact that they can more easily be persuaded by others to participate in the program.

Self-Esteem and Self-Concept

While the impact of the attitudes of others toward visual impairment might explain difficulties that visually impaired persons have in forming a positive and an accurate self-concept, these problems might also be understood in the light of Stotland and Canon's (1972) theories about the development of self-esteem. Among other factors, Stotland and Canon felt that a person's sense of competence or self-esteem can be affected by the person's perception of the effectiveness of his own actions, his perceived freedom to select from a number of possible actions, his sense of similarity with others, and the communications he receives from others about his own competence. Considering these factors in relation to the task of independent movement, it is easy to see how the immobile person or the person who must depend on others can end up with a poor self-concept. Coopersmith (1967) found that boys who started walking earlier had a higher sense of competence when they were 8-10 years old than did boys who started walking at a later age. Their early walking also opened up many other possible activities and the opportunity to experience even greater success. In general, Coopersmith found that the more children are able to act effectively in their environment, the higher is their self-esteem.

To the extent that a person has a repertoire of actions to choose from in attaining goals, he is also likely to develop more effective and efficient actions and thus greater self-esteem. In traveling, the visually impaired person who has the options of moving independently or going with a guide has more opportunity to respond to each day's challenges in a variety of ways that contribute to his sense of competence. If he is limited to responding to opportunities only when he has a guide available, his choices are limited.

Recently Delafield (1974) reported that visually impaired people who obtain their first dog guide experience an increase in self-esteem and that this increase has a relatively long-term effect. Similar studies for persons receiving other forms of mobility training are needed.

Stotland and Canon (1972) reviewed research that indicated the effect of the ratings of experts and others on the self-esteem of individuals. People were found to be quite susceptible to the opinions of others, especially when these others were considered expert in the area of being evaluated. When the visually impaired person travels independently, he usually receives positive reactions and support, since this is a skill that sighted people generally do not expect from visually impaired persons. This feedback from others and these ratings of success can have a very positive effect on the self-concept of the visually impaired person.

The interaction between the self-concept and independent travel with reduced vision is complex and reciprocal. If the person has developed a negative self-concept as a result of some of the natural reactions associated with visual loss in our culture, this attitude may reduce the likelihood that the person will aspire to the achievement of success in independent travel. Either his poor self-concept prevents him from beginning the training, or his self-esteem will not sustain him through the initial frustrations and the anticipated fears. This lack of success will further reinforce his negative self-concept or result in some other defense mechanism that protects him from a negative self-evaluation.

On the contrary, if the individual can be helped to experience success in the tasks of independent movement and can be rewarded for this success in the context of an accepting relationship with the mobility specialist, then perhaps the visually impaired peson can begin to feel more positive about himself and continue to improve in these feelings throughout the training sequence.

Baker (1973) extends this type of interactive model one step further by including the attitudes and behaviors of other people in this process. As implied in the discussion so far, there appears to be a circular relationship among several of the variables discussed. The attitudes of others toward visual impairment and visually impaired people affect their behavior toward visually impaired people. This behavior very much affects the perceptions that visually impaired people develop about themselves, that is, their self-concepts. The self-concept has been shown to be a major influence on the behavior of visually impaired people, as it is for everyone. However, the behavior of visually impaired people can also have an impact on the attitudes of sighted people.

If Baker's model or one similar to it does represent accurately the socialization process experienced by visually impaired persons, then it also suggests a variety of alternatives for dealing with difficulties that visually impaired people experience as a result of this process. If the relationships are circular, then the helpful intervention might come at a number of different points on the circle. For example, a psychotherapeutic intervention in the area of the visually impaired person's self-concept may effect a change at that point that would go on to affect the other components in the system. A public education model would attempt through various means to improve the attitudes of sighted people, with the hope that these improvements would also go on to affect the other components. In still another approach, rehabilitation training, the appropriate intervention might be to effect a change in the behaviors of the visually impaired person first, and hope that those changes would have the effect of improving the other aspects of the system.

Actually, efforts should be made to improve all aspects of the system at the same time. The model suffers because the effects of one variable upon the other is not only in the clockwise direction, but can also be in the reverse direction. Improvements in the behavior of the visually impaired person will probably have a positive impact on the self-concept of the person independent of the attitudes and behaviors of others. The model is helpful, however, in demonstrating that improvements in the functioning and behaviors of visually impaired persons such as those affected by mobility training and other rehabilitation activities can have an important impact on the psychological and social experiences of such people.

FAMILY RELATIONSHIPS

The previous discussion focused on the impact of the attitudes of significant others, especially family members, on the self-concept of the visually impaired person. However, the person's relationship with his family has a much broader and far-reaching effect on adjustment to visual loss and on success in orientation and mobility. As with the other psychosocial variables, the interaction between the family and the behaviors of the visually impaired person are reciprocal and complex. The attitudes and behaviors of family members can be a positive force toward successful rehabilitation or can produce a negative effect. The person's success or lack of it in independent functioning can have both positive and negative effects on the attitudes of family members. To further complicate this, it appears that many of the psychosocial variables already discussed can be understood as intervening variables between the attitudes of family members and the success of the visually impaired person. The person's motivation, anxiety, sense of independence, and self-concept may each reflect the impact of his family's feelings and attitudes.

Lindenberg (1976) has reviewed the role of the family in rehabilitation generally. A number of studies were cited, such as Neff (1954), McPhee and Magelby (1960) and Weiner (1964), which indicated a correlation between success in rehabilitation and stable family relationships. Studies by Olshansky and Beach (1975) and Wardlow (1974) indicated an association between lack of success in rehabilitation and poor or disrupted family relationships. Studies were also cited which indicated that, for some families, the entry of the disabled person into the rehabilitation program may precipitate a crisis due to the importance of the dependency of the disabled member to the dynamics of that family. This was the conclusion of studies by Klausner (1969), Rosenstock and Kutner (1967) and Fordyce (1971).

Other reports and studies cited by Lindenberg (1976) discussed the active inclusion of families in rehabilitation. Galloway and Goldstein (1971) reported on the positive effect of family therapy on the work performance and adjustment of rehabilitation clients. Hurwitz (1971) reported his work with the parents of deaf young adults in a rehabilitation program. Also Nau (1973) and Bellis and Sklar (1969) reported on the involvement of parents and family members in rehabilitation activity.

The effect of family members on the successful adaptation of visually impaired persons has not been overlooked in the literature related to visual loss. The majority of the references are concerned with the interaction between visually impaired children and their parents. A major study was done by Sommers (1944), who focused on the effect of parental attitudes and behaviors on the personality development of visually impaired adolescents. Sommers related five categories of parental reactions to the handicap of their children to five types of adjustive behavior on the adolescents. She concluded that the way to effect more satisfactory personality development in visually impaired children is to build up in the parents of such children more wholesome attitudes toward the handicaps of their children.

Cowen, Underberg, Verrillo, and Benham (1961) did not find any relationship between the attitudes of mothers and the adjustment of visually impaired children. They did note that a high degree of parental understanding, as measured by a parent's ability to predict a child's test behavior, correlated consistently and significantly with good adjustment. Cowen and his collaborators felt that the ability to predict apparently indicated an empathy and a reality perception which they felt were essential for a child's good adjustment. More recently, Hall (1974) and Froyd (1973) have discussed the role of parents and families in the education and adjustment of visually impaired children. Bauman and Yoder (1966) have reviewed a number of studies from the blindness area and beyond, which focus on the interaction between the feelings and behaviors of parents and the adjustment and achievement of children.

Families' Reactions to Rehabilitation

The interaction between visually impaired persons and their families in relation to rehabilitation has also been studied. Krause (1962) presented data in support of the theory that part of the good effect of a residential rehabilitation center was that it removed visually impaired persons from the dependency relationships they experienced at home and exposed them to the therapeutic environment of the rehabilitation setting. Bauman and Yoder (1966) reported that the most successful group of visually impaired persons in their study of vocational success generally have better home and family situations than did the two groups who were less successful. The successful subjects were less dependent, more likely to be married, and reported more enjoyment of family life.

There has been very little systematic study of the effect of family relationships on success in orientation and mobility. Graham (1965) studied the mobility activities of blinded male veterans and concluded that one of the significant factors which separated the most and the least successful groups was a supportive and stable family condition. A review of related research by Warren and Kocon (1974) led them to conclude that the families of successfully mobile children would be supportive and encourage the individual's attempt to become independently mobile.

While there has been little formal research on this topic, there are a number of apparent connections between family relationships and success in orientation and mobility that might contribute to a mobility specialist's understanding of the dynamics behind the behavior of a particular client. In many cases some of the psychosocial variables previously discussed could be understood as intervening variables between a visually impaired person's experience with his family and his behaviors in the mobility situation.

The person's motivation to enter mobility training as well as his interest in later using his skills in his home area may be affected positively or negatively by his relationship with family members. Literature already reviewed suggests that the willingness of a visually impaired child to explore and move freely through his environment is determined to a large extent by the behaviors of his parents. Similarly, an adventitiously blinded person's desire to enter rehabilitation training or to begin to move independently through the home environment can result from the encouragement and expectation of family members. On the negative side, either the family's lack of knowledge about what is possible with reduced vision or its desire to keep the visually impaired dependent relationship may lead to explicit or subtle pressure against independent functioning. Some families discourage the visually impaired person from seeking independence because of the family's need to keep the person in the "sick role."

When the visually impaired person returns home from the rehabilitation program or completes mobility training, the encouragement and support of the family is usually quite helpful and necessary in transferring the skills to the home area. Members of the family should have a basic knowledge of the level of skill that the person has achieved, so that they can encourage and reward his attempts to perform independently in appropriate situations. Many clients fail to use their skills fully after completion of training because families do not understand what is possible and they fail to communicate expectations that are similar to those of the training program or consistent with the person's level of skill.

The interaction between the person's motivation and feelings of independence or dependence in relation to his family is complex. The person may be strongly motivated toward independent mobility if he perceives himself as the head of the household on whom the family depends, or as a significant contributor to the welfare of the family. Another person may see himself as dependent on his family and, perhaps unconsciously, realize that increased independence carries with it a threat to his position in the family. Once the person returns home and begins to function more independently, this new behavior may precipitate a crisis to the extent that the visually impaired person's dependency was significant for the dynamics of the family. Prior discussions of the person's possible independence may not have communicated to the family the nature of the problem as forcefully as does the actual mobility of the rehabilitated person. This may be the first manifestation of a problem that had not surfaced earlier.

The anxiety and fear that visually impaired persons experience may have been influenced by similar fears and concerns felt by family members. The parents who feel responsible for a child often have stronger fears for his safety than the child does. The visually impaired person may have never experienced the dangers of stairs or streets, but may have developed anxiety in relation to these concepts due to the frequently expressed admonitions of family members. Wilson (1967) expressed the conclusion that much of the fear in blind children is parental fear communicated to the child.

Including Family in Program

If it is true that the fear and anxieties of family members can affect the experience of the visually impaired person during and after mobility training, this variable must be considered and dealt with by persons responsible for delivering mobility services. In some instances, this difficulty can be lessened through information provided to the family. It is helpful for most families to observe a number of mobility lessons at various stages in the training so that they can have a better understanding of what skills are being developed and the types of solutions that are available for various problems. Observing actual lessons also provides family members with an opportunity to question the mobility specialist and to express some of their concerns. This opportunity should be available, both in the presence of the visually impaired person and privately, since some people may be reluctant to express their fears for the visually impaired family member to hear.

The concept of including family members in the rehabilitation program to provide them with necessary information and an opportunity for discussion has been implemented in the Veterans Administration blind rehabilitation training program. The content and the purposes of these programs have been described by Ault (1968), Blakeslee (1976), and Acton (1976). In some instances, education and information are sufficient to help family members adjust to the new skills and behaviors of the visually impaired person. In other cases, however, the problems may be complicated and require more extensive services from other professionals or even from other agencies.

The concepts discussed earlier, related to the importance of a developmental sequence of lesson plans and the relationship between the instructor and the client for dealing with the psychosocial variables, also relate to the interactions with family members, particularly when they are not enthusiastic about the person becoming more independent. The mobility specialist should be aware of this possibility and try to pull the family members into the planning and activity of the mobility training as much as the setting allows. Wright (1960) has offered suggestions for the worker that appear to contribute to building a better relationship with the parents of visually impaired children. Wright suggests that the parents must feel 1) the worker is not working against them, but that together they are seeking solutions to the problems; 2) the worker likes the child and sees him as an individual, not just another blind child, and 3) the worker appreciates the parents' strengths and their efforts to do the best they can for their child.

In elaborating these points, Wright noted that the parents are likely to view the rehabilitation worker as the authority who is in a position to pass judgment on the success or failure of the parents' efforts to help their child develop. The parents may enter the relationship with the worker with a fear that they will be blamed for the child's difficulties or that the worker will make new demands on the parents that they cannot meet. They may also fear that the worker will shatter their "strands of hope" that their child will be able to be helped to function. The parents may fear that the child may become too attached to the worker. The worker can add to these difficulties if he possesses attitudes such as that expressed by the sentence, "The trouble with children is their parents." Another harmful attitude on the part of the worker is the feeling that his job is to provide answers. Progress toward a good working relationship with parents will be made to the extent that the worker is sincerely open to hearing the parents' viewpoints and allowing them a full share in the decision-making about their children.

While Wright was focusing on the interactions between workers and parents of children with impairments, the concepts might also apply to dealing with the families of adults who enter rehabilitation programs. Little attention has been given to this area.

INTERACTIONS WITH THE PUBLIC

In discussing the self-concept as an important psychosocial variable, the point was made that the attitudes and behaviors of significant others play an important role in determining the feelings a person develops about himself. While the role played by the attitudes of the general public was minimized in the discussion of the self-concept, these attitudes and the behaviors which they generate do have an impact on the psychosocial aspects of independent travel for visually impaired persons.

Many visually impaired persons are stigmatized when they travel in public. The concept of stigma is not used in the sense of its primary meaning as a mark of infamy or disgrace, but rather it is used in a more general sense as a mark, label, or behavior which indicates some deviation from a norm or standard, a deviation that does not necessarily indicate a negative evaluation. Some persons are stigmatized by their appearance resulting from the eye condition that led to the loss of vision, while others are stigmatized by the equipment that they use or the behaviors that they adopt to offset the fact of the vision loss. Some low vision persons only become stigmatized when they are forced to solicit assistance in a situation where a person with normal vision would be able to function independently.

The fact that many visually impaired persons are stigmatized elicits particular types of reactions and behaviors from people with whom the stigmatized person must interact. These reactions and behaviors elicited from others, in turn, may affect the self-concept and other attitudes of the stigmatized person or may lead to changes in his own behavior. The visually impaired person, or for that matter any handicapped person, must learn to cope with the reactions of people to stigma if he is going to be able to move independently through the environment.

The perspective taken in this discussion, similar to that which has influenced the discussion of the other psychosocial variables, is one which emphasizes the reciprocal interdependence between the variables involved, that is between the attitudes and the behavior of the visually impaired person and the attitudes and the behaviors of the members of the public. Wright (1960) pointed out that the reactions that an impaired person has to an exchange with members of the public can be influenced by how he perceives himself and his disability, that is, by his self-concept. However, the form that his reaction takes may itself go a long way toward making the exchange worse or controlling it or even turning it into a positive experience for both parties, thus influencing the attitudes and future behaviors of the non-stigmatized person. Moreover, these events can also have important consequences for the visually impaired person's self-concept.

The fact that people treat differently persons who are stigmatized by a disability, or by information about a disability, has been documented in a number of empirical studies. Farina and Ring (1965) and Farina, Holland, and Ring (1966) demonstrated how the perception of a person as mentally ill can influence the behaviors and attitudes of those who interact with that person. It was found that when a co-worker is viewed as mentally ill, subjects prefer to work alone rather than with him and blame him for experimentally manipulated inadequacies in the joint performance.

In another series of investigations, Kleck, Ono, and Hastorf (1966) studied the effects of physical deviance on face-to-face interactions. The results indicated that subjects interacting with a physically disabled stimulus person: 1) tended to demonstrate less variability in their behavior than did subjects interacting with a physically normal person; 2) tended to terminate the interaction sooner than did subjects in the non-disabled interaction; 3) expressed opinions which were less representative of their actual beliefs than were those expressed by subjects in the non-disabled group.

Stigma Theories

Goffman (1963), Davis (1961), and Friedson (1965) have theorized about the effects of stigma on human interactions. In all of their theories, it is clear that the problem does not reside in the person who possesses the stigma nor entirely in the persons who react to the stigma, but in the interaction between these two sets of actors and in the nature of their interactions.

There are three theoretical concepts that appear particularly useful in understanding the psychosocial experience of visually impaired persons in relation to the general public. These are the concepts of the *new psychological situation, overlapping roles,* and *passing.* The first two of these originated in some of the early work of Lewin (1936) and were first applied to the situation of disabled persons by Barker, Wright, Meyerson, and Gonick (1953). They have been elaborated by Meyerson (1963). The concept of passing which will be discussed with particular application to low vision people was developed by Goffman (1963).

A *new psychological situation* is one in which the location of positive goals and the path by which they can be reached are not clearly perceived by the person, as opposed to an old situation in which both the positive and negative goals and the behavioral possibilities are well known. Entering a new psychological situation both attracts and repels a person, because of the uncertain location of a positive goal. A person will engage in trial and error behavior and will experience a certain amount of vacillating as he strives to discover the location of the goal and how to achieve it. The person in the new situation will experience frustration as a result of the searching and the trial and error behavior, and this frustration may lead to the experience of anxiety and the disruption of behavior. The person will be in conflict as he simultaneously tries to reach the goal of the new situation and then withdraw to the safety of the old situation.

Visually impaired persons, along with other physically disabled persons, more frequently experience new psychological situations than do non-impaired persons. This is true for congenitally disabled persons to the extent that they have been overprotected and/or deprived of some of the common experiences of non-disabled persons. Some situations are new for all disabled persons to the extent that they lack a necessary tool for dealing with this situation. Vision is a tool that people use to learn about changes in the environment and to inform themselves of the need for changes in common behavior patterns. Without vision, the person enters more situations in which he may not have information about changes that have taken place. Some situations are new for the disabled person as a result of the stimulus value that the disabled person represents for the non-disabled persons who are present. According to Meyerson, "Disability has many meanings to others. The disabled person often does not know when he enters a social situation whether he will be an object of curiosity, pitied, sympathized with, helped, patronized, exhibited, praised for his spunk, avoided, or actively rejected" (Meyerson, 1963, p. 41). What is reasonably certain is that the disabled person will elicit a strong reaction of some sort, but what is uncertain is the direction and type of reaction to expect and how to cope with it.

The experience of interacting with a disabled person is also often a new psychological situation for the non-disabled person. The infrequency of this experience along with the strong stimulus that the disabled person represents, signals to the non-disabled person that this is a different situation which he may not know how to handle. For the non-disabled as well as the disabled person, the new psychological situation is likely to give rise to trial-and-error searching for the right behavior and the frustration that accompanies this. It is also likely to lead to anxiety and the disruption of normal behavior patterns and eventually to conflict about interacting or leaving the situation.

The remedy for the psychosocial problem that emerges from this type of situation lies in reducing the newness of the situation through information and the rehearsal of appropriate behavior patterns for a number of possible situations. More will be discussed about this as a solution later in this section.

Overlapping Roles

The concept of *overlapping roles* arises from the realization that each person belongs to many different groups simultaneously and must play multiple roles. As Meyerson (1963) notes, many overlapping roles are *compatible,* so that it is possible for an individual to be a son, a brother, a college student, a football player, an English major, and a musician at the same time without any conflict. Some overlapping roles may be *interfering,* such as belonging to the university football team and the marching band at the same time. This conflict is resolved simply by choosing one or the other of these roles. Some overlapping roles are *antagonistic,* as in the case of the young man who brings his fiancee home for a visit where his doting mother treats him as a child. In this instance, the individual is under pressure to choose one or the other role, either the mature adult who is about to become married or the dependent child and dutiful son. Responding to one of the roles automatically rules out the other. Frequently, visually impaired persons have to choose between the antagonistic roles of either being a dependent person who relies on help or an independent person who functions without help. Sometimes it is difficult to get just a little help without being compelled to take more than is actually needed.

A fourth type of overlapping role is that of *excluding* roles. In this situation a person rejects a role that is open to him in favor of a role that he cannot reasonably attain because of a lack of ability or because of social barriers. The disabled person finds himself torn between the role of the disabled person and that of a physically normal person. There are strong cultural forces acting upon the disabled person to act and appear as normal as possible. However, the role of the disabled person excludes that of the normal person in every situation in which the disability makes a difference. If the person acts appropriately for a disabled person in that situation, for example, using a cane for mobility, he will automatically surrender the possibility of being considered a non-disabled person. This conflict most frequently surfaces in social situations where the rewards for being a "normal" person are greatest and the negative effects for deviating from the norm are most potent.

The Phenomenon of "Passing"

There are strong forces acting upon people in our society to act as if they are not disabled and not impaired. The struggle to resolve this conflict can put the visually impaired person under considerable strain and can lead to strong resistance to being identified as a disabled person in public situations, particularly through the advertisement of a long cane. The pressures associated with trying to resolve the conflict of excluding overlapping roles may often result in the phenomenon of "passing." Passing has been discussed by Goffman (1963) as behavior by a person designed to conceal a salient aspect of his identity. This may be particularly true for low vision persons who are frequently able to conceal their vision loss.

Goffman discusses the stages of passing that some people experience as they first discover that they have passed accidentally by realizing that people have treated them as not having the disability they do actually possess. The stages progress through passing for the "fun of it," passing on vacations, passing in situations involving people with whom one interacts frequently, and finally passing completely and being able to conceal the problem identity entirely. Goffman also discusses some of the strains and difficulties associated with passing. He particularly notes the anxiety associated with always having to be alert to all of the details of a situation which might otherwise be responsible for unveiling the identity. There is also the strain associated with explaining the ruse when the true identity of the person comes to be revealed one way or another.

Passing, of course, is something that is done in relation to other people, and it is during the time that a visually impaired person must interact with other people that the threat associated with passing is most severe and the anxiety is highest. The concept of "passing" applies most frequently to low vision persons. For many low vision persons, the disability is not obvious. It becomes apparent in some situations or at certain times. This variability leaves them with decisions to make concerning how they present themselves. If they emphasize the disability component of their identity, then they expose themselves to the demeaning aspects of that identity at times when they might otherwise be spared those difficulties. This choice also creates problems when low vision persons are noticed functioning visually by persons who perceived them as lacking vision. If low vision persons choose to conceal the disability components of their identity, they are spared some of the difficulties in those situations in which their vision loss does not matter. However, when they encounter situations in which they cannot function visually, their inability to function or their need for assistance may then stigmatize them and cause interaction problems.

For persons who have chosen the first alternative, that of identifying themselves as visually impaired in mobility situations, it has frequently been recommended that this can be most effectively accomplished through the use of, or merely carrying, a long cane, usually of the collapsible variety. This results in their being identified as visually impaired persons more than is necessary, but when they do need assistance, their reason for asking is obvious to others. For those who choose to remain unidentified, they can frequently be helped to develop ways of approaching others in situations where help is needed. These strategies, such as preceding a request for information by acknowledgement of the vision loss, usually require some revelation that a disability is present, but this can be done in a more focused and less public way than by carrying the cane. Persons choosing either alternative might also benefit from the opportunity to role play and rehearse responses for those situations when the alternative aspect of the identity they are emphasizing is discovered in a social situation. The person who is carrying a cane but is confronted about his obvious ability to function visually in some situations should be ready with an easy explanation of his complicated circumstances that will quickly dispose of a potentially troublesome interaction. Similarly, the person who presents himself as non-disabled, but is found to be unable to perform certain functions without assistance should be able to handle the confusion and emotions that may accompany it.

It is not the role of the mobility specialist to decide for the low vision person how he wants to present himself. This can be decided only by the person himself. The mobility specialist does have a responsibility to be certain that the person has considered all of the factors associated with one approach versus the other in travel situations. These include both psychosocial and physical safety factors. The mobility specialist may be able to help the person consider all of the complex components in making his decision on travel method. Once the client has made a decision, or is in the process of trying to make a decision, the mobility specialist should expose the low vision person to the full range of possible situations he will encounter. He should also structure learning and practice opportunities during which the client can try out a variety of solutions to the safety, the psychosocial, and the orientation problems that are involved in his circumstances. The criteria of what will be the best solution for each individual must include consideration of his psychosocial functioning along with the other variables involved.

Uncovering Conflicts

For many visually impaired persons mobility training and independent travel first bring some of these conflicts to light. Before learning to travel independently, the expectation that comes as part of mobility training is that the visually impaired person will contact people in public places. He may not have had many experiences of this nature. A congenitally blind child may have been protected from these encounters by parents and family members, or through social and play experiences only with friends and neighbors who are "in the know." The adventitiously blinded person may have also been restricted in his social experiences or protected by members of his family who always "run interference" for him in social situations. These persons, by always being with the visually impaired person, prevent others from approaching and offering assistance or expressing curiosity. However, mobility training eventually will require that the visually impaired person move through populated environments on his own at a distance from the instructor and at the mercy of interactions with the public.

When discussing the interactions between visually impaired persons and members of their families, it was suggested that family members could be involved in rehabilitation activities and helped to change their expectations of and be-

8

haviors toward the visually impaired person. This solution does not apply to problems associated with interactions with the public. While public education efforts may help ameliorate the situation somewhat, on the whole they are not effective in bringing about changes in the behaviors of the public. This leads to the conclusion that any efforts to improve the interactions between the visually impaired person and the public must focus on the visually impaired person and his behaviors and reactions in these situations.

Mobility training deliberately exposes the client to situations in which he will be approached by and have to interact with members of the public representing a wide range of attitudes toward visual impairment. The mobility specialist will be with the client during most of these encounters and will be in a position to observe how the client handles the interaction and to give some feedback and advice on how to handle the situation differently when necessary. The frustrations associated with unpleasant examples of these encounters may be very discouraging for the visually impaired person, and may result in his experiencing more acutely this type of excluding overlapping roles discussed above. This, in turn, may lead to his traveling less and less independently or terminating his lessons if still in training. Because of this, the mobility specialist must be sensitive to how the client is coping with this aspect of the mobility training, and must be ready to modify the lesson plans if necessary or to arrange the sequence of lessons along a gradient of involvement with other persons in order to assist clients with the difficulties associated with such interactions.

Problematic Interactions With Public

The most frequent interaction has to do with offers to help. There are three types of offers, those which are unsolicited and unnecessary, those which are unsolicited and necessary, those which are solicited. Each of these types of offers may or may not have an effect on the visually impaired person depending on how he is coping with his identity as a person with a disability. The person who is feeling the confict of excluding overlapping roles is likely to be further frustrated by any offer of help, whether needed or not, whether accepted or not. Such a person is also less likely to solicit assistance when it is needed which may further aggravate a frustrating situation. In a similar way, the person who reacts to new psychological situations with a great amount of anxiety or emotion may be more upset by offers of help and less likely to solicit assistance when needed because of the implications of entering a new situation.

Both of these types of persons may be helped in coping with offers of assistance from the public through role playing a variety of situations that occur during travel and rehearsing different responses to each of these situations. Being prepared for these situations and having confidence in the effectiveness of certain responses will help to reduce the newness of new psychological situations and thus reduce the anxiety associated with them. This type of learning may also help the person struggling with excluding overlapping roles. Having effective responses to use in interactions with the public may help the person to better maintain his self-esteem as a disabled person, become more comfortable in the role of the disabled person where it is unavoidable, and reduce the conflicts associated with struggling to function as a non-disabled person in situations where the disability does exclude normal functioning.

Certain responses to unnecessary and unwanted offers of help are more effective than others in getting rid of the help. An effective response for one client may be ineffective for another client. The mobility specialist's role is to discuss the variety of responses that are possible and to assist the visually impaired person to select those which he will prefer to use in future situations. Part of this decision process will be based on feedback that the specialist provides the client as he observes him interacting with people in real travel situations during training.

Extracting necessary assistance from sighted pedestrians once a contact has been made is an associated skill. Since this is usually a new situation for the sighted person, he may not know what information will be useful, or because of his anxiety, he may make rather basic errors. The visually impaired person must learn how to "take charge" of the interaction to assure that he gets the information he needs. He must learn how to ask specific questions that will elicit responses from the sighted person other than "yes" or "no." He must able to break down requests for orientation information into manageable units that the sighted person can respond to in a way that will assure the visually impaired person of getting thorough information. This structuring of the interaction by the visually impaired person will take some of the "newness" and uncertainty out of it for both persons, which will result in less anxiety and frustration for both.

Another problem associated with offers of help is less open to management by the visually impaired traveler. Some "would-be" helpers communicate in their offers their attitudes of superiority and their true motivation, the inflation of their own egos, and their own self-aggrandizement. Many disabled persons properly resent this type of assistance, and some experience conflicts about how to terminate such interactions. Some feel that a remark in response to such a patronizing tone is both cathartic and justified, but they worry that they will create future problems for themselves and for other disabled persons who may someday need assistance from the person they have insulted. Even the person who presents such an insensitive attitude has the potential for learning and changing. This change may be better accomplished by a firm and confident refusal of assistance and subsequent exhibition of successful independent behavior than by a curt remark.

Other types of interaction also can be problematic. Persons may approach the visually impaired person with expressions of curiosity or sympathy. These experiences can produce anxiety and frustration to the extent that the visually impaired person is unprepared to cope with them. Since these situations are likely to occur in mobility lessons, the instructor must be prepared to help the client cope with the emotions that these events may generate and to assist the client through discussion and perhaps role playing to be able to cope with these situations when they occur. If the client can keep these events in a proper perspective and understand them in the total context of how disability is perceived by and misunderstood by non-disabled persons, he will be better able to prevent the negative impact of these experiences on his self-concept and his attitude toward moving independently through the community.

In summary, the interactions with members of the public can have a negative effect on the attitudes and emotional well-being of the visually impaired person. As a result they can have a negative impact on his willingness and ability to travel independently. However, if these events and interactions are capably handled, they can permit the person to experience fuller independence and can contribute positively to his acceptance of his identity as a person who has a disability but who can manage to function in spite of it.

PROBLEM SOLVING

The final variable is more of a cognitive variable than a psychosocial variable, but it is considered here because of its close association with the other variables discussed. One of the prerequisites for independent movement through the environment is the ability to solve problems and to make decisions. This is true for every person who moves through the environment because areas change and various types of barriers or blockades make usual routes impassable. This is even more true for the visually impaired traveler who receives less information from the environment both about blockages and about alternative solutions to problems encountered. In addition, the task of orientation with reduced vision or no vision is more problematic than with full vision. Information is less reliable and less specific than visual clues, and the visually impaired traveler has to make more judgments and decisions and do more interpreting of the clues presented.

The congenitally visually impaired person who has not had as many opportunities to travel independently also has not had many opportunities to make decisions about his orientation and about reaching certain destinations. As with other skills, those associated with problem-solving are not innate but develop through practice and successful use. It is not uncommon to observe deficiencies in the problem-solving abilities of congenitally impaired persons in mobility training.

Adventitiously visually impaired persons may also experience difficulties in this area. This can happen when visual loss is experienced by a person who was not very adept at problem-solving as a sighted person. It also happens as a result of the anxiety or other adjustment problems the person is experiencing related to his sight loss, especially if the loss is sudden. Emotional trauma can interfere with this area of functioning as witnessed by the difficulties that each of us experiences in settling important matters during periods of stress. Some of these problems in adventitiously visually impaired persons may also relate to the person's lack of confidence in basing decisions on information received through sense systems other than vision. Prior to vision loss, the person used his vision as the major channel of information and even to verify information obtained through other channels. Now he must learn to rely on these other channels to a much greater extent, and this can lessen his confidence in the decisions he makes based on this information.

For these reasons, it is likely that the person who enters mobility training may not have a high degree of problem-solving ability or may not have confidence in what ability he does have. This lack of ability or lack of confidence can cause deficiencies in the person's self-esteem, can create additional anxiety, can prevent the emergence of independent functioning, and may be the basis for family members distrusting this person's potential for responsibility for himself in travel situations. For these reasons as well as because this ability is necessary in actual travel situations, mobility instruction must deal directly and systematically with the skill of problem-solving and decision-making.

Cofer (1966) suggested that the stages of problem-solving are: 1) recognition that a problem does exist, 2) elaboration of the alternative hypotheses and possible solutions, and 3) the selection and verification of an effective solution. This process is integrated into the entire mobility training continuum and is approached in the same developmental sequence described earlier.

Problem Solving in Lesson Plans

From the earliest lessons in the sequence, the mobility student is exposed to problems of orientation and is asked to solve them. Initially they are simple and basic problems related to remaining oriented while traveling with a sighted guide, but as training progresses, they become more complex. Once the student begins to travel by himself he is required to make more decisions on his own and to cope with the consequences of these decisions, including the new problems that wrong decisions bring.

The mobility specialist attempts to control the complexity of the problems that the client must deal with through the structuring of the lesson plans and through his own decisions about when to step into a situation and provide additional assistance. The instructor has wide discretion relative to how complex the problems of the client become. He must decide when to terminate a lesson and when to let it continue. Through the close working relationship that the mobility specialist tries to develop with the client, he is able to evaluate how much frustration a client can tolerate. This relates to the earlier discussion of the effect of level of aspiration on the experience of success. It is unlikely that the client will develop more confidence in his ability to solve problems if the problems presented do not represent a reasonable challenge. The specialist must monitor the lessons closely to be certain that the challenges do not extend beyond the client's current ability leading to further frustration and a possible set-back in his progress.

The drop-off lesson described earlier is an important technique available to the mobility specialist in helping the client develop problem-solving abilities. The drop-off lesson can be modified by the instructor to make it suitable to a particular client's level of ability. For example, some clients may be given one or more items of information about the starting point for the drop-off lesson. They will be expected to complete the route to the objective once they have determined the other dimensions of their starting point that are relevant. This type of modification can be made more simple or more complex depending on the particular client's needs and state of development in problem solving. The mobility specialist can help the client become aware of and develop a variety of strategies and solutions from which to choose in problem situations.

Success in the problem-solving activities that occur throughout the lesson plan sequence as well as in the drop-off lessons can have an important impact on the person's confidence in his own abilities. This success can also have an important impact on the person's self-concept, his sense of independence, and his motivation to continue in training and to transfer his skills to new areas.

PSYCHOSOCIAL ASPECT OF THE TRAINING SITUATION

Finally, it is important to consider the psychosocial dimensions of the mobility training situation itself. The manner in which mobility training is offered, through individualized instruction in real environments, leads to the possibility of certain relationships and situations which can cause their own difficulties.

Most of the problems in this area have to do with the close relationship between the mobility specialist and the client. Early in the discussion and throughout, reference has been made to the role that this relationship plays in helping the client cope with many of the negative aspects of the psychosocial components presented. As with all human relationships, however, such a close association between instructor and student is subject to misunderstanding and conflict which may interfere with the purpose of the relationship.

It was pointed out that the relationship between the instructor and student may be responsible for helping the student through a period of necessary dependency on the instructor, to independence. Also, the instructor's expectations can become an important motivator and reinforcer for certain clients. Just as these observations are true, so is the possibility that the relationship can lead to excessive dependency on the instructor and on the approval of the instructor. If this happens, it is possible that the client will not perform adequately outside the training situation and will not learn skills that are useful later.

Another problem that may develop in the relationship is that the instructor will overidentify with the client to the point that he will not be able to make objective judgments or hard decisions about him (Schulz, 1972). The mobility specialist may have difficulty communicating and enforcing clear and appropriate expectations for certain clients.

An opposite problem may be that the mobility specialist could develop an unpleasant or antagonistic relationship with a client, or have a bias or prejudice against clients with certain characteristics. Such negative feelings can work themselves out as unfair expectations or unreasonably negative evaluations. The effect of these on the client may be that he is not helped to develop a realistic self-concept of his ability and is probably not motivated to continue in training.

Importance of Adequate Supervision

One possible safeguard against many of the difficulties that might arise in a close relationship of this type is the use of appropriate supervision or by soliciting judgments and evaluations about particular clients from other mobility specialists. Supervision is particularly necessary in any situation in which a professional attempts to use himself in close relationships to assist clients to change and develop. There is a history of supervision in counseling, social work, psychotherapy, and similar disciplines. Unfortunately, the short history as well as some of the circumstances of service delivery in orientation and mobility make the use of supervision very difficult in many situations where mobility instruction is offered.

Related to the concept of the relationship between the mobility specialist and the client are the difficulties that may be associated with the "weaning process," an important part of mobility instruction for many clients. When this is done improperly, or when it is not well-timed, a number of difficulties can arise. The person may experience an increase in anxiety rather than being able to handle the next stage. The client may act as if the instructor is always close, by attempting to talk with him during the lesson to verify certain information. The person may also give evidence of being slow to recognize problems and to implement any problem-solving strategies. As suggested earlier, the instructor may be ready to move into a new segment of the mobility lesson plan that implies more independent functioning. The client may not yet be ready for that stage perhaps because the instructor has not been clearly communicating his expectations for independent functioning at each prior stage.

In some situations the instructor's reactions to the sighted public, particularly those which he expresses in the presence of the client can create additional difficulties. The instructor may lose his patience with persons who interfere with his client or with the lesson. He may lead the client to be predisposed toward considering the sighted public as stupid or inconsiderate as a result of his expressions of impatience. This could lead to similar expressions by the client or, more important, it could interfere with the client's being able to rely comfortably on the assistance of the public if and when needed.

The reaction of the instructor is particularly poignant in those situations in which the visually impaired person is insulted or treated poorly by a member of the public. The instructor's tendency may be to step in and defend the client. It is important to consider, however, the message that such a defense might convey to the client himself. For some clients, such an event might communicate that the client is indeed a helpless person who must be defended by others. As discussed above, it is not possible to change very effectively the attitudes and behaviors of the general public. There will continue to be people in the community who will have negative, stereotypical reactions to visually impaired persons. The visually impaired person must learn how to cope with this type of situation on his own, since his defender the mobility specialist, will not always be present. Perhaps role playing and rehearsing effective responses in such situations does more good than the interference of the specialist.

The Blindfold

An important psychosocial concern in planning lessons for low vision persons centers around the use of the blindfold. The previous chapter presented a number of the issues related to the use of the blindfold in mobility training for low vision persons. While the blindfold may have some usefulness in helping low vision persons learn to use their other senses more effectively, the psychosocial components of its use must also be considered. For many persons with partial loss of sight, perhaps the strongest fear is the possible loss of the remaining vision. Some low vision persons resist the use of the blindfold because of the stimulus value that the blindfold has for them in causing them to try to function without any vision. It forces them to think too much about a situation that they fear very much.

For those people who fear the possibility of total sight loss, the mobility instructor's explanation that the blindfold is being used only to help the person learn how to use other sense systems to supplement his vision may not be credible. The emotional stimulus related to eventual total blindness dominates and the person becomes unable to tolerate the mobility training and leaves. For this reason, the use of the blindfold must be approached with extreme caution and a clear commitment to a use of the blindfold only if the client is in agreement with this procedure. Even this approach does not eliminate the problems since many clients as a result of their past experiences with authority figures still feel that they cannot really refuse to work with the blindfold, and they may perceive their only recourse as flight from the mobility training situation.

SUMMARY

The major thrust of this chapter has been to establish the psychosocial functioning of visually impaired persons as an important component of their ability to function independently in orientation and mobility. Difficulties in the psychosocial area can be as detrimental as are hearing losses, posture and gait problems, lack of concepts, and deficiencies in other sense systems. In the same way, successful functioning in the psychosocial area is an important foundation for successful mobility.

The analysis of the variables that are involved with this topic has been approached with two goals in mind. The first goal has been to demonstrate the complexity and the idiosyncratic nature of these variables. It is impossible to establish many axioms or principles of behavior that will apply without exception to all or even most clients. Instead, the mobility specialist should be aware of all of the variables that might possibly influence a person's experience as he attempts to understand the experience and functioning of each individual as a unique entity.

The second goal has been to demonstrate the interactive nature of these variables. To the extent, for example, that the self-concept, if deficient, can prevent successful orientation and mobility, it is also true that success in orientation and mobility can have a positive effect on the self-concept. This understanding of psychosocial variables leads to an approach that does not focus on the minimum levels of a particular ability or characteristic that is necessary before instruction can be begun or can be useful. Instead, the approach that emerges is one that begins with each individual at his own level of functioning on these characteristics, and structures situations and learning experiences to help the person improve in each of these areas.

The mobility training experience depends quite a lot on the understandings associated with the variables discussed. Mobility training could be improved as a result of systematic research on these variables to test out some of the theoretical understandings that have been suggested. It is also possible that this research even though focused on the reactions of visually impaired persons may contribute to broader applications and understanding of these variables with other disability groups or with people in general. In this way, it is hoped that knowledge and information developed in this area will begin to interact more with the knowledge that is developing in other areas related to psychosocial functioning.

Bibliography

Acton, J. J. Establishing and maintaining a therapeutic environment in a residential rehabilitation center for the blind. *New Outlook for the Blind*, 1976, **70**, 149-152.

Adler, A. *The Practice and Theory of Individual Psychology*, New York: Harcourt, 1924.

Ault, C. Social work essentials in severe visual impairment and blindness. *Program Guide to Social Work Service*, Washington D. C.: Veterans Administration, 1968.

Baer, D. M. A technique of social reinforcement for the study of child behavior: Behavior avoiding reinforcement withdrawal. *Child Development*, 1962, **33,** 847-858.

Baker, L. D. Blindness and social behavior: A need for research. *New Outlook for the Blind,* 1973, **67,** 315-318.

Bandura, A. & Walters, R. H. *Adolescent Aggression*. New York: Ronald, 1959.

Bandura, A. & Walters, R. H. *Social Learning and Personality Development*. New York: Holt, 1963.

Barker, R. G. & Wright, B. The social psychology of adjustment to physical disability. In J. F. Garrett (Ed.). *Psychological Aspects of Physical Disability*, Dept. of Health Education and Welfare. Office of Vocational Rehabilitation, Rehabilitation Services Series No. 210, 1952.

Barker, R. G., Wright, B. A., Meyerson, L., & Gonick, M. R. *Adjustment to Physical Handicap and Illness: A Survey of the Social Psychology of Physique and Disability*. New York: Social Science Research Council, 1953.

Barry, J. R., Dunteman, G. H. & Webb, M. W. Personality and motivation in rehabilitation. *Journal of Counsel Psychology*, 1968. **15,** (13), 237-244.

Bauman, M. K. & Yoder, N. M. *Adjustment to Blindness Re-Viewed*. Springfield, Ill.: Charles C Thomas, 1966.

Bellis, J. & Sklar, N. The challenge of adjustment of retarded adolescents in a workshop. *Journal of Rehabilitation*, 1969 (May-June), 19-22.

Bice, H. Some factors that contribute to the concept of self in the child with cerebral palsy. *Mental Hygiene*, 1954, 120-131.

Blakeslee, R. The role of the social worker in a rehabilitation center for the visually handicapped. *New Outlook for the Blind*, 1976, **70**, 69-71.

Blank, R. Psychoanalysis and blindness. *The Psychoanalytic Quarterly*, 1957, **26,** 1-24.

Cairns, R. B. The influence of dependency inhibition on the effectiveness of social reinforcers. *Journal of Personality*, 1961, **29**, 466-488.

Calloway, J. P. & Goldstein, E. *Some Influences of Family Group Therapy on the Rehabilitation Potential of Clients*. New Orleans: Delgado Junior College, 1971.

Campeau, P. Test anxiety and feedback in programmed instruction. *Journal of Educ. Psychology*, 1968, **59**, 159-163.

Carkhuff, R. *Helping and Human Relations*. New York: Holt, Rinehart and Winston, 1969.

Carkhuff, R. New direction in training for the helping professions: Toward a technology for human and community resource development. *The Counseling Psychologist*, 1972, **3** (3), 12-30.

Carroll, T. J. *Blindness: What it is, What it Does, and How to Live With it*. Boston: Little, Brown & Co., 1961.

Cholden, L. S. *A Psychiatrist Works With Blindness*. New York: American Foundation for the Blind, 1958.

Cofer, C. N. Reasoning as an associate process. III. The role of verbal responses in problem-solving. In R. C. Anderson and D. P. Ausubel (Eds.), *Readings in the Psychology of Cognition*. New York: Holt, Rinehart and Winston, 1966.

Coopersmith, S. *The Antecedents of Self-Esteem*. San Francisco: Freeman, 1967.

Cowen, E., Underberg, R., Verillo, R., & Benham, F. *Adjustment to Visual Disability in Adolescence*. New York: American Foundation for the Blind, 1961.

Crandall, V. J., Preston, A., & Robson, A. Maternal reactions and the development of independence in young children. *Child Development*, 1960, **31**, 243-251.

Cutsforth, T. D. Personality and social adjustment of the blind. In A. P. Zahl (Ed.) *Blindness: Modern Approaches to the Unseen Environment*. Princeton, N.J.: Princeton University Press, 1950.

Davis, C. J. Development of the self-concept. *New Outlook for the Blind*, 1964, **58,** 49-51.

Davis F. Deviance disavowal: The management of strained interaction by the visibly handicapped. *Social Problem*, 1961, **9,** 120-132.

Davis, F. *Passage Through Crisis: Polio Victims and Their Families*. Indianapolis: Bobbs, Merrill Co., Inc., 1964.

Delafield, G. L. Adjustment to blindness, *New Outlook for the Blind*, 1976, **70**, 64-68.

Delafield, G. F. *The Effects of Guide Dog Training on Some Aspects of Adjustment in Blind People*. Unpublished Doctoral Dissertation, Nottingham University, 1974.

Diamond, M. D., Weiss, A. J., & Grynbaum, B. The unmotivated patient. *Archives of Physical Medicines and Rehabilitation,* 1968, **49,** 281-284.

Diethelm, O. & Jones, M. Influence of anxiety on attention, learning, retention, and thinking. *Archives of Neurology and Psychiatry,* 1947, **58,** 325-336.

Easterbrook, J. A. The effect of emotion on our utilization and the organization of behavior. *Psychological Review,* 1959, **66,** 183-201.

Ekehammer, B. Interactionism in personality from a historical perspective. *Psychological Bulletin,* 1975, **81,** 1026-48.

Endler, N. S. & Hunt, J. Generalizability of contributions from sources of variance in the S-R inventories of anxiousness. *Journal of Personality,* 1969, **37,** 1-24.

Endler, N. S. & Hunt, J. S-R inventories of hostility and comparisons of the proportions of variance from persons responses and situations, for hostility and anxiousness. *Journal of Personality and Social Psychology,* 1968, **9,** 309-315.

Endler, N. S. & Hunt, J. Sources of behavioral variance as measured by the S-R inventory of anxiousness. *Psychological Bulletin,* 1966, **65,** 336-346.

Farina, A., Holland, C. H., & Ring, K. Role of stigma and set in interpersonal interaction. *Journal of Abnormal Psychology,* 1966, **71,** 421-428.

Farina, A. & Ring, K. The influence of perceived mental illness on interpersonal relationships. *Journal of Abnormal Psychology,* 1965, **70,** 47-51.

Fluharty, W., McHugh, J., McHugh, M., Willits, P., & Wood, J. Anxiety in the teacher-student relationship as applicable to orientation and mobility instruction. *New Outlook for the Blind,* ,1976, **70,** 153-156.

Fordyce, W. Behavioral methods in rehabilitation. In W. Neff (Ed.) *Rehabilitation Psychology,* Washington D. C.: American Psychological Assn., 1971.

Friedson, E. Disability as social deviance. In M. Sussman (Ed.) *Sociology and Rehabilitation,* Washington D. C.: American Sociological Association, 1965.

Fromm, E. *Escape from Freedom.* New York: Rinehart, 1941.

Froyd, H. F. Counseling families of severely visually handicapped children. *New Outlook for the Blind,* 1973, **67,** 251-257.

Galloway, J. P. & Goldstein, H. K. *A Follow-Up Study of the Influences of Group Therapy with Relatives on the Rehabilitation Potential of Rehabilitation Clients* (Final Report) Delgado Community College, New Orleans, La. 1971.

Goffman, E. *Stigma.* Englewood Cliffs: Prentice-Hall, Inc., 1963.

Graham, M. D. Wanted: A readiness test for mobility training. *New Outlook for the Blind,* 1965, **59,** 157-162.

Grayson, M. Concept of acceptance in physical rehabilitation. *Journal of the American Medical Association,* 1951, **45,** 893-896.

Haggard, E. A. Psychological causes and results of stress, *Human Factors in Undersea Warfare.* National Research Council, 1949.

Hall, G. C. *Parent's Role—Report to Boston Center for Blind Children.* Boston: Boston Center for Blind Children, 1974.

Hallenback, P. A. *Dogmatism and Visual Loss.* New York: American Foundation for the Blind, 1967.

Havens, L. L. Dependence: Definitions and strategies. *Rehabilitation Record,* 1967, **8** (2), 23-28.

Heathers, G. Acquiring dependence and independence: A theoretical orientation. *Journal of Genetic Psychology,* 1955, **87,** 227-291.

Hendrick, I. Instinct and ego during infancy. *Psychoanalytic Quarterly,* 1942, **11,** 33-58.

Horney, K. *Neurosis and Human Growth.* New York: Norton, 1950.

Horney, K. *Our Inner Conflicts.* New York: Norton, 1945.

Hurwitz, S. N. *Habilitation of Deaf Young Adults.* St. Louis: Jewish Employment and Vocational Services, 1971.

Hyman, M. Social psychological determinants of patient's performance in stroke rehabilitation. *Archives of Physical Medicine and Rehabilitation,* 1972, 217-226.

James, W. *Principles of Psychology.* New York: H. Holt and Co., 1908.

Jervis, F. A comparison of self concepts of blind and sighted children. *Guidance Programs for Blind Children,* Watertown, Mass.: Perkins School for the Blind, 1959.

Klausner, S. J. *Disabled Families: A Study of a Link Between the Social Contributions of the Disabled and the Retardation of Their Rehabilitation in the Family Context.* Washington, D.C.: Health, Education and Welfare, 1969.

Kleck, R., Ono, H., & Hastorf, A. The effects of physical deviance upon face to face interaction. *Human Relations,* 1966, **19,** 425-436.

Krause, E., Dependency and the blind: Family vs. therapeutic work setting. *New Outlook for the Blind,* 1962, **55,** 352-357.

Krider, M. A comparative study of the self concepts of crippled and non-crippled children. *Easter Seal Research Foundation*, 1959, **32.**

Langer, J., Wapner, S., & Werner, H. The effect of danger on the experience of time. *American Journal of Psychology*, 1961, **74,** 94-97.

Levy, D. M. *Maternal Overprotection.* New York: Columbia University Press, 1943.

Lewin, K. *Principles of Topological Psychology.* New York: McGraw-Hill, Inc., 1936.

Lindenberg, R. E. Perspectives on Work With Families in Rehabilitation. Paper presented at American Personnel and Guidance Association Convention, Chicago, April, 1976.

Loshkin, H. Psychological factors in casework with blind older persons. *New Outlook for the Blind*, 1957, **51,** 1-8.

Lukoff, I. et al. *Attitudes Toward Blind Persons.* New York: American Foundation for the Blind, 1972.

MacDonald, A. P., Jr. Internal-external locus of control: A promising rehabilitation variable. *Journal of Counseling Psychology*, 1971, **18,** 111-116.

MacDonald, A. P., Jr. & Hall, J. Internal-external locus of control and perception of disability. *Journal of Counseling and Clinical Psychology*, 1971, **36,** 338-343.

MacDonald, A. P., Jr., & Hall, J. Perception of disability by the non-disabled. *Journal of Consulting and Clinical Psychology*, 1969, **33,** 654-660.

MacGuffie, R. A., Janzen, F. V., Samuelson, C. O., & McPhee, W. M. Self concept and ideal self in assessing the rehabilitation applicant. *Journal of Counseling Psychology*, 1969, **16,** 157-161.

MacMillan, D. The problem of motivation in the education of the mentally retarded. *Exceptional Children*, 1971, **37,** 579-586.

Mandler, G. Anxiety. *International Encyclopedia of the Social Sciences*, 1968, Vol. I, 356-365.

Mandler, G. & Sarason, S. A study of anxiety and learning. *Journal of Abnormal and Social Psychology*, 1952, **47,** 166-173.

Maslow, A. H. *Motivation and Personality.* New York: Harper, 1954.

McPhee, W. & Magelby, F. L. Success and failure in vocational rehabilitation. *Personnel and Guidance Journal*, 1960, **38,** 497-499.

Mead, G. H. *Mind, Self, and Society,* Chicago: University of Chicago Press, 1934.

Meighan, T. *An Investigation of the Self Concept of Blind and Visually Handicapped Adolescent.* New York: American Foundation for the Blind, 1971.

Meyerson, L. Somatopsychology of physical disability. In Wm. Cruickshank (Ed.) *Psychology of Exceptional Children and Youth*, Englewood Cliffs, N. J.: Prentice-Hall, Inc., 1963.

Mittleman, B. Mobility in infants, children and adults. *Psychoanalytic Studies of Children*, 1954, **9,** 142-177.

Monbeck, M. *The Meaning of Blindness.* Bloomington: Indiana University Press, 1973.

Murphy, T. J. Motivation for mobility. *New Outlook for the Blind*, 1965, **59,** 178-180.

Nau, L. Why not family rehabilitation? *Journal of Rehabilitation*, 1973, **39** (May/June), 14-17, 42.

Neff, W. *Psychological Aspects of Disability.* Washington: American Psych. Assn., 1970.

Neff, W. R. *Success of a Rehabilitation Program: A Follow-Up Study of the Vocational Adjustment Center.* Monograph 3, Chicago: Jewish Vocational Center, 1954.

Olshansky, S., & Beach, D. Special report. *Rehabilitation Literature*, 1975 (August).

Palermo, D. S. Relation between anxiety and two measures of speed in a reaction time test. *Child Development,* 1961, **32,** 401-408.

Phares, J. E. *Locus of Control in Personality.* Morristown, N. J.: General Learning Press, 1976.

Rheingold, H. L. The modification of social responsiveness in institutional babies. *Monograph in Sociological Research in Child Development*, 1956, **21,** (2).

Rogers, C. *Client-Centered Therapy.* Boston: Houghton Mifflin, 1951.

Rosen, B., and D'Andrade, R. The psycho-social origins of achievement motivation. *Sociometry*, 1959, **22,** 185-218.

Rosenstock, F., & Kutner, B. Alienation and family crisis. *Sociological Quarterly*, 1967 (Summer), 397-405.

Ryan, E. D. Effects of stress on motor performance and learning. *The Research Quarterly*, 1962, **33,** 111-119.

Sassenrath, J. M. & Knight, H. R. Anxiety, anxiety-reduction and motivating instructions in human learning and performance. *Psychological Reports*, 1965, **16,** 243-250.

Schulz, P. J. Psychological factors in orientation and mobility training. *New Outlook for the Blind.* 1972, **66,** 129-134.

Scott, R. *The Making of Blind Men.* New York: The Russel Sage Foundation, 1969.

Sears, R., Macoby, E. E., & Lerien, H. *Patterns of Child Rearing.* Evanston, Ill.: Row, Peterson, 1957.

Secord, P. F. & Jourard, S. M. The appraisal of body cathexis: Body cathexis and the self.

Journal of Consulting Psychology. 1953, **17**, 343-347.

Shedletsky, R. & Endler, N. S. Anxiety: The state-trait model and the interaction model. *Journal of Personality*, 1974, **42**, 511-527.

Siller, J., Ferguson, L., Vann, D., & Holland, B. Structure of attitudes toward the physically disabled. *Studies in Reactions to Disability XII*, New York University, Nov. 1967.

Skinner, B. F. *Science and Human Behavior*. New York: Macmillan, 1953.

Smith, M. B. Competence and adaptation. *American Journal of Occupational Therapy*, 1974 (Jan.) **28** (1), 11-15.

Sommers, V. S. *The Influence of Parental Attitudes and Social Environment on the Personality Development of the Adolescent Blind*. New York: American Foundation for the Blind, 1944.

Spielberger, C. D. Anxiety as an emotional state. In C. D. Spielberger (Ed.) *Anxiety: Current Trends in Theory and Research Vol. I*, New York: Academic Press, 1972.

Spielberger, C. D. The effects of anxiety on complex learning and academic achievement. In C. D. Spielberger (Ed.) *Anxiety and Behavior*. New York: Academic Press, 1966.

Stotland, E. & Canon, L. K. *Social Psychology: A Cognitive Approach*. Philadelphia: W. B. Saunders Co., 1972.

Sullivan, H. S. *The Interpersonal Theory of Psychiatry*. New York: Norton, 1953.

Taylor, J. A personality score of manifest anxiety. *Journal of Abnormal and Social Psychology*, 1953, **48**, 285-290.

Wardlow, D. A Nine Month's Drop Out Study. Hot Springs Rehabilitation Service. In B. Cobb (Ed.) *Special Problems in Rehabilitation*. Springfield, Ill: Charles Thomas, 1974.

Warren, D. H. & Kocon, J. A. Factors in the successful mobility of the blind; a review. *American Foundation for the Blind Research Bulletin*, 1974, **28** (Oct.), 191-218.

Weinberg, J. R. A further investigation of the body cathexis and the self. *Journal of Consulting Psychology*, 1960, **24**, 277-281.

Weiner, H. Characteristics associated with rehabilitation success. *Personnel and Guidance Journal*, 1964, **42**, 687-694.

White, R. W. Motivation reconsidered: The concept of competence. *Psychoanalytic Review*, 1959, **66**, 297-333.

Whiteman, M. & Lukoff, I. A factorial study of sighted people's attitudes toward blindness. *Journal of Social Psychology*, 1964a, **64**, 339-353.

Whiteman, M. & Lukoff, I. Attitudes toward blindness in two college groups. *Journal of Social Psychology*, 1964b, **63**, 179-191.

Whiteman, M. & Lukoff, I. Attitudes toward blindness and other physical handicaps. *Journal of Social Psychology*, 1965, **66**, 134-145.

Whiting, J. W. M. & Child, I. L. *Child Training and Personality*, New Haven: Yale University Press, 1953.

Wilson, E. L. A developmental approach to psychological factor which may inhibit mobility in the visually handicapped person. *New Outlook for the Blind*, 1967, **61**, 283-289, 308.

Wolpe, J. *Psychotherapy by Reciprocal Inhibition*. Stanford, Calif.: Stanford University Press, 1958.

Wright, B. *Physical Disability—A Psychological Approach*. New York: Harper and Row, 1960.

Concept Development

Everett Hill and Bruce B. Blasch

A visually impaired person experiences three basic losses (Lowenfeld, 1948). They are not distinct categories but overlap. The first loss, control of the environment and self in relation to the environment, may affect the information received in social interactions. The individual may be unable to determine when another person leaves or enters the room or walks away from a group. The visually impaired person may not know whether another person is talking to or listening to him because he cannot see facial expression and hand gestures, or use eye contact.

The second loss is mobility. While the degree of this loss may be lessened by rehabilitation, a visually impaired person will never completely compensate for this loss. There may be difficulty in learning a new geographic area without some assistance or locating a specific landmark with which there has been only verbal familiarization. Unless he regains vision, he will not drive a car which is critical for mobility in many areas.

The third loss is the limitation of the range and variety of concepts. For the adventitiously visually impaired person, there is difficulty in updating concepts, such as technological developments, fashions and fads, and environmental changes. This loss is a major problem affecting most aspects of the congenitally blind person's life because the development of concepts is the foundation of academic, social, and psychomotor learning.

While the sighted individual develops and verifies many concepts informally, the visually impaired person must have a structured presentation of most concepts to insure accurate development of these fundamentals.

Traveling without vision requires the acquisition of certain basic concepts. The necessary basic concepts related to mobility are body awareness, which includes body schema, body concepts, and body image (Frostig, 1969); body planes and parts; and laterality and directionality (Cratty, 1967). Some concepts, such as positional and relational concepts as well as concepts of shapes, measurements, and actions, are necessary for orientation. The individual must also have accurate concepts of the environment, topography, textures, and temperature.

The mobility specialist must know the range of necessary concepts, be able to define them, and understand how they are developed by the sighted individual. There must also be an understanding of how visual impairment affects the normal development of concepts, and how problems arise for the visually impaired individual. Familiarity with assessment instruments will enable the mobility specialist to assess a visually impaired person's level of concept development in order to begin teaching at the appropriate level for that person.

It is important to understand basic prerequisites for normal motor development, and the perceptual-motor theories relating to cognitive development. Thus, this chapter builds on the basic developmental information presented by Hart in Chapter 2.

CONCEPT DEFINED

The term "concept" is commonly used and has assumed a variety of meanings. Basically, a concept is a mental representation, image, or idea of what something should be. It is formed by classifying or grouping objects or events with similar properties. For example, a person can have a concept of dogs even though all dogs are not alike. Most people who see an English Bulldog, a Cocker Spaniel, and a Golden Retriever have little difficulty detecting distinct differences among these three animals, yet these dogs have certain characteristics in common that serve as a basis for conceptual grouping. Most concepts are associated with a general descriptive name or label or, stated another way, are represented by words. Concepts may range from very concrete or real objects such as dog, table, or cane; to abstract or more intangible ideas such as beauty, love, or justice.

The ability to perceive and discriminate similarities is a perceptual process, and is therefore *fundamental for concept development*. Because of the importance of perception to concept development it is important to briefly consider perception itself. Gibson (1967) describes perception as a dynamic process by which we obtain first hand information about the immediate environment through the use and integration of the functional sensory receptors. The ability to abstract information from the environment has several aspects, including the organism's awareness of events presently occurring in the immediate environment and a discriminative, selective response to the immediate environment. Perception is, by nature, selective. There is rather gross selectivity at birth which becomes progressively refined with development, experience, and learning.

Environmental stimulation is so vast and varied that the individual receives more information than he is able to process. There is no correlation with ongoing events or with qualitative or quantitative differences in stimuli without a discriminative response. In other words, sensory information is meaningless without the ability to determine similarities or differences in stimuli. While perception may be interpreted as an end result, it appears more productive to consider perception as a dynamic process in the sense of exploring and searching.

Viewing perception as a way of information extraction in man's adaptive behavior relates to the general problem of cognitive development and a full understanding of the nature of reception, acquisition, assimilation, and utilization of concepts. From this point of view, perception becomes the core process in the acquisition of concepts.

The formation of concepts is accomplished in two ways: by abstraction and generalization. The first process involves the ability to perceive, discriminate, and abstract similarities from a variety of objects and attach a word or label to the idea or abstracted similarities.

The second process in forming concepts is generalization. Generalization entails applying the similarities or abstracted properties to a new exposure of the concept involved. For example, the concept "dog" can be generalized to include a particular type of animal, such as a Bedlington Terrier, even though in this particular instance the dog resembles a lamb.

In a discussion of concepts by Zweibelson and Barg (1967), they cite three levels of attainment:

1. Concrete—the ability to identify specific characteristic(s) of an object.

2. Functional—to identify what the object does or what one does with the object.

3. Abstract—the summarization of all major characteristics of the object.

Considering these three levels under the previous discussion on the development of a concept by abstraction, the concrete and functional levels are then steps in developing the completeness of the concept via abstraction.

LIMITING VARIABLES

The above discussion of concept formation describes abstracting information via the senses, discriminating similarities and differences, categorizing the information, and then labeling the concept. The effectiveness of an individual's ability to form concepts is dependent in part upon the richness and variety of perceptions available to him. For better understanding and fostering of concept development it is necessary to consider the factors that may limit perceptions and development of concepts, particularly in dealing with visually impaired persons.

Combs (1952) has discussed some limiting variables that apply to perception and concept development in general; limitations that also apply to persons with visual impairment. The first limitation to perception and concept development is physiological: developmental disabilities; sensory losses such as blindness; physical handicaps such as loss of locomotion, use of arms or hands; malnutrition; and chronic fatigue. Certain physical factors seriously affect the ability of the individual to make adequate differentiations and discriminations when acquiring information.

Vision plays a primary role as a source of stimulation and integration of other sensory information in normal development. It is maintained by some (Gesell, Ilg & Bullis, 1949; Getman & Kane, 1964) that the human is the most vision-oriented of all living creatures, and that approximately 80 percent of learning occurs through vision. Similarly, Telford and Sawrey (1977) state that "the educational experiences occurring in a typical classroom are estimated to be 85 percent visual in nature." These statements about the relative importance of vision for learning are interesting yet questionable, as the percentages are not based on any systematic investigation or appropriate data. Although the figures may never be substantiated, the importance of vision in most aspects of learning is not in question. Vision enables an individual to gather direct sensory input at a distance from an object, to comprehend a total image of an object, and to process sensory information rapidly. Indeed, some very important concepts such as color can only be developed through vision.

Vision plays an important role in motivating an infant's environmental exploration. Scott (1969) discusses the emergence of differences in the development of the normal and visually impaired child as the sighted child becomes aware of and attracted to his environment and begins to have direct sensory experience with it. Scott further explains that the part of the environment which is available to the visually impaired child does not have the same stimulus and motivational value that it has for the sighted child. Therefore, the environment which is available for the visually impaired child is limited and is less motivating. The development of visually impaired and sighted infants is quite similar in the early months, but diverges when the sighted infant begins to reach for external objects (Warren, 1977).

Cratty (1978) stated that because visually impaired children lack efficient spatial receptors they must substitute hearing, touch, action, and thought to acquire critical spatial concepts and percepts. Fraiberg, Smith, and Adelson (1966a), in their research with blind infants, found that sound was not an efficient substitute for sight in stimulating blind children to reach for objects. Whereas sighted children generally begin to develop normal eye-hand coordination around 4-6 months, blind children were found to develop the corresponding ear-hand coordination around 10-12 months (Fraiberg, et al., 1966a). Furthermore, Fraiberg found blind infants, compared to their counterparts, to be delayed in motor behavior and interacting with the environment.

A second factor discussed by Combs (1952) is environmental richness. Differentiations in environmental richness may be divided into two categories, actual/concrete and symbolic/vicarious. Limited exposure to actual environmental events may be inherent in a given physical environment. For example, a child in the South may not know snow or a child from the North may not be familiar with palm trees. Other environmental factors of this sort include rural, urban, near water (ocean or lake), inland, mountains, plains, etc.

Limitations in exposure to symbolic or vicarious events also cause deprivations. Individuals may develop perceptions and concepts from reading, movies, television, radio, conversation, and other such forms of communication. Individuals whose environments provide little in the way of reading materials or conversation are very restricted.

Exposure to events does not necessarily determine or guarantee the perceptions an individual will make. Exposure to an event, either actual or vicarious, is only one factor in determining what perceptions are developed. Two individuals exposed to the same event or individuals exposed to events at different times perceive quite different aspects of the event. This does not necessarily mean that one individual makes fewer perceptions than another individual, but that he makes different ones.

Time may also limit perception. Discrimination requires time. The richness of an individual's perception is in part a function of how much time the person has to experience the event. If it is true that a perception is possible only when an individual is exposed to an experience, it is also true that this exposure must be long enough to make differentiation possible.

The amount of time it takes to make a differentiation is obviously not a constant and varies from individual to individual. Some of the limiting factors on perception can interact with time also. For example, a person with a physiological limitation such as low vision may take longer to scan the environment to locate the stimulus, while another individual may immediately locate the stimulus and, therefore, make the discrimination more quickly. Previous experience and exposure to various events also influence the time it takes to make differentiations.

An individual's goals and values may also limit perception. They may be explicit or implicit, simple or complex, but they vary from individual to individual. While there is a certain amount of stability in the general goals and values of a particular individual, there may be fluctuations in the perception of events from time to time with changing emphasis on certain goals and values. For example, some individuals place a high value on learning about the environment along a route and tend to seek out and attend to various aspects of it. Another individual may only be concerned about getting from place A to place B and regard information about the route as distracting and unimportant.

Self-concept may also limit perception. Perception is a selective process and the concept one holds of oneself is a vital factor in determining the richness and the variety of the perception selected. For example, an individual who feels he is not very good at learning new environmental concepts may avoid situations involving new environments. This attitude may then become a self-fulfilling prophecy where the individual tells himself he is not good at learning about the environment, avoids situations in which he can learn new information, and therefore has difficulties with new environmental concepts.

Another factor which may limit perception is threat. When an individual feels threatened, there is a tendency to narrow the perceptual field to the object or event that threatens. For example, a person might not hear anything but a truck approaching. A threatening or anxiety-producing situation not only narrows the field of perception but also reduces the possibility of being receptive to different or new perceptions in addition to those already held. Therefore, under threat, behavior becomes rigid and the possibility of perceptual change is reduced and the opportunity for new perceptions or learning is greatly reduced.

The social environment can also limit exposure to a variety of concepts. A common cause of this limitation is the overprotectiveness of parents. For a variety of reasons, parents tend to protect their blind child from bumps and bruises, from getting dirty, lost, or hurt, or from the comments of others. This protectiveness prevents a child from experiencing other types of stimulation and acquiring a variety of new concepts. Only recently have materials been developed that parents may use to provide varied stimulation to help blind children develop concepts.

CONCEPT DEFICIENCIES IN VISUALLY IMPAIRED CHILDREN

Several studies support the hypothesis that visually impaired children have deficiencies in concept development. Garry and Accarelli (1960) studied the way blind children link words with experiences and develop a meaningful language base. In data obtained from a Spatial Relation Performance Test administered to a group of 70 totally blind children between the ages of 5 and 15 they found evidence that about 50 percent of the group, regardless of chronological age or intelligence quotient, had difficulties in understanding and applying spatial concepts, which resulted in poor orientation, lack of manipulative skills, and limited interest in the environment. This data was also substantiated by direct observation and reports from school personnel. Hapeman (1967) stated that, "blind children tend to lack the necessary concrete knowledge of their environments. . . ."

Kephart, Kephart, and Schwarz (1974) stated that, "the manner in which blind children are processing personal and environmental information appears to result in fragmented and distorted understandings of simple, straightforward concepts. The blind child in the early years must rely on receiving information from persons whose primary frame of reference is a visual one. These results seem to indicate that blind children are not understanding what they encounter."

In the conclusion and implications of his study, Lord (1969) said, "study should be directed to the many aspects of concept formation of the blind child relative to object and space. Significant concepts should be delineated and plans for systematic instruction established."

Piaget (1960) postulated a hierarchical sequence of stages and concepts within stages through which children progress in the process of cognitive development. These stages are sensori-motor, preoperational, concrete operating, and formal operations. It appears that visually impaired children go through the same stages of cognitive development, but at a much slower rate. Studies by Simpkins and Stephens (1974) have shown that blind children demonstrate a lag of as much as four to eight years in the developmental stages postulated by Piaget. Other studies based upon the developmental levels of Piaget have supported the findings of Simpkins and Stephens (Friedman & Pasnak, 1973: Gottesman, 1973; Higgins, 1973; and Tobin, 1972).

Finally, in a study by Hartlage (1968) dealing with spatial ability, the results indicated, "there was a significant difference between blind and sighted S's performance on spatial questions, but not on non-spatial questions. Blind S's performance on the spatial half of the test was significantly lower than their performance on the non-spatial half."

The mobility specialist must be able to identify the range and variety of concepts that appear to be lacking in many visually impaired children and the terminology that confuses the visually impaired child. The following treatment of concepts and terminology does not focus on the entire range of concepts that might be affected by lack of vision, but emphasizes those that are most significant for mobility.

BODY CONCEPTS

Developing concepts of space and objects in space depends greatly on the relationship of the object to the observer. The individual is always the center of his orientation and perceives objects in relationship to himself or from this egocentric view (Blasch, Welsh, & Davidson, 1973) using terms such as above, below, in front, or to the left side. This perception of objects in relation to self, which might be considered the first orientation ability to develop, depends on accurate development of body awareness. Perception of the relationship of the body to an object or objects is developed through vision as well as through haptic exploration, proprioception, and audition. In defining body awareness, Frostig and Horne (1964) discuss three elements—body image, body concept, and body schema—and maintain that if any of them are disturbed, a child's perception of spatial relationships is also disturbed.

Frostig discusses body image in terms of a person's subjective experience of his own body (i.e., his feeling about it). This subjective impression involves such feelings about himself as attractive, too short, overweight, muscular, shapely, graceful, etc. Body image is based upon emotional factors, peer group and other social interactions, specific career or social aspirations, and various cultural values. A person's self-image may differ considerably from his actual image. For example, an adolescent may have only a small facial blemish but feel that his entire face is covered with ugly pimples that everyone notices.

Body concept is the knowledge the person has of his body, acquired through a conscious learning process. Information the child acquires in developing a body concept includes the ability to identify parts of the body, legs, arms, knees, nose, ears, hair, etc., and knowing the location and functions of the various body parts.

Frostig and Horne (1964) differentiate body schema from body image and body concept. Body schema is unconscious and changes from moment to moment. It is derived from stimulations produced within the body, known as proprioceptive sensations. This information is used to regulate the body—the position of the different muscles and parts of the body in relation to each other and in relation to the pull of gravity. A person's balance is dependent upon body schema. If a person's body schema is disturbed, difficulty in making coordinated movements such as walking, sitting down, or bending over would result.

A person's knowledge of body schema and body concepts forms the basis of spatial and directional concepts. Adequate knowledge in these areas may be viewed as central to the development of concepts and to the process of orienting oneself to the environment and to being mobile.

The term body image used by Cratty and Sams is similar in meaning to the term body concept used by Frostig and Horne (1964).

In a test of blind children's body image, Cratty and Sams (1968) evaluated five components. The first, body planes, included the ability to identify the front, back, sides, top and bottom of one's body. The evaluation also included having the individual place body planes in relation to external surfaces, as well as placing objects in relation to body planes.

The second included the identification of body parts. The third concerned body movement, including gross movements in relation to body planes and limb movements.

The fourth component, laterality, determined not only whether a blind child could accurately identify his left and right body parts, but also how well he could move himself so that his left or right side or hand were nearest to objects, and conversely how well he could place objects in relation to his left and right sides while remaining in one place.

The fifth component of body image, directionality, determines how well a child could identify the left and right sides of objects and of other people.

For accurate development of body concepts it is important to know the significant body-related terms. Body parts, examples of body functions, body surfaces, and examples of the relationship of body parts and of the movement of body are included in the following concept lists:

Head	Trunk	Limbs and Appendages
hair	shoulders	arms
scalp	back	biceps (muscle)
forehead	spine	elbows
face	chest	forearms
eyebrows	breasts	wrists
eyes	stomach (belly, tummy)	hands
eyelashes	belly button	palms
eyelids	waist	fingers
nose	sides	index (pointer,
nostrils	hips	first, braille)
cheeks	rear (seat, bottom, rump)	little (baby, pinkie)
mouth	genitals	middle (big)
lips	groin	ring
teeth		thumb
gums		fingernails
tongue		fingertips
jaw		knuckles
chin		legs
ears		thighs
neck		knees
throat		kneecaps
		calves
		shins
		ankles
		feet
		heels
		arches
		toes
		toenails

When the visually impaired child is able to identify parts it is important also to describe the functions of the body parts. Examples of body functions are as follows: ears—enable one to hear sounds, speech; hands—used to grasp, hold, and manipulate; legs—support the standing body and help with walking and running, etc.; teeth—used to bite and chew food; nose—enables one to breathe and smell.

Another body concept that is important is the knowledge of the following body surfaces: anterior or front, posterior or back, lateral or side(s), superior or top, inferior or bottom.

Examples of the relationship of body parts reinforce the functional knowledge of these parts: hair is on top of the head, knee is above the shin, nose is in the center of the face, forearm is between the elbow and wrist, and chin is below the mouth.

Another important aspect is the movement of body parts or surfaces: bend your arm at the elbow, rise up on your toes, bend your body slowly forward, walk backwards, place your hands on your hips.

SPATIAL CONCEPTS

As an individual develops more knowledge of his own body, forming an accurate body concept, information is also gathered about positional and relational concepts. For the visually impaired child it is particularly important to learn how body parts are positioned and how they relate to one another so that positional and relational concepts can be transferred to the external environment (Hill, 1970).

The following list illustrates the wide range of positional/relational spatial concepts:

Anterior—front, in front of, face, facing, forward, before, ahead
Posterior—back, behind, rear, backward, after
Superior—top, above, over, up, high, upward
Inferior—bottom, below, under, down, low, downward, beneath, underneath
Lateral—next, next to, beside, right, left, sideways, alongside of
Proximics—next, next to, beside, away, distant, far, close, near, here, there, against
Internal—into, in, inside, within, inner, inward
External—out, outside, out of, outer, outward
Other—clockwise, counterclockwise, opposite, across from, parallel, perpendicular, around, toward, upside down, middle, between, in between, center, on, off, anterior, posterior, superior, inferior, interior, adjacent, medial, median, northeast, northwest, southeast, southwest (north, south, east, west . . . bound, . . . erly, . . . ward, . . . ern), diagonal, horizontal, vertical, uppermost.

Also included in the range of spatial concepts are shapes. Concepts of shape become extremely important when the visually impaired individual begins to identify objects and work with mobility concepts such as street configurations, grid patterns, building layouts, etc. The following is a list of important shapes:

Primary—round, triangle, circle, rectangle, square, oval, loop
Secondary—sphere, octagon, hexagon, pentagon, cylinder, figure 8, ellipse, cube (cubical), cone, rectangular solid, pyramid, rhombus, trapezoid, parabola, parallelogram
Descriptive Terms—rectangular, rounded, circular, squared
Shapes of Particular Objects—pear shaped, rain drop, tear drop, heart shaped, ring shaped, box shaped, diamond shaped
Letters Used to Describe Shapes—T-Intersection, H, L, O, S, T, V, U, X, Y.

Concepts of measurement are also extremely important in daily living and for orientation and independent mobility. Obviously, many of the following spatial concepts are not specific to mobility but are important in many facets in the life of a visually impaired child:

Distance	Amount	Time	Weight and Volume	Width, Length, and Size
inch	whole	second	ounce	wide
foot	half	minute	pound	narrow
yard	quarter	hour	pint	thick
block	full	day	quart	thin
degrees	empty	week	liter	

Distance	Amount	Time	Weight and Volume	Width, Length, and Size
mile	shallow	month	milliliter	tall
millimeter	less	year		short
centimeter	least	today		long
meter	more	tomorrow		big
kilometer	most	yesterday		vast
	all	quarter-hour		large
	none	half-hour		huge
	some	time/distance		great
		per second		small
		per minute		little
		per hour		tiny
		morning		
		afternoon		
		evening		
		night		

Another important category is that of action concepts. Obviously, in mobility it is important to understand various terms related to movement. These concepts are employed in a variety of ways including giving directions, in describing various movements, in maintaining orientation, to mention a few. The following terms are spatial concepts dealing with action:

Turns—45° turn, ¼-turn, 90° turn, right-angle turn, 180° turn, half turn, whole turn, about face, 360° turn, full turn, pivot, U-turn

Action—move, scoot, creep, crawl, roll, stretch, bend, lie, sit, stand, squat, kneel, stoop, position, drift, angle, veer, walk, run, jump, hop, skip, gallop, climb, march, leap, forward movement, backward movement, sideways movement, upward movement, downward movement, jay walk, put, place, grasp, push, pull, swing.

Movement through the environment requires not only an understanding of the body and basic spatial concepts, but also an awareness of what exists in the environment and how it can be used, as well as overall descriptions of the environment.

ENVIRONMENTAL CONCEPTS

Lists of environmental concepts can be long and seemingly endless. However, the emphasis in this section will be on environmental concepts directly related to travel. Certain terms may be specific to certain geographic areas, for example, water fountain, drinking fountain, and bubbler. The following list is intended to be comprehensive in terms of environmental concepts of objects (some are object related) related to pedestrian mobility, but is not an attempt to list all synonymous terms relative to a specific concept:

universe	traffic light
planet	stop and go light
continent	red light
country	scatter light
state	pedestrian traffic control device
county	split cycle
city	traffic
business district	traffic jam

273

semi-business district
residential district
city blocks
neighborhood
freeway—1, 2, 3, etc. lanes
tollroad—1, 2, 3, etc. lanes
highway—1, 2, 3, etc. lanes
road
street (one way, two way)
roundabout
layby
circular drive
grid pattern
intersection
offset-intersection
irregular-intersection
T-intersection
Y-intersection
traffic lanes
feeder or turning lanes
crown of the street
camber of the road
divider line
solid line (white, yellow)
broken line (white, yellow)
double solid lines
   (white, yellow)
double broken lines
   (white, yellow)
broken and solid lines
median strip
safety island
street corner
crosswalk
through street
two-way stop
three-way stop
four-way stop
shoreline
grassline
grass
lawn (yard)
tree-lawn area
hedges
dirt
tree line
bush
shrub
flower
weed
fence
path
landmark

*traffic surge
*car idle
*reviving motor
*traffic patterns
curbs
blind curb
wheelchair ramp
gutter (storm sewer)
grates
alley
driveway
boulevard
parkway
parking lot
railroad track/crossing
park
playground
city property
house
store
building
floor, story, level
lobby, foyer, entryway
door (doorway)
hallway
stairs (step)
wall
room
radiator
ceiling
floor
mat, rug, carpet
window (screen)
vent
roof
chimney
elevator
escalator
revolving door
manhole cover
trash can
park bench
bus bench
bus shelter
street furniture
street sign
bus stop
bus (city, school)
fire engine
truck
car, police car
cab stand
taxi stand

telephone pole (guide wire)
fire hydrant
parking meter
lamp post
newspaper rack
telephone booth
water fountain
bubbler
drinking fountain

ambulance
limousine
van
train
plane
boat
ship
subway
elevated train
terminal
pedestrian
*right of way
crowd
*crowd surge

*Environmental concepts are not necessarily objects

Concepts of topography may be used not only to foster understanding of the environment, but also to serve as landmarks. For example, when a person reaches an incline in the middle of a block it can serve as a landmark for locating a specific sidewalk. The following are environmental concepts relating to topography:

side
border
edge
seam
joint
perimeter
end
corner
angle
ridge
hill (hilly, mountainous, rolling)
ramp
slope
dip
decline
incline
raised
tilt

lean
flat
level
straight
line
curved (curve)
crooked
irregular
off-set
catty-cornered
intersection
gridwork
point
reference point
focal point
open
closed
arc

Environmental concepts of texture are also extremely important. Textural concepts are used in school, in daily living activities, in employment, and in many other situations including mobility. Various texture concepts become very important in considering the effect of the various textures when using a cane. The resonance, sound, amount of sticking, and the modification of the touch technique depend on surface texture. The following are some of the more common textural concepts:

pavement
cement
asphalt
stone
gravel

slick
silky
icy
slippery
coarse

275

cobblestone	fine
slate	sharp
brick	dull
tile (rough, smooth)	rough
wood	jagged
glass	bumpy
plastic	smooth
hard	torn
soft	grassy
wet	sticky
dry	

Finally, concepts of the environment would not be complete without mention of the temperature concepts particularly as they relate to mobility. Based on information about temperature the traveler can plan for appropriate clothing but should also be aware of the effects of the temperature on textures. If it is very hot, asphalt may be soft and sticky. If, on the other hand, it is cool and has rained, the person may want to avoid the slate sidewalk on a hilly surface because of slippery and hazardous conditions. The following list represents important temperature concepts:

hot	sweltering
cold	muggy
warm	humid
cool	dry
mild	centigrade
chilly	Fahrenheit
brisk	

The above lists represent a variety of concepts relating to the environment. In some cases more than one term with the same meaning has been listed. However, this was not done for all concepts and the mobility specialist should not regard the lists as all-inclusive or exhaustive.

ASSESSMENT OF CONCEPT DEVELOPMENT

When the mobility specialist begins to teach mobility to young children in particular, it is first necessary to establish the student's abilities and deficiencies in order to plan appropriate remediation of conceptual learning and/or appropriate mobility instruction. Proceeding without basic assessment often leads to teaching or learning problems because of poor concept development.

The mobility specialist must be able to differentiate between a verbalism of a concept, and a concrete understanding of a concept. Harley (1963) states that a verbalism may be the result of inaccurate and/or vague concepts resulting from insufficient sensory experience. When asked to describe a concept, a student may give a very adequate definition of the concept (verbalism) which he has memorized, yet not be able to use the concept functionally. A student with an inadequate concept of a city block perhaps would not be able to walk around the block because he does not realize the size of a block, that four turns have to be made, and that street crossing is not necessary. It is, therefore, extremely important that the mobility specialist assess not only the verbal understanding of a concept but also obtain a behavioral response that indicates a valid concept.

CONCEPT ASSESSMENT INSTRUMENTS
The Body Image of Blind Children (BIBC, Cratty & Sams, 1968)

This instrument can be used to assess a child's ability to identify his body parts;

the left-right dimensions of his body and his body parts; his body planes (sides, back, front, etc.); ability to respond to requests for specific body movements; and the ability to discern the movements of a person who is touching him. In addition to assessing an individual's ability to make right-left discriminations about his own body, questions are used to assess the ability to differentiate between another person's left and right body parts. Finally, the extent to which the child can accurately judge the location of objects relative to his body, and the manner in which he can accurately place his body relative to objects may also be assessed.

Section I, *Body Planes*, contains three subsections of five items each, such as: touch the top of your head, lie down on the mat so that the side of your body is touching the mat, place the box so that it touches your side.

Section II, *Body Parts*, contains 20 items in four subsections, such as: touch your arm, touch your ear, touch your wrist, hold up your thumbs.

Body Movement contains 15 items in three subsections. Examples of the subsections are: bend your body slowly backwards (or "away") from me, walk forward toward me, bend one arm at the elbow.

The fourth section, *Laterality*, contains 15 items in three subsections. Examples of the subsections are: touch your right knee, place the box so that it touches your right side, touch your right hand with your left hand.

The final section, *Directionality*, contains 15 items in three subsections. Examples of the subsections are: tap my left shoulder, touch the right side of the box, (tester is seated facing the child; the child's hands are placed on the tester's shoulders) am I bending to my right or left?

The assessment instrument was based on a 16-step body-image training sequence for sighted children (Cratty, 1967). The BIBC is designed for use with visually impaired children and is individually administered. Little experience is required for the administration of this instrument but the complete manual should be read.

The strength of the instrument is that it attempts to assess the body-image of blind children in a systematic fashion. In addition, it goes beyond just asking a child to name body parts. There are also implications for training and working tasks. Its major weakness lies in the limited data on reliability and validity. The pass-fail grading system, while easy to administer, does not give any value to approximations of a correct response. For example, if a child touches his right forearm (rather than his wrist) with his left hand there would be no credit given even though the child appears to have the concept of laterality.

The sequence of body planes and then body parts is questionable because the use of some body parts is in the body plane section. Therefore, a child could fail the section on body planes because of not knowing body parts. An item such as "Bend your body slowly backwards (or away from me)," may be difficult to score because of the inclusion of multiple concepts. If the child did not respond, the examiner would not know whether the child understood the concepts of bend, slowly, or backwards.

Orientation and Mobility Scale for Young Blind Children—Short Form (Lord, 1969)

This scale was developed to assess the relevant behavioral skills in orientation and mobility of visually impaired children. It contains 24 items relating to directions and terms, movement in space, and self-help. The items have five levels of performance for the examiner to check. These items were selected from an original 124 items (Lord, 1969) and administered to 173 blind children ranging in age from 3 to 12 years. All of the children were either totally blind or, at most, had light perception, and had no other limitations that might interfere with performing the task. Norms expressed in percentage of children at each age level who performed the task are available (Lord, 1969). Two examples from the Direction and Turns section are:

Responds Correctly to a Command to Turn Left.
Procedure: Take the child to open doorway. Say, "Let's look at this doorway." Allow him to explore the opening.
Examiner stands approximately three feet from opening. Say, "Now come back here where I am. I want you to go out of the door and turn left. Keep walking until I tell you when to stop."
Score: Makes left turn correctly. Walks several steps.

Travels a Route with One Turn Described in Terms of Cardinal Directions.
Procedure: Use a short hallway in school building or the sidewalk in front of the building. Face the child to the south. Say, "You are now facing south. Walk until I say 'turn'—then turn to the east." Score: Child makes correct directional turn.

The short form of the test is comprised of the following items:

1. Directions, Turns
   Responds correctly to a command to turn left.
   Correctly describes a familiar route in terms of right and left turns.
   Points out cardinal directions in a familiar setting.
   Travels a route with one turn described in terms of cardinal directions.

2. Movement in Space
   Walks with weight properly distributed.
   Walks with relaxed gait.
   Walks up steps alternating forward foot, one foot per tread.
   Walks down steps, alternating forward foot, one foot per tread.
   Hops on one foot.
   Hops, alternating feet.
   Gallops.
   Skips.
   Runs freely by himself.
   Jumps off low wall or bench.
   Jumps, coordinating other body movements.

3. Self-Help
   Locates and demonstrates working parts of doors.
   Uses key to lock and unlock doors.
   Puts on sweater unassisted.
   Buttons sweater.
   Puts on sweater (presented with one sleeve turned).
   Puts on belt and fastens buckle correctly.
   Dials telephone numbers successfully.
   Identifies simple tools.
   Uses helping hand efficiently.

This developmental scale offers some guidance to the mobility specialist when assessing a limited group of behaviors directly related to mobility. Many of the tasks are of a higher level without testing prerequisite concepts. Instructions for administering the device should be understood thoroughly before being used by mobility specialists.

Performance Test of Selected Positional Concepts for Visually Handicapped Children (Hill, 1971)

This performance test was developed to assess spatial concepts (positional terms) of visually impaired children ages 6-14. This performance test consists of 75 items divided into three parts. Selected positional-spatial concepts are tested in different ways in each part. In the first part, the child identifies the correlation of various body parts as he follows spoken directions to move and position those parts; touch the *front* of your leg, touch the *back* of your neck, touch the *left* side of your body.

In the second part, the child is tested in the same way for "self" in relation to environmental objects: place yourself in *front* of the chair, put the chair in *back* of you, move the chair so it is on your *left*.

The third part consists of manipulatory moving of objects in relation to each other: put the block in *front* of the cup, put the stick in *back* of the block, put the block to the *left* of the stick.

The items are scored: 0 (does not complete task), 1 (approximates task), and 2 (successfully completes task). An administration and scoring manual is available.

This instrument is similar to *The Body Image of Blind Children* assessment by Cratty and Sams but is presented in a more sequential fashion and generally has more items specifically related to orientation and mobility. While assessing a child's ability to use prerequisite orientation and mobility concepts in a variety of ways, it assumes that the child has a knowledge of basic body parts.

The Stanford Multi-Modality Imagery Test (SMIT, Dauterman, 1972)

William Dauterman designed this test to assess the functional imagery of blind persons. Its "multi-modality" aspects rest on the nature of the tasks to be performed in Phases I and II. During these phases, haptic (tactile and kinesthetic) and verbal stimuli involving geometric patterns are used for imagery stimulation. The test has three phases, the first two of which are the learning phases and involve the subject in the construction of simple three-sided and four-sided figures by placing rubber bands around a rectangular shaped board. Phase I of the test, "Comprehension and Following Instructions," familiarizes the subject with the apparatus by practice exercises on the rectangular board. The three items in Phase I are:

1. Using the notches as guides in which to place the rubber band, I want you to place the rubber band around the board so that it makes a line from the middle of the top side to the middle of the bottom side. I will be using a stopwatch during all phases of the test but take as much time as you need.

2. Now take that line off. Next place the rubber band around the board so that it makes a line from the upper left corner to the lower right corner.

3. Now take that line off. From now on I will tell you to draw a line instead of mentioning the rubber band. Next draw a line from the lower left corner to the middle of the top.

Phase II, "Conceptualizing Spatial Relations," is intended to be a teaching and verifying situation. The four items in Phase II are:

1. Draw a line from the middle of the left side to the middle of the right side and from the middle of the top to the middle of the bottom. Do the figures created by these lines have three sides or four sides or are there both kinds of figures?

2. Now take those lines off. Next draw a line from the lower left corner to the middle of the top, and from the middle of the top to the lower right corner. Do the figures created by these lines have three sides or four sides or are there both kinds of figures?

3. Now take those lines off. Next draw a line from the upper left corner to the middle of the bottom, from the middle of the bottom to the upper right corner, from the lower left corner to the middle of the top, and from the middle of the top to the lower right corner. Do these figures created by these lines have three sides or four sides or are there both kinds of figures?

4. Now take those lines off. Next draw a line from the upper left corner to the middle of the right side and from the middle of the top to the middle of the bottom. Do these

279

figures created by these lines have three sides or four sides or are there both kinds of figures?

In Phase III, ''The Multi-Modality Imagery Test,'' the rectangular board and rubber bands are not used, but questions are asked; for example:

Imagine a rectangle the same size as the one with which you were working. Now imagine a line drawn from the lower left corner to the upper right corner. How many three-sided and how many four-sided figures would this make?

Imagine a rectangle with a line drawn from the middle of the left side to the middle of the right side and from the middle of the top to the middle of the bottom and from the lower left corner to the upper right corner and from the lower right corner to the upper left corner, from the middle of the top to the lower right corner and from the middle of the bottom to the upper right corner with a vertical line drawn from the top to the bottom through the point of intersection of the last two lines. How many three-sided and how many four-sided figures would this make?

The standardization studies were based on a sample of 200 legally blind individuals; 170 were 16 years of age or older, while the remaining 30 were 14 and 15 years of age.

Many tasks are extremely complex and not applicable to young visually impaired children. Also, the relationship of the tasks to orientation and mobility is questionable.

The SMIT manual gives specific directions for administration and needed materials, and the test may be administered by mobility specialists.

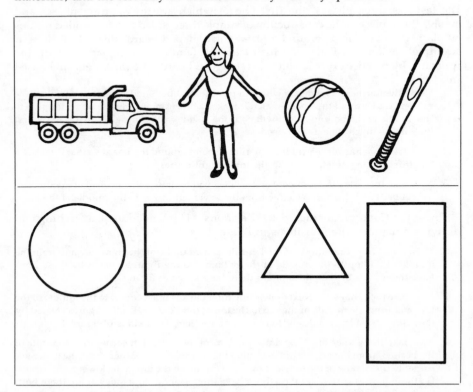

Figure 1-9. A tactile analog for a concept on the BTBC and TTBC. (Reproduced from the *Boehm Test of Basic Concepts* © 1967-1970 by the Psychological Corporation. Reproduced by special permission.)

Tactile Analog to the Boehm Test of Basic Concepts—Form A (TTBC, Caton, 1976)

The *Boehm Test of Basic Concepts* (BTBC) is designed to measure children's mastery of concepts that are considered necessary in the first school years. The test, read aloud by the teacher, is used with sighted children in kindergarten, 1st and 2nd grades. The purpose of the test is to identify children whose overall level of concept mastery is low and who, therefore, may need special attention. It is also used to identify individual concepts with which large numbers of children in a class may be unfamiliar (Boehm, 1971). Form A of the BTBC was translated into a haptic format, the *Tactile Test of Basic Concepts* (Caton, 1976), to be used with visually impaired children who require braille and other haptic media for their educational program.

The BTBC consists of a series of 50 picture items. The TTBC is composed of 50 plastic sheets on which 50 items of the BTBC are presented in raised outline drawings. The outline drawings represent the same concepts in the same context and order as those in the BTBC. In some cases, single geometric forms are used to represent the concepts (Fig. 1-9).

The following concepts are tested:

top	whole	beginning	separated
through	nearest	other	left
away from	second	alike	pair
next to	corner	not first or last	skip
inside	several	never	equal
some, not many	behind	below	in order
middle	row	matches	third
few	different	always	least
farthest	after	medium-sized	
around	almost	right	
over	half	forward	
widest	center	zero	
most	as many	above	
between	side	every	

The study which developed the analog to the BTBC (Caton, 1977) field tested 75 visually impaired students (braille or eventual braille users), 25 each from kindergarten, first, and second grade.

This test may be administered by the mobility specialist, but the *Tactile Test of Basic Concepts Test Manual* (Caton, 1976) should be used. The print form of the BTBC may be used with any low vision children without modifications. The major weakness of this instrument is the lack of validity, therefore it should be used as a criterion reference test.

The Basic Concept Inventory (BCI, Engelmann, 1967)

A series of concepts are tapped by this criterion-referenced inventory, subjectively selected as being basic for success in first grade. The inventory purports to evaluate the instruction in certain beginning academically-related concepts as well as the instruction given an individual child. The BCI is designed for sighted children who are preparing for beginning academic tasks. It is primarily intended for culturally disadvantaged preschool and kindergarten children, slow learners, emotionally disturbed, and mentally retarded children.

The BCI consists of three parts. In the first part, Basic Concepts, the child is shown a series of nine picture cards (used in the first part only) to evaluate degree of understanding of common words and word combinations. In the second part,

Statement Repetition and Comprehension, the child is required to repeat statements, some of which are nonsense statements. The third part, Pattern Awareness, includes imitation of movement patterns and digit sequences and some sound blending.

The instructions for administering and scoring the measure are explicit, detailed, and item specific. Much of the manual is devoted to classroom applications of the inventory. This inventory is designed for sighted children, so adaptations for visually impaired children are necessary. However, some low vision children may use it without modification. Its major weakness is lack of validity and reliability information.

The various tests discussed here are some of the more commonly used instruments. There are many such assessment tools designed for sighted children (Buros, 1972), and others for the visually impaired such as the Kephart Scale (Kephart, Kephart, & Schwarz, 1974). There are also many mobility checklists and teacher-made devices not necessarily intended for distribution but very useful. Some of these concept assessments are designed for the specific population and/or situation with which the mobility specialist is working.

Whatever concept assessment instruments are used, they only assess a limited number of the concepts needed for independent travel. It is therefore extremely important that the mobility specialist observe mobility lessons conscientiously, and discuss them with the student. This is very important because it determines the ability of the student to translate a verbal, abstract concept into a behaviorally functional concrete situation. The various assessment devices and analytic observations dictate what is needed for concept development and the method of presentation.

TEACHING OF CONCEPTS

After the mobility specialist completes the assessment, strategies for teaching concepts may be characterized by one or a combination of several approaches, depending on the age of the child and the teaching situation.

For younger children, appropriate concepts should be geared to the developmental level of the child by referring to any one of a number of developmental norms established for normal children. The mobility specialist should be particularly aware of the level of mobility at a specific age. This involves a task analysis of the many environmental concepts used at that level. One should not make an assumption of the child's level of concept knowledge nor accept only a verbal description of the concept. Rather, the mobility specialist should require a physical demonstration of concept understanding from the child.

A second approach is to present the conceptual learning activities in the context of mobility instruction as the need or occasion arises, relying on the mobility situation to elicit the concept deficiency. This requires that the mobility lessons utilize a wide variety of concepts. It is also important to discuss the mobility lessons with the student in order to assess understanding. Difficulty with a lesson may include problems with cane technique, with orientation, or a problem with concepts. Unless the specific concept deficiency is dealt with, the problems will continue.

Another method of teaching concepts is a class focusing on concept attainment. This differs from the first method which focuses primarily on children and developmental concepts such as body awareness. In a concept class, students of all ages may participate. The types of concepts which could be discussed are: right turn on red, location of bus stops and the various types of buses, specific street configurations or peculiarities, and layouts of stores or shopping centers.

A final method of concept teaching is the integration of concept-learning activities with other activities involving teachers, staff, and family to allow for systematic reinforcement of concepts in other contexts by individuals other than the mobility specialist. By teaching significant others the importance of explaining new concepts, the student will be exposed to a greater range and variety of concepts that should be continued after the student finishes the mobility training program. Also, it sensitizes family members, teachers, and other staff to the importance of concepts for mobility and provides them with some strategies for explaining such concepts.

Parents are now being encouraged to allow their visually impaired children to participate in physical activities, exploring the environment, playing catch, going for walks, etc. But just engaging in these activities is not enough; the visually impaired child must be encouraged to use as many types of stimulation as possible. Textures of surfaces, inclines, declines, curves, temperature changes, discernible odors or sounds, etc., should be pointed out to the child with sufficient verbal information accompanying the actual physical experience. Frequently an adult does not take time to find out what the child knows about the particular experience or to verify an accurate understanding of the verbal description. There is often lack of attention to the appropriate verbal labels given to the experience by the adult. A poor choice of labels, ones which have other meanings or no real meanings at all, does not help the child. It is important that the adult and visually impaired child understand each other. Whenever possible, a verbal concept should be verified by a concrete activity.

It is important for the mobility specialist to emphasize to teachers and parents of visually impaired children that many of these concepts can be introduced and integrated into their normal routine without a great deal of extra time. For example, while riding in a car to the grocery store, a parent could ask the child to keep track of left and right turns. Or a teacher in a classroom situation (during a question and answer session) might ask children to raise their right hands, left hands, or touch the top of their heads if they know the answer.

While the concept teaching methods were presented in four distinct forms, one or a combination of these methods may be used. The ideal situation is to incorporate as many methods as are appropriate to the mobility student's program. Again, the type of situation in which mobility is taught, the age of the student, the student's background and attitude toward blindness, are all variables that must be considered.

METHODS AND MATERIALS

With a variety of methods and materials available for teaching concepts, it is important that an appropriate selection be made to gear the methods to the age and motivation of the learner and the concept to be taught. Talking down to a student can be demeaning and counterproductive. It is important, especially with adults, to try to relate new concepts to those already known. Similarly, it is important not to present materials at too high a level—talking over the student's head. New concepts are sometimes related to ones the student is already *assumed* to have.

Systematic analysis of the full range of concepts associated with a particular object or situation is important. An example of such a teaching outline is used in the explanation of the concept of a reclining chair:

Identification of Parts—arms, footrest, seat, etc.
Function—to sit in, to lean back in, to rest or sleep in
Object Surfaces—top, bottom, sides, front, back
Relationship of Object Parts—the seat is between the arms, the footrest is below
   the seat, the arms are parallel to one another

Movement of Object Parts or Surfaces—the chair can be turned to face west, the footrest can be pushed back, the chair can be turned upside down, etc.

Relationship of Object and Other Objects (not essential to general concept of reclining chair)—the chair is next to the couch, the lamp is to the right of the chair, the rug is under the chair, etc.

An example of an analysis of teaching the relationship of self to the environment is:

Self to Objects—I am north of the school, I am perpendicular to the door, I am 20 feet from the building, etc.

Object to Self—The chair is to the left of me, the ceiling is above me, the table is near me, etc.

Movement of Self in Environment—I am stretching my arms toward the ceiling, I have turned so my side is next to the door, I am walking parallel to Elm Street, etc.

Movement of Environment—The traffic is moving towards me, the chair was turned to face me, the person walked behind me, etc.

Presentation

After a concept assessment has been made and a teaching outline developed, the mobility specialist should select an appropriate method of presentation. The most frequently used is verbal presentation. While verbal presentation is readily available, it was pointed out earlier that there may be deficiencies in concept understanding because concept terms are not thoroughly understood. In spite of this limitation, verbal presentations such as those used in many mobility lessons are extremely useful and effective.

A second method is the use of games. Games may vary from such activities as Simon Says, treasure hunt, or follow the leader; to commercial games such as chinese checkers, and construction toys such as Leggos, etc. Games provide an opportunity to teach, reinforce, and employ a variety of concepts, and at the same time maintain a high level of motivation. Games are generally used with visually impaired children and not with adults.

The third method involves the use of schematics and models. A thorough presentation of a variety of schematics and models is in Chapter 10 by Bentzen. Their strengths and weaknesses are also presented and should be considered when teaching concepts.

Finally, a fourth method used to teach concepts is concrete experience, one of the basic principles upon which the success of orientation and mobility instruction is based. While all of the other methods offer certain advantages they are basically supplemental, a replacement for direct experience. Obviously, direct experiences are not always possible and other activities must be employed. In some instances, a student may be unable to conceptualize the cartographic schema of a city by direct experience. In such cases one or all of the other methods, games, verbal presentations, and schematics and models, may be used in conjunction with mobility experiences in the real situation.

Table 1-9 presents many frequently used concepts that are prerequisite to the process of orientation and are built upon a foundation of previously learned concepts.

Just as orientation requires many prerequisite concepts, mobility also requires many concepts. It is not enough to be ambulatory or just possess good cane skills. Balance, coordination, dynamic posture, gait, dexterity, stamina, and reaction time are an integral part of the mobility process. Mobility requires the visually impaired individual to be able to maintain a straight line of travel, execute various turns, and utilize available sensory systems efficiently. Examples of prerequisite

TABLE 1-9.
Orientation Concepts and Prerequisites.

Orientation Concepts	Concept Prerequisites
Landmarks	Awareness of the existence of objects; awareness of the nature of fixed, movable and moving objects; awareness that objects are three-dimensional; ability to identify, recognize, and discriminate objects by their size, shape or form, position, texture, and function; ability to determine an object's distance and direction, its relationship to other significant things in the environment; to be able to determine an object's transference value to corresponding areas
Cues	Ability to identify, discriminate, and interpret environmental stimuli through various sensory modalities; awareness of body position in relationship to cue; awareness of temporal relationships; concept of a straight line; distance awareness; concept of parallel and perpendicular
Numbering Systems	Spatial concepts, such as middle, end, side; environmental concepts such as street, block, intersection, gridwork, etc.; ability to generalize and transfer concepts of odd and even numbers, ordering and patterns; measurement concepts, such as distance and time; ability to use environmental cues and directions; knowledge (environmental) of sources to solicit specific information
Measurement	Body awareness, object identification; functional knowledge of body as a measuring device—arm span, waist high, pacing, etc.; knowledge of the relationship and movement of self to environment; specific spatial terms such as long, short, wide; knowledge of standard increments of measurement and quantitative concepts
Compass Directions	Positional (egocentric) concepts, such as left, right, front, back, center, middle; object to object relationships; understanding of right angle, perpendicular, and parallel.

mobility concepts are italicized in two mobility techniques. Concepts that are repeated are not italicized a second time.

Use of Sighted Guide (Hill & Ponder, 1976)
1. With the *back* of his *hand* the guide contacts the student's *arm* (implied knowledge of body parts of another person, movement of body parts, and knowledge of one's own body parts)

2. The student *moves* his hand *up* the guide's arm to a *position* just *above* the *elbow*

3. The student's *thumb* is positioned just above the elbow *on* the *lateral side* of the guide's arm with the remaining four *fingers* on the *medial* side, *in* a grip that is secure yet comfortable for the guide (implied knowledge of another's body planes)

4. The student's upper arm is positioned *parallel* and *close* to the side of his body

5. The student's *upper* and *lower* arm form an *angle* of approximately 90° with the *forearm pointing forward* (implied relationship and movement of one's own body parts)

6. The *shoulder* of the student's grip arm is directly *behind* the shoulder of the guide's arm (implied—relationship of one's own body parts to those of another)

7. The student remains approximately *one-half-step* behind the guide (implied—relationship of one's own body planes to those of another).

Touch Techniques (Hill & Ponder, 1976)

1. The *cane grip* rests *in* the *mid-line* of the *base* of the *palm* with the *back* of the *hand facing laterally,* (implied—identification of object parts [cane grip]; relationship of body parts; knowledge of body planes)

2. The *index finger* is *extended downward along* the *flat side* of the grip, (implied—movement of body parts; knowledge of object planes [side])

3. The *thumb* is *positioned over* and *around* the grip with the remaining fingers *flexed* around the *bottom* of the grip so that the crook is in an *inferior* position, (implied—relationship of self to environment; relationship of object parts)

4. The *wrist* should be *centered* at body mid-line and *out* from the body at a *point* where the *arm*-cane combination forms a *straight line*

5. Wrist *movement* is from side to side, (implied—movement of body parts)

6. Utilizing the proper wrist movement, the cane tip is moved to a point contacting the *ground one* inch *beyond each shoulder* (implied—object to object relationship; environment concept [ground])

7. At the *height* of the *arc,* the cane tip is one inch *above* the ground

8. The student moves in a rhythmic manner so that the cane tip and the *heel* of the *opposite foot* contact the ground in unison.

As demonstrated in these examples, the importance of establishing a foundation of basic concepts is therefore fundamental to both orientation and mobility, and explains why mobility specialists have been particularly interested in this aspect of the development of visually impaired people. As programs develop further, however, it is expected that assistance with concept development will be provided more and more by classroom teachers of the visually impaired and other types of special education or rehabilitation staff prior to, or in conjunction with, orientation and mobility instruction.

Bibliography

Apple, M. Kinesic training for the blind: A program. *Education of the Visually Handicapped,* May, 1972.

Atkins, L. *A study of spatial conceptual abilities tests with blind subjects.* A Project Submitted to the Department of Occupational Therapy, Virginia Commonwealth University, May, 1974.

Ayres, J. A. *The Ayres Space Test.* Beverly Hills, Calif.: Western Psychological Services, 1962.

Ball, T. S., & Edgar, C. L. The effectiveness of sensory-motor training in promoting generalized body image development. *Journal of Special Education,* F, 1967.

Berla, E. Effects of physical size and complexity on tactual discrimination of blind children. *Exceptional Children,* 1972.

Bishop, V. E. *Teaching the visually limited child.* Springfield, Ill.: Charles C Thomas, 1971.

Bitterman, M.E., & Worchel, P. The phenomenal vertical and horizontal in blind and sighted subjects. *American Journal of Psychology,* 1953.

Blackhurst, A. E., Marks, C. H., Tisdall, W. J. Relationship between mobility and divergent thinking in blind children. *Education of the Visually Handicapped,* May 1969, **1**(2).

Blasch, B., Welsh, R., & Davidson, T. Auditory maps: An orientation aid for visually handicapped persons. *The New Outlook for the Blind,* 1973, **67**(4), 145-158.

Boehm, A. E. *Boehm Test of Basic Concepts: Test manual.* New York: The Psychological Corporation, 1971.

Braley, W., Konicki, G., & Leedy, C. *Daily sensori-motor activities—A hand book for teachers and parents of preschool children.* Freeport, N.Y.: Educational Activities, 1968.

Brown, J. The use of educational toys in the training of blind pre-school children. *American Journal of Occupational Therapy,* 1951.

Buros, O. K. *The seventh mental measurements yearbook.* Highland Park, New Jersey: The Gryphon Press, 1972.

Carr, H. A. *An introduction to space perception.* New York: Hafner Publishing Company, 1966.

Caton, B. J. *Concept development: North American Conference on Visually Handicapped Infants and Preschool Children.* American Foundation for the Blind, May 22-25, Minneapolis, Minnesota, 1978.

Caton, H. R. The development and evaluation of a tactile analog to the Boehm Test of Basic Concepts, Form A. *Journal of Visual Impairment and Blindness,* 1977, **71**(9), 382-386.

Caton, H. R. *The Tactile Test of Basic Concepts: Test manual.* Louisville, Ky.: American Printing House for the Blind, 1976.

Church, J., & Stone, J. L. *Childhood and adolescence.* New York: Random House, 1966.

Combs, A. W. Intelligence from a perceptual point of view. *Journal of Abnormal and Social Psychology,* 1952, **XLVII**, 662-673.

Cone, J. The effects of blindness on children's development. *New Outlook for the Blind,* 1966, **60**(5).

Cratty, B. J. *Development sequences of perceptual motor tasks.* Freeport, N.Y.: Educational Activities, 1967.

Cratty, B. J. *Movement and spatial awareness in blind children.* Springfield, Ill.: Charles C. Thomas, 1971.

Cratty, B. J., & Sams, T. A. The body image of blind children. New York: *American Foundation for the Blind Research Bulletin* No. 17, July, 1968.

Cratty, B. J., & Williams, H. G. Accuracy of facing movements executed without vision. *Perceptual and Motor Skills,* 1966, 23.

Cutsforth, T. D. *The blind in school and society.* New York: American Foundation for the Blind, 1951.

Cutsforth, T. D. An analysis of the relationship between tactual and visual perception. *American Foundation for the Blind Research Bulletin,* No. 12, January 1966.

Dauterman, W. L. *Manual for the Stanford Multi-Modality Imagery Test.* New York: American Foundation for the Blind, 1972.

Davey, B. L. *The teacher's role in orientation and mobility.* Norfolk, Va.: Old Dominion University, 1970.

Davis, C. J. Development of self-concept. *New Outlook for the Blind,* 1968, **58**(2).

del Campo, A. Blind can 'see' the shape of things. *Medical World News,* 1966, **7**(37).

Dickinson, R. *Mobility training for the visually handicapped: A guide for teachers.* Springfield, Ill.: Illinois Office of the Coordinator of Visually Handicapped Services, 1968.

Dickinson, R. *Orientation and mobility for the visually handicapped: A guide for parents.* Springfield, Ill.: Illinois Office of the Coordinator of Visually Handicapped Services, 1968.

Dokecki, P. R. Verbalism and the blind. *Exceptional Children,* April, 1966.

Drever, J. Early learning and the perception of space. *American Journal of Psychology,* 1955.

Duggar, M. P. What can dance be to someone who cannot see? *Journal of Health, Physical Education and Recreation,* 1968, **39**(5).

Duncan, B. K. A comparative study of finger maze learning by blind and sighted subjects. *Journal of Genetic Psychology,* 1934.

Early, G. H. *Perceptual training in the curriculum.* Columbus, Ohio: Charles E. Merrill, 1969.

Eichorn, J., & Vigorosa, H. Orientation and mobility for pre-school blind children. *International Journal for the Education of the Blind,* 1967, **XVIII**(2).

Eichorn, J., & McDade, P. *Teaching orientation and mobility to the mentally retarded blind.* Chestnut Hill, Mass.: Boston College, 1969.

Eisenberg, R. A. Concept development in preparation for the cane or dog. *Long Cane News,* 1968, **2**(4).

Eliot, J., & Salkind, N. J. *Children's spatial development.* Springfield, Ill.: Charles C Thomas, 1975.

Engelmann, S. E. *The Basic Concept Inventory, field research edition.* Chicago, Ill.: Follett Educational Corporation, 1967.

Fields, J. E. Sensory training for blind persons. *The New Outlook for the Blind,* 1964, **58**(1).

Fisher, G. H. Spatial localization by the blind. *American Journal of Psychology,* 1964, 77.

Forgus, R. H. *Perception.* San Francisco, Calif.: McGraw-Hill, 1966.

Foulke, E. A multi-sensory test of conceptual ability. *The New Outlook for the Blind,* 1964.

Foulke, E. The role of experience in the formation of concepts. *The International Journal for the Education of the Blind,* 1962.

Fraiberg, S., Smith, M., & Adelson, E. An educational program for blind infants. *Journal of Special Education,* 1966, **3**(2).

Fraiberg, S., Siegel, B. L., & Gibson, R. *Sound in the search behavior of a blind infant, the psychoanalytic study of the child.* New York: International Universities Press, 1966.

Friedman, J., & Pasnak, R. Attainment of classification and concepts by blind and sighted subjects. *Education of the Visually Handicapped,* 1973, **5,** 55-62.

Frostig, M., & Horne, D. *The Frostig program for the development of visual perception: Teachers guide.* Chicago: Follett Publishing Co., 1964.

Frostig, M., & Maslow, P. *Move-grow-learn (teacher's guide).* Chicago: Follett Educational Corporation, 1969.

Garry, R. J., & Ascarelli, A. Teaching topographical orientation and spatial orientation to congenitally blind children. *Journal of Education,* 1960.

Gesell, A. *The first five years of life: A guide to the study of the preschool child.* New York: Harper, 1940.

Gesell, A., Ilg, F., *The child from five to ten.* New York: Harper, 1946.

Gesell, A., Ilg, F., & Bullis, G. *Vision: Its development in infant and child.* New York: Paul B. Hoeber, Inc., 1949.

Gibson, E. J. *Principles of perceptual learning and development.* New York: Appleton-Century-Crofts, 1967.

Gibson, J. J. *The senses considered as perceptual systems.* Boston: Houghton Mifflin Co., 1966.

Gockman, R. L. Orientation and mobility skills for children. *Long Cane News,* 1969, **3**(2).

Gockman, R. L. The importance of parental influence upon a program of orientation and mobility for children. *Long Cane News,* **1**(4).

Gottesman, M. A. A comparative study of Piaget's developmental schema of sighted children with that of a group of blind children. *Child Development,* 1971, **42,** 573-580.

Gottesman, M. A. Conservation development in blind children. *Child Development,* 1973, **44,** 824-927.

Graham, M. D. Wanted: A readiness test for mobility training. *The New Outlook for the Blind,* 1965, **58**(5).

Graham, M. D. *Multiply-impaired blind children: A national problem.* New York: American Foundation for the Blind, 1968.

Gregory, R. L., & Wallace, J. G. *Recovery from early blindness: A case study.* Experimental Psychology Society Monograph, No. 2, 1963.

Guldager, V. *Body image and the severely handicapped rubella child.* Watertown, Mass.: Perkins Publications, No. 27, 1970.

Hackett, L. C., & Jensen, R. G. *A guide to movement exploration.* Palo Alto, Calif.: Peek Publications, 1967.

Hall, E. A conversation with Jean Piaget. *Psychology Today,* 1970.

Hart, V. *The multi-impaired visually handicapped in the residential school. A look at the child.* Selected Papers Association for the Education of the Visually Handicapped, 1970.

Halliday, C. *The visually impaired child—growth, learning, development, infancy to school age.* Louisville, Ky.: American Printing House for the Blind, 1970.

Hapeman, L. Developmental concepts of blind children between the ages of three and six as they relate to orientation and mobility. *International Journal for the Education of the Blind,* 1967, **27**(2).

Harley, R. K. *Verbalism among blind children.* New York: American Foundation for the Blind, Research Series No. 10, 1963.

Hartlage, L. C. Deficit in space concepts associated with visual deprivation. *Journal of Learning Disabilities,* 1968, 1.

Hartlage, L. C. The role of vision in the development of spatial ability. Unpublished doctoral dissertation, University of Illinois, 1968.

Haupt, C. Improving blind children's perceptions. *The New Outlook for the Blind,* 1964, **58**(6).

Held, R., & Rekosh, J. Motor-sensory feedback and the geometry of visual space. *Science,* August, 1963.

Hermelin, B., & O'Connor, N. Spatial coding in normal, autistic and blind children. *Perceptual and Motor Skills,* 1971.

Hetherington, F. F. Elementary school travel program. *International Journal for the Education of the Blind,* 1955, **5**(1).

Higgins, L. C. *Classification in congenitally blind children*. New York: American Foundation for the Blind, 1973.

Hill, E. W. The formation of concepts involved in body position in space. *Education of the Visually Handicapped*, 1970, **12**(2).

Hill, E. W. The formation of concepts involved in body position in space, Part II. *Education of the Visually Handicapped*, 1971, **3**(1), 21-26.

Hill, E. W. Mobility and concept development for low vision children. *Low Vision Abstracts*, 1971, **1**(1).

Hill, E. W., & Ponder, P. T. *Orientation and mobility: A guide for the practitioner*. New York: American Foundation for the Blind, 1976.

Hoffman, M. L. & Hoffman, L. W. *Child development research*. New York: Russell Sage Foundation, 1964.

Hoop, N. Haptic perception in preschool blind children. *The American Journal of Occupational Therapy*, 1971, **25**(7).

Howard, I. P. & Templeton, W. B. *Human spatial orientation*. New York: John Wiley and Sons, 1966.

Hunter, W. F. An analysis of space perception in congenitally blind and sighted individuals. *Journal of General Psychology*, 1964, **70**(2).

Illingworth, R. S. *The development of the infant and young child—normal and abnormal*. Baltimore: The Williams and Wilkins Co., 1966.

Illinois Visually Handicapped Institute and Western Michigan University. *Proceedings: Parameters of posture and mobility in the blind*. Kalamazoo, Mich.: Western Michigan University, 1969.

Instructional Materials Center for the Visually Handicapped. *Toys for early development of the young blind child.* Springfield, Ill.: Author, 1971.

Johnson, O. G., & Bonimarito, J. W. *Tests and measurements in child development: A handbook*. San Francisco, Calif.: Jossey-Bass, Inc. Publishers, 1976.

Juurmaa, J. *An analysis of the components of orientation, mobility and mental manipulation of spatial relationships*. Helsinki, Finland: Report from the Institute of Occupational Health, No. 28, August, 1965.

Kephart, J., & Kephart, C. *Kephart Scale: A means to assess the personal and environmental awareness of young blind children*. Curriculum Materials Clearing House, 1973.

Kephart, J. G., Kephart, C. P., & Schwarz, G. C. A journey into the world of the blind child. *Exceptional Children*, March, 1974.

Kephart, N. C. *Slow learner in the classroom*. (2nd ed.) Columbus, Ohio: Charles E. Merrill Publishing Co., 1971.

Knickerbocker, B. A central approach to the development of spatial and temporal concepts. *Learning Disorders*, 1968.

Laurendeau, M., & Pinard, A. *The development of the concept of space in the child*. New York: International Universities Press, Inc., 1970.

Leonard, J. A. *The concept of the minimal information required for effective mobility and suggestions for future non-visual displays*. Department of Psychology, University of Nottingham, England, 1970.

Leonard, J. A. & Newman, R. C. Spatial orientation in the blind. *Nature*, 1967, 215.

Lord, F. E. Development of scales for the measurement of orientation and mobility skills of young blind children. *Exceptional Children*, 1969, **36**(2).

Lord, F. E., Manshardt, C. E., Adams, G. S. & Bailey, M. J. Identification of Orientation and Mobility Skills Relating to Developmental Tasks for Young Blind Children. U.S. Dept. HEW, Office of Education, Grant No. 5-0980-4-11-3. Los Angeles, Calif.: California State College at Los Angeles, Dept. of Special Education, 1967.

Lowenfeld, B. Effects of blindness on cognitive functions of children. *Nervous Child*, 1948, 7.

Lowenfeld, B. *Our blind children, growing and learning with them*. (2nd ed.) Springfield, Ill.: Charles C Thomas Publisher, 1964.

Lydon, T., & McGraw, M. L. *Concept development for visually handicapped children*. New York: American Foundation for the Blind, 1973.

McDade, P. R. Teaching orientation and mobility to mentally retarded blind. *Long Cane News*, 1967, **2**(3).

Metheny, E. *Body dynamics*. New York: McGraw-Hill, 1952.

Michigan School for the Blind. *Pre-cane mobility and orientation skills for the blind*. Lansing, Mich.: Author, nd.

Miller, C. K. Conservation in blind children. *Education of the Visually Handicapped*, 1969, **12**, 101-105.

Mills, R. Orientation and mobility for teachers. *Education of the Visually Handicapped*, 1970, **II**(3).

Mills, R. Orientation and mobility for teachers. *Education of the Visually Handicapped,* May, 1971.

Mills, R., & Adamshick, D. The effectiveness of structured sensory training experiences prior to formal orientation and mobility instruction. *Education of the Visually Handicapped,* 1969, **I**(1).

Moor, P. M. Blind children with developmental problems. *Children,* 1961.

Napier, G., & Weishahn, M. *Handbook for teachers of the visually handicapped.* Louisville, Ky.: American Printing House for the Blind, 1970.

New Outlook for the Blind, The. Basic concepts of blind children. New York: Author, 1965, **59**(10), 341-343.

Norris, M. What affects blind children's development. *The New Outlook for the Blind,* Sept. 1956.

Ohio Department of Education. *Guiding the development of the young visually handicapped child: A selected list of activities.* Ohio: Author, 1969.

Piaget, J. *Psychology of intelligence.* Paterson, N.J.: Littlefield-Adams, 1960.

Piaget, J., & Inhelder, B. *The child's perception of space.* New York: W. W. Norton and Co., Inc.: 1948.

Randolph, L. G. Don't rearrange the classroom: Why not? A proposal for meaningful classroom mobility. *Long Cane News,* 1971, **4**(3).

Raynor, S., & Drouillard, R. *Get a wiggle on.* Mason, Mich.: Ingham Intermediate School District, 1975.

Rice, C. E. Early blindness, early experience and perceptual enhancement. *American Foundation for the Blind Research Bulletin, No. 22,* Dec., 1970.

Roach, E. G., & Kephart, N. C. *The Purdue Perceptual Motor Survey.* Columbus, Ohio: Merrill, 1966.

Royster, P. M. Peripatology and the development of the blind child. *The New Outlook for the Blind,* 1964, **29**(5).

Rubin, E. J. *Abstract functioning in the blind.* New York: American Foundation for the Blind, 1964.

Scott, R. A. *The making of blind men.* New York: Russell Sage Foundation, 1969.

Simpkins, K., & Stephens, B. Cognitive development of blind subjects. *Proceedings of the 52nd Biennial Conference of the Association of the Education of the Visually Handicapped,* 1974, 26-38.

Stephens, B. Cognitive processes in the visually impaired. *Education of the Visually Handicapped,* 1972, **4,** 106-111.

Telford, C. W., & Sawrey, J. M. *The exceptional individual,* (2nd ed.). Englewood Cliffs, N.J.: Prentice-Hall, 1977.

Tisdall, W. J., Blackhurst, A. E. & Marks, C. H. *Divergent thinking in blind children.* Lexington, Ky.: Kentucky University, Project R-012 (10-21) Grant No. 32-27-0350-6003, 1967.

Tobin, M. J. Conservation of substance in the blind and sighted. *British Journal of Educational Psychology,* 1972, **42**(2), 192-197.

Trevena, T. M. *The role of the resource teacher in mobility instruction.* Hayward, Calif.: Alameda County School Dept., 1971.

Vigoroso, H. R. Concept development—thinking out loud. *Long Cane News,* 1969, **3**(1).

von Senden, M. *Space and sight: The perception of space and shape in the congenitally blind before and after operation.* Glencoe, Ill.: Free Press, 1960.

Wardell, K. T. Assessment of blind students' conceptual understanding. *New Outlook for the Blind,* 1975, **69**(10), 445-446.

Wardell, K. T. Preparatory concepts of orientation and mobility training. *Education of the Visually Handicapped,* 1972, **4**(3).

Warren, D. H. *Blindness and early childhood development.* New York: American Foundation for the Blind, 1977.

Webster, R. A concept development program for future mobility training. *New Outlook for the Blind,* 1976, **70**(5), 195-197.

Weisgerber, R. A., & Hall, A. P. *Environmental sensing skills and behaviors.* Palo Alto, Calif.: American Institutes for Research, 1975.

Whitstock, R. Orientation and mobility for blind children. *The New Outlook for the Blind,* 1960, **24**(3).

Wolf, J. *The blind child with concomitant disabilities.* New York: American Foundation for the Blind Research Series, No. 16, 1967.

Worchel, P. Space perception and orientation in the blind. *Psychological Monographs,* 1951.

Zweibelson, I., & Barg, C. F. Concept development of blind children. *The New Outlook for the Blind,* 1967, **61**(7).

Orientation Aids

Billie Louise Bentzen

Orientation aids are tools to be used by visually impaired persons to develop or enhance their understanding of basic spatial relationships, to facilitate their comprehension of specific travel environments, to refresh their memory of routes and areas, to further their skill in independent route planning, to enable them to travel independently in unfamiliar areas, and to add to their knowledge and enjoyment of physical space.

Mobility specialists convey most spatial information to their students or clients through spoken explanations and descriptions during lessons, and by means of direct familiarization. In some learning situations, for some visually impaired persons, these techniques alone are either inadequate or inefficient and the visually impaired person cannot acquire the concepts and cognitive maps of the environment that make independent travel possible.

Leonard and Newman (1970) found that subjects with no travel vision using one of three types of portable route maps traveled a new route with fewer orientation ("map") errors than a control group who relied only on memory of verbal instructions. The three types of route maps were a disc with a braille code, an auditory map, and a graphic map. Instruction in use of any of the three maps occupied considerably less time than was required for control group subjects to be sure they understood and could remember the verbal directions.

The following are examples of situations in which spoken explanations and direct familiarization may be inadequate or inefficient techniques:

1. A student has had little concrete experience with objects in the environment. Although he uses spatial and positional terms, he is lacking in many concepts necessary for making intelligent decisions about travel

2. A student has difficulty in recalling descriptions or instructions either while on a lesson or during subsequent independent travel

3. A student has difficulty understanding complex spatial relationships such as irregular placement of driveways, walks, and buildings on a campus. He cannot plan new routes in this environment. It may be neither desirable nor practicable for him to learn each route that he may wish to travel as a route, per se

4. A student has difficulty because of a hearing, a perceptual, or a language problem, in processing spoken information. He has limited understanding of spoken explanations, descriptions, and instructions

5. A student has only limited time with a specialist to acquire information about a new area in which he is to travel independently

6. A student who has completed a program of instruction in orientation and mobility at a school or rehabilitation center away from his own community and does not have access to a specialist for help in efficient acquirement of accurate and relevant information for independent travel in his home area.

CATEGORIES

In such situations, orientation aids may help to clarify concepts, assist recall, organize spatial information, supplement and complement spoken information, or present new information not directly available from an instructor.

There are three categories of aids which may be used either separately or in combination.

Models—three-dimensional representations of real objects or groups of objects found together in the environment.

Graphic aids—tactile, visual, and tactile-vision diagrams or maps having information perceptible to touch, vision, or to both touch and vision.

Verbal aids—(auditory, braille, and print). Specific types of spoken or written descriptions of the environment (area maps) and/or ways to travel within the environment (route maps).

Table 1-10 describes sample learning situations and indicates the category or categories of orientation aids which could assist in students' efficient acquisition and utilization of skills or concepts. The aids do not substitute for instruction by a mobility specialist. Suggested aids would be used primarily by visually impaired persons who are receiving instruction or who have already completed a course of instruction in independent travel skills.

Orientation aids are appropriate for many students and many learning situations. However, aids are not a panacea, and should not be used as ends in themselves. The decision to use an aid must be based on the specialist's actual knowledge of whether a student needs it, and whether he can use it.

The need for an aid will be apparent to the specialist when a student fails to progress using the commoner teaching methods of spoken explanation and description, and direct familiarization. The specialist should, however, know his students well enough to anticipate their problems and use appropriate aids before failure leads to discouragement.

Whether or not a student can use an aid in a particular situation often depends on the flexibility, imagination and skill of the specialist in choosing an appropriate aid, making correct decisions about the design of the aid, making the aid, and teaching the student to use the aid. The student must be able to receive, perceive, and decode the symbols and to conceptualize information presented through the medium chosen.

All categories of aids have some characteristics in common, but some have special characteristics of their own.

Characteristics in Common

1. Decisions about information content and the design for its representation on an aid can best be done by a mobility specialist who knows what information, in what situation, is necessary and useful for a particular student and a particular learning need. All categories of aids, however, can be prepared by specialists, volunteers, or family members.

2. Some aids in each category can be prepared, added to, or altered by visually impaired users.

3. Commercially available materials and systems exist for the preparation of aids in all categories.

4. Commercially available materials and systems are flexibly designed within each

---

TABLE 1-10
Learning Situations and Suggested Aids

Situation	Aid
Client does not understand relationship of floors in school/ agency building	Model
Does not understand permanent and moveable features of a room	Model
Has difficulty understanding where he is, when he veers while crossing a street	Graphic (tactile and/or visual), and/or model
Does not understand configuration of a complex intersection	Graphic (tactile and/or visual), and/or model
Wishes to travel many different routes infrequently but independently	Graphic (tactile and/or visual); verbal (auditory or braille)
Wishes familiarization to unfamiliar metropolitan area	Graphic (tactile and/or visual); verbal (auditory or braille)
Cannot remember more than one-step directions	Verbal (auditory)
Cannot remember route from home to workshop	Graphic (tactile and/or visual), or verbal route (auditory)
Cannot understand verbal route instructions on lessons	Graphic (tactile and/or visual)
Cannot verbalize route to specialist before traveling it; needs system to to let specialist know where he is going	Graphic (tactile and/or visual)
Client with severe hearing loss needs familiarization to new nursing home	Graphic (tactile and/or visual)
Because of impaired tactile sensitivity (palsy or peripheral neuropathy) client needs a memory aid for independent and repeated use	Verbal (auditory)
Needs for a portable route-memory aid useful in cold weather	Verbal (auditory)

category so that specialists may make modifications for specific students and situations.

5. Specific aids within all categories are portable enough to permit reference by the visually impaired person while en route to a destination, although models are not usually designed with this characteristic in mind.

6. Aids within all categories can be developed for the repeated use of one or a number of visually impaired persons.

7. Aids within all categories permit some degree of user control over the rate at which information must be attended to, and the amount which will be attended to at any one time.

Special Characteristics of Models

When made to high standards of scale, texture, and color, models are more realistic than graphic or verbal aids. They may thus excel in situations where the primary problem is a conceptual deficit.

SPECIAL CHARACTERISTICS OF GRAPHIC AIDS
Tactile

1. Tactile graphic aids excel at representing environmental configurations such as intersections, floor plans of buildings, campus layouts, city street patterns, and the relationships between public transportation systems and the areas they serve.

Visual

1. Visual graphic orientation aids may be simultaneously read by blind and sighted persons, facilitating assistance with reading by specialist or non-specialists.

2. They may be inconspicuous because they are similar to orientation aids (maps) used by sighted persons.

3. They can be made inexpensively, both for single and multiple copies.

Tactile-Visual

1. Tactile-visual graphic aids have all the characteristics of tactile graphic aids.

2. They also permit simultaneous reading and assistance with reading by specialists or non-specialists.

3. In addition, they enable the person who can perform some near vision tasks, but who can also profit by tactile input, to make maximum use of both senses and permit him to determine which input he will use for the task at hand.

Verbal (Auditory)

1. Recorded verbal aids present environmental information, routes to be traveled, and areas in which to travel, in terms which the visually impaired person has already learned to recognize. He does not need to learn any new perceptual or conceptual skills, but only the mechanics of operating the tape recorder.

2. The tape recorder itself, although it may be heavier and more cumbersome than some graphic aids, can be carried by a neck or shoulder strap while communicating information, leaving both hands free. The recorder is inconspicuous as it is relatively common for sighted persons to carry tape recorders, and it can be operating while the listener travels.

3. Auditory maps are the least limited in terms of the amount and detail of information they can convey and still be portable (Blasch, Welsh & Davidson, 1973). Detailed information about landmarks, suggestions for the use of specific techniques for specific travel situations, and historical, cultural and esthetic enrichment information can be more easily included on recorded aids than on graphic aids.

4. Auditory maps do not require braille skills or sufficient vision to read print.

5. Auditory maps can be listened to simultaneously by the visually impaired student and his instructor.

Braille

1. Blind persons, themselves, can make permanent braille memory aids or descriptions of geographic areas by brailling those portions of verbal explanations and directions which are necessary to them, or by writing down information about a route or an area which is obtained by independent exploration.

Print

1. Print verbal orientation aids share the characteristics of braille aids, but do not require the specialized skills and equipment to produce braille.

2. In addition, print permits simultaneous reading and help by either a specialist or non-specialist.

The materials and design of any aid must be able to convey the information needed. In addition, decisions about design and materials should be based on general considerations, singly or combined as they apply to each situation and each individual (Table 2-10).

These considerations and the criteria for aid materials and designs which they necessitate, should be kept in mind during the reading of subsequent sections. Specific design factors and particular properties of materials will be discussed under the categories of models, graphic aids, and verbal aids.

MODELS AS AIDS FOR TEACHING SPATIAL CONCEPTS

As presented in the chapter on concept development, visually impaired persons must understand many spatial concepts in order to be maximally independent travelers. The following is a discussion of some of the models that can be used in teaching specific spatial concepts related to independent travel.

Congenitally visually impaired persons may frequently have difficulty forming complete and accurate concepts of components of the environment such as different kinds of buildings, vehicles and intersections which are too large for them to see in detail or encompass totally through haptic exploration. Adventitiously visually impaired persons may have incomplete, and inaccurate or outdated concepts. Models can be useful aids for the learning of such concepts.

The best models are those which are most like the thing they represent, yet no model conforms totally to the original. Selection or construction of a model is always a compromise in which attributes like the original are chosen because they are important to the acquisition of a complete and accurate concept, and unlike attributes are chosen because they facilitate observation and understanding. Other unlike attributes may be permitted because they do not present a significant obstacle for the specific learning need. Some attributes to be considered in model selection and their implications for the acquisition of concepts are presented in Table 3-10.

TABLE 2-10.
General Considerations for Choice of Design or Materials

Consideration	Criteria for Design or Materials
What information must be conveyed to satisfy the need of the learning situation?	Include only that information which is essential for the purpose of the aid.
How much information can a person or group of persons perceive and comprehend on a single aid?	The aid should not exceed the perceptual and conceptual skills and abilities of the person or group of persons by including too much information or by having too high an information density.
What materials can best convey the desired concept or information to the particular person or group of persons?	Materials for a particular person or group of persons should be pleasing to them, appropriate for their level of functioning and easy for them to use.
Is the aid to be temporarily used by one person?	It may be highly specialized for that person's needs and abilities. It should be easy and inexpensive to make. It need not be durable.
Is the aid to be repeatedly used by one person?	It may be highly specialized for that person's need and abilities. It should be relatively inexpensive to make. It should be durable.
Is a single aid to be repeatedly used by many persons?	Both design and materials should be appropriate for the range of needs and abilities of the entire group. Expenditure of considerable time and money may be warranted. It must be durable.
Are many persons to have their own copies of the aid?	See above criteria. The aid must be capable of reproduction at reasonable cost and with good quality.
Is the aid to be used while the user is stationary, in a comfortable environment?	It need not be portable or weatherproof.
Is the aid to be used while the user travels outdoors?	It must be portable (lightweight, easy to carry, inconspicuous), weatherproof, and easy to use while traveling. Its usefulness should not be affected by adverse weather. It is helpful if it has some system for the user to mark his current location.
Is it desirable for a visually impaired person to be able to give feedback by adding to or altering the aid?	The aid must permit such addition or alteration.
Is it desirable for a visually impaired person to be able to make similar aids by himself, either to give feedback to the specialist, or for personal use, independent of an instructional situation?	Materials must be available to visually impaired persons, and techniques of construction must be within their skill level.
Is the aid to be used during an extended time period?	It should be possible to update the aid to reflect changes in the environment with reasonable expenditure of time and money.

TABLE 3-10.
Considerations for Selecting or Constructing Models

Attribute	Implications for Concept Acquisition
Size	The chief reason for making many models is to make spatial, structural features or details, either very large or very small, perceivable by haptic exploration. In actual practice, a good size for a particular need can usually be determined empirically if the model designer has several persons perform haptically the tasks expected of students. (Modifications should be made where there are significant differences between designer and student, in haptic sensitivity or in physical size.)
Scale (relative proportions of parts of a model to each other)	Wherever possible, scale should be consistent throughout a model. There is always conceptual distortion when relative proportions of parts of a model are not consistent. For example, model cars should be proportional to the width of streets they are to be driven on, the height of curbs, and the size of model pedestrians. Whenever scale is inconsistent, it is important to be sure that the student understands the inconsistency. However, where one wishes to convey relative physical dimensions of similar objects, such as sizes of buildings or widths of streets, the haptic perception of these relative dimensions is influenced by the Steven's power function (see Chapter 5, Pick) which indicates that some systematic variation in scale of model parts may enhance the accuracy of haptic perception of size differences.
Texture	Textures which are the same as, or similar to, those they represent will be most readily associated with the real object. Textures must be selected haptically, not visually. For example, visual selection of a rough textured green rubber mat to represent grass for a totally blind student, might be inferior to the selection of a napped fabric such as velveteen.
Density	Models which are made of materials quite unlike those of the original may be so different in density that association with the original may be difficult. Flexible, compressible rubber cars may be difficult to associate with real cars. Metal dolls may be more difficult to associate with real persons than flexible, compressible dolls.
Color	Models for low vision students should be of a color readily associated with the object they represent.
Completeness of detail (presence of the detail, and its ability to function as in the original)	Exact, small or large scale replicas of original objects are usually very expensive, hard to find, and tedious to make. In selecting or making a model, choose those details which are most relevant to what is being taught. For example, a staircase is an essential detail in a model of a two-story house used to teach the concept that stairs are the usual route from one floor of a house to another.

There are some common environmental elements or concepts that are difficult to perceive without full vision:

Buildings
   Walls (interior and exterior)
   Ceiling
   Roof
   Windows
   Doors (interior and exterior)
   Different floors—connected by stairs
   Rooms (shape, function and placement in relation to each other)
   Permanent and moveable features
   Placement of furniture in relation to function
   Utilities
   Characteristics of a house in relation to sidewalk, street, driveway, yard, garages, neighbors, etc.
   Features which distinguish buildings used for different purposes from one another.

Vehicles
   Front, back, sides, top, bottom
   Doors
   Windows
   Seats
   Position of driver
   Engine
   Different vehicles—relative sizes, shapes and characteristics, in relation to function and particular style.

Neighborhoods
   Block (square block vs. linear block)
   Street Corner
   Intersection
   Sidewalk
   Driveway
   Curb
   Gutter
   Alley
   Buildings (relative size and position in relation to the foregoing)
   Other obstacles or landmarks (their sizes, shapes, expected locations, and functions) such as poles (street signs, traffic lights, utility poles, other traffic controls)
   Differences between neighborhoods, such as residential and commercial.

Models of the above may be helpful in teaching the following orientation systems:

Topocentric—relation of objects in the environment to each other

Cartographic—recognizable organizational patterns of environment, such as grid patterns, floor plans, and address systems

Polarcentric—use of compass directions for specifying a particular position in space or for relating relative positions or routes between positions.

Acceptable models for the teaching of some of these concepts can be purchased from toy and educational equipment suppliers, and others can be obtained from the American Printing House for the Blind.

Many of the best models are constructed by a mobility specialist who selects exactly those attributes which contribute the most to his student's acquisition of a desired concept. In a situation in which many students need instruction in the same concepts, it might be worthwhile to invest relatively large amounts of time, effort, and money to construct models which have many attributes of the objects they represent. Some excellent, portable models made by teachers are available on loan from local or regional resource leading centers.

ENVIRONMENTAL CONCEPTS, ROUTES, AND AREAS

Graphic orientation aids add several dimensions to the mobility specialist's basic techniques of verbal description and direct familiarization. The term *graphic aids* is used here to mean aids in which ideas are expressed "by means of lines, marks or characters . . . on a surface" *(Webster's New Collegiate Dictionary)*. Graphic aids that are perceptible by haptic exploration will be referred to as *tactile graphic aids*. Those perceptible through vision will be referred to as *visual graphic aids*. Aids perceptible both tactually and visually will be referred to as *tactile-visual graphic aids*.

Graphic aids excel in the presentation of information about environmental configurations such as complex intersections or irregular street patterns, even though verbal aids can include greater detail and more varied information. Knowledge of environmental configurations is essential to independently planned travel. For example, aspects of the environmental configuration of a small business area which the visually impaired traveler needs to know in order to plan varied routes include:

1. Which are the primary business streets?

2. In what direction/s do they run?

3. Do they have significant curves in the distance to be traveled?

4. How many streets intersect the primary business streets?

5. Are there other streets parallel to the primary business streets? (How many? Where?)

6. What is the configuration of each intersection?

If the visually impaired traveler combines this information with a knowledge of address systems and with good mobility skills, he can travel effectively to and from any destination in the area. Such information can be presented by many tactile and visual graphic techniques. Those unaccustomed to using graphic information may need to learn special skills to obtain maximum benefit from such aids. However, Kidwell and Greer (1973, p. 16) state that: "Although it may be that the physical-spatial map initially places greater perceptual demands on the user than either the brailled or taped sequential map, its potential benefits are far greater for the highly motivated and mobile blind traveler."

Some environmental configurations are too complex to be easily described verbally, but they can be constructed and perceived graphically. The configuration of a campus in which the vehicular and traffic pattern is based on irregular, winding driveways and walks which are neither parallel nor perpendicular to them could be represented graphically. This complex configuration, presented graphically, could be supplemented by verbal information about landmarks and other orientation clues.

Some extensive environments such as entire cities can be constructed and perceived on small-scale maps more readily than they can be described verbally.

Such maps can be supplemented by specific verbal information about features which are helpful or those that are difficult for the visually impaired traveler.

Some students, often those with prior visual map reading experience, understand the environment more readily if it is portrayed graphically, in a form they can utilize, than if it is portrayed verbally (Bentzen, 1972).

It has been experimentally demonstrated that some people having little or no useable vision, who have good independent travel skills, can independently choose and travel routes on a totally unfamiliar campus solely on the basis of a tactile map (Bentzen, 1972). Other research demonstrated that adult blind subjects who used a tactile map concomitantly with verbal directions were able to travel a life-sized maze in less time and with fewer errors than subjects using verbal directions alone (Maglione, 1969).

Graphic aids can facilitate communication between teacher and student when there is a language barrier, either because both are not fluent in the same language, or because the student has a receptive or expressive language impairment.

With graphic aids, students can set their own pace in acquiring information, and choose the order in which they will attend to aspects of the environment represented by the aid. A student who is highly motivated to get from his house to a friend's may first discover this route on a neighborhood map, and later fill in what he may perceive as less significant bits of information, such as street names and traffic control systems, as they assume importance to him in actual travel. He does not have to accept the specialist's priorities, as he does with verbal presentation alone. (Specially prepared braille, print, or auditory verbal aids can also facilitate acquisition of information at the student's own pace, but he has less control over the order in which information is presented.)

Both graphic aids and verbal aids can be used repeatedly either to refresh memory or to enable observation of details. Both can help in the discovery of new routes, and enrich total knowledge of an area.

Graphic aids allow the experience of a great variety and number of model problem-solving situations to occur in safety and comfort. For example, an aid depicting a plus intersection is a lesson on analysis of possible veers in street crossings. Many students never experience all possible veers at a plus intersection, but in a single lesson using a graphic aid, they can consider the consequence of all veers and relate all possible reorientation information to each one. Such model problem-solving experiences should be used to complement the actual experiences that each student has while receiving instruction, both to alleviate emotional stress (Fluharty, McHugh, McHugh, Willits, & Wood, 1976) and to offer the broadest possible range of experiences.

TACTILE GRAPHIC AIDS

The *design* of tactile aids is "made difficult by the following paradox. In comparison to that of vision, the perceptual span for touch is extremely limited making the task of reading maps far more difficult and prolonged. Consequently, tactual maps should be as small as possible. In comparison to that for vision, tactual acuity is much more coarse requiring tactual figures to be much larger than visual figures in order to be discriminated. This requires tactual maps to be much larger than visual maps if the same information is to be presented" (Nolan & Morris, 1971, p. 75).

There are some principles and hypotheses that should govern the design of tactile aids. Undocumented suggestions are based on the author's own experience and not on experimental evidence. Areas of tactile aid design to be considered are: information content, scale, size, choice of symbols, information density, labelling and indexing, and provision of supplementary verbal information. Decisions about all of them must be based on the designer's knowledge of what is to be communicated to whom, as well as on what is known about the relationship between each of these areas and the perceptual capacity of the haptic system.

Information Content

The first major problem is to decide what the aid should portray. Information content is dependent on both what one wishes to communicate and to whom.

There are no cardinal rules about what information is necessary. Obviously they will vary with the aid user and the need that the aid is designed to satisfy. Selected information should be that which the user needs in order to function in a particular situation. Landmarks shown should be ones that have an excellent chance of being located. The choice of landmarks will differ, somewhat predictably, depending on whether the aid user travels with a cane, with a dog, or has some vision. Individual differences in detecting landmarks, such as ability to detect a slight slope, can suggest the inclusion of particular kinds of landmarks for each person.

There are two basic rules concerning information content; include only information that is absolutely necessary, and, err on the side of providing too little.

The amount of useable information on a tactile map is less than the total amount which can be haptically recognized (Angwin, 1968). The user may be able to identify all of the symbols on a map, but if much more information is presented than is needed in order for the user to perform the necessary tasks with the map, relevant information and important relationships may be obscured. Information to be included should be selected by personal inspection of the area by someone experienced in selecting those elements of the environment that are of greatest significance for the visually impaired traveler (Wiedel & Groves, 1969). Persons having more experience traveling with the aid of maps are able to use maps with more detail (Wiedel & Groves, 1969). Therefore, maps designed for experienced map users can generally have greater information content than maps designed for persons without experience. Kidwell and Greer (1973) found, in evaluating their highly complex map of the Massachusetts Institute of Technology (Fig. 1-10), containing information represented by 28 different kinds of symbols, that sophisticated users favored the inclusion of too much information rather than too little.

When presenting complex and extensive information to persons with little experience in using tactile orientation aids, it is practical to present the information in a series of maps (Fig. 12-10) having increasing information content, but produced at the same scale (Bentzen, 1972). The first map presented should contain basic information about environmental configurations. Subsequent maps should add details to this base.

The scale at which a particular aid is to be constructed is also based on the designer's knowledge of what the aid is to communicate and to whom.

SCALE

The scale of an aid is an expression of the relationship between the size of features as depicted on a map or model, and the actual size of those features. On a large-scale map, (Fig. 2a-10) for example, a plus intersection occupies more space than the same intersection occupies on a small scale map (Fig 2b-10).

Although visually impaired persons can probably acquire a more accurate cognitive knowledge by use of an aid in which every feature is shown at the same scale, it is fortunately not essential for the scale to be absolutely the same in all parts of a map for it to be useful. Several limitations of the haptic system (Chapter 5) and the haptic abilities of different students make some aids or parts of aids having consistent scale illegible (two lines may be too close together to be

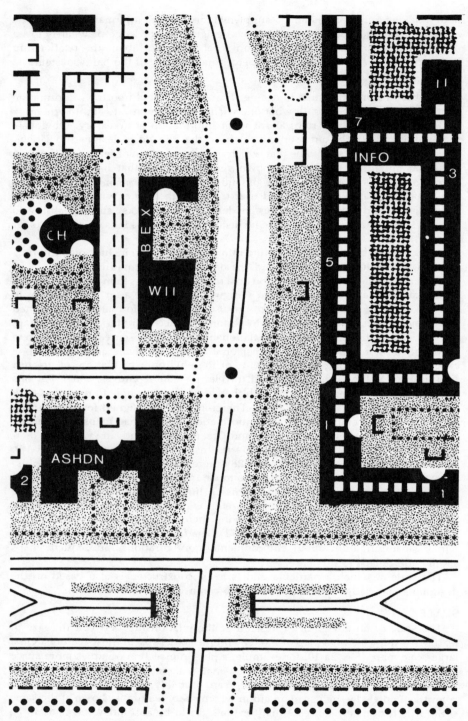

Figure 1-10. Tactile-visual map of MIT campus (actual scale) illustrates information that can be included on a useable map. (Produced by Howe Press, Perkins School for the Blind. Cartography by Kidwell and Greer.)

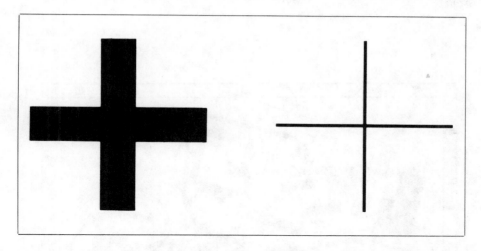

Figure 2a-10. Plus intersection, large scale.   **Figure 2b-10.** Plus intersection, small scale.

perceived as two separate lines). This is especially true for aids having high information content. Some problems are:

1. Fixed dimensions of braille may preclude use where it is needed for labelling

2. There must be some distance between two symbols for them to be recognized as two discrete symbols

3. The optimal width of line symbols for maximum traceability

Fortunately several investigators have demonstrated that absolute consistency in scale is not essential to the usefulness of all maps, notably Armstrong (1973), Bentzen (1972), James (1972), and Kidwell and Greer (1973). Wiedel and Groves (1969b) found that subjects were more confused by large-scale maps having inconsistent scale than by small-scale maps having inconsistent scale. Therefore, large-scale maps should be more consistent in scale than small-scale maps.

In applying the principle of Weber's Law (see Chapter 5, Pick) it appears that features portrayed on a tactile map (or symbols selected to represent those features) must vary from one another in size by 25 percent to 30 percent to be haptically perceived as different by 90 percent of users. Inconsistencies in scale may, therefore, be necessary in order to make differences in sizes of tactile symbols haptically perceptible.

Amendola (1973) contends that schematization is more important than consistency of scale or accuracy of direction. He emphasizes such geometric aspects of environmental configurations as symmetry, oppositeness, parallelism or perpendicularity by purposeful variations in scale. Such schematization probably facilitates the initial cognitive mapping of an area, although it is limited in accuracy. Figure 3a-10 is a map of Brandeis University Campus, which is schematically expressed in Fig. 3b-10.

Graphic Abstraction

James (1972) theorizes that, as the blind traveler judges distance primarily by the time it takes him to complete a journey and by the number of landmarks he contacts, it may be preferable to design route maps with varying scales in which relatively uneventful sections (which may be perceived as shorter by the blind

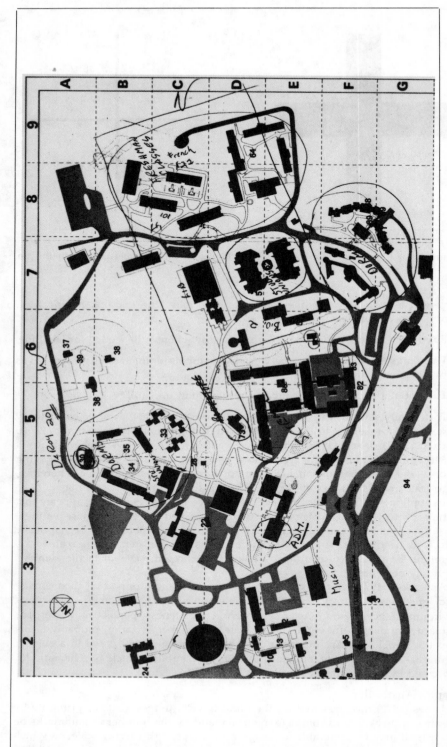

Figure 3a-10. Brandeis University, campus map.

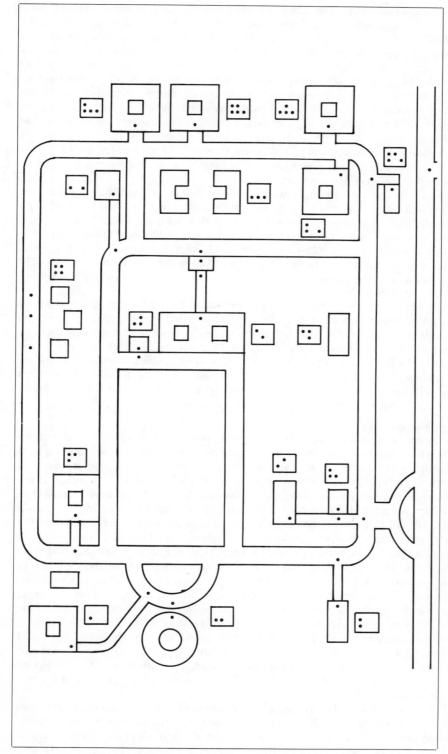

Figure 3b-10. Schematic representation of Fig. 3a-10 by R. Amendola. Original map road width is 0.25 in. (0.6 cm).

traveler) are shown as shorter than sections having many important landmarks.

One determinant of scale is the level of graphic abstraction meaningful to the student. Students whose grasp of environmental concepts is not yet adequate for intelligent travel planning may work best with large-scale aids such as models which have rather literal representations of features of the environment which they are trying to utilize. For example, a student who is having difficulty understanding the predictable useful, relationships between streets, curbs, sidewalks, and inside guidelines, may benefit greatly by a model on which the sidewalks are as wide as his gait (so that with a comfortably based stride he encounters either the inside guideline or the curb with each step), a curb, which in width and height is proportional to the sidewalk, and a street which is also proportional to the sidewalk. The student, by extending his feet and/or cane, can perceive the parallel relationship between each feature shown.

The same student, having grasped these concepts but still having difficulty understanding, for example, that he could travel east or west on the same sidewalk, may then effectively use a much smaller-scale aid (tactile and/or visual map), showing a street, curbs, sidewalks and inside guidelines. On this map, the sidewalk might be 1 in. (2.54 cm) wide, and other features shown in proportional scale. A doll 1½ in. high (3.8 cm), with an easily recognizable front, could be positioned on the sidewalk by the student so that it was, for example, traveling east on the north side of the street.

Another determinant of scale is the tasks that the student is to perform using the aid. In the example above, if the student really needed to move the doll along the sidewalk in order to solve tasks leading to an understanding of possible directions of travel along a sidewalk, the aid would need to be large enough to be proportional to the doll, and large enough so that he could manipulate the doll on it. Students must perform tasks using an aid, in order to learn from it. A consideration of the tasks to be performed with the aid should therefore guide decisions about the design of the aid, such as scale.

Shape Recognition

One of the most difficult haptic tasks to be performed on a tactile map is shape recognition, whether the shape is an enclosed figure such as the outline of a building or the shape of an intersection. Most persons find shapes easier to recognize in relatively small scale than in relatively large scale. Therefore, if the primary purpose of an aid is to demonstrate a shape, it should be no larger than necessary for good discrimination. The small-scale map of a plus intersection in Fig. 2-10 would be more readily recognized as a plus by most users than the larger-scale map would be. Two examples (reproduced here in print) depict the same interconnected building complex on Perkins School campus in actual scale (Fig. 4-10). The small-scale map, which is also simplified by the deletion of information not essential to independent travel, is readily perceived as a variation of a print "U". The large-scale map requires tedious haptic exploration of a larger area than the small scale map, as well as more sophisticated schematization, for the same building to be perceived as "U" shaped. The larger-scale map of the building contained no information about walks leading to entrances or about the location of entrances. The small-scale map as shown in Fig. 5-10, however, contained information about walks and entrances that made it an effective aid for independent route planning (Bentzen, 1972). The smaller scale did not prohibit the inclusion of essential information.

The choice of scale is ultimately dependent on the aforementioned principles and considerations, plus the complex interaction between information content, symbol size, and the limitations imposed by production materials and techniques. The least important considerations should be production materials and

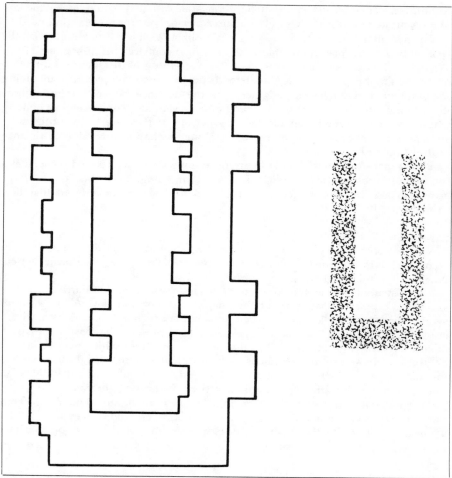

Figure 4-10. Portions of two tactile maps.

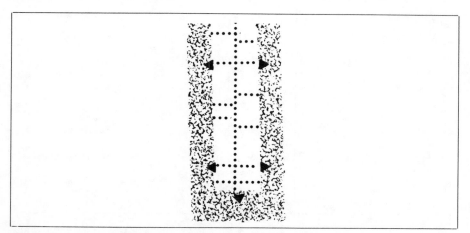

Figure 5-10. Map in Fig. 4-10 showing walks and main entrances.

techniques. They *should not* predetermine scale, as they could make the aid inappropriate both for the visually impaired person and for the learning need.

The overall *size* of a tactile graphic aid is probably best if it is not larger than the span of two hands placed together with the fingers outstretched (Shepherd, 1967; Wiedel & Groves, 1969b; Armstrong, 1973). Perception of distance and direction on tactile graphic aids is little understood, but is a very complex task involving increasingly difficult haptic judgments as the distance between informational items being attended to increases. Therefore, one should err on the side of making maps too small, rather than too large, especially if they are to be utilized by students who have not had experience in making fine haptic judgments of distance or directionality.

Larger maps can undoubtedly be used by some visually impaired persons and for some purposes (Kidwell & Greer, 1973; Armstrong, 1973). Sections of large areas can also be represented on separate sheets which are indexed together. (Armstrong, 1973).

SYMBOLS

The symbols for a particular aid should be those that are discriminable and recognizable to the person who is to use the aid. There are three basic symbol types: point, line, and areal.

Point symbols show the location of a landmark, clue, or particular travel situation, but say nothing about the shape or dimension (Fig. 6-10). A point symbol may show the location of a certain landmark such as a specific pedestrian-crossing light-control, or may be generic and represent the position of each pedestrian-crossing light-control in the area shown. Clues which may be shown are fixed sources of sounds or smells. A travel situation which might be shown is the location of an traffic light at an intersection. The symbol would indicate an intersection with a traffic light not the location of a traffic light pole.

Line symbols convey information that is linear in nature (Fig. 7-10). They indicate both location and direction. They do not necessarily convey information about the width or height of what is represented, although they may be modified to do so, especially in situations where a student's conceptual level requires

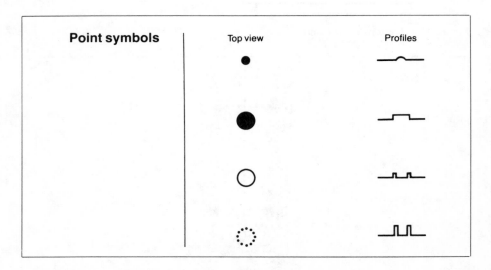

Figure 6-10. Point symbols. (Drawn by S. Emrich.)

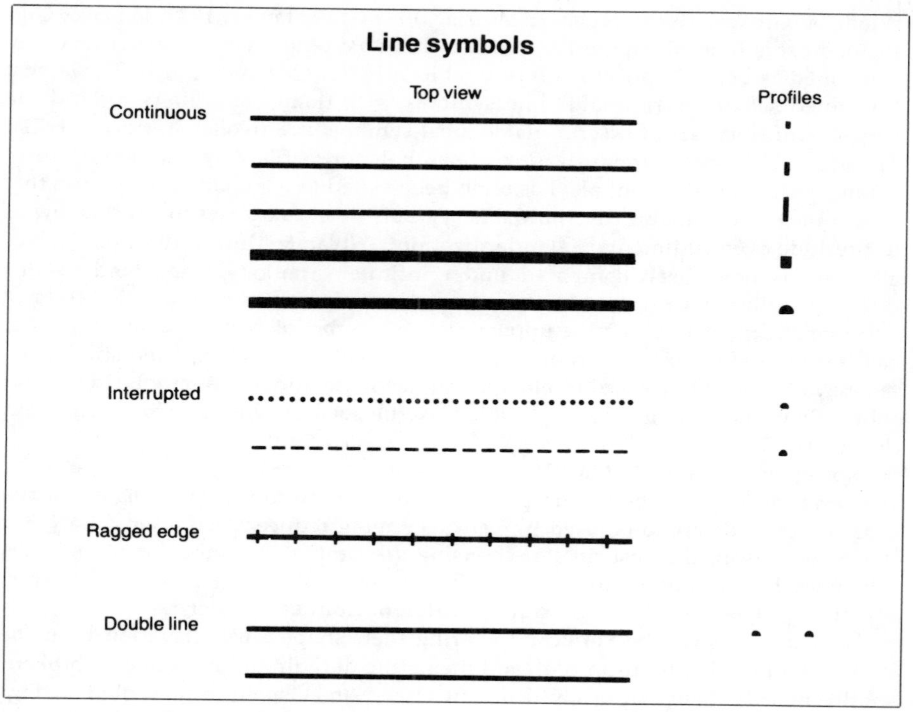

Figure 7-10. Line symbols. (Drawn by S. Emrich.)

somewhat literal representations. A line symbol may represent the location and direction of a specific linear feature such as Pleasant St., or a particular line symbol may be generic and represent the location and direction of each heavily traveled street in the area shown.

Areal symbols convey information about the location of a feature and its shape and size as seen from above (Fig. 8-10). A particular texture may represent the location, shape, and size of one building on a campus; the same texture may be used in different locations, and in varying shapes and sizes, for all buildings on a campus.

Symbols which are to be used together on an aid should differ from each other in as many ways as possible, to be most discriminable (Schiff & Isikow, 1966; Leonard, 1966a; Wiedel & Groves, 1969b; Nolan & Morris, 1971). Choice of symbols which are maximally different from each other requires consideration of the dimensions along which each kind of symbol can be varied. These are discussed on succeeding pages.

Choice of symbols which are easily associated with what they represent will assist aid users in remembering symbol meanings, thus decreasing the need for reference to a key (see Chapter 5, Pick).

Haptic qualities of all three types of symbols produced by different processes and in different materials may be very different, although dimensions and visual characteristics are identical. Therefore, symbols for tactile graphic aids should be chosen by haptic inspection.

For the past two decades, investigators have attempted to identify sets of discriminable symbols of each type (Heath, 1958; Morris, 1961; Schiff, 1966;

Wiedel & Groves, 1969b; Nolan & Morris, 1971; Gill & James, 1973; James & Gill, 1975). At this time, the largest set of discriminable point symbols experimentally confirmed as being haptically discriminable is 13 (Gill & James, 1973). The largest confirmed set of discriminable line symbols is 10 (James & Gill, 1975), and the largest confirmed set of discriminable areal symbols is 8 (Nolan & Morris, 1971). Therefore, although standardization of symbols for tactile maps (assigning fixed meanings for specific symbols) has often been stated as a goal, it now appears that "the number of available discriminable symbols in all categories may be so few as to preclude even rudimentary standardization" (Nolan & Morris, 1971, p. 73). Not all symbols have been compared under infinite variations, and standards for discriminability have been arbitrarily set by investigators, so these figures do not necessarily represent either the upper or lower number of symbols of any type that can be successfully combined on one aid for a particular person. The studies, so far, have been more helpful in elucidating factors to enhance symbol discriminability than in establishing replicable, useful sets of symbols for tactile aid designers.

No research has related tactile sensitivity, per se, especially as it is affected by temperature or peripheral neuropathy, to the recognition of symbols on tactile aids. Where aids are to be used by persons having reduced tactile sensitivity, for whatever reason, the best rule for choosing discriminable symbols is to use ones which are larger, higher, and rougher than those on aids for persons with normal sensitivity. They should be maximally different from each other.

Point symbols can be varied by altering their shape, size, elevation from the background (and/or their profile), and the nature of their outline (smooth, broken, solidly raised). Four haptically different circles are visually represented in Fig. 6-10. If two circles are to be used as point symbols on the same map, they should differ from one another in two or three characteristics. Other point symbols on the map can also differ in shape. Point symbols should fit under the reader's fingertip, but be large enough to be haptically discriminable. Nolan (1971) found that a set of point symbols approximately 0.20 in. (5.1 mm) on each side were more discriminable by blind students than the same symbols reproduced at approximately 0.15 in. (3.8 mm) on each side. Symbols within his sets differed from each other only in shape and/or the nature of their outline. There was no significant grade difference in students' abilities to discriminate symbols at each size. Gill and James (1973) in a test of discriminability of point symbols where all symbols were approximately 0.20 in. (5 mm) in their largest dimension, found that adult braille reading subjects made significantly more errors in point symbol discrimination than subjects who were school children.

In the practical application of this research data, it now seems that if shape and nature of outline are the only variables in point symbol construction, the optimal size may be approximately 0.20 in. (5.1 mm) on each side. However, varying point symbols in size, elevation, and/or profile, as well as in shape and nature of outline may contribute to optimum discriminability of symbols on any one aid.

Line symbols can be varied by making them continuous or interrupted, thick or thin, smooth edge or ragged edge, and single or double (multiple). Height and profile of lines can also be varied. (See Fig. 6-10.) In choosing line symbols, it is important to consider the tasks for which they will primarily be used, as well as their discriminability. For example, the line symbol which will be used for the greatest number of tracing tasks on an aid should be the one having the best traceability. Unfortunately, little research has been conducted to date to indicate which lines are optimal for such tasks as recognizing the presence or shapes of intersections, curves, or angles, which are often the primary tasks on orientation aids.

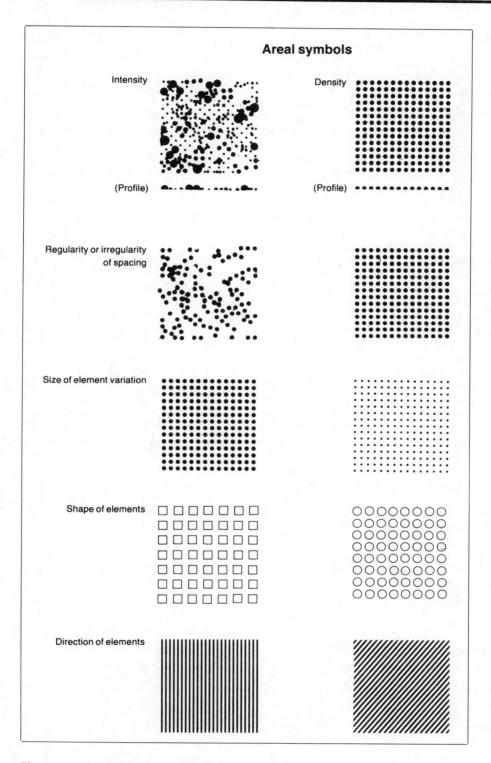

Figure 8-10. Areal symbols. (Drawn by S. Emrich.)

Line Characteristics

Characteristics of lines which contribute to traceability have been the subject of several studies by different investigators, who came to somewhat different conclusions. Broken lines are thought to be easier to trace than smooth lines (Angwin, 1968; Leonard, 1966a; Wiedel & Groves, 1969b), perhaps the best being a line with approximately 20 raised-dots-per-inch.

Amendola (1973) contends that any line symbol should be a track or furrow in which there are two parallel lines or edges. This, he suggests, holds the finger better than any single-line symbol, thus increasing speed and accuracy in tracing. For optimal traceability according to Amendola, the two lines or edges should be 0.20 to 0.25 in. (5.1 to 6.35 mm) apart. The two lines can have various other characteristics, as long as the spacing is correct. Gill, however, (1973) timed 15 subjects on a tracing task on two maps which varied only in that one represented roads with a smooth single line and the other represented roads with a smooth double line 0.16 in. (4.0 mm) between lines. He found that the mean tracing time for the single-line map was shorter than for the double-line map. Because the spacing between Gill's double lines was other than that advocated by Amendola, his findings do not necessarily contradict those of Amendola. Nolan (1971) found that raised lines 0.125 in. wide (3.175 mm) produced better results than incised lines (or tracks) of the same width in a task involving tracing.

In a related study Berlá and Butterfield (1977) compared speed of performance on tasks involving recognition of closed but adjacent shapes (states) by tracing their outlines, which were produced as smooth thin raised lines 0.048 in. (0.12 cm), smooth broad raised lines 0.254 in. (0.635 cm) and smooth broad incised lines 0.254 in. (0.635 cm). Speed and accuracy were not significantly different between subjects using the thin raised-line map and subjects using the incised-line map. Mean scores for subjects using the wide raised-line map indicated greater speed and accuracy with this design. The authors interpret the results as indicating that subjects tracing thin raised lines, as well as those tracing broad incised lines are more likely to be confused by the intersection of other lines than those tracing broad raised lines, because a finger tracing one edge of a broad raised line outlining a shape will not encounter intersections. While this appears to be true, and indicates that boundaries on political maps should probably be broad raised lines, they should probably be avoided on orientation aids in which recognition of a pattern formed by intersecting lines is frequently more important than shape recognition.

Research is currently being conducted by the author, with the assistance of Boston College peripatology students, to find out which of these lines currently favored by other investigators are best for various tasks involved in reading a tactile orientation aid.

Optimal Tracing Qualities

An initial experiment was designed to further knowledge about optimal line qualities for line tracing. Test materials were prepared using the Tactile Tracing Kit. The lines used were:

1. A double smooth line (track) have 0.25 in.(6.35 mm) between lines

2. A double rough line (track) having 0.25 in. (6.35 mm) between lines and consisting of 20 dots-per-inch

3. A single smooth line identical to one half of the double smooth line

4. A single rough line identical to one half of the double rough line.

On a task involving tracing the lines through comparable series of angles and curves, both single lines were traced significantly faster and with fewer behaviors (finger movements other than those involved in a continuous forward tracing of the line from one end to the other) than both double lines (tracks). There was no significant difference in time or number of behaviors between single rough and single smooth lines or between double rough and double smooth lines. Thus, if an aid is designed with one line and no intersections, either a single rough or single smooth line is preferable to a double line. Most aids, however, are not so simple.

When similar lines were placed in a pseudomap where each line intersected each other line, tracing took significantly longer and there were significantly more behaviors for all line types. A common occurrence was for subjects encountering an intersection of the single line with a double line, to interpret the first encountered side of the double line as the continuation, in a new direction, of the line they were tracing. In numerous instances, subjects "lost" the line they were tracing and had to have help to complete the task. This occurred more frequently when subjects were attempting to trace single lines than when attempting to trace double lines.

The apparent inconsistency in these results could be predicted if the double lines act, not as better finger guides than single lines (as argued by Amendola), but if their helpful function is to present redundant information. That is, double lines are traced more slowly because there is more information for the perceiver to attend. This additional information helps to improve accuracy when the tracing task includes intersections of lines which differ from one other. From this limited study it appears that aid designs in which single lines intersect double lines should be avoided.

Continuing research will attempt to discover which lines are most effective in communicating information such as the shape of an intersection or the extent and direction of curvature of a street, and which lines convey the most memorable image. It has been assumed that whatever lines are most discriminable and most easily traced will also produce the most memorable images and will function best to convey information about shape and directionality. There has been no research to support this assumption. It seems axiomatic that a line must be traced before it can communicate anything, but lines which do not communicate well may not be worth tracing.

There are factors other than traceability which should be considered in choosing between single- and double-line symbols. Double lines may be preferred because a student is on an elementary conceptual level and needs somewhat literal representations of the environment, or because they are more suggestive of linear features such as roads, which have two sides (Gill, 1973a). Double lines also enable the portrayal of more detailed information, such as the shapes of curbs or islands. It should be kept in mind, however, that where width between double lines representing roads is varied to represent varied road widths, the traceability of the line symbol will vary, and a change in width between the two lines may cause the line to be perceived and interpreted as an entirely different symbol.

Single lines occupy less space, thereby making possible the reduction of overall size, scale, and information density on aids which otherwise might be too cluttered, or too large in size or scale.

There are several guidelines to aid in selection of discriminable line symbols. Primarily, differences in line construction should be maximized, as was true for point symbols. Lines that will be used in short spaces should consist of small elements (dots, dashes, etc.) closely spaced, as discriminability of a broken line is related to the number of symbol elements that are present in the length of line actually displayed. Minimum discriminable line lengths may be 0.5 in. to 1.0 in. (12.7 mm to 25.4 mm), depending on the pattern of the symbol (Nolan & Morris,

1971). The spacing between dots in a line distinguishes one dotted line from another, but the spacing between dashes in a line is not a distinguishing characteristic (James & Gill, 1975).

Structure

Where line symbols are to cross one another, they are thought to be best recognized if they are very different in structure, and one of the lines is broken at the intersection (Schiff & Levi, 1966).

Areal symbols may be used to differentiate adjacent areas on a map so that the user does not have to trace an outline to determine whether he is "in" or "out of" a particular area. Areal symbols may differ from each other in density of texture elements (spacing between), intensity or sharpness (rough vs. smooth) of the haptic sensation produced, regularity of element spacing, size of elements, shape of elements, direction of elements, and relative height in relation to surrounding areas (Fig. 8-10).

Differences in intensity make symbols highly discriminable (Levi & Schiff, 1966), and are easily achieved in some techniques by the use of different grades of sandpaper combined with many of the materials suggested below. Four different grades of standard sandpaper reproduced in vacuum-formed plastic can be readily discriminated in areas 0.75 in. (19.05 mm) square (Levi & Schiff, 1966), and sandpaper copied by this process is more pleasant to touch than sandpaper itself.

Variations in density of texture elements have greater distinguishing characteristics than differences in the shape or orientation of the elements (Levi & Schiff, 1966). Differences in size of elements can be distinguishing characteristics (Nolan & Morris, 1971).

Large-scale areal symbols (those with large elements or large spaces between elements) cannot be recognized in sizes as small as small-scale areal symbols (Levi & Schiff, 1966; Morris & Nolan, 1963). One of the problems in research to find discriminable symbols is that a majority of symbols tested were of relatively large scale. Even though a specific large-scale symbol may be highly discriminable, it may be nearly unusable because the greater need is for a variety of areal symbols which are discriminable in very small sizes.

Overuse of areal symbols may obscure more relevant information on a tactile graphic aid. Use of areal symbols where not absolutely necessary may create "tactile noise" (Berlá & Murr, 1975), that can result in decreased speed and accuracy in such tasks as locating point symbols or tracing lines. Textures should, therefore, be avoided on areas where line or point symbols are needed to represent significant information or on aids where line tracing is the major component of tasks to be performed with the aid.

Differences in *elevation* within and between symbol types are known to enhance symbol legibility for various tasks (Schiff & Isikow, 1966; Wiedel & Groves, 1969b; Nolan & Morris, 1971; Gill, 1973a). Wiedel and Groves specifically suggested producing braille at a height of 0.02 in. (0.51 mm), line and areal symbols at a height of 0.04 in. (1.02 mm), point symbols at 0.06 in. (1.52 mm). Nolan and Morris have done the most elaborate research on the effects of differences in elevation on location of point, line, and areal symbols, and on speed of tracing line symbols (Nolan & Morris, 1971). They found that performance of 126 blind school children on pseudomaps having areal symbols elevated 0.015 in. (0.38 mm), line symbols elevated 0.025 in. (0.635 mm), and point symbols elevated 0.035 in. (0.89 mm), was better for location of point symbols and tracing of a line symbol than pseudomaps having all symbols of equal heights or of two different heights above the surface. Gill (1973) had 15 blind adults rate maps produced with point and line symbols at various elevations, on comfort, distinctness, and ease of scanning. Mean scores of his subjects for all three criteria indicated a preference for line symbols elevated 0.032 in. (0.85 mm), combined with point symbols at a height of 0.05 in. (1.24 mm). (Although these symbols were higher than those of Nolan and Morris, they were not the highest in Gill's test materials; comfort, distinctness, and ease of scanning declined for higher symbols.) No systematic study has yet been done on the effects of variation in elevation within symbol type, on aids having more than one symbol type, although Schiff and Isikow (1966) demonstrated that accuracy of identification of areal symbols was enhanced by variation in elevation as well as intensity, where the aid consisted entirely of areal symbols. All of this research indicates that the height of symbols should be varied between and/or within symbol types to enhance discriminability on tactile graphic aids.

Two specific symbol uses have been the subject of much practical development and some controlled experimentation. These are symbols for steps and for direction. The most important information to be conveyed about steps is the direction in which they go in relation to one's direction of approach, and whether they go up or down. Wiedel and Groves (1969b) developed a symbol for steps (Fig. 9-10) which indicated both the orientation of steps and whether they went up or down from the present level, on a map in which the direction of approach was apparent, as in approaching a building. In this instance the bar indicates the top of steps. The symbol needed modification before it could be used where the direction of approach was uncertain, such as in the midst of a shopping mall or subway station. James and Gill (1974) modified Wiedel's symbol by changing its profile (Fig. 10-10), so that it was useable in any context. This step symbol scored better than any other symbol in their study of learning and retention of symbol interpretations.

Polarcentric concepts need to be conveyed in a variety of contexts on graphic orientation aids. The use of a compass rose in tactile form is not effective. Wiedel and Groves (1969b) recommended marking the entire north edge of a map with a distinctive line. James (1975) included a line suggested for this use in the Kit of Map Making Parts. Sometimes it is desirable to indicate one-way linear direction, such as direction of traffic flow or direction of slope. Schiff (1965) designed a tactile line symbol (Fig. 11-10) that is relatively smooth when traced in one direction and relatively rough when traced in the opposite direction. It can indicate the direction of traffic flow, the direction one should travel, or a gradient. Such a line, having a

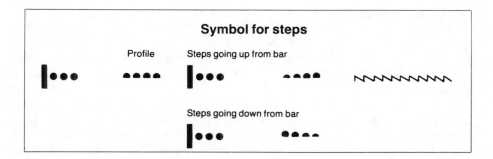

Symbol for steps

Profile   Steps going up from bar

Steps going down from bar

Figure 9-10. Symbol for steps. (Weidel & Groves, 1969b.)

Figure 10-10. Symbol for steps where bar indicates the direction from which the steps are approached. (James & Gill, 1969b.)

Figure 11-10. A directional line. (Shiff, 1965.)

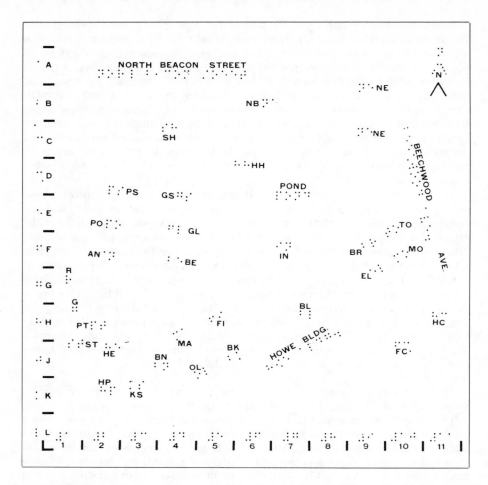

Figure 12a-10. Labels and marginal grid, campus map of Perkins School for the Blind. (Drawn by R. Cruedale.)

saw-toothed profile necessary to convey direction along its entire length, is difficult to produce in most materials. Schiff used a specially produced wheel (produced by Howe Press) for embossing into foil masters. Excellent saw-toothed directional lines can be produced by the computer aided design and production system developed by Gill (1973a; 1973b; 1974).

Symbol Density

Information density for a particular aid should be determined by consideration of several factors. The user's haptic acuity and haptic perceptual ability should be considered. A person whose haptic acuity is reduced by environmental (cold) or physical (peripheral neuropathy; calluses) conditions, will be best able to use an aid having maximum spacing between all symbols. A person whose haptic perceptual ability is limited (one who has difficulty haptically isolating figure from ground) needs aids with minimal information density.

Symbols placed closer together than 0.125 in. (3.175 mm) tend to be perceived as parts of each other rather than as separate symbols. It is therefore recommended that no two symbols be placed closer together than 0.125 in. (3.175 mm). Nolan and

Morris (1971), in a controlled experiment with 126 blind school children who performed a point-symbol location task on pseudomaps having minimum symbol separation of either 0.09 in. (2.29 mm) or 0.15 in. (3.8 mm), found "the wider spacing resulted in significantly more subjects locating all the points."

Information density will be influenced by other design factors such as information content, scale, size, symbols, and construction materials. There are some techniques for reducing information density, which may be appropriate for specific situations:

1. Use the smallest discriminable symbols

2. Use single line symbols rather than double lines or tracks

3. Increase the scale, which will also increase the size unless information is deleted

4. Delete unnecessary information, such as borders around maps

5. Place keys on a separate page

6. Place some information on an overlay or underlay.

Overlays

An overlay for a tactile graphic aid consists of two pages attached at the top which are carefully aligned so that information on the overlay is directly over related information on the aid itself. The reader places one hand on the overlay and the other hand on the page below to read related information. An underlay is made

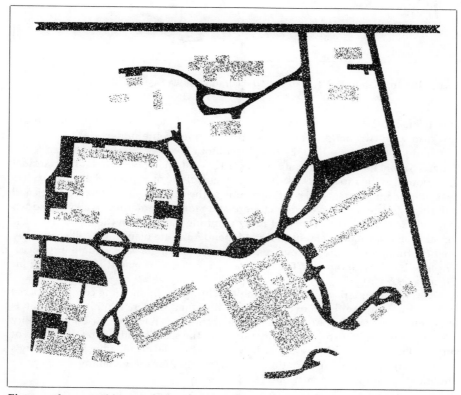

Figure 12b-10. Building and paved areas (driveways and parking lots). (Drawn by R. Cruedale.)

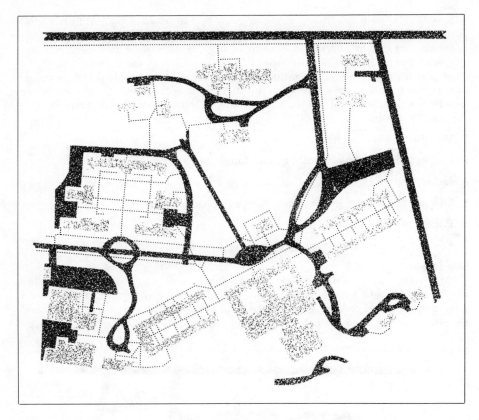

Figure 12c-10. Map in Fig. 12b-10 with the addition of walks. (Drawn by R. Cruedale.)

with related information shown on the under side of the same sheet. Underlays are also read with two hands, one on the top and one on the underside.

The line drawings in Fig. 12-10 represent four levels or overlays of a map of the Perkins School for the Blind campus. Level 12*a* contains braille labels and marginal grid, bound at the top so it can be used over any of the map pages. Level 12*b* shows basic dominant features and configurations of the campus such as paved areas and buildings. Subsequent levels depict more and more information. Walks are added to Level 12*c* to teach the process of route planning based upon the map. Level 12*d* contains all information essential for independent route planning to all commonly used destinations on the campus: paved areas, buildings, walks, main entrances, fences or barriers, and pond. The original tactile maps measured 11 in. by 11½ in. (28 cm x 29.5 cm).

Overlays or underlays are also suitable techniques for showing complex spatial interrelationships without overwhelming information density in a way that is comprehensible for the blind reader. These techniques have been used in mobility maps to show relationship of different floors of the same building; relationships of subway lower level, subway upper level, and street level; relationship of a city's streets to its public transportation system. Suggestions for making overlays or underlays are found in Armstrong (1973).

Braille Labels

Adding *labels* to tactile aids often increases the problems of information density, scale, and choice of symbol size. Braille labels are most legible if they are horizontal, although many aid users can read labels placed in other directions. Where labels are to be abbreviated, abbreviations should consist of a minimum of two braille cells, and they should be mnemonic, for example, "ps" for Potter Schoolhouse on the map in Fig. 12a-10. Labels reduce the need for reference to an index. On any one aid, each label should consistently be placed in a position relative to its subject.

A solution to clutter or added density by the use of braille labels is to put them on an overlay (Angwin, 1968; Wiedel & Groves, 1969b) or underlay (Kidwell & Greer, 1973). The author recommends the use of underlay labels with conceptually sophisticated users only, because a mirror-image cognitive map may be developed by a student who becomes familiar with the aid by studying it with the label side facing up, towards him. This is a great temptation for persons who are more accustomed to reading braille than to learning from tactile graphics.

Tactile grid

On a map of an extended area, it is often desirable to have a tactile grid to facilitate locating specific points given in a verbal index. This system is used on print maps with indexes. Lines run at regular intervals from side to side and from top to bottom on the map to form grids that are either numbered or lettered in sequence in the margins. A destination listed in the index can be located on the map in the rectangle formed by the intersection of the space labelled E and the

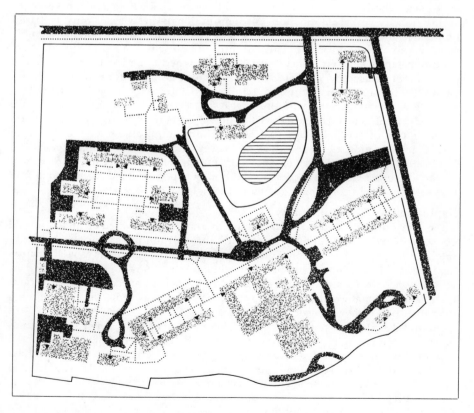

Figure 12d-10. Paved areas, buildings, walks, main entrances (arrows), fences, barriers (solid line), and pond. (Drawn by R. Cruedale.)

space labelled 6. Haptic scanning (or scanning with low vision) is much more time consuming than visual scanning with unimpaired vision. Therefore, it is important to provide what assistance is possible to help a visually impaired user to narrow the field that must be searched to find a destination on a map. A tactile grid can be provided along the margins of an aid only, or a complete raised grid can be provided on an overlay or underlay (Armstrong, 1973). (See Fig. 12a-10.)

If a tactile graphic aid is needed for independent travel in a unfamiliar area, verbal (auditory, braille, or print) information can be provided along with the tactile map (Bentzen, 1972; Kidwell & Greer, 1973).

VISUAL GRAPHIC AIDS

Little research has been done on the design of graphic orientation aids for low vision persons. Therefore, it is not possible to be as exact in specifying design criteria for visual graphic aids as for tactile graphic aids. One reason for lack of research is that many low vision persons use the same techniques and low vision aids that enable them to read regular print, to use graphic aids prepared for fully sighted persons. Another reason is related to the wide variability of visual conditions and visual efficiency among low vision persons. Actual or statistical experimental control of these crucial variables with large enough populations of low vision persons to make results significant is difficult.

The issues in designing graphic aids for low vision persons are similar to those which must be resolved in designing tactile graphic aids: information content, scale, size, choice of symbols, information density, labelling, and provision of supplementary verbal information. Also, resolution of these issues must be based on the designer's knowledge of what is to be communicated to whom, and on his specific knowledge of each student's abilities. Because of the variability of visual conditions and visual efficiency, visual aids designed to be ideal for one student often cannot be used by other students. Tactile aids designed for persons with less variability in haptic sensitivity may be useful to a greater number of students.

All low vision persons who are *unable to use regular print graphic aids* have reduced visual acuity, impaired visual fields, or both. The two most common visual effects of eye pathology that have definite implications for the design of visual graphic aids are reduced visual acuity and impaired visual fields. The implications mentioned here, except where noted, are based on conjecture formed by the author's practical experience, and not on experimental data. Research into these issues would contribute greatly to the field.

Implications of Reduced Acuity

For persons with reduced visual acuity, information presented on an aid should be large and/or have high contrast with the surroundings, and perhaps the information should be presented through other perceptual systems as well, such as haptic or auditory. Figure-ground discrimination problems are often concomitant with low acuity, so aids should not be cluttered with unnecessary information. Experienced visual graphic aid users can probably utilize more information on a map than inexperienced users.

Reduced acuity will probably not be a determinant of scale, per se, but symbols must be large enough and far enough apart to be perceived. Shapes and spatial relationships may be more discriminable to persons having reduced acuity if they are depicted in larger scale than must be used on aids for persons having normal acuity. Use of larger symbols widely spaced may necessitate increased size. It may then be preferable to make several large-scale but small-size maps if information content is high. Informal experimentation with this concept by the author and Boston College peripatology students seemed to suggest that the optimal size for low vision maps was between 6 in. and 12 in. (15 and 30 cm) square.

Implications of Visual Graphic Symbols

In general, visual graphic symbols for low acuity should be larger than those for normal acuity. The same possibilities exist for varying visual symbols as for varying tactile symbols, with the following exceptions. Height off base and varied profile are not possible with visual symbols but color is an excellent means of making symbols different. Combining symbols on the same aid which differ from each other in as many ways as possible is probably the best means to assure discriminability in low acuity. Symbols that have some visual resemblance to what they represent or which are already familiar to a user in other ways have better association than abstract shapes frequently used in tactile aids. A visual symbol which looks somewhat like steps, or the print letter S, may be better symbols for stairs than the solid dot tactile stairs' symbol in Fig. 9-10.

Letters and numerals are more versatile symbols on print graphic aids because print which is less than 24-point type occupies less space than comparable braille letters and numerals. In addition, single print letters and numerals can be read without some of the confusion and ambiguity which may arise from the use of single cell braille characters. The 26 letters of the alphabet, both capital and lower case, plus numerals one through nine, provide 61 symbols discriminable to most low vision readers, when reproduced in a space less than that occupied by one braille cell.

Type Size

Aids prepared for an individual user should, of course, be labeled with the print size, boldness, and style best for him. There is some evidence that 18-point type may be legible for more low vision children than larger or smaller sizes (Nolan, 1959). Therefore, on aids for an unknown population of low vision children, 18-point type may be optimal. Somewhat larger type may be appropriate for adults who no longer have the powers of accommodation to achieve adequate enlargement by bringing print very close to their eyes. Enlargement much beyond the size necessary for the type to be seen is unlikely to increase legibility for continuous reading, but it may make labels consisting of small groups of letters easier to locate. Increasing the boldness of type improves legibility for most partially sighted readers (Shaw, 1969).

Type Face

Type style (face) probably effects legibility, but the evidence is inconclusive. Nolan (1959) found a serif face slightly more legible than sans serif, but Shaw's (1969) results are in conflict. (A serif is the terminal stroke finishing off certain main strokes of a type face.)

In regard to information density, a minimum spacing of 0.125 in. (3.175 mm) between adjacent symbols is acceptable to most low vision persons. A practical means to reduce density is to place different types of information on different overlays. Placing labels and a grid reference system on an overlay enables the low vision person to attend to the print only, to scan for a particular label, and to attend only to graphic display when he does not need the identification provided by labels. Increasing the space between the letters and words, between words only, or between lines only, does not appear to increase legibility (Shaw, 1969).

IMPLICATIONS OF VISUAL FIELD LOSS

Persons who have a reduced peripheral field but who have normal acuity in their remaining central field may be able to use regular print graphic aids. However, there are some problems. The information portrayed may not be that information in the environment which is the most visible or useful to the person. For example, it may be more helpful in some situations for him to know the color of the largest building at each intersection than to know the name of each street.

Grid Reference

It may be very difficult for someone with peripheral field loss to locate desired information on a map, especially a large one. Most commercially available print maps have a grid reference system to help users locate specific features. In reduced peripheral field, the use of a grid reference can eliminate the need for much tedious scanning. Difficulty in scanning visually across grid lines can be alleviated by visually locating the letter and the numeral in the margins, placing an index finger on each, then moving each finger either horizontally or vertically on the map until their paths intercept near the location of the desired feature.

Even those who can use regular print maps may sometimes prefer maps having only that information appropriate to their needs, that have symbols or labels slightly larger than necessary for legibility, for ease in location and compact size.

Scale

The scale for persons with impaired fields should be small enough so that the user does not have to scan the aid unnecessarily in order to recognize shapes and relationships. Shapes are probably recognized most efficiently if they are small enough to require a minimum number of fixations.

Size

The optimal size of a visual graphic aid for a person having impaired fields should be relatively small, probably between 6 and 12 in. (15 and 30 cm) so the user will not have to attend to a large stimulus field. Tasks which require visual tracking and integration are more difficult if the stimuli are spread over a large field than a small field.

Density

Aids with high information density may not prove to be difficult for persons with reduced peripheral fields to use, as they will be more efficient in relating symbols to each other when the need for scanning and tracking is minimized because the symbols are close together. They should be encouraged to hold the aid as far as possible from the eyes when performing tracking and integration tasks, for effective reduction of the percentage of the visual field occupied by the stimulus.

Recognition of symbols larger than necessary may require more scanning than recognition of smaller symbols, so very large visual symbols should be avoided on aids for people with field defect.

Supplementary verbal information about landmarks, structural details, suggested routes, cultural and historical features, and other may be produced in whatever reading medium is best for a particular client, and may substantially increase the usefulness as well as enjoyment of the aid.

Color Coding

Color is an important means for symbol coding on visual graphic aids, and probably makes the number of visual graphic symbols discriminable to low vision persons greater than the number of tactile graphic symbols discriminable to blind persons. There have not been specific studies on best use of colors on low vision graphics but one investigation (Greenberg & Sherman, 1970) has indicated that white lines on a black background are more legible to low vision persons than black lines on a white background.

The most common form of color-deficient vision is red-green color blindness (Vaughan, Asbury, & Cook, 1971). To minimize the possibility that symbol identification would be made difficult by color-deficient vision these colors should not be combined on the same aid.

Dependence on color as the distinguishing feature of symbols on maps to be used by persons with a central scotoma should be avoided as they have impaired color vision.

Glare can be minimized on graphic aids for low vision persons by the use of matte-finish materials and inks.

Some people have reduced acuity as well as field defects. Some implications of reduced acuity in design of graphic aids are in the direction of increasing size or scale of information on aids, while field defects necessitate aids with relatively small symbols, size, and scale. In designing aids for persons who have both problems the mobility specialists should start with relatively small symbols, small scale, and small size. If the user has difficulty, the specialist might first make the symbols more bold, then increase the distance between the symbols, and last of all, make the symbols and the aid larger in size and scale.

GRAPHIC TACTILE-VISUAL AIDS

It has been suggested during the past decade (Sherman, 1965; Angwin, 1968; Wiedel & Groves, 1969b) that graphic aids for visually impaired persons should have both tactile and visual information coding systems. The following arguments have been used:

1. Inclusion of print on tactile graphic aids facilitates assistance by a sighted person

2. Tactile-visual graphic aids used by both blind and low vision persons make a more economically viable market for commercially produced aids

3. For commercial production of graphic aids for low vision persons, the ideal would be production of each aid in a variety of sizes, scales, and symbols so that each person could make maximum use of visual abilities. This is not a feasible production system. However, production of tactile-visual graphic aids will enable users who cannot see all of the information presented visually to acquire the same information presented haptically. Therefore, one tactile-graphic aid design will serve a more varied group of low vision persons than any visual graphic aid.

Low vision persons who have access to aids which are both raised and printed have been found to use aspects of both coding systems according to their visual and haptic abilities (Bentzen, 1977). Those who have low acuity but full visual fields may, for example, choose to scan the aid visually first to get an overall impression of the structure and information content, and then confirm their observations or read detailed information haptically. Conversely, persons who have reduced peripheral field but good acuity may choose to scan the aid to obtain an overall impression haptically, and then seek detail visually.

There appears to be enough similarity in criteria for tactile graphic aids for blind persons and visual graphic aids for low vision persons to make the design of tactile-visual graphic aids possible. Optimum information content, scale, size, symbols, information density, labelling, and provision of supplementary verbal information appear to be affected by many of the same variables, with similar decisions resulting from considerations of these variables. It is also technologically feasible by both hand and commercial means to make aids having tactile and visual coding systems. Indeed, it is commonplace to see geographic, especially topographic relief, maps for sighted users which are raised as well as printed.

For those reasons, all commercially produced graphic aids for visually impaired persons should be *tactile-visual aids*. Teacher-produced aids should also be tactile-visual to have the greatest possible usefulness.

A good subject for study would be the determination of the relative ease of reading by low vision subjects of tactile-visual graphic aids in which:

1. Visual information is presented on the same page as tactile information

2. Visual information is presented on an overlay, over tactile information

3. Tactile information is presented as an underlay, on the back side of a page having visual information

4. Visual and tactile information are presented side by side (on two pages).

MATERIALS AND PRODUCTION TECHNIQUES

Materials and techniques for the production of tactile or tactile-visual graphic aids should be selected on the basis of certain criteria. There follows a description of materials and techniques, their sources, and particular advantages and disadvantages. Selection of appropriate materials and techniques should be considered in light of the following factors:

1. The perceptual and learning characteristics of the student who is to use the aid

2. The particular learning situation that the aid will facilitate

3. The design criteria most appropriate for the student and the learning situation. Particular materials solely for the production of visual graphic aids will not be discussed here. Appropriate pens, inks, and papers are available widely from drafting, and arts and crafts suppliers.

COMMERCIAL TACTILE AND TACTILE-VISUAL AIDS

Chang Tactual Diagram Kit

A black Velcro pile board, 24 in. x 18 in. (61 cm x 46 cm) that can be folded in center to give 12 in. x 18 in. (30.5 cm x 46 cm) work space, 104 yellow, flat geometric forms of 27 different shapes and sizes, backed with Velcro hook; 27 additional Velcro hook strips for making other shapes and materials, two modeled stickmen; instructional guide; carrying case (Fig. 13-10). (Chang & Johnson, 1968.) It can be obtained from the American Printing House for the Blind, price $52.00, with carrying case.*

Advantages. The kit has high visual contrast, it is easy for teacher or student to manipulate, and is pleasant to touch. It is possible to make the streets wide enough to have students "drive" cars on them, and its large size may be an advantage in representation of a large area.

Disadvantages. The large overall size is cumbersome for carrying while on a lesson and it may be difficult for students to integrate parts into whole if they have limited visual field or use tactile input only. Width (scale) of streets can be varied, but blocks are fixed sizes (if used with streets shown wide, streets and blocks will be inconsistent in scale, which may lead to misconceptions). It is limited to two areal symbols. Stick men are much too large to achieve consistent scale. Their height is equal to or greater than length of most "blocks" supplied.

Suggestions for Use. The kit is good for teaching concepts of intersection configuration, for analysis of veers, and for understanding corrections at crossings for students at low conceptual level. The shapes supplied with kit can be cut to different sizes and shapes. To modify kit for more varied symbols, glue line and point symbols onto cardboard "blocks" supplied; glue Velcro hook onto point and line symbols to be placed directly onto Velcro pile; make other sizes, textures, shapes, and colors of blocks out of cardboard with Velcro tabs.

---

*Prices for all aids are as of publication date and may change.

Hook and Loop Board

Black loop, 17 in. x 11 in. (43 cm x 28 cm), plus a quantity of cardboard in assorted colors for teacher construction of symbols. It may be purchased from DeSigns Company, 2473 Fletcher Drive, Los Angeles, CA 90039, for $11.00.

Advantages. The same advantages apply as for the Chang Kit. The small size is portable and easier to scan and trace. It contains materials for teachers to adapt for varied symbols, sizes, and shapes.

Disadvantages. The Hook and Loop Board does not contain ready-made interchangeable parts, and has no carrying case.

Suggestions for Use. The uses are the same as for the Chang Kit.

Mag-Stix

A green, iron-core board, 24 in. x 18 in. (61 cm x 46 cm), with black, fine-line, painted grid. It has brown, magnetic rubber strips: 4 ft (1.2 m) of 1-in. (2.5-cm) wide strip, and 12 ft (3.6 m) of ¼-in. (0.62-cm) wide strip; brown cord—12 ft (3.6 m); yellow sheet—7 in. x 11 in. (18 cm x 28 cm), available from Howe Press for $16.25.

Advantages. Mag-Stix are durable, pleasing to touch, easy for teacher or student to manipulate. It is possible to make streets wide enough for students to "drive" cars on them. The tactile grid may help students to align magnetic strips. Additional rubber strips and other miscellaneous magnetic symbols are available from Howe Press. Other magnetic symbols are available at graphics display outlets.

Disadvantages. The visual and texture contrasts are minimal. The overall size is large. The magnetic symbols can easily be moved accidentally.

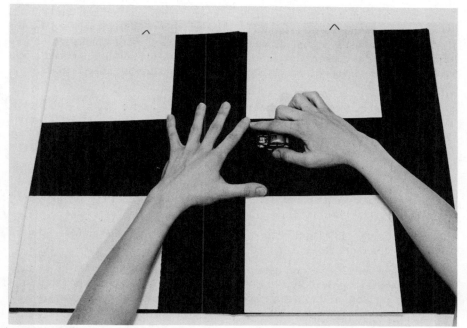

Figure 13-10. Chang Tactual Diagram Kit with student demonstrating possible motions of car at intersection. (Photography by R. Friedman.)

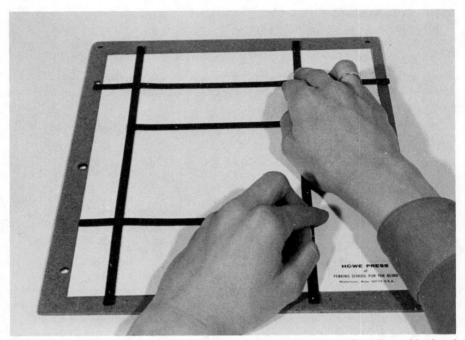

Figure 14-10. JR Mag-Stix with student determining configuration of small neighborhood intersections. (Photography by R. Friedman.)

Suggestions for Use. Mag-Stix are useful for teaching basic positional and directional concepts, concepts of intersection configuration, and neighborhood street patterns. Symbols in varied sizes, shapes, colors, and textures can be made by gluing small pieces of magnetic rubber to other materials selected by the designer. Materials, as supplied, are usually used to represent streets, with raised lines and blocks as background (conceptually opposite to reality), but raised blocks can be made of cardboard, etc., if student has difficulty with raised streets.

JR Mag-Stix

A white, washable, magnetic board 9 in. x 11 in. (23 cm x 28 cm), with brown, magnetic rubber strips—4 ft (1.2 m) of 1-in. (2-5 cm) wide strip, and 8 ft (2.4 m) of ¼-in. (0.6-cm) wide strip; brown cord—6 ft (1.8 m); yellow sheet—5.5 in. x 7 in. (14 cm x 18 cm), (Fig. 14-10). Available from Howe Press, $6.25.

Advantages. JR Mag-Stix have the same advantages as Mag-Stix. The white surface provides good contrast with dark brown rubber. The small size is more portable and easier to scan and trace. A washable felt marker or china marker can be used for visual information.

Disadvantages. JR Mag-Stix are of poorer magnetic quality than Mag-Stix, and their surface is more easily damaged.

Suggestions for Use. Same uses apply as for Mag-Stix. They can be used for visual or tactile graphic aids, and used as holders for Brailon or paper map to be carried on a lesson, and to mark current position with the small magnets.

Raised Line Drawing Kit

A dense rubber board, 8½ in. x 11 in. (22 cm x 28 cm), sold by the American Foundation for the Blind, at $13.95.

10

Raised Line Drawing Board

A board, 11½ in. x 11½ in. (29 cm x 29 cm), with 100 Mylar sheets, ruler and pencil stylus, (Fig. 15-10). Sold by Howe Press, for $16.00.

Advantages.   Can be used to produce upright raised image. The chief difference between the two boards is the way in which the plastic film is attached to the rubber-faced drawing board. The AFB Board holds the film with spring clips on two corners. The film is attached to the Howe Press Board by large knurled washers at four corners. The accessories of the Howe Press model make it a good aid for measuring, and for mathematical drawing. They are portable and relatively easy for teacher or student to manipulate (congenitally blind students, unaccustomed to a pen, may find it difficult to maintain an upright angle of the pen with sufficient pressure to produce lines with good haptic quality). Relatively high information density (much information in a small space) is possible.

Disadvantages.   The boards offer no visual contrast and have high glare (inappropriate for students who have useful near vision). The sheets are easily punctured, detached, or wrinkled. Line symbols can be varied only by having single or multiple lines. It is difficult to produce varied point symbols or labels on them.

Suggestions for Use.   The boards are especially good for graphic communication on a lesson with an adventitiously blind student who is accustomed to drawing, and are particularly useful for familiarization to street patterns (grids and their variations).

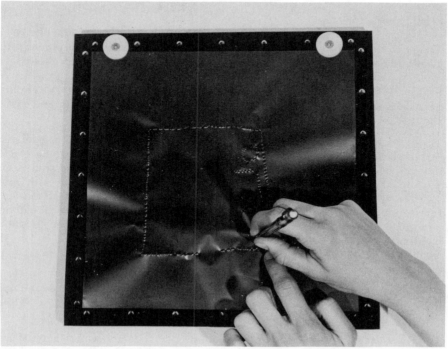

Figure 15-10. Raised Line Drawing Board (Howe Press) with student drawing a conceptualization of a room shape and positions of furniture in room. (Photography by R. Friedman.)

327

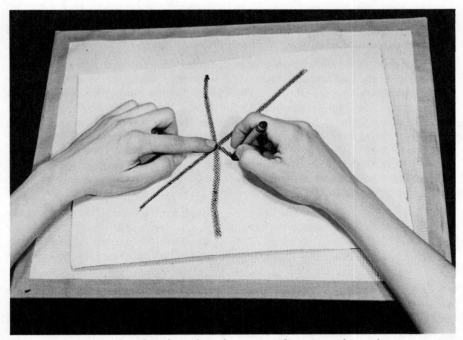

Figure 16-10. Screen board with student drawing configuration of complex intersection. (Photography by R. Friedman.)

Plastic Sheets for Maps

These are colorless, textured, translucent plastic that is adhered to white paper along two sides. A sketch of what is to be produced on teacher-made aid, or print as additional aid for a low vision person, can be inserted between plastic and backing paper. An upright raised image is produced by drawing with pencil or braille stylus. Its source is De Blindas Forenings Forsaljningsaktiebolag, Sandsborgsvagen 50, S-122 33 Enskede, Sweden. 25 Sw. Cr./50 sheets, and cost is about $5.75.

Advantages.　These sheets have a more pleasant "feel" and have less glare than that of plastic supplied with raised line drawing boards, and they need no special drawing board. The braille stylus may be easier for congenitally blind students to learn to draw with than a pen. It is easy to add visual information with good contrast by drawing with a felt pen on the plastic or by inserting a drawing between the plastic and backing. They are stiff enough to be read without additional backing. The map sheets are portable and easy for teacher or student to manipulate. Relatively high information density is possible, and they can be labelled with brailler or slate and stylus. A backing sheet makes the maps more durable than Mylar sheets.

Disadvantages.　Line symbols can·be varied only by using single or multiple lines, and it is difficult to produce point symbols. The haptic quality of lines is only fair.

Suggestions for Use.　The map sheets are used in the same way as a raised line drawing board and are for neighborhood maps in which the street pattern is the primary information content.

Freund Longhand Writing Kit (Screen Board)

The writing kit (Fig. 16-10), is a wire screening mounted on masonite with a newsprint tablet, on which crayon is used to write. The kit is sold by the American Printing House for the Blind for $17.50.

Advantages. These materials are relatively easy for teacher and student to manipulate. The cost per copy is very low. Relatively good visual contrast is possible.

Disadvantages. The overall size is large, and the tactile image is not durable. It rubs out easily, and paper is easily torn. The line symbol is limited to one kind, that is not highly traceable. The point symbol is also limited to one kind of a small, not very distinctive size. The paper cannot be labelled with braille, and small-scale and high-information density is not possible.

Suggestions for Use. This screen board is often helpful for a student who has a good mental image of spatial relationships but who has difficulty verbalizing to an instructor.

Tactile Tracing Kit

This is a set of key-tracing templates for mobility maps containing: 11 point symbols; 6 special-use point symbols with braille labels; 9 basic-line symbols (which can be varied to provide additional symbols); 7 basic-areal symbols; various curves to combine with straight lines; regular and jumbo braille cells for composing labels or textures; embossed print alphabet; two special embossing tools; kneaded rubber eraser; braille stylus; 2 translucent plastic layout grids (based on finger track spacing); 2 translucent plastic layout grids (based on braille spacing); a supply of opaque white and translucent plastic sheets; and instructions for use (Fig. 17-10). Additional components (purchased separately) are a photo-mechanical thermo-master consisting of the same components as in the template, that can be used to compose maps (or master copies for vacuum formed maps) out of raised movable images; backing sheets for use with photo-mechanical thermo-master; and special purpose (non-mobility) templates. The manufacturer is Gilligan Tactiles, Inc., 68 Lindbergh Avenue, West Newton, Massachusetts. The approximate cost is $29.50 for the basic kit.

Advantages. The kit contains a large variety of point, line, and areal symbols, as well as regular and jumbo braille. The small size of individual aids makes them highly portable. The translucent and white plastic provided is tactually pleasing. The kit makes possible the design of aids of relatively small scale, with high-information density. If well designed, individual aids have good haptic properties, and are relatively durable. The template design facilitates production of uniform, highly traceable line symbols. Additional components are available for production of vacuum-form copies of maps that are nearly identical to single-copy maps. The materials are relatively easy for a sighted person to manipulate.

Disadvantages. Visual contrast is not an inherent characteristic of these materials.

Suggestions for Use. This kit is especially suited to produce schematized (simplified) representations of neighborhoods, campuses, or public transportation routes. Visual contrast can be added with a felt tip pen, a pencil or wax pencil on the back or front of the aid, or the tactile aid can be overlaid on (and adhered to) a visual aid.

Kit of Map Making Parts

The kit consists of ten 10½ in. x 10½ in. (27 cm x 27 cm) cellulose sheets backed

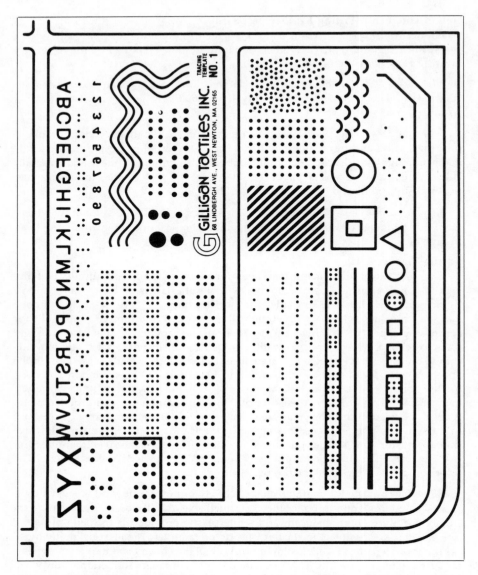

Figure 17-10. Tactile Tracing Kit shown actual size in inset. (Designed by R. Amendola.)

with Twin-stick; 30 sets of plastic point symbols (12 symbols in each set); 6 rolled solder-line symbols, approximately 150 ft (43 m); 4 sheets of areal symbols; ballotine-glass powder to negate sticky surface after all symbols are adhered (Fig. 18a-10). The kit makes masters for vacuum-formed maps (Fig. 18b-10). They are made by Blind Mobility Research Unit, Nottingham, England, and distributed in the United States by Howe Press, at $16.00.

Advantages. The kit parts are suitable for very small-scale, high-information content maps. Individual copies of aids are relatively durable and highly portable. All symbols in the kit can be combined on the same aid, to produce an aid that has

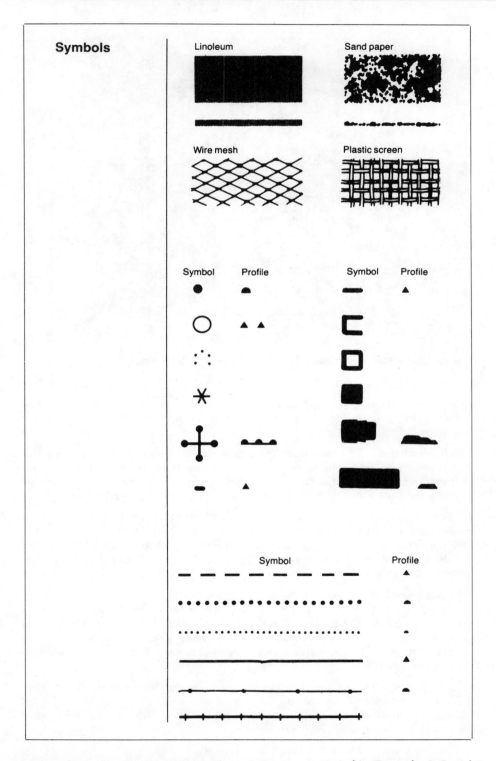

Figure 18a-10. Kit of Map Making Parts, symbols same size as in kit. (Drawn by S. Emrich.)

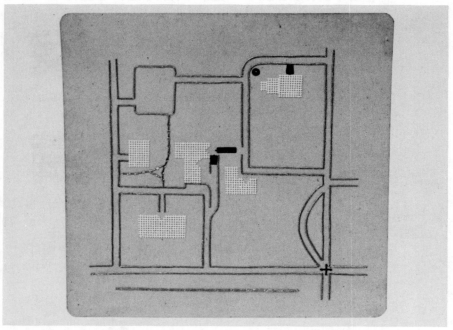

Figure 18b-10. Map master made from kit. (Photography by R. Friedman.)

varied information content. Line and point symbols have been tested for discriminability (James, 1975). The kit produces from 5 to 100 copies relatively inexpensively.

Disadvantages.   The map making parts are suitable only for master copies of vacuum-formed aids. The materials are relatively time consuming to use and difficult to manipulate. It is difficult for visually impaired persons to make or alter masters for aids. For less than five copies of an aid, the cost is relatively high.

Suggestions for Use.   These materials are especially suitable for maps of neighborhoods, business areas, or campuses, where high-information content is desired in an aid of small size, in the range of 5-100 copies. Additional symbols can be incorporated by the designer (see James, 1975, for additional specific suggestions for use).

The Sensory Quill

This is a raised line writing and drawing instrument for producing 11 in. x 11½ in. (28 cm x 29 cm) tactile aids. It is available from Mechstat, Inc., 830 N.E. Loop 410, Suite 210, San Antonio, Texas 78209. The cost of the Personal Model is $295.00. The Institutional Model (which can prepare aluminum masters for vacuum forming) is $745.00.

Advantages.   The Sensory Quill produces upright raised images, and also can be used to produce lines varying in texture and elevation. It is easier for an inexperienced user to produce consistently legible lines with this than with other means of producing upright raised images.

Disadvantages.   The initial investment is expensive. There is no visual contrast. It is a cumbersome but delicate instrument and should be used on a sturdy table.

Suggestions for Use. The instrument can be used for teacher preparation of simple aids for use in lessons, and for student graphic feedback to the instructor. Visually impaired persons can make their own individual maps of routes or areas with which they have become familiar.

Multiple copies of aids made with several of the foregoing sets of materials can be produced by vacuum forming. Many schools and agencies have a vacuum-forming machine (such as Thermoform), used primarily for reproduction of braille reading materials in a textured, cream-colored plastic (Brailon), available in two weights. Although less expensive plastics can be used in this machine (Gill, 1973a), heavy Brailon (about fifteen cents a sheet) produces some of the best results for pleasing texture, good symbol definition, and durability for outdoor use. Materials that can be used for master copies of Thermoformed maps are: Hook and Loop Board, JR Mag-Stix, Portable Mobility Kit, Tactile Tracing Templates Kit, and Kit of Map Making Parts (Table 5-10). All Brailon aids can be given visual contrast by coloring on the symbols with a felt pen after vacuum forming, or by silk-screening or offset printing before vacuum forming (Gill, 1973a). Size of individual aids is limited to 11 in. by 11.5 in. (27.9 cm by 29.2 cm) unless separate sheets can be combined to make larger aids. The map in Fig. 19-10 was produced by B. Bentzen and Boston College peripatology students using the Kit of Map Making Parts. Copies were first offset printed in black ink on Brailon and then thermoformed. The illustration is reduced for publication.

Many commonly available materials can be used to produce either single-use aids, repeated-use aids, or masters for vacuum-copied tactile or tactile-visual aids. There are two primary techniques that are used with a variety of materials. In one,

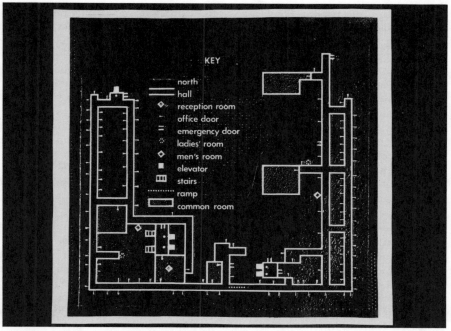

Figure 19-10. Master for floorplan of Massachusetts Commission for the Blind headquarters, produced using Kit of Map Making Parts. (Designed by B. Bentzen and Boston College peripatology students.)

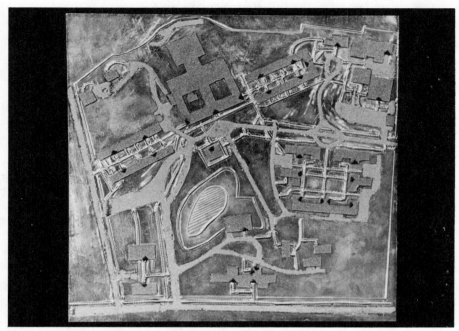

Figure 20-10. Master of map in Fig. 12d-10 (By B. Bentzen.)

raised images are produced by debossing symbols using various tools. In the other, raised images are produced by adhering various materials to a backing sheet. The two techniques are often used in combination. When symbols are debossed, debossing from the back side of the base material is necessary to produce an embossed image on the front side. In the second technique, materials (symbols) are adhered to the front of the base material, directly producing an upright image. If the two techniques are combined, it is helpful to first deboss information on the back and then adhere additional information to the front. Figure 20-10 is a photograph of a map master produced by using both techniques. Symbols for sidewalks, fences or barriers, and pond were debossed into aluminum foil. Symbols for paved areas, buildings, and entrances were adhered to the front surface. The master map was vacuum formed.

Tables 4-10 and 5-10 list materials commonly available for the construction of debossed and adhered aids.

Three publications are useful as handbooks of specific techniques for making graphic aids. *Handbook on Mobility Maps* (James & Armstrong, 1976) is the most comprehensive guide available for the production of graphic and verbal aids of all kinds. It includes specific instructions for use of the Nottingham Kit of Parts for Mobility Maps. *Tactual Mapping*, (Wiedel & Groves, 1971b) is the most complete discussion of techniques for making debossed Thermoform master copies for maps. "The Use of Aluminum Sheets in Producing Tactual Maps for Blind Persons" (Craven, 1972) describes specific techniques for producing high quality debossed Thermoform master maps, using scrap materials.

COMMERCIAL PRODUCTION OF TACTILE OR TACTILE-VISUAL MAPS

Commercial production of orientation maps for visually impaired persons,

TABLE 4-10.
Common Materials for Debossed Aids

Base Material	Tools	Special Qualities
Writing paper	Tracing wheel	Quick production for a simple but not very durable aid.
Braille paper (or similar weight paper)	Tracing wheel Braille writer or slate	More durable than writing paper (can be vacuum formed). A braille writer enables a visually impaired person to construct simple, upright maps with regular grid patterns and braille labels.
Brailon, light or heavy weight	Tracing wheel, braille writer or slate.	More durable and more expensive than braille paper (original cannot be vacuum formed).
Heavy aluminum foil, (available at craft stores, or American Printing House for the Blind, fifty—10½" x 10½" sheets, $5.00)	Tracing wheels, leather working tools, mimeograph stencil tools, braille stylus, teflon braille eraser, ball point pen	Variety of symbols possible. Can be vacuum formed.
Offset printing plate (they can be used plates)	Same tools as for aluminum foil	Variety of symbols possible. Can be vacuum formed. Symbols not as sharp as in aluminum foil, but base material may be available free (Craven, 1972).

TABLE 5-10.
Common Materials for Adhered Aids

Base Material	Adhered Materials	Use
Braille paper Lightweight cardboard Textured cardboard Old x-ray plates	Line symbols 　String, yarn, rope, wire, solder, tape, pipe cleaners, stirring sticks Point symbols 　Buttons, tacks, paper fasteners, beads Areal symbols 　Sandpaper, emery cloth, fabric, wire or plastic screening, linoleum, cardboard Labels 　Braille paper, Dymo tape in braille slate, aluminum Dymo tape (for vacuum forming).	Many combinations are possible. Imaginative use of combinations of these materials, chosen according to good design criteria, produces simple or highly complex maps appropriate for many students and many learning situations. Many of these aids are easy to produce, relatively durable, and very interesting to students. Many can be vacuum formed, if there are no undercut symbols (symbols in which the top surface is larger than the surface that is adhered to the base), and none of the materials melt with the heat of the vacuum forming process.

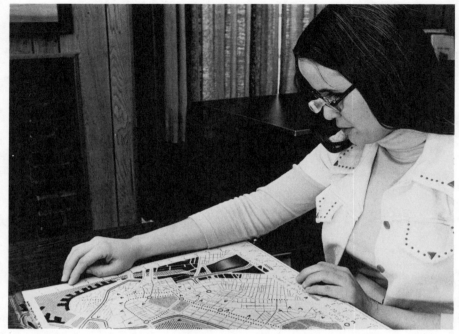

Figure 21a-10. Locating the coordinates in margin, layer 2. (Photography by R. Friedman.)

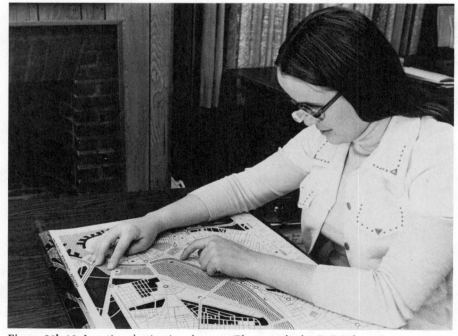

Figure 21b-10. Locating destination, layer 2. (Photography by R. Friedman.)

unlike commercial production of such geographic maps, may never become common because the number of visually impaired persons able to use and interested in orientation maps for any given area usually makes production costs prohibitive, on a per unit basis. Nevertheless, at least three commercial methods have been used to produce tactile or tactile-visual orientation maps during the period 1971-1976.

Polyvinyl chloride has been used in a patented process to produce maps with a larger number of symbols and greater information content and information density than any other material or technique (Kidwell & Greer, 1973). Conventional drafting techniques produce art work that is the master copy for a photo-engraved plate from which a master surface mold is prepared. This mold determines the form of a layer of pigmented vinyl permanently affixed to the base. Characteristics of maps so produced are that symbols are at multiple heights, everything which is printed is also raised (and vice versa, so that print numbers are also raised and braille numbers also printed), the maps are durable and highly flexible, and overlays and/or underlays can be used. The maps are expensive to design and to reproduce. Only two colors are used on maps produced by this technique. ITK Plastics Inc. (49 Salem Street, Salem, Massachusetts) is the only manufacturer that has attempted to produce maps using this technique.

Boston Cambridge Map

A tactual map of Boston and Cambridge produced in polyvinyl chloride (Fig. 21-10), contains a great amount of information, depicted at relatively small scale, 1 in. = 1000 ft (2.54 cm = 30 m), relatively large size, 17.5 in. x 23.5 in. (44 cm x 60 cm), with high information density. The map has four layers of information. Layer 1 (overlay) is a transparent flat map of the cities, printed in black. Layer 2 (overlay) is a raised and printed map of the cities. Layer 3, on the back of the second layer (underlay), contains braille labels for major streets and rapid transit stations. Layer 4 is a map of the public transportation system serving the cities.

The map is registered with the maps of the cities. It was designed by K. Lieneman, and produced by Howe Press of Perkins School for the Blind.

A client locates her destination coordinates in a braille directory, and, in turn, locates the coordinates, C-16, haptically in the margins of Layer 2 of the map (Fig. 21a-10). Although the student can perceive all the information visually on the transparent overlay (layer 1), she is able to scan more quickly using the tactual information.

Figure 21b-10 shows the client moving her right index finger horizontally across the map from letter C while moving her left index finger vertically up from number 16, using vision through her normal lenses to keep directions straight. Where her fingers meet is her destination, The Museum of Science, confirmed by viewing through her bioptic lens.

Sliding her left hand between the two layers of the map, the client scans the underside (Fig. 21c-10) to find the location of the rapid transit station nearest to the Museum of Science (as nearly underneath as possible). The right index finger is kept on the V indicating the location of the Museum on layer 2. With her left index finger, she finds that the Science Park Station is slightly east of the Museum on the street where the Museum is located. By combining the information from these two layers, she determines that in order to reach the Museum from the Station, she must travel west on the south side of the street, that her destination is within the first block she will walk, and that its main entrance faces the street.

Using both hands on layer 4 for haptic tracing of the route on public transportation from Kenmore Square (the station nearest her residence) to Science Park Station (Fig. 21d-10), the student knows from the open raised-circle symbol that Kenmore Square is underground, and that Science Park Station is above

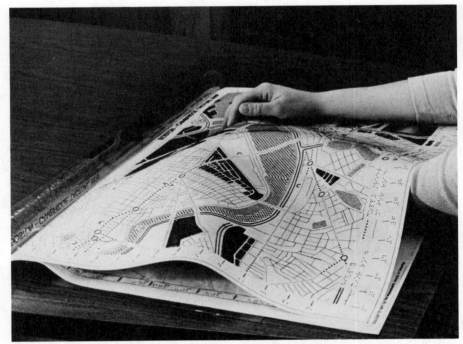

Figure 21c-10. Locating transit station (underlay), layer 3. (Photography by R. Friedman.)

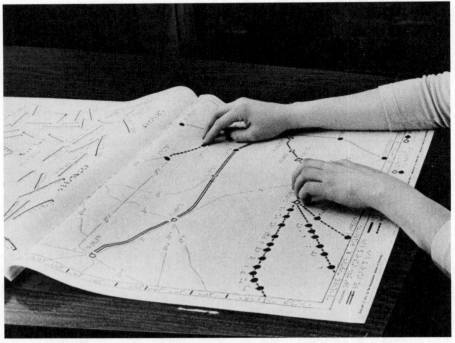

Figure 21d-10. Haptic tracing of transportation route, layer 14. (Photography by R. Friedman.)

ground from a solid raised-circle symbol indicating its location. She guides her finger visually, looking through her regular lenses, along the line indicating the subway route.

An embossed translucent plastic is being used in maps designed by Robert Amendola and produced by Gilligan Tactiles, Inc. (Bentzen, 1977). Commercially produced maps have been made of the MBTA Transit System (Boston) and downtown Philadelphia as of June, 1976. These maps are tactile and visual, and are highly schematic and trackable. However, they do not have detail as fine as those produced in polyvinyl chloride, nor the variety of symbols. Multiple heights are said to be possible, but the maps which have been commercially produced by this process to date have had only one elevation above the base. Not all raised information needs to be printed, nor printed information raised. Production is less expensive than the polyvinyl chloride system, and multicolored maps are being produced.

Specifications of maps produced by these two systems are available in "Orientation Maps for Visually Impaired Persons (Bentzen, 1977).

Computer Design and Production

Application of the computer to design and production of tactile-graphic orientation aids for visually impaired persons has been pioneered by John Gill, Ph.D., Warwick University, Coventry, England (1973a, 1973b). Design of the aid is accomplished by tracing the outline of the graphic display with a coordinate table linked to a computer, and then positioning standard symbols as desired, using a joystick. Sizes and heights of symbols are variable, and labels can be typed in on a keyboard, converted to Grade 1 braille by the computer, and positioned by moving the joystick. A visual display unit enables continuous monitoring of input. When the display is satisfactory, output is produced on a digital plotter, magnetic tape, or punched paper tape. A negative master is produced in laminated plastic by a routing machine guided by the computer tape. A positive copy is produced in epoxy resin, and used as the master copy for vacuum formed maps. Characteristics of aids produced by this system are exceptionally fine, uniform symbols of varying heights.

Although necessary equipment is costly, it can be shared with other manufacturing, business, research, or cartographic uses to make the actual running cost of such a system reasonable. The computer aided system is far more economical in design time than the two previously mentioned systems. Aids can be modified or updated quickly without the need for costly art work. If the aids are to be both tactile and visual, they can be printed by either silk screening or photo-offset prior to vacuum forming. Not all raised information needs to be printed, nor printed information raised. This system is probably the most economically viable for the production of high-information content, excellent quality, tactile or tactile-visual graphic aids in quantities of 10-100 copies (Fig. 22-10).

Development of computer-aided design and production techniques for tactile aids is being continued in the United States by John Sherman, Ph.D., Dept. of Geography, University of Washington, Seattle, WA., Joseph Wiedel, Ph.D., Dept. of Geography, University of Maryland, College Pk., MD., and Emerson Foulke, Ph.D., Perceptual Alternatives Laboratory, University of Louisville, Louisville, KY.

Other commercial systems for producing tactile aids are described in Gill (1974). None of these other systems are as appropriate for the production of tactile graphic orientation aids as those described here, although there are other commercial techniques for the production of tactile geographic aids.

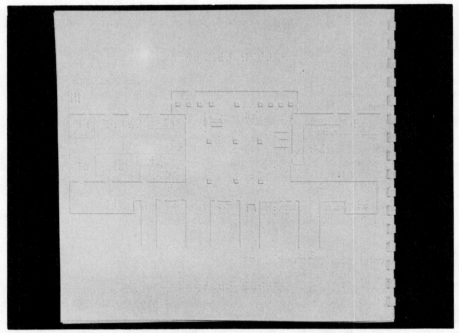

Figure 22-10. Map of Euston Square produced using the computer aided design and production system developed by J. Gill. (Photography by R. Friedman.)

USING GRAPHIC ORIENTATION AIDS

Visually impaired persons must develop some specific concepts and skills in order to comprehend and be able to use to best advantage the orientation information conveyed in any graphic aid. Requisite concepts are:

1. That a line conveys linear continuity

2. A symbol usually represents a real object

3. Size at which information is portrayed on the map is related in an understandable way to real size of objects (concept of scale)

4. Shape can be understood by relating the shape of an enclosed graphic figure to a known shape

5. Relative locations of things portrayed on a map indicate relative locations of those things in reality (distance and direction in relation to each other)

6. Actual location on the earth of things portrayed on a map can be understood by relating their location on the map to compass directions and by converting distance on the map to actual distance, using the scale. For example, the campus map user can find his destination, Moore Hall, on the map. He can also find his current location on the map. If Moore Hall lies directly south (on the map) of his present location, he knows that if he faces south (on the earth) he will be facing his destination. On the map, his destination is 2 in. (5.1 cm) from his current location. He knows that the map scale is 1 in. to 100 ft (2.5 cm to 30 m). He is therefore able to determine that Moore Hall is 200 ft (60 m) directly in front of him.

Requisite skills are:

1. Scanning in a systematic pattern to locate graphic symbols
2. Identifying (discriminating) graphic symbols
3. Tracing graphic line symbols
4. Shape of recognition, which combines tracing and discriminating.

Problem solving with the use of a graphic orientation aid, even at its simplest level, involves the integration of concepts with skills. A student does not need to have all of the concepts and skills listed in order to utilize some graphic aids to advantage. Best use of complex mapped information to facilitate independent travel requires the use of all these concepts and skills.

Some students will have acquired map concepts and skills before onset of visual impairment. They may need to learn to use haptic information instead of visual information, to use low vision aids in order to exercise the same skills they have previously developed, or to apply previously developed skills to maps which simplify the perception of visual graphic information for them. Low vision persons may learn all three sets of skills, and use them to supplement one another.

Other students will have previously acquired map concepts and skills by learning to use geographic maps for visually impaired persons. Maps for visually impaired school-age students are typically of poor quality and limited in information content. They have frequently not been designed with knowledge and application of principles that facilitate haptic perception or visual perception by persons with low vision. Current research is directed toward the production of higher quality geographic as well as orientation maps.

A curriculum and materials specifically for teaching map reading concepts and skills to young blind students are currently in the final stages of development and evaluation under the direction of Frank Franks at the American Printing House for the Blind. Students having completed this program will more likely be well prepared for the use of graphic orientation aids. A preliminary report notes that "Totally blind students as young as six years of age were able to 'read' a simple map after completing the 80 lessons" (American Printing House, 1975).

It may be desirable, but it certainly is not necessary, that students have at least some of the requisite skills and concepts before using a graphic aid with an orientation and mobility specialist. Blind subjects, ages 10 to adult, with some map reading training were more successful than subjects with no training in experimental map reading tasks, especially those involving orientation and route finding (Wiedel & Groves, 1969b). But the same study also indicates that map reading ability is positively correlated with amount of mobility instruction and with actual travel proficiency. Congenitally blind subjects had greater difficulty than adventitiously blinded subjects in map reading tasks.

Teaching map reading concepts and skills to visually impaired persons differs little from teaching the same concepts and skills to persons without a visual impairment. Following are some general suggestions drawn from personal experience in teaching these concepts and skills. Materials for each technique should be selected or designed according to the visual and/or haptic and cognitive abilities of the students. Some specific impairment-related suggestions are made. Otherwise, it is to be assumed that suggestions apply equally to teaching blind students to use tactile maps, teaching low vision students to use specially prepared visual or tactile-visual maps, or teaching low vision students who read regular print to use regular print maps.

TEACHING MAP READING CONCEPTS

Linear Continuity

A line conveys linear continuity. To isolate this concept for evaluation or teaching, an aid should be presented to the student in a form that can be readily perceived and manipulated, consisting of one straight line about two in. (5.08 cm) long. The aid should be placed in front of the student with the line running toward and away from him. The student should be told that the line says something about where he is going, and asked what he thinks it says. Most students are able to generalize that the line means they will go straight ahead, in the direction they are then facing. Then a similar line can be connected to the far end of the first line turning to the left. The student may be helped, if necessary, to understand that he will then turn left and walk straight ahead in the new direction. The lesson continues, with teacher and student taking turns drawing and interpreting routes consisting of straight lines and 90° turns. Curved lines, and turns of other angles can then be used. Later, this understanding of the directional quality of linear information is related to objects, such as walls, streets, or sidewalks.

Symbolic Representation

A symbol can represent a real object. Students who have some symbolic communication system, whether it is oral, written, or manual, usually do not have difficulty, if materials and expectations are geared to their abilities, in associating graphic symbols with real objects. Very low functioning, nonverbal low vision students may begin by associating photographs with real objects (perhaps travel destinations in their school building). Then progression can be made to drawings of those objects and to more abstract symbols, through repeated association of the symbol (a red dot for the classroom having a red door) with going to the destination.

When the student has acquired this concept, he will have little difficulty, if the situation arises, in learning that a graphic symbol may also occasionally be used to represent other kinds of information, such as a place to observe caution, a fixed sound source, or a point at which to solicit aid.

Size and Scale

Size at which information is portrayed on the map is related in an understandable way to real size of objects (concept of scale). To relate the general concept of scale to mobility in a practical way, it is possible to use the same materials and essentially the same techniques used to teach linear continuity. To teach scale, the teacher should begin with two lines going toward and away from the student, a short line and a long line. The student should be asked which line is longer, and which line would mean a long walk. It is helpful to coordinate this generalization by actually walking different distances in a straight line, and having the student portray each trip graphically. When the generalization is established, the lesson continues, with teacher and student drawing short, medium, and long walks, to give practice in comparing lengths of lines which may or may not be close together or going in the same direction.

The mathematical concept of scale such as 1 in. = 100 ft (or metrically, 1 cm = 1 m), is taught only after the student has some familiarity with estimating actual distances of travel and has the arithmetical skill necessary to relate the numerical value of scale to actual distance to be traveled. Many students use maps very well without ever learning to convert scale to actual distance, but relative distance, is a necessary concept for the understanding of nearly all maps, "First I travel a long block, and next, a short block."

Shape

Shape can be understood by relating the shape of an enclosed graphic figure (outline or the edge of an areal symbol) to a known shape. In teaching this concept, it can be helpful to begin by having students match drawings of shapes with corresponding plane shapes. The task is easiest if the drawings and plane shapes are at a scale of 1:1, if the shapes fit easily into one hand, and if they are presented in the same orientation. The student may then match drawings with larger planes, in different orientations, and next match drawings with objects having a dominant (top) plane surface of a simple shape, such as jar lids and box tops. Later the student can match drawings with larger objects such as tables, which he must walk around in order to understand their shapes. At a more advanced stage, he can relate drawings to rooms or to small buildings which he can walk all the way around, observing their shape through the integration of visual and/or haptic information.

The greatest difficulty in teaching this concept will generally arise with congenitally low vision students. The convention of mapping areas and the objects in these areas, is usually to draw these as seen from a position directly above each object without showing any information about features in the vertical plane, or about functions of objects. The convention of drawing things as seen from above must be specifically taught to some students. For example, one low vision student drew a map of a classroom which showed doors as concentric arcs. He drew the bookcases as he saw them in the vertical plane, and the doors as he experienced them. It is therefore helpful, in all shape recognition tasks leading up to map reading, to work with plane figures or objects which have a prominent, obviously top, plane surface. Low vision students may need to have attention called to this top surface.

Relative Locations

Relative locations of things portrayed on a map indicate relative locations of those things in reality. In teaching this concept it is helpful to work in a small, simply furnished room that will be mapped cooperatively by teacher and student. Materials for the map might include a base (magnetic or other board or tray) which has the same shape and relative dimensions as the room, and an assortment of symbols or pieces resembling the furnishings in a scale relative to the map base and to each other in shape, as seen from above, and perhaps in regard to other characteristics. The student should first explore the room, noting its shape and the furnishings that will be represented on the map, with the starting point for observations along one wall. When finished, he should sit at the starting point facing the opposite wall, and relate the base map to the shape of the room, positioning it so that the side faced is farthest from his body. He should then make tentative selections from available materials of symbols to be used to represent furnishings. If necessary, guidance should be given in choosing symbols appropriate in size and shape to what they represent. This is very reinforcing to the learning of concepts of symbolic representation, size and scale, and shape. The student should arrange the symbols along the opposite wall on his map, in positions corresponding to his memory of their relative positions. Accuracy can be confirmed by another trip to explore the opposite wall, paying more attention, if necessary, to relative distances between furnishings. The walls to the right and left can be mapped in the same way. Pointing to actual objects as their symbols are placed on the map helps to further connect map location with actual location.

It can be helpful to have the student change perspective before he maps the wall against which he was originally seated. He should sit against the wall which he was previously facing, facing the original starting point. The map should remain oriented correctly in relation to the room, that is, the side farthest from his body is not yet mapped. The student should again point to symbols on the map and to the furnishings each represents. He should notice that he points generally left for things which are shown on the left side of the map and recall that he pointed generally to the right to point at these same objects before he changed his position. An important generalization to help the student make at this point is that he turned neither the room nor the map. When the student has mapped furnishings along the walls, he may add central furnishings.

Concluding tasks would involve planning routes on the map, verbalizing them, and traveling them from various starting points. Each trip will further confirm the relationship between location of things on the map and things in reality. This is an excellent lesson to combine with actual room familiarization.

Compass Orientation

Actual location on the earth, of things portrayed on a map can be understood by relating their location on the map to compass directions and by converting distance on the map to actual distance. The student who has fully grasped the concepts involved in the preceding tasks needs to add an understanding of compass directions as they are shown on a map, and the arithmetic necessary to convert distance on a map to distance on the earth. This should be taught in conjunction with actual travel in which compass directions are being learned, and it can complement such lessons. Important points to remember are that the map must have a north indicator, preferably a distinctive north edge. This should be interpreted as "toward the north," not as a point or even a side which *is* north. All travel which moves from the side opposite the north edge, towards this north edge, is generally going north. The north side of an east-west street is that side (of the two sides of the street which should be shown on a map for this purpose) which is nearest to the north edge. The northwest corner of an intersection is that corner which is closest to both the north and west edges of the map.

In using the map during actual travel, it is helpful, at least initially, to keep the map oriented so that the north edge is always toward the north. What is farthest from the student on the map will be that which is in front of him. What is on the left side will be to his left, etc. The student should understand that it is he who is turning, not the area in which he is travelling, or the map. Frequent touching of symbols on the map and then pointing to objects they represent will reinforce this concept as well as the ability to relate what is shown on a map to actual body position within the area mapped.

TEACHING MAP READING SKILLS

In all map reading tasks with low vision persons, there should be glare-free lighting. Each kind of task should be tried with and without any optic aid normally used for near work. The specialist should remember that tasks especially requiring acuity, such as the identification of small symbols, may be easier with various aids. Tasks facilitated by a full field, such as gaining a general idea of the utilization of space or relating widely separated areas of the map to each other, may be easier without aids that magnify but also reduce the user's field.

Systematic Scanning

Scanning in a systematic pattern to locate graphic symbols is, regardless of the type of impairment, essentially the application of organized search procedures to the graphic aid. In teaching the skill, graphic aids having few and highly discriminable symbols should be used. First, the student should be shown an isolated sample of the symbol. Then the graphic aid should be systematically searched for examples of the symbol, using a side-to-side, or top-to-bottom pattern. It may be helpful for the student to use markers such as his hands, a card, or a ruler.

Research by Berlá (1972) indicates that the most efficient strategy for the haptic location of point symbols is to use two hands moving in vertical patterns. The index and adjacent two fingers of each hand are placed side by side in the upper left corner of the aid. These six fingers travel down the page, next to one other, completely scanning a vertical section of the aid as wide as the user's six fingers. The two hands then move to the right along either the top or the bottom edge of the aid, a distance equal to the width of the six-finger span. This can be accomplished either by estimating the distance and sliding both hands directly across, or by first placing the fingers of the left hand to the right of the fingers of the right hand, and then placing the fingers of the right hand to the right of the left hand. The six fingers then move either up or down the aid to scan a vertical path adjacent to the first. The process is repeated until the entire aid has been scanned.

Systematic scanning of an entire map (tactile and/or visual) should give the reader some idea of the size of the map, information density, concentrations of information (if any), and symbols used. Subsequent haptic or visual scanning for specific symbols may start, and go outward from an easily recognized feature on the map, rather than an arbitrary edge or center. Easily recognized tactile features are the highest or roughest features on a map. Students should learn to find such features readily.

Mounting print maps, especially large maps, on a wall sometimes facilitates scanning by low vision readers by permitting better illumination (e.g., from a window), and requiring less awkward or tiring postures for the reader to get close enough to all parts of the map. Other low vision readers may prefer to move the map, instead. Those who use optic aids for near viewing should be encouraged to try scanning each map both with and without the optic aid. Depending on the map, the circumstances of viewing, and the tasks to be performed, scanning may be facilitated by a full field (without the aid), while identifying may require the use of the aid.

Symbol Identification

Identifying of (discriminating) graphic symbols uses haptic acuity, visual acuity or both. In teaching students to identify symbols, the teacher should begin with aids having few, highly discriminable symbols. The student should be able to identify readily each symbol used, before being given tasks requiring the combination of symbol identification with other information gathering techniques. A perceptually and conceptually easier task than the foregoing is to isolate symbols on individual cards which can be paired, sorted, or identified by the meaning associated with the symbol.

There is some evidence that haptic readers perform best on discrimination tasks when the index fingers only are used (Foulke, 1964; Lappin, & Foulke, 1973; Berlá & Butterfield, 1977; Hill, 1973).

Specialists who have low vision students perform symbol identification tasks should be certain that optic aids, if any, are properly focused for maximum acuity, and that the map is held at the best distance from the eyes for fine discrimination.

Tracing Line Symbols

Visual tracking or haptic tracing of line symbols may be facilitated by using one index finger as a reference, positioned or traveling after each successive haptic or visual fixation along the line. This will make both correction, if one "gets off the track," and return to a starting point easier.

Berlá (1973) found that in a haptic tracing task, the most successful readers were those who used both index fingers only. Berlá's experimental tasks involved tracing for the purpose of recognizing enclosed shapes (outlines). Intersecting lines were irrelevant information. This author believes that in haptic tracing tasks on orientation maps in which the recognition of intersecting lines and adjacent point symbols is frequently a part of the tracing task, the use of the index and middle fingers may give better performance. The index fingers will actually trace the line, while the middle fingers will notice intersecting lines and adjacent point symbols.

As discussed in Pick, Chapter 5, the direction of motion of the hand as it explores a tactile line appears to influence the perception of the direction of that line in space. Thus, in teaching map reading, it is important to encourage students to hold maps squarely in front of their bodies in order to perceive the directions of lines most accurately.

Shape Recognition

Ability to recognize a shape requires the skills of tracing haptically, or visually tracking the outline of the shape, recognizing a distinctive feature or features of that shape, and comparing the distinctive feature or features of the shape with remembered features. Both haptic readers and persons with reduced visual fields may need practice in combining these skills into shape recognition.

Errors in judgment of relative lengths of visual or tactile lines, as in determining whether a city block is square or rectangular, may be influenced by the horizontal-vertical illusion (see Chapter 5, Pick) where sides of a block are defined by tactile lines that differ from one another in texture, the length of the fine-textured line may be overestimated and the length of the coarse-textured line may be underestimated (see Pick, Chapter 5.)

It is of critical importance that such readers have a system for shape recognition tasks, as the relationship of distinctive features (hence shape) may appear different if each feature is not perceived, and perceived in the same order each time the reader looks at the same shape (Gibson, 1966).

Berlá and Butterfield (1977) demonstrated that shape recognition and speed and accuracy of locating shapes could be improved by giving students who were braille readers specific instruction in haptically tracing a raised line (outline of a shape) and in recognizing distinctive features. Students were trained to trace a shape with the index finger of their preferred hand, while using the index finger of their other hand as a reference. Tracing began and ended at the reference finger. Students were trained to recognize distinctive features such as "parts that stick out, parts that are pointed, parts that go in, parts that are curved."

Lesson Plan Suggestions

A suggested lesson plan follows, using a graphic orientation aid to assist self-familiarization with a small residential neighborhood: (It is assumed that the student has at least elementary knowledge of the concepts and skills mentioned in the foregoing sections, such as the easy reading of labels.)

1. Tell the student what the map represents. (Exploration of a graphic aid haptically or with limited vision is too complex to make a guessing game any fun.)

2. Hand the map to the student "right" side up. (The orientation of the map should correspond to reality. If, for some reason such as the easy reading of labels, you want a particular side to be "top," seat the student opposite that side. Don't turn the map.)

3. Allow the student to explore the aid freely. (He should have time to experience and ask questions about its qualities such as the construction materials, size,

weight, flexibility, and information coding system before he is asked to make specific observations.)

4. Encourage the active use of both hands (especially both index fingers) and/or of any residual vision. (Encourage low vision students to experiment with their optic aids for near, altering the lighting or altering the distance or angle of the map from their eyes.)

5. Teach a systematic scanning strategy if the student has not already learned it.

6. Have the student discover the content and structure of the map by locating a sample of each symbol that is used; giving a prominent "reference point," and having him return to it after looking at other parts of the map; answering questions which relate symbols to one another; answering questions which relate the map to reality, such as direction and relative size and distance of what is portrayed on the aid; planning and describing a route and alternate routes using the aid; and providing ample opportunity for review and rehearsal (Pick, Chapter 5).

7. Take the student and map "on location" and locate tactile, visual or auditory clues that show what is represented on the aid is an accurate, smaller scale, representation of reality.

8. Have the student travel the route he has planned, perhaps keeping track of his progress by marking the aid.

9. If the student is disoriented, have him use clues from the aid to reorient himself.

10. Review the lesson by having the student trace on the aid the route he has traveled. Have him give verbal information about specific landmarks, useful clues, or problem areas which were not apparent from the map.

11. If desired, add additional information as discovered by the student.

VERBAL MAPS

Little actual research, but some development has been done on verbal maps as orientation aids for visually impaired persons. Auditory maps of routes and of areas have been made, used, and described in the literature (Leonard & Newman, 1970; Blasch, Welsh, & Davidson, 1973; James & Armstrong, 1976). Many visually impaired persons make written braille or print notes about routes or areas they travel. A few specific techniques have been developed and described in the literature for making verbal route memory aids. This section will discuss variables affecting the choice of information for auditory and written maps, and some techniques for effectively incorporating the information into useable aids. Some specific techniques and materials for verbal route memory aids will be described.

Information Content

The amount and type of information in a verbal map can vary greatly depending on what is to be communicated to whom. In choosing information for a verbal map, as for a tactile, visual, or tactile-visual map, it is important to select landmarks which are perceptible to the user's remaining senses and/or which have a high likelihood of being located with that particular travel aid.

All verbal maps will have some kind of an orientation system which will influence the amount and type of information contained. Four orientation systems which may be used separately or together are:

TABLE 6-10.
Examples of Verbal Aids for Various Learning Situations

Learning Situation	Aid Type	Information Content
1. Client needs memory aid to limit need for instructor intervention for travel on residential-small business route on which he is currently receiving instruction.	Auditory route map (to be carried on lesson).	Specific route instructions, including side of street to travel on and specific instructions for each crossing, if necessary. Broken into small segments, each ending at landmark readily perceived by student. Gives specific directions for soliciting aid at complex crossings such as, "You are now facing Trapelo Rd., Common St. is beside you on the left. The Exxon station is behind you. Get help for crossings." Tells what technique to use for each segment and exactly how to locate and recognize the destination. Similar instructions for return trip.
2. Client needs orientation and memory aid for medium sized business area to which he is being familiarized and which he will frequently use after completion of orientation and mobility program.	Auditory area map (to be listened to before the trip).	Names of main streets, their directions related to compass, and relative sizes, presented systematically: north to south, then east to west, including direction of traffic flow, and configuration and control of each intersection of the main streets. Systematic listing of each business, in order going away from the center of the business area, with description of tactile, proprioceptive, auditory, and olfactory landmarks for recognizing each, such as "The entrance to Joe's Barber Shop is immediately preceded by a barber pole, about 12″ (30.48 cm) in diameter, located along the building line, extending from the sidewalk to head height. The wide recessed entrance is carpeted and slopes up. On warm days the door may be open, and recorded music and the scents of soaps and powders may be perceptible from a short distance outside the shop."
3. Client needs orientation aid to an unfamiliar college campus.	Auditory area map (an aid to route planning and overall comprehension & appreciation of the area).	Location of campus within urban area, using cartographic and polarcentric terms. Main public transit access routes to the campus. Names, locations and directions of streets bounding the campus. Systematic description of main vehicular and/or pedestrian traffic routes, including detail sufficient to enable student to confirm his location, if desired, when passing near each building. Specific routes which this student is likely to use may also be described.

TABLE 6-10.
Examples of Verbal Aids for Various Learning Situations

Learning Situation	Aid Type	Information Content
4. Client needs orientation and memory aid for route planning of public transportation trips.	Written or auditory (can be used before or during trip).	Name, direction, stops and end points on each line. May also have detailed route or area descriptions of stations, especially ones frequently used, or where one can transfer from one line to another.
5. Client needs memory aids for routes traveled independently but infrequently, in piano tuning business.	Written or auditory (can be used before or during trip).	Information selected entirely by client. Minimal information needed to reach and return from each destination, such as "Red line to Harvard. Waverley trolley to Payson St. Cross Payson. Payson Church is first building set back from sidewalk." Return. "Turn left on leaving the church. Go three blocks east to traffic light at Belmont and School Sts. Cross Belmont. Trolley stops just right of cross walk. Take trolley to Harvard. Red line to Central Station."
6. Client needs system for making brief memory aid for route described verbally by an untrained person.	Auditory (can be used before trip or during trip).	As visually impaired person listens to verbal directions, he tape records himself repeating the salient points. Actual content may be similar to that of Example 5.
7. New clients traveling to agency for visually impaired persons need orientation information sufficient to enable them to choose and travel a route from subway station to agency, with minimal need for assistance.	Auditory (can be used before trip and relevant information abstracted in written or auditory form for use on trip).	Information should first include systematic overall description of area involved. General description of subway station, levels and line, and names of main streets and their directions. Detailed description of route should not be specific but should include sufficient information about all types of landmarks to enable each traveler to select the route and landmarks he will use.

1. Egocentric, in which the traveler relates the environment to his own body using such terms as left, right, in front, behind
2. Topocentric, in which the traveler relates himself to landmarks and landmarks to each other
3. Cartographic, in which the traveler relates himself and landmarks to organized structures of the man-made environment such as grid patterns, building structures, and address systems
4. Polarcentric, in which the traveler uses the universal abstract method of orientation based on the earth's rotational axis, compass directions.

The orientation system or systems used in a particular verbal aid must be understood by the person using the aid. Aids constructed for the use of a varied group of persons should use both a lower and a higher level orientation system throughout (Blasch, Welsh & Davidson, 1973 pp. 147-149).

The range of complexity in information content is illustrated in Table 6-10, which gives examples of students, their learning needs, appropriate types of verbal aids, and suggested types of information for each student and his needs.

Characteristics of Verbal Aids

Some of the special characteristics of auditory, braille and print aids were described earlier. Additional considerations are given below.

Any visually impaired person who can understand either spoken or written language is a potential user of verbal aids. The use of verbal aids, whether tape recorded, in braille, or in print, may be a natural extension of the use of the person's already developed information gathering and memory techniques. In conventional orientation and mobility instruction, visually impaired persons receive and will be learning to use and to organize verbal information throughout their course of instruction. Thus, the presentation of such information in an auditory or written form with which the user is already comfortable, may place fewer new processing demands on the user than models or graphic aids.

Verbal aids, whether brief and simple, or lengthy and complex can be prepared in auditory or written form by a student or a specialist. The specialist who uses such aids in instruction should always include opportunities for his student to make similar aids for himself, and to update or revise existing aids to enhance usefulness.

The choice of medium for verbal aids is based partly on the need for special equipment and on the verbal skills of the student. Auditory maps do not require that the user read braille or print, but they do require special equipment to produce and use. Braille aids require simpler and less expensive equipment to produce, but they also require that the student read braille, and the majority of blind people do not read braille. Print aids require no special equipment to produce, but they do require that the user read print.

All verbal aids can use various kinds of orientation reference systems, and are thus adaptable for persons with varied levels of sophistication, from egocentric to the use of polarcentric directions.

Verbal Maps, Materials and Techniques

Helpful specific suggestions for specialists who design and produce verbal maps are included in Blasch, Welsh, and Davidson (1973) and James and Armstrong (1976).

Rapidly changing designs and features of portable cassette tape recorders make it pointless to suggest the use of any one recorder. The optimal qualities of a recorder for auditory maps to be used while traveling are:

1. Portability—small (preferably pocket size), lightweight, good strap, does not need to be carried in the hand

2. Ease of operation—one handed

3. Durability—weatherproof and shockproof

4. Ear piece for privacy

5. Beep index capacity for easy return to specific passages

6. Rechargeable batteries.

Braille or print maps can be made on paper normally used for the purpose, on file cards, or in a notebook. Braille maps can also be written directly on waterproof Brailon (Thermoform Corporation, Box 125, Pico Rivera, CA 90660).

Specific Techniques—Verbal Route Memory Aids

A coding system first developed by J. Alfred Leonard (1970) has been further developed in braille and print as a route memory aid (Armstrong, 1973, p. 8). It is used primarily in England. The basic coding system is:

Code Letter	Braille	Meaning
c		Cross here and carry straight on.
r		Turn right before crossing.
l		Turn left before crossing.
s		Cross here and turn right on upkerb.
p		Cross here and turn left on upkerb.
e		End.
d		Take special care here.
o		Roundabout.
x		Left hand side of street.
y		Right hand side of street.

This code can be used either on a plastic, pocket size memory disc with a metal place marker (Fig. 23-10), on strips of heavy aluminum foil attached to the cane or on file cards (Armstrong, 1973). Discs are available from Mickleborough Engineering Co., Ashfordby Street, Leicester, England.

The chief advantages of this simple special verbal memory aid are that they make minimal demands on the perceptual and manipulative skills of users, minimal time is needed to perceive all information given for each section of a trip, and all of these aids can be produced by either the specialist or the visually impaired user.

AIDS AND THE MOBILITY SPECIALIST

Each mobility specialist should be thoroughly familiar with orientation aids, design principles, materials available for production, and techniques for their use to enable streamlining and individualizing of teaching concepts and skills necessary to independent travel.

Specialists should be involved in the design of permanent or special-purpose orientation aids for schools, agencies, metropolitan areas, transit systems, that wish to provide mobility maps to visually impaired persons using their facilities. A responsible and informed specialist is the person most capable of judging which information, for what purpose, displayed using what techniques, is most appropriate to promote independent travel in any situation. Any specialist participating in the design of such an aid should be certain that the aid will be made available in ways to facilitate its optimum use and best understanding.

Specialists who wish to contribute to the availability of orientation aids as resources for visually impaired persons in a community or geographic area, can train volunteers to assist in the production of such aids, which can then be available for purchase or on loan from the volunteer group or agency; a system widely used and highly successful in England.

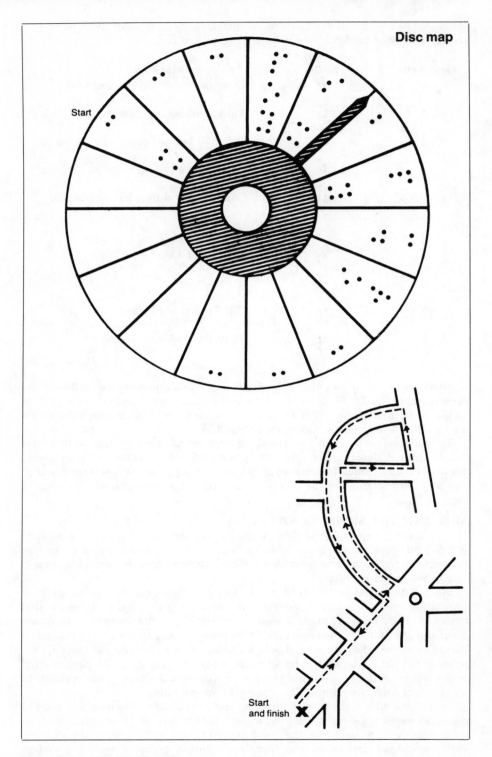

Figure 23-10. Memory disc map.

It is essential that mobility specialists work in cooperation with persons who are currently doing basic and applied research into the design and production of orientation aids. Only through such cooperation will needed aids be designed, produced, and used. Involvement of mobility specialists is essential to the development of commercially produced orientation aids.

Mobility specialists should, themselves, take an active role in research, development, and controlled evaluation of all aids designed to facilitate the acquisition of orientation concepts, skills and information by visually impaired persons.

Bibliography

Amendola, R. Practical considerations in tactile map design. *Long Cane Newsletter,* 1976, **9**(2), 22-24.

American Printing House for the Blind. *Education Research, Development and Reference Group, Report on Research and Development Activities—Fiscal, 1975.*

Angwin, J. P. B. Maps for mobility—1. *New Beacon,* 1968, **52,** 115-119.

Angwin, J. P. B. Maps for mobility—2. *New Beacon,* 1968, **52,** 143-145.

Armstrong, J. D. (ed.) *The design and production of maps for the visually handicapped.* Mobility Monograph No. 1, Blind Mobility Research Unit, Department of Psychology, University of Nottingham, Nottingham, England, 1973.

Bentzen, B. L. Orientation maps for visually impaired persons. *Journal of Visual Impairment and Blindness,* 1977, **71,** 193-196.

Bentzen, B. L. Production and testing of an orientation and travel map for visually handicapped persons. *New Outlook for the Blind,* 1972, **66,** 249-255.

Berlá, E. P. Behavioral strategies and problems in scanning and interpreting tactual displays. *New Outlook for the Blind,* 1972, **66,** 272-286.

Berlá, E. P. Strategies in scanning a tactual pseudomap. *Education of the Visually Handicapped,* 1973, **5,** 8-19.

Berlá, E. P. Effects of physical size and complexity on tactual discrimination of blind children. *Exceptional Children,* 1972, **39,** 120-124.

Berlá, E. P., Butterfield, L. H., & Murr, M. J. Tactile political map reading by blind students. A videomatic behavioral analysis. *Journal of Special Education,* 1976, **10,** 266-276.

Berlá, E. P., Butterfield, L. H., & Murr, M. J. Tactile political map designs for blind students. In Nolan, C.Y. (Ed.) Facilitating the education of the visually handicapped through research in communications, Part 3. *Facilitating Tactile Map Reading—Final Report.* Grant # OEG-O-73-0642, Department of Health, Education, and Welfare, Bureau of Education for the Handicapped, 1976.

Berlá, E. P. & Butterfield, L. H. Tactile political maps: Two experimental designs. *Journal of Visual Impairment and Blindness,* 1977, **71,** 262-264.

Berlá, E. P., & Murr, M. J. The effects of noise on the location of point symbols and tracing a line on a tactile pseudomap. *Journal of Special Education,* 1975, **9,** 183-190.

Blasch, B. B., Welsh, R. L., Davidson, T. Auditory maps: An orientation aid for visually handicapped persons. *New Outlook for the Blind,* 1973, **67,** 145-158.

Borish, I. M. *Clinical Refraction.* Chicago: Professional Press, 1949.

Chang, C. & Johnson, D. E. Tactual maps with interchangeable parts. *New Outlook for the Blind,* 1968, **62,** 122-124.

Craven, R. W. The use of aluminum sheets in producing tactual maps for blind persons. *New Outlook for the Blind,* 1972, **66,** 323-330.

Fluharty, W., McHugh, J., McHugh, M., Willits, P., & Wood, J. Anxiety in the teacher-student relationship as applicable to orientation and mobility instruction. *New Outlook for the Blind,* 1976, **70,** 153-156.

Foulke, E. Transfer of a complex perceptual skill, *Perceptual and Motor Skills,* 1964, **18,** 733-740.

Gill, J. M. Design, production and evaluation of tactual maps for the blind. Unpublished doctoral thesis. University of Warwick, Coventry, England, 1973.

Gill, J. M. Method for the production of tactual maps and diagrams. *American Foundation for the Blind Research Bulletin* No. 26, 1973b, 203-204.

Gill, J. M. Tactual mapping, *American Foundation for the Blind Research Bulletin* No. 28, 1974, 57-80.

Gill, J. M. & James, G. A. A study on the discrimination of tactual point symbols, *American Foundation for the Blind Research Bulletin* No. 26, 1973, 19-34.

Gilson, C., Wurzburger, B., & Johnson, D. E. The use of the raised map in teaching mobility to blind children. *New Outlook for the Blind*, 1965, **59**, 59-62.

Gibson, J. J. *The senses considered as perceptual systems.* Boston: Houghton Mifflin, 1966.

Greenberg, G. L. Map design for partially seeing students: An investigation of white versus black line symbology, Unpublished doctoral dissertation, University of Washington, Seattle, Washington, 1968.

Greenberg, G. L. & Sherman, J. C. Design of maps for partially seeing children, *International Yearbook of Cartography*, **10**, 1970, 111-115.

Heath, W. R. Maps and graphics for the blind. Some aspects of the discriminability of textural surfaces for use in areal differentiation. Unpublished doctoral dissertation, University of Washington. Ann Arbor, Mich: University Microfilms, 1958, No. 69-829.

Hill, J. W. Limited field of view in reading lettershapes with the fingers. In F. Geldard, (Ed.) *Cutaneous communication systems and devices.* Psychonomic Society, 1973.

James, G. A. Problems in the standardization of design and symbolization in tactile route maps for the blind. *New Beacon,* 1972, **56**, 87-91.

James, G. A. Kit for making raised maps. *New Beacon,* 1975, **59**, 85-90.

James, G. A. & Armstrong, J. D. An evaluation of a shopping centre map for the visually handicapped, *Journal of Occupational Psychology*, 1975, **48**, 125-128.

James, G. A. & Armstrong, J. D. *Handbook on Mobility Maps,* Blind Mobility Research Unit, Department of Psychology, University of Nottingham, Nottingham, England, 1976.

James, G. A. & Gill, J. M. Mobility maps for the visually handicapped: Study of learning and retention of raised symbols. *American Foundation for the Blind Research Bulletin* No. 27, 1974, 87-98.

James, G. A. & Gill, J. M. Pilot study of the discriminability of tactile areal and line symbols for the blind. *American Foundation for the Blind Research Bulletin* No. 29, 1975, 23-31.

Jansson, G. Symbols for tactile maps. In B. Lindqvist & N. Trowald (Eds.) *European Conference of Educational Research for the Visually Handicapped.* Project PUSS VIII. Report No. 31, 1972, 66-73.

Kidwell, A. M. & Greer, P. S. The environmental perceptions of blind persons and their haptic representations. *New Outlook for the Blind,* 1972, **66**, 256-276.

Kidwell, A. M. & Greer, P. S. *Sites, perception and the nonvisual experience; Designing and manufacturing mobility maps.* N.Y.: American Foundation for the Blind, 1973.

Lappin, J. S. & Foulke, E. Expanding the tactual field of view. *Perception and Psychophysics.* 1973, **14**, 237-241.

Leonard, J. A. Aids to navigation; a discussion of the problem of maps for the blind traveller. Paper presented at St. Dunstan's International Conference on Sensory Devices for the Blind, London, 1966(a).

Leonard, J. A. Experimental maps for blind travel. *New Beacon,* 1966b, **50**, 32-35.

Leonard, J. A. & Newman, R. C. Three types of "maps" for blind travel. *Ergonomics,* 1970, **13**, 165-179.

Levi, J. M. & Schiff, W. Study of texture discrimination. Appendix B. of Development of raised line drawings as supplementary tools in the education of the blind. Final report, September, 1966, Project No. RD-1571-S, Department of Health, Education and Welfare, Vocational Rehabilitation Administration.

Maglione, F. D. An experimental study of the use of tactual maps as orientation and mobility aids for adult blind subjects. Unpublished doctoral dissertation, University of Illinois, 1969.

Morris, J. E. Discriminability of tactual patterns. Unpublished master's thesis, University of Louisville, 1961.

Morris, J. E. & Nolan, C. Y. Minimum sizes for areal type tactual symbols. *International Journal for the Education of the Blind,* 1963, **13**, 48-51.

Mumford, D. O. Sequential maps: Tactile. Mobility Map Conference. Nottingham, England. Sept. 1972.

Nolan, C. Y. A study of pictures for large type textbooks. *International Journal for the Education of the Blind,* 1960, **9**, 67-70.

Nolan, C. Y. Teacher preference for types of illustrations in large type text books. *International Journal for the Education of the Blind,* 1961, **10**, 112-114.

Nolan, C. Y. Illustrations and educational devices for the blind. *Proceedings of the American Association of Instructors of the Blind,* 1964, **47**, 54-68.

Nolan, C. Y. Relative legibility of raised and incised tactual figures. *Education of the Visually Handicapped,* 1971, **3**, 33-36.

Nolan, C. Y. Readability of large types: A study of type sizes and type styles. *International Journal for the Education of the Blind,* December, 1959.

Nolan, C. Y. & Morris, J. E. Improvement of tactual symbols for blind children. Final report, 1971. Project No. 5-0421; Grant No. OEG-32-27-0000-1012, Louisville, Ky.: American Printing House for the Blind.

Schiff, W. Manual for the construction of raised line diagrams. Appendix JJ of Development of raised line drawings as supplementary tools in the education of the blind. Final report. September, 1966, Project No. RD-1571-S, Department of Health, Education and Welfare, Vocational Rehabilitation Administration.

Schiff, W. Research on raised line drawings. *New Outlook for the Blind*, 1965, **59**, 134-137.

Schiff, W. & Isikow, H. Stimulus redundancy in the tactile perception of histograms. Appendix C. of Development of raised line drawings as supplementary tools in the education of the blind. Final report, September, 1966, Project No. RD-1571-S, Department of Health, Education and Welfare, Vocational Rehabilitation Administration.

Schiff, W. & Levi, J. Development of raised line drawings as supplementary tools in the education of the blind. Final report, September, 1966. Project No. RD-1571-S. Department of Health, Education and Welfare, Vocational Rehabilitation Administration.

Shaw, A. *Print for Partial Sight*. London: The Library Association, 1969.

Shepherd, O. Map work with blind students. Paper presented at the meeting of the International Council of Educators of Blind Youth, Watertown, MA.: August, 1967.

Sherman, J. C. Needs and resources in maps for the blind. *New Outlook for the Blind*, 1965, **59**, 130-134.

Vaughan, D., Asbury, T. & Cook, R. *General ophthalmology*, 6th Ed. Los Altos, CA.: Lange Medical Publications, 1971.

Wiedel, J. W. & Groves, P. A. Designing and reproducing tactual maps for the visually handicapped. *New Outlook for the Blind*, 1969a, **63**, 196-201.

Wiedel, J. W. & Groves, P. A. Tactual mapping: Design, reproduction, reading and interpretation. Final report, 1969b, University of Maryland, Project No. DR-2557S, Department of Health, Education and Welfare, Vocational Rehabilitation Administration.

Mobility Devices

Leicester W. Farmer

Many ways and means have been used by visually impaired persons to satisfy the basic desire to be mobile. From earliest times, animals, sighted people, and devices (such as sticks or canes), have been used to achieve varying levels of mobility. Today, there are basically three (possibly four, if electronic travel aids are considered) common ways of getting about. The first is the use of a sighted human guide. The other two most accepted and proven methods are with canes of varying lengths and dog guides.

CANES

Several types of canes and walking aids are manufactured to meet the varied needs and demands of visually impaired persons. The long cane, a folding or collapsible cane, a white wooden cane, or a support or orthopedic cane are most commonly used. They are fabricated from wood, aluminum alloy, fiberglass, plastic, and stainless steel.

In addition to enabling a person to become mobile and travel independently and extensively through space, a cane provides a measure of protection and travel safety. The distinction between the provision of protection and of safety by the cane, as two separate (although related) entities, may be questioned by some specialists, but one need only imagine the long cane in the hands of a trainee just learning to use the aid as opposed to one who has completed a comprehensive training course. If both had to travel in a large city, the cane would afford even the trainee some measure of protection against collision with obstacles and pedestrians. However, of the two users, only the person who had successfully completed mobility training would be equipped to use the cane safely in confusing, complex, and often dangerous travel situations.

The cane extends the tactual sense of the user to the length of the cane shaft or tip to provide information about the environment. In addition, the cane identifies the user as handicapped or visually impaired and, in some cases, provides physical support.

THE LONG CANE

After the work done with the cane by Richard E. Hoover at Valley Forge, agencies and mobility specialists themselves for many years fabricated or bought canes without any standard specifications. The need for uniformity in an acceptable long cane was apparent. Under the leadership of Russell C. Williams, the Veterans Administration (1964) published *Specifications for the Long Cane (Typhlocane)*, which helped to establish a model long cane (Appendix A).

Although this publication of specifications for the long cane was very useful, it was still not an adequate set of requirements or characteristics. In September, 1971, a group of scientists, administrators, technologists, and mobility specialists met to draw up standards and specifications for the long cane and to develop acceptable techniques for its use under a variety of conditions (National Research Council, 1972).

Specifications

The cane is composed of four parts: the crook, the grip, the shaft, and the tip.

Specifications for the Long Cane (Typhlocane) defines the *crook* as the upper end of the cane which is curved to form an arc or "hook"; the *grip* as that portion of the cane which has been adapted for grasping by covering with leather, plastic, rubber, or other suitable material; the *shaft* as the main part of the cane that extends from the base of the crook to the tip end of the cane; the *tip* as the element at the lower end of the cane that normally contacts the ground. Outside diameter of the tubing is 0.500 in. (13 mm), wall thickness is 0.062 in. (1.6 mm), and inside diameter 0.375 in. (9.5 mm).

The 1971 National Academy of Sciences (NAS) conference in Washington, D.C. adopted physical and functional characteristics for the crook, the grip, and the tip, as well as for the shaft of the long cane. Desirable design features are:

1. Straight vertical axis of shaft

2. Slight taper of shaft from grip to tip

3. Various lengths to fit height of individual user

4. Sufficient length to provide the user with essential information in ample time to react to it but not to inhibit the user's physical freedom (ideally to extend from the ground at the side of the foot in forward position to 1½ in. [3.8 cm] above the bottom of the breast bone)

5. Weight as light as possible without affecting balance or sacrificing other requirements, depending on length, 6 to 8 oz. (0.168 to 0.224 kg)

6. Low wind resistance

7. Enough rigidity to enable user to establish accurate distance and position of object detected without excessive whip or bend, maintaining original shape under stress

8. Must not conduct significant amounts of thermal or electrical energy

9. Adequate transmission of vibrations from the tip to the grip to provide best tactile and aural stimulus

10. Sufficient durability to withstand hard bumps and constant usage without bending, shattering, or posing other hazards if it should break

11. High visibility to motorists and pedestrians

12. Makes minimal noise without artificial dampening devices

13. Good balance so that it is self-aligning when allowed to rest lightly in the palm of the hand

14. Acceptable appearance.

Although some agencies make their own long canes, many are purchased from commercial establishments. Various types are listed in the *International Guide to Aids and Appliances for Blind and Visually Impaired Persons* and *Aids and Appliances for the Blind and Visually Impaired* (American Foundation for the Blind, 1977; 1977-78).

11

Advantages

The long cane is the most effective and efficient mobility aid yet devised for safe, independent travel by the majority of visually impaired people. The scanning system in which the user operates the cane supplies echo-ranging cues and force-impact data that give vital information about immediate environment. It informs the traveler about the nature and condition of the surface underfoot, gives sufficient forewarning of downsteps or dropoffs to prevent falls or injury, and protects the lower part of the body from collision. The cane informs the user about various ground-surface textures which can be related to specific areas and destinations. It is a highly maneuverable aid that allows investigation of the environment without actual hand contact. The long cane is reliable, long lasting, and somewhat unaffected by unfavorable weather and temperature conditions. Most require no accessories, and virtually no maintenance except occasional replacement of a worn tip. The cane can be accommodated to most users' physical specifications and, in some instances, their disabilities.

Disadvantages

There are, however, some disadvantages peculiar to the long cane and its use. Primarily it does not provide adequate protection against collision to the upper part of the body. The long cane is non-collapsible, and storing it at social gatherings, in public or private transportation, or when following a sighted guide presents a problem. There is also the danger of tripping pedestrians in congested areas. Cane tips do break or wear out and must be replaced. High winds sometimes interfere with maneuverability of the cane, and the long cane is not a weight bearing or support cane. Although the scanning process employed is functional, the length of the cane limits the range and amount of information transmitted to and received by the user. In addition, learning to use the long cane requires extensive training.

FOLDING OR COLLAPSIBLE CANES

Many efforts have been made to develop a satisfactory folding or collapsible cane. The first collective effort to discuss status, make recommendations, and set tentative standards was made by mobility specialists, researchers, and mobility consumers at a Mobility Research Conference of the Massachusetts Institute of Technology in 1963. The Conference, sponsored by the American Foundation for the Blind, the Office of Vocational Rehabilitation, Seeing Eye, the Massachusetts Institute of Technology, and the Veterans Administration, resulted in a project aimed at development of a collapsible or folding cane (Bauman, Gerstley, Neuman, & Ochsner, 1963).

Specifications

The following standards were established for the folding cane:

1. Weight not to exceed 1 lb (0.45 kg)

2. Folded cane must fit into a coat pocket 5 in. x 10 in. x 0.62 in. (13 cm x 25 cm x 1.6 cm)

3. Aside from collision damage, the cane must survive 5000 fold-extend cycles based on one year of use by an active blind traveler

4. Assembled unit must provide a handle and tip with "feel" and sound generating capabilities comparable to the long cane

5. While extended length cannot be changed by user, design must include

provisions for supplying cane assembly in 2-in. (5-cm) increments of length over a range of 36 in. to 70 in. (91 cm to 178 cm)

6. Should be easy to open and close

7. One-handed operation should be possible in opening, closing, locking, and storing procedures

8. Simple overall design with assembly of component parts that do not require specialized techniques

9. A realistic mass market price of under $10.00.

Other requirements for consideration are:

1. Closest possible mechanical equivalent to the conventional long cane when extended (Massachusetts Institute of Technology, 1965)

2. Ability to be collapsed and expanded quickly

3. Tip should be sensitive, durable, and constructed so as not to stick or catch in cracks or on rough surfaces

4. Reasonable freedom from operational failure

5. Should be well balanced so as to center and align easily

6. Joints should be self-cleaning

7. A continuous metallic path along the cane axis, to provide the same vibrotactile information capabilities as a one-piece unit

8. Should not require retraining to use.

Types

The two basic types of collapsible canes are the folding cane and the telescopic cane. Each has two generally accepted classifications, the standard and the heavy duty.

The standard folding cane has a single inner elastic cord with a series of reductions in cane diameter from top to bottom. For example, the Mahler cane is 0.500 in. (13 mm) in diameter at the top, then 0.437 in. (11 mm), 0.375 in. (10 mm), to 0.312 in. (9 mm) at the bottom. While the standard cane is light and compact, its single elastic cord does not permit as good tactile response as the heavy duty canes because the cane is held together less firmly. The tension in some cases is diminished to the point where a person with normal dexterity can fold the cane very easily, but tactile response is reduced. The elastic cord can be tightened, but then the life of the elastic is shortened particularly when the cane is folded and unfolded frequently.

Although there are folding canes composed of seven and eight sections, a four section cane is practical and convenient, and folds to fit into a standard brief case. With seven or eight sections, the cane will be more compact when folded but less rigid and durable. Folding canes with single inner elastic cords include: the *Rigid-Fold Cane* (Fig. 1-11), made of 0.500-in. (13-mm) aluminum tubing, has four sections with three joints, a flat side on the grip as a reminder, and a tip that can be oriented by rotating it 90° from the reminder grip (Noble, personal communication, 1977); the *Mahler Standard Folding Cane* (Fig. 2-11); and the *Hycor Autofold Cane* (Fig. 3-11).

The Mahler Heavy Duty Cane has a double band of elastic rather than the single elastic found in the standard folding cane. The two elastic cords provide greater tension, holding the cane together more securely. They also provide a safety factor in that it is unlikely that both bands of elastic will break at once. It is made of 0.500-in. (13-mm) aluminum tubing and while it is stronger throughout, it is less compact. The joints are designed differently than those of the standard model.

The Hycor Cable Cane (Fig. 4-11) is also heavy duty, and features a plastic sheathed stainless steel cable instead of an elastic cord. It has six sections but because of the steel cable is very rigid when assembled. A toggle clamp inside the handle is used to apply tension to the cable in the fully extended position. The complicated handle sometimes gets out of alignment, or the tension has to be readjusted with an Allen wrench.

Hycor's Autosupport Cane is a larger diameter folding orthopedic or support cane intended for older people and those with low vision who will not use a long cane but still need some kind of aid or identification (R. Stanton, personal com-

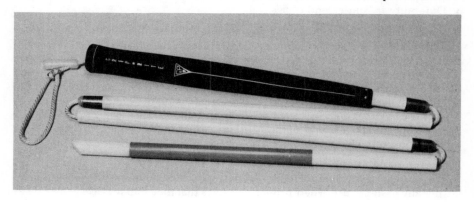

Figure 1-11. Rigid-Fold Cane. (Courtesy Wayne Noble, President, Rigid-Fold Inc.)

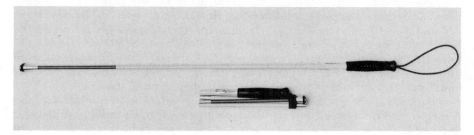

Figure 2-11. Mahler Standard Folding Cane. (By permission Mahzell Precision Products.)

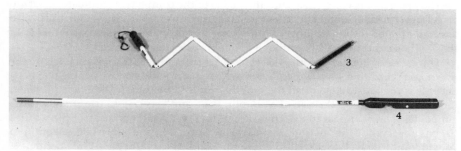

Figure 3-11. Hycor Autofold Cane.   **Figure 4-11.** Hycor Heavy Duty Cable Cane.

munication, October 1, 1976). It folds into four sections, is self-opening, and capable of supporting considerable weight.

The diversity of collapsible canes offers a greater opportunity for prescribing a cane for a specific individual, based on several variables:

1. The type of person to whom the cane is issued or sold

2. The kind of treatment the cane is expected to receive

3. Degree of visual impairment

4. Degree of traveler's activity

5. Number of sections and joints in the cane

6. Durability in fold-extend cycles.

A telescopic or heavy duty cane would be more serviceable if the cane is to be roughly handled and subject to undue impact loading (cumulative effects of percussion to joint and cable). If the user is very tall, or simply prefers a longer cane, a heavy duty cane might be more appropriate; or if the traveler is short or prefers a shorter cane, and compactness and lightness of weight are important, the standard cane might be the answer. Some people with residual vision tend to be more careful in using the cane, making relatively few contacts with obstacles. They may feel more comfortable with the features of the standard cane, and the single inner elastic cord cane would probably suffice.

Advantages and Disadvantages

Some collapsible canes are more expensive, have no better tactile response, and are not any easier to use. Their primary virtue is that they fold for ease in storing or carrying when not in use.

Some think that the folding cane has been fabricated to replace the long cane, but judgment of its advantages and disadvantages must be made on a comparative basis. Sometimes collapsing and extending the cane is difficult and time consuming, and the tension in the elastic or cable is difficult to control and maintain. The collapsible cane is not as sturdy or rigid as the long cane. In addition, hinge and cable life are vulnerable under prolonged use because of the force necessary to extend the cane. Even though greater force is required to extend the cane, it is still under a certain amount of force or pressure in the extended state.

Frequently, when sections of a folding cane get bent, the joints are also damaged, and if the elastic in a standard folding cane tears, it could be difficult or impossible to use. If, on the other hand, a long cane is bent, the traveler can usually straighten it out for immediate emergency use.

SUPPORT OR ORTHOPEDIC CANES AND CRUTCHES

The specialist is concerned with the needs of the completely ambulatory person traveling crowded areas and complex areas in towns and cities, but must also assume greater responsibility for supplying appropriate and supportive aids to those whose ability to walk or move about is restricted or limited.

The cane, or the use of cane-like objects for support, has been with us since the dawn of civilization and is a common walking aid within most people's experience. It is the most likely of all the mobility tools to be underestimated and taken for granted. Teaching the use of a support cane and learning to use it are not the simple tasks they appear to be. There are proper techniques and safety procedures to be observed. The reason for using a support cane must be taken into consideration as well as selection of the cane and its tip (Murphy, 1965; Bennett & Murphy, 1977).

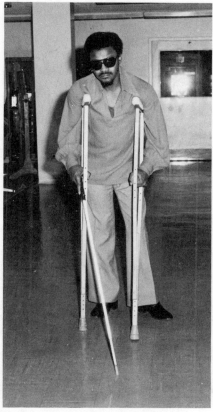

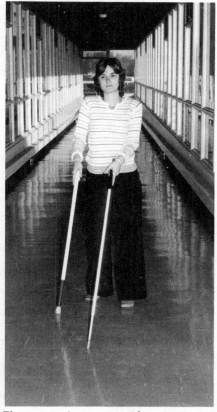

Figure 5-11. Long cane with crutches.   **Figure 6-11.** Long cane with support cane.

Advantages

A support cane should provide assistance to mobility by broadening a person's base of support, and improving balance. It provides some degree of sensory feedback by detecting irregularities of the walking surfaces, and offering increased stability on varying grades of surface (Murphy, 1965). It may help to prevent or alleviate a limp, and also can help to make walking less tiring and energy consuming.

The long cane can be used in concert with a support cane, crutches, or other mobility aids, including electronic aids (Figs. 5-11, 6-11)

Disadvantages

A disadvantage of the support or orthopedic cane is that it cannot be used if a person requires underarm support or is unable to bear weight on the hands. There are few other disadvantages; its purpose is to afford support to the user, which it does in a very practical and efficient manner.

Specifications

A support or orthopedic cane must be durable and long lasting, light in weight, and be the proper length or adjustable. In addition, it should have a safe, firm, comfortable gripping surface, and a safety non-skid tip. It must be easy to handle, with maneuverability within the capabilities of the user, and be capable of supporting the necessary weight without breaking or shattering.

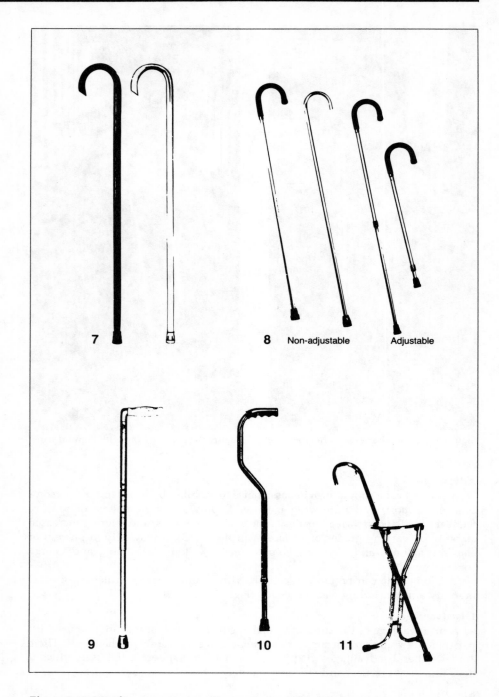

Figure 7-11. Wooden support cane. (By permission C.J.A. Preston Corp.)
Figure 8-11. Adjustable and nonadjustable aluminum canes. (By permission C.J.A. Preston Corp.)
Figure 9-11. Straight handle adjustable cane. (By permission C.J.A. Preston Corp.)
Figure 10-11. Adjustable offset cane. (By permission C.J.A. Preston Corp.)
Figure 11-11. Cane-seat. (By permission C.J.A. Preston Corp.)

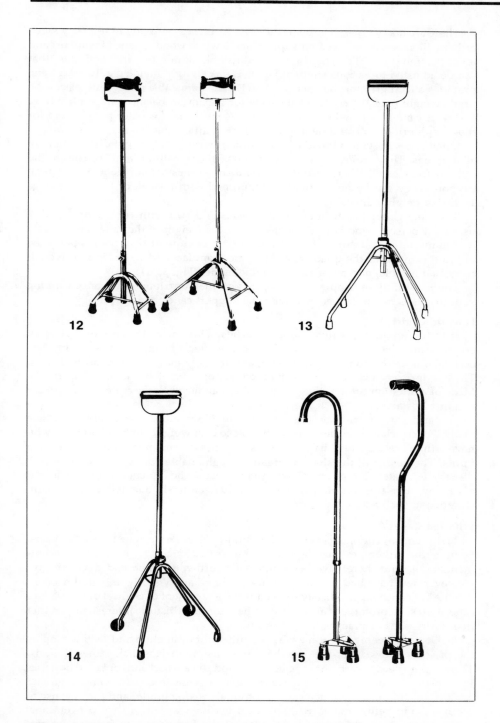

Figure 12-11. Quad canes, small and large base. (By permission C.J.A. Preston Corp.)
Figure 13-11. Height adjustable quad cane (By permission C.J.A. Preston Corp.)
Figure 14-11. Cane glider. (By permission C.J.A. Preston Corp.)
Figure 15-11. Tripod and offset tripod cane. (By permission C.J.A. Preston Corp.)

There are many types of support canes and crutches presently in use. A wooden orthopedic cane may be used for support and a white wooden cane for support and identification (Fig. 7-11). There are non-adjustable aluminum canes and those that can be adjusted to various lengths (Fig. 8-11). A straight handled adjustable cane provides a firm grip for the user (Fig. 9-11). The adjustable offset cane places the user's weight over the center of the cane for maximum balance and control (Fig. 10-11). A cane-seat may be useful for cardiac sufferers, for older people, and for those with orthopedic and neuromuscular disabilities (Fig. 11-11).

Quad canes provide a broad base of support with equal weight distribution on all four legs. They are frequently used to make the transition from crutches to the cane or from parallel bars to the cane, and sometimes for supplementary lateral support. They can be non-adjustable, equipped with a small or large base (Fig. 12-11), or height-adjustable (Fig. 13-11).

The cane glider has two legs with wheels and two with rubber tips, and is useful for persons who have difficulty lifting the weight of the cane (Fig. 14-11).

Aluminum tripod canes offer a larger surface of support than the support cane but not as much as the quad cane. They are manufactured in a standard model, height-adjustable, and an offset adjustable model (Fig. 15-11).

The possibility of tripping over the legs of quad or tripod canes or of tripping pedestrians is much greater than with the support canes and crutches.

Forearm Crutches

In addition to the conventional crutches, aluminum forearm or Canadian crutches may be used by persons who do not require underarm support. The crutch cuffs are contoured to fit the forearm to allow more freedom of the hands. The handgrips can be released without danger of the crutches falling (Fig. 16-11). Made of aluminum tubing, they have rubber handgrips, large crutch tips, and are height adjustable.

Forearm trough crutches (Fig. 17-11) provide a more comfortable and safe method of crutch walking for persons unable to bear weight on their hands, or who have arthritic or deformed hands, triceps weakness, forearm fracture, or extensive burns. The design of the shaped forearm trough enables body weight to be well distributed. Safety straps on the trough can secure the crutches to the forearm if necessary, but this attachment could be dangerous if one fell with forearm strapped to such a long lever arm.

Wheeled Canes

Many unconventional canes for the blind have been designed over the years. Some of the prototypes have been turned over to agencies for evaluation, recommendations, and there have been grants for further research and development. However, few have had any merit for use by blind and visually impaired people.

One old concept periodically revived is the attachment of a wheel or wheels to a cane. Two such prototypes are described here for their historic interest only, rather than for reasons of practicality and utility.

In 1963, the Seeing Eye Cane was submitted for evaluation and field testing by the patients and staff at the Veterans Administration Hospital, Hines, Illinois. There was no need to carry the cane because it rode on a wheel and contacted obstacles in its path. Its purpose was to enable the user to maintain contact with the ground surface, to eliminate the touch cane technique, the dog guide, and the expense of acquiring and being trained with either. The cane was longer than conventional canes to help the user to avoid kicking it and also having to lean forward at street intersections, stairwells, and similar situations. Among the obvious disadvantages were that if the cane was leaned on, it would roll out from under the user, it was not practical in snow, ice or sleet, or other unstable environments and, because of

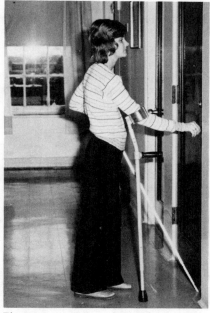

Figure 16-11. Forearm (Canadian) crutch.

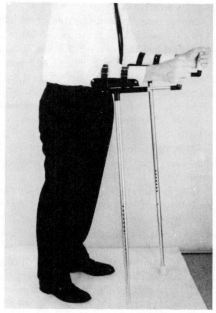

Figure 17-11. Forearm trough crutches. (By permission C.J.A. Preston Corp.)

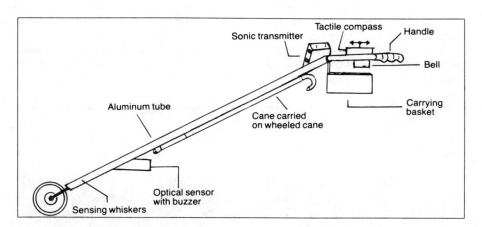

Figure 18-11. Wheeled cane.

its length, it got in the way of other pedestrians.

Another wheeled cane to be pushed in front of the user was submitted for evaluation to NASA, George Marshall Space Flight Center (Martin, 1970). In addition to being on wheels, this cane could carry other useful devices such as a tactile compass, a bell or horn to alert others, hooks upon which to hang packages, and a carrying basket. An additional wheel could be mounted beneath the handle assembly for additional weight support. More sophisticated devices such as miniature sonar transmitters and side-mounted sensing whiskers could be carried on the cane (Fig. 18-11 is an artist's conception of the cane).

High Visibility Canes

Some canes have been designed to provide visibility for the user during travel at night and under hazardous weather conditions such as rain, fog, and snow. Two examples are the Pathom Lucite Tube Cane and the Louchek Cane.

The Pathom Lucite Tube Cane was designed to be used in hazardous weather such as fog, rain, and snow, and to be more clearly visible at night. Made of aluminum stock, it had a flashing light encased in Lucite above a fluorescent impact-resistant tubing that extended to within 7 in. (18 cm) of the bottom of the cane. An electromagnetic button in the handle of the cane vibrated when the light was flashing.

The red fluorescent glow in the Lucite tube reportedly could be seen by motorists more clearly and at a greater distance than the fluorescent tape on other canes.

The Louchek Cane (Louchek Products, 1976) is intended for use as a second cane for night travel (Fig. 19-11). The plastic tube contains a light bulb that shines down the length of the translucent cane. The bottom 5 in. (13 cm) of the shaft is painted red. The device is powered by two penlight AA batteries in the top of the cane. An on-off switch is countersunk 6-¾ in. (17 cm) from the top of the cane.

The Louchek cane is heavier but considerably more flexible than a conventional long cane, a characteristic which seems to cause mobility specialists some concern but appears not to bother blind people who use it. Sunlight and artificial light render the cane light invisible, but it is effective in dark areas and can easily be seen by motorists at a distance.

WALKERS

An important aid in rehabilitative, postoperative and convalescent activities of many people is the walker (Fig. 20-11). It is commonly used in early stages of mobility training if one or both legs are so disabled that full weight bearing is not possible. Adult- to child-size adjustable walkers are available. The aluminum tubing frame with plastic handgrips and rubber-tipped legs is light enough for most people to lift. Walkers can also be used in conjunction with electronic travel aids.

Some currently produced walkers found in a well-equipped facility include those illustrated here (J. A. Preston Corp., 1974).

A push-button adjustable folding walker has an aluminum tubing frame with a single push-button control for folding (Fig. 21-11).

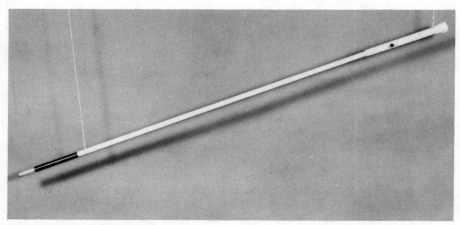

Figure 19-11. Louchek Cane.

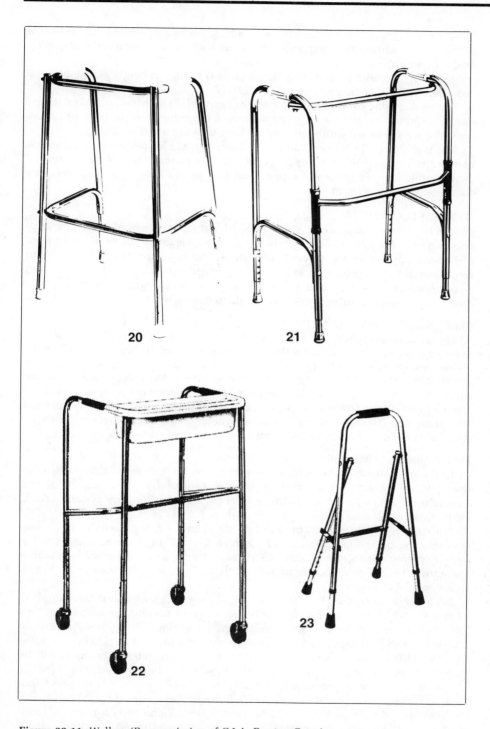

Figure 20-11. Walker. (By permission of C.J.A. Preston Corp.)
Figure 21-11. Push-button adjustable folding walker. (By permission of C.J.A. Preston Corp.)
Figure 22-11. Walking aid with wheels. (By permission of C.J.A. Preston Corp.)
Figure 23-11. Walker-cane combination. (By permission of C.J.A. Preston Corp.)

A walker with crutch attachments is an adjustable folding walker that has a pair of removable, adjustable crutch attachments with arm pads to be used in very early stages of ambulation training. (See Appendix C.)

A walking aid with wheels is designed for easy rolling, is height adjustable, and has a removable plastic utility tray (Fig. 22-11).

The walker-cane combination is made of lightweight aluminum, folds flat, and has push-button height and angle adjustments. It combines the features of a quad cane and walker to constitute an intermediate walking aid (Fig. 23-11).

The Walkamatic Reciprocal Motion Walker is an aid for relearning a reciprocal gait before using crutches, a support cane, or a long cane. The walker has special swivel joints to allow reciprocal action. Each side moves forward alternatively in a controlled pattern (Fig. 24-11).

OTHER SPECIALISTS

It is important that mobility specialists, who are inexperienced in the prescription and use of support canes, crutches, and other walking aids, seek advice from orthopedists, physiatrists, physical therapists, and corrective therapists who can recommend the appropriate aid for the particular disability. They can also recommend conditioning and reconditioning exercise programs that will avoid damaging or overstraining weak and debilitated muscles.

ELECTRONIC TRAVEL AIDS

However resourcefully and widely the long cane is used, it does have disadvantages, the commonest of which is the inability of the touch technique to scan all the space through which the body travels. The body from the waist up is vulnerable to physical contact with objects or people (Suterko, 1967). More important is that the information the cane provides is transmitted at the moment of contact—not before! The mobility specialist must be aware not only of the virtues of the long cane but also recognize its shortcomings to seek remedies and supplements. Electronic travel aids (ETAs) and sensory systems offer some answers and alternatives.

History and Development

In the past, inventors sometimes designed devices that were decades ahead of the state of the art and technology. Several historical reviews document the research and development of electronic travel devices and sensory systems (Zahl, 1962; Bliss, 1966). One of the best is by Nye and Bliss (1970).

Noiszewski's Elektroftalm, built in 1897 (Starkiewicz & Kuliszewski, 1963), and D'Albe's Exploring Optophone, in 1912 (Nye & Bliss, 1970), remarkable as they were, represent unorganized, random attempts by talented, visionary men working under the technological limitations of their times to try to contribute to the well-being of the blind.

As a result of studies by the Office of Scientific Research and Development during World War II, the first serious collective effort was made to develop ETAs and sensory systems (Zahl, 1950; Dupress, 1963). Haskins Laboratories, Stromberg Carlson, Brush Development Company, Hoover Company, the Franklin Institute, and the United States Army Signal Corps, were the research centers involved. In 1945 the National Academy of Sciences (NAS)—National Resource Council (NRC) took over the task of improvement and development of sensory aids for blind and visually handicapped persons (NAS, 1968). Support was assumed by the Army and the Veterans Administration. In addition to the central laboratory for research and evaluation at Haskins Laboratories, mobility studies continued. Work was done on reading aids by Naumberg and Radio Inventions, and by Radio Corporation of America (RCA). Dartmouth Eye Institute, Perkins Institute, and Franklin Institute developed magnifiers for the partially sighted.

In 1950, before the Korean conflict, the Veterans Administration (VA) contracted with Haverford College to field test 25 models of a Signal Corps sensory aid (a large hand-held device) designed by Lawrence Cranberg and produced by RCA (Benham, 1952; Benham & Benjamin, 1963). The contract called for an evaluation of the device and recommendations for the development of an improved ETA (Benjamin, 1968). Based on the recommendations, further laboratory investigation was conducted by Biophysical Instruments, Inc. (later Bionic Instruments, Inc.), initially as a subcontractor under a VA contract with Haverford and later as a direct VA contractor. This research and development project produced successive models, including the intermediate C5 Obstacle Detector evaluated under VA contract by TRACOR (Deatherage, 1965) and culminated in the production model C5 Laser Cane.

Since the early 1960s many conferences and meetings have been held at which electronic travel devices and sensory aids were discussed and demonstrated and many other factors in the environment-user-device interface widely explored. Examples are: in June 1962, the International Congress on Technology and

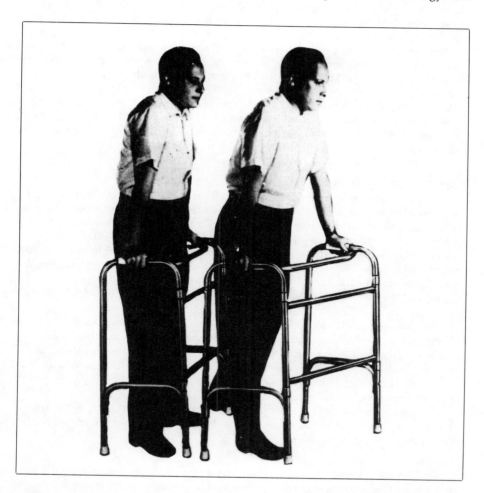

Figure 24-11. Walk-A-Matic Reciprocal Motion Walker. (By permission of C.J.A. Preston Corp.)

371

Blindness in New York; in August 1964, the Rotterdam Mobility Research Conference; the Conference on the Ultrasonic Spectacles for the Blind, Chicago, 1970; the Conference on the VA-Bionic Instruments, Inc., C4 Laser Typhlocane, Hines, Illinois, 1970; and the Conference on Travel in Adverse Weather, Minneapolis, 1975.

Following World War II, many sensory aids were built and exhibited representing various principles and systems. Some devices, such as "Optar" (Kallman, 1950, 1954), were *passive* aids which "peered" into space and responded to ambient light reflected from objects within range. However, most of the ETAs were active systems that radiated a beam or cone of electromagnetic or acoustic energy into the environment and operated when the reflected signal or echo was detected by the receiving mechanism of the device. At the present time in the evolution of sensory aids, it is estimated that more than 30 devices have been built or designed. Of these, only a small number have survived beyond the prototype stage and fewer still have survived to the field testing phase.

Three ETAs that showed promise in the 1950s and 1960s, the Lindsay Russell Pathsounder, the Bionic Laser Typhlocane (C5 Laser Cane), and the Sonicguide, have been field tested, used in training programs, and shown to be useful in dynamic travel situations.

Sensory aids are not the answer to all the problems that the blind or visually impaired traveler encounters. With one exception, the laser cane, ETAs are secondary devices designed to be used in conjunction with the only proven and accepted primary modes for independent travel, a dog guide or long cane. The user of an ETA must not expect the device to compensate for liabilities such as lack of orientation, or poor cane technique and travel skills. A candidate for a sensory aids program should be one who has successfully completed formal training at a dog guide school, or an orientation and mobility training course in a blind rehabilitation center or agency (Miyagawa, 1974; Thornton, 1975).

DEFINITION AND PURPOSE

An ETA may be described as a device that sends out signals to sense the environment within a certain range or distance, processes the information received, and furnishes the user with certain relevant bits of this information about the immediate environment. The device should probe the immediate area, sense the situation, and present the detected information to the traveler in an intelligible and useful manner. An ETA should, either of itself or in concert with a cane or dog guide, inform the traveler of objects in the travel path from the ground to the vicinity of the head, as well as forewarn of any surface discontinuities that might constitute a safety hazard (Farmer, 1975).

With the dog guide and long cane proven, accepted, and used extensively and effectively, why is so much money and effort spent on the research and development of sensory aids—particularly when specialists who are involved in the training and use of ETAs report that experience, evaluation, and consumer interviews show that demonstrating further improvement in mobility performance can sometimes be very difficult?

The answer lies in two separate but related areas; the functions that the aid was engineered to perform for the consumer, and the benefits that consumers feel they receive from using the device.

Function

An ETA can provide a degree of sensory insight into the environment which, even under the most ideal circumstances, would not be possible using only a long cane or dog guide. A sensory aid detects and locates objects, provides information that allows the user to determine (within acceptable tolerances) range, direction, dimension and height of objects. It makes noncontact trailing and tracking possible, enabling the traveler to receive directional indications from physical structures that have strategic location in the environment. With the Sonicguide it is even possible to achieve a degree of primitive object identification because the timbre of the auditory signal may give clues about the nature of the surface being detected (Farmer, 1975).

Benefits

ETA users with long cane experience particularly appreciate the early warning nature of the laser cane and experience fewer collisions (Advisory Panel for Evaluation of the Laser Cane, 1974). Some say the additional detection range of the beams is a convenience in searching for landmarks or scanning the environment. Many have a greater sense of well-being and believe that because they feel safer and more secure, they move about with less tension. Some indicate that for the first time in their experience as travelers they have the option to avoid or make contact with objects, or just use them for orientation or reference points. There are many times when contact *is* desirable and it is gratifying to know when one is within range of the target and can follow the electronic beam to within cane reaching or hand touching distance.

Airasian's (1973) evaluation of Binaural Sensory Aid trainees reported that although use of the device did not seem to increase independent travel, shorten travel time, or improve travel patterns, it was rated quite favorably as a mobility aid. Trainees reported better mobility on a wide range of travel skills with reduced travel stress, and travel in a wider variety of areas than before training. Trainees claimed a better understanding of the environment, more accurate location and identification of objects, and better distance determination.

A blind man interviewed by Farmer (1975) on laser cane use reported that being adventitiously blind, he had had to learn to listen more carefully and that there were gaps in his ability. He felt that the ETA tended to fill in the gaps in his hearing so that he was more than twice as efficient in traveling with the aid than he had been without it.

Guidelines

Before 1970, some investigators and developers went their separate ways without much communication and cooperation with mobility specialists. Many sensory devices designed failed to meet even the most fundamental travel needs of visually impaired consumers because of a lack of uniform guidelines.

While sensory devices differ in principle, design, display, and output, there are many like functions that they must perform as secondary travel aids. At present no one device meets all of the requirements for an ideal aid but guidelines for such an ETA can be set forth.

Benham (1952, 1953, and 1954) and Benjamin (1968) suggested that a device should detect obstacles, and indicate their approximate location and distance. It should detect downsteps and holes, upsteps and low obstacles, be small, lightweight, easily stored, and easily picked up and put down. Dupress (1963) felt that the readout from the device should be synchronized with other cues, that it should give the traveler additional navigation and orientation information, and that the data from the device should be simple enough for quick interpretation without extensive training. He also felt that the device should give no false cues and the traveler's attention be readily secured without fatigue or accommodation.

Farmer (1975) stated that an electronic travel device must serve its intended purpose of helping and not hindering the basic mobility process. It should have specifications that manufacturers are required to meet. It must not, in any way, interfere with natural sensory channels or association with the environment. The aid should have a minimum of accessories, boxes, and connecting cords with the option of an auditory or tactile output; or a combination of these and other possible future outputs. It must be reliable and durable, reflecting good quality control that guarantees interchangeability among models of the same generation without ill effects. Parts should be interchangeable among modified versions of the same generation of models. Updated models should not render standard parts or batteries obsolete or unusable. Repairs should be infrequent but, when necessary, should be done quickly. The ETA should be waterproof and operate well in abnormal environmental conditions. The device should be designed to make the use of a wireless telemetry system (useful in mobility training and research contexts) economically feasible.

Rechargeable batteries should be accessible for removal or replacement. Batteries should have serial numbers and be dated. They should be capable of running continuously for five hours or more and should have a life of from three to five years. Chargers should be completely automatic, capable of charging at least two batteries simultaneously, and have audible controls (vibratory or tactile for persons with hearing impairments) which, when activated, would indicate whether the batteries were fully charged, charging, or completely flat.

Finally, but by no means least important, ETAs must be cosmetically acceptable!

Candidate Requirements

Whenever ETAs are discussed at conferences and workshops, participants frequently want to know the requirements for entry to a sensory aids program, and if any prescriptive criteria for matching a person with an aid have been developed. At present, there is no standard list of requirements for participation, although agencies with ETA programs usually have their own guidelines by which they determine the eligibility of applicants for those programs. Little work has been done in developing criteria for matching a person to an aid.

The Veterans Administration orientation and mobility research specialists use a general set of guidelines for candidate selection to acquaint blinded veterans, their families, and VA personnel with the ETA program and to help referring agents who serve the veterans (see Appendix B). The candidate who has light projection or less seems to profit most from the use of ETAs and is given priority in VA programs. However, it is likely that certain visually impaired persons with diabetes, retinitis pigmentosa, glaucoma, uveitis and possibly others, could benefit from the use of ETAs.

Selection Considerations

When a mobility specialist screens, accepts, and undertakes to train a candidate to use an ETA, he must consider the travel history of the candidate, past and present level of competence and confidence with the primary travel mode, current and future travel needs, and whether travel is in unfamiliar as well as familiar areas. The mobility specialist must consider degree of activity or inactivity, and whether the activity is occupational, recreational, civic, or other. If occupational, is the person a professional person, or a factory, office, or farm worker, or perhaps a student?

The mobility specialist must find out how the traveler feels about the device. Is he sensitive to public reaction to the device? Is the device cosmetically acceptable? Is the signal output sufficiently private and personalized? It is valuable to learn the attitudes and reactions of family members, friends, and neighbors. These attitudes are very important to some visually impaired people.

Of major importance is the geographical area in which the individual lives and travels. Whether the area is urban, rural, residential, industrial, farm land, a new development, or a combination of these, careful consideration must be given to select a device that will enable the user to cope most effectively with that environment.

A person might have the ability and physical attributes to use a particular ETA well, but might not be able to tolerate the kind of display peculiar to that aid. The individual might prefer one output over another, or one which does or does not continuously monitor the environment. One user may want a play-by-play audio-tactile inventory of environmental events along the route while another might wish to be informed only about objects in the direct travel path.

The obvious factors to be considered in matching a person to an aid are auditory and visual acuity, motivation, and cost benefit to the individual in terms of time, effort, and money.

Although some ETAs are designed to respond to ambient light reflected from detected objects, most of the attention is presently focused on active energy radiating systems. The energy used by these aids is either acoustic or electromagnetic.

Display of Environmental Information

Two opposing viewpoints about device display and output have been expressed by Russell (1965), developer of the Lindsay Russell Pathsounder, and Kay (1974), developer of a binaural sensory aid, the Sonicguide Mark II. Both devices use ultrasonic acoustic energy for object detection and environmental sensing.

Russell believes that an aid should not burden the user with complex sounds. It should simply display information indicating to the traveler whether the travel path is or is not clear; a "go-no go system." The Pathsounder, therefore, strips away all complexity from the signal by processing or codifying the echoes it receives. Russell refers to the display concept as a "language system," because the presentation consists of a language of discrete sounds. He suggests that it is a question of giving either the headlines or the text; he has chosen to give the headlines.

Kay's approach, on the other hand, has been to design an aid that displayed the maximum amount of environmental information the auditory sensory channel could effectively transmit, and do this in such a way that the user could readily disregard both redundant and unwanted information merely by focusing attention on pertinent information (analog system).

Benjamin and his staff developed the laser cane, which employs electromagnetic (light) energy. While the Russell and Kay devices irradiate the forward and peripheral fields with an inherently wide ultrasonic cone to get environmental information, the laser cane emits three pencil-thin beams of invisible infrared (IR) light for target detection.

An Eyeglass Mounted Mobility Aid (Mims, 1972a) using an infrared source—a light emitting diode (LED)—has been fabricated and evaluated on a small scale. This device, along with other active and passive aids, will be discussed later.

THE LINDSAY RUSSELL E MODEL PATHSOUNDER

The Pathsounder was invented by Lindsay Russell while a consulting engineer with the Sensory Aids Evaluation and Development Center (SAEDC) at MIT. Much of the early testing of the device as well as development of the tactics for its use was done by John K. Dupress (Russell, 1965). Dupress was then with the American Foundation for the Blind, and later with the SAEDC. The first Pathsounder field tested was the H Model (Russell, 1969). In 1968, eleven Pathsounders were built, most for the three VA Blind Rehabilitation Centers (Russell, 1970). In 1974, the present E Model Pathsounder (Fig. 25-11) was made for distribution by the three VA Blind Rehabilitation Centers. It is a small, battery-operated sonar device

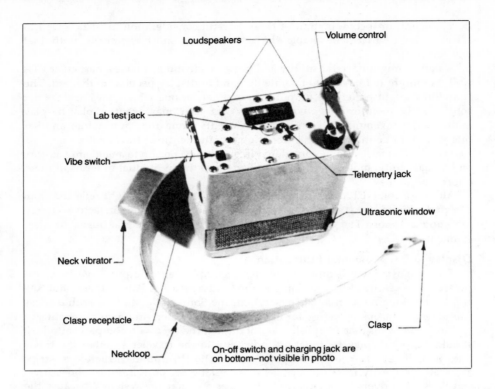

Loudspeakers

Volume control

Lab test jack

Vibe switch

Telemetry jack

Ultrasonic window

Neck vibrator

Clasp receptacle

Clasp

Neckloop

On-off switch and charging jack are
on bottom–not visible in photo

Figure 25-11. E Model Pathsounder.

designed as a secondary ETA—to complement, but not replace, the long cane.
Chest mounted, it warns the user of objects within the field of view above and
below the waist, just outside shoulder width, and in the direct travel path. The
Pathsounder emits bursts of ultrasonic waves into space 15 pulses-per-second with
a maximum diameter sonic cone of approximately 20-24 in. (50-61 cm) at a distance
of 6 ft (182 cm) from the traveler's chest. The E Model Pathsounder, unlike its
predecessor, the H Model, has two output signals—vibratory (tactile) and auditory.

With this device if there is no reflecting surface within the irradiated zone, and
hence no echo, there is no output. When the traveler is within 6 ft (182 cm) of an
object, echoes from objects within the outer protection zone, 31-72 in. (79-182 cm),
are detected by the receiving transducers of the Pathsounder. (Transducers are the
electronic components which convert one form of energy to another, as a
microphone converts sound energy to electrical energy or a LED converts electrical
energy into light energy.) The information is processed or coded and displayed to
the user by means of an output which can be auditory, vibratory, or both. The
auditory output, while the target is in the outer protection zone, is a buzzing
sound that changes to a high-pitched beeping sound when something appears
within the 32-in. (81-cm) inner protection zone. Echoes from objects further out
than 6 ft (182 cm) are excluded from presentation by timing circuits. In accordance
with the "go-no go" concept, no special electronic status is given to objects of
varying size, and all echoes are reduced to a uniform level by the use of a circuit
limiter.

Vibratory signals are available to indicate the presence of objects in the same zones. When an object is detected in the outer protection zone, the entire unit vibrates rapidly on the chest (chestvibes), and when the object appears in the inner protection zone, the chestvibes stop and a neckstrap vibrator activates a vibration against the back of the neck (neckvibes).

The vibratory system was incorporated to serve the hearing-disabled blind person, to replace an auditory signal in a noisy location where masking of sounds might take place, and as an inconspicuous private signal (Russell, 1974).

The ultrasonic waves that detect objects are emitted through the screened ultrasonic window or opening in the front of the Pathsounder and must never be blocked by clothing. The unit does not usually hang vertically on a person's body but tilts upward, and tilt allowance is incorporated in the design. An arrow on the left side of the device indicates the direction of maximum sensitivity for a person of normal build and posture, and should point horizontally ahead. The device may be returned to the manufacturer for adjustment to accommodate postural differences.

The pathsounder also has a simple ranging capability called "ramp," that produces a buzz when an object approaches or is approached, at first faint, then growing louder and louder. When operating in a noisy environment, this feature should be set at full volume.

The external rubber sonar horns which transmitted the ultrasonic pulses and received the echoes from objects on the H Model Pathsounder were considered cosmetically unsightly by some users. The E Pathsounders have rubber horns too, but they are now inside the unit. The cosmetic improvement makes the unit less sensitive to close objects such as clothing and other poor reflectors.

Factory Modifications

The E Model Pathsounder is still of experimental design but has been developed

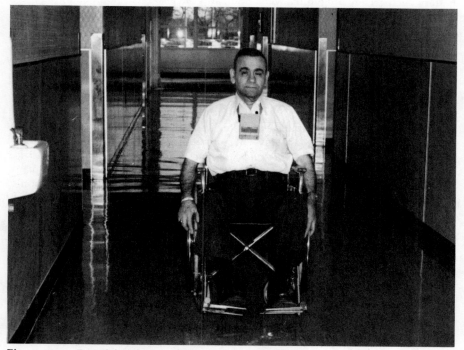

Figure 26-11. E Model Pathsounder in use with wheelchair.

so that quick modifications can be made. For instance, the heavy clothing can block chestvibe signals, so the outer zone pickup can be connected to the neck vibrator to make the neckvibes stronger for inner zone objects.

Although the Pathsounder was developed to supplement the long cane, by providing protection to the upper part of the body and head by giving a distant early warning, the aim has never been fully realized. Perhaps the restricted range, limited production units, and the fact that it is usually chest mounted are contributing factors against wide use in a dynamic travel setting. However, it can be a versatile and useful device to enable blind persons confined to wheelchairs (Fig. 26-11), who need upper-body protection, or those who must use crutches or walkers, to achieve varying levels of independent navigation.

THE SE PATHSOUNDER

Three prototype Pathsounder Special E (SE) units were delivered to the VA in 1975 (Russell, 1975), intended for use by multiply handicapped blind persons. The SE Model operates in the same way as an E Pathsounder but consists of two units, a headset and a control box connected by two cables (Fig. 27-11).

The headset assembly is worn just *above* the ears, and the control unit may be held in a pouch or affixed to a wheelchair. By putting the transducers in the headset (transmitter in the right and receiver in the left), the scan and search patterns are easily performed by a head motion in a natural manner. The two output modes in the SE Pathsounder are the auditory signals emitting from miniature loudspeakers inside the headpieces and a vibrator located in the control unit.

Pathsounders have an internal nickel-cadmium battery that operates for from two to five hours, depending upon usage. The E and SE Pathsounders' battery chargers have battery status capability that automatically adjusts charge time to battery needs. They plug into a wall outlet, and can also be used for charging the H Model Pathsounder.

Limitations

The present Pathsounders are not waterproof, and if exposed to heavy rain they will not function. The aid can be restored to normal operation by being allowed to dry out for a day. There are no particular problems associated with hot weather use, but the battery loses strength rapidly at very low temperatures.

Training Methods

The Pathsounder is simple to operate, and should take only 20-40 hours of training to achieve an acceptable level of competence. Training methods and travel tactics are presented in the *Pathsounder Instructor's Handbook, Operating Instructions for the E and SE Model Pathsounder,* and are appropriate for basic lesson plans. Baird (1977) discusses potential applications of the Pathsounder for exploration of the environment to help bridge developmental gaps in a blind child's life. Use of the Pathsounder seems effective for nonambulatory blind people and for training formats. See Appendix C for use with wheelchairs, crutches, and walkers.

For the past two years, a mobility specialist at Perkins has been using the Russell Pathsounder with a 30-year old deaf blind, spastic quadraplegic woman who uses a walker with wheels (C. Morse, personal communication, November 19, 1976). Before using the aid, she used to bump into people and obstacles, and had to be escorted everywhere. She is now employed at Howe Press and has a degree of mobility and independence not possible before. Morse made certain adaptations to the aid, such as attaching a longer neck strap, so that it could detect furniture, low objects, and small children. The Pathsounder was also adjusted so as not to detect anything closer than one foot, such as the bar of the walker.

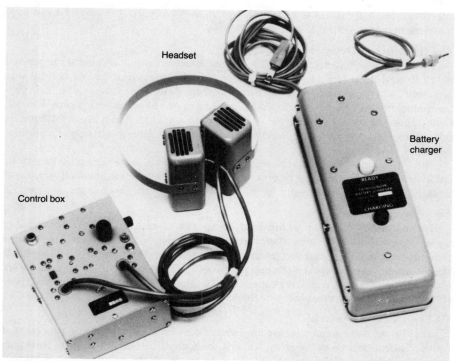

Figure 27-11. SE Model Pathsounder.

Baird (1976) has done some imaginative work with children using the Lindsay Russell Pathsounder. In working with small children, one of the best ways to communicate with them is to humanize and personalize the aid by giving it a name such as Mr. Pathsounder. Outdoor settings were chosen, when possible, to eliminate or reduce feedback, and familiar sound-producing objects used to sensitize the children to the signals of the device and to prepare them for constant signal output in congested areas.

In addition to being a good tool for concept development, the Pathsounder gave them confidence and motivated introduction to the long cane. Also, the vibratory mode gave sensory input to the deaf blind child and motivation to explore. The device was excellent for beginning orientation and mobility activities with a view to graduating to the Sonicguide.

LASER CANES AND OTHER AIDS

The Laser (*Light Amplification by Stimulated Emission of Radiation*) Cane, developed and manufactured by J. Malvern Benjamin and his colleagues of Bionic Instruments, Inc., is a product of the combined efforts of private enterprise and government. It evolved from a series of efforts using optical principles implemented with progressively better components.

United States Signal Corps Obstacle Detector

Lawrence Cranberg designed a hand-held sensory aid for the United States Signal Corps in 1943, employing the principle of optical triangulation with light from an incandescent lamp to detect objects and determine their range and azimuth. RCA manufactured 25 of these experimental devices (Fig. 28-11). Thomas A. Benham (1952) evaluated them in 1950, and his recommendations became the specifications for the G5 Obstacle Detectors subsequently developed by Bionic Instruments, Inc. for the VA.

The G5 Obstacle Detector

The G5 Obstacle Detector (Fig. 29-11) had a tactile output and three ranges of 5 ft, 10 ft, and 35 ft (1.5 m, 3 m, and 10.5 m). The stimulator in the handle was activated whenever an obstacle came within detection range. The aid was incapable of step-down detection, and would have to be used with a cane if at all. Occupying the free hand of the traveler over an extended period of time is undesirable, so the optical triangulation system was later built into a cane-like device.

The "flashlight" detector, the last of the hand-held aids designed by Biophysical Instruments, had a range of only 6 ft (182 cm), and was not practical as a travel device. However, it was useful in the development of the laser canes.

Early Laser Canes

Technical advances in minimized components such as integrated circuits; small Fresnel lenses; smaller batteries; and especially intense solid-state, room-temperature, gallium-arsenide lasers (which increased the light availability 1,000 times) made very compact housing possible. As a result, by 1966, the C3 Laser Cane became the first true laser cane and an evaluation by 50 blind users and their trainers led to the development of the improved C4 Laser Cane (Fig. 30-11).

C4 Laser Cane Evaluation

In 1971, an Advisory Panel for the Evaluation of the C4 Laser Cane was created by the Subcommittee on Sensory Aids of the Committee on Prosthetics Research and Development, Division of Medical Sciences, National Research Council, National Academy of Sciences, funded by the VA, to develop a protocol for

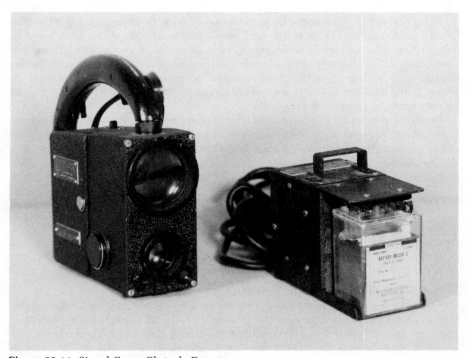

Figure 28-11. Signal Corps Obstacle Detector.

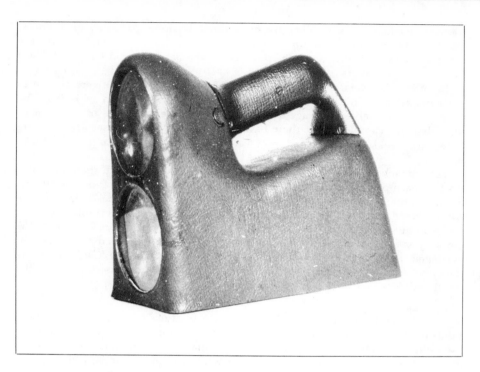

Figure 29-11. Bionic G5 Obstacle Detector.

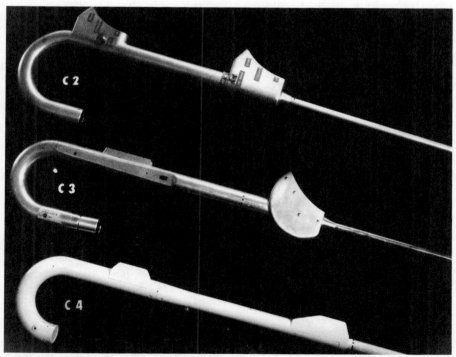

Figure 30-11. C2, C3, C4 Bionic Laser Canes.

training, evaluation, and follow-up procedures (National Academy of Sciences, 1973). Training and follow-up activities of the study were conducted by the orientation and mobility research specialists at the Palo Alto and Hines VA Blind Rehabilitation Centers.

Eight blinded veterans (four each from Hines and Palo Alto) were chosen as participants in the training and follow-up phases of the study in 1971-1972. The candidates were above-average travelers with travel experiences of one year or more beyond completion of their basic mobility training course. The training lasted five weeks, and at the end, each veteran was issued a C4 Laser Cane to take home.

Periodic telephone contacts were made with each veteran, and there were two visits to each participant's home, one after 4 to 6 months and the final one after 12 or 13 months. During the home visits, selected items from a questionnaire were administered, interviews taped, and video tapes made of travel performances with and without the experimental device and in familiar and unfamiliar areas. VA mobility specialists and private agency staff rated and evaluated the tapes and evaluated the travel performances. Evaluation results of the C4 Laser Cane (National Academy of Sciences, 1973) formed the basis for the development of the improved, less bulky C5 Laser Cane (Fig. 31-11).

The C5 Laser Cane

The C5 Laser Cane is essentially a long cane (and used in the same way) with built-in secondary electronic detection capabilities for distant early warning or "shorelining." The cane was designed to enhance the environmental-probing ability of the long cane to reduce tension while traveling, enabling the user to make more graceful progress.

The C5 Laser Cane has three miniature solid-state gallium-arsenide (GaAs) room-temperature injection lasers which omit 0.2-microsecond pulses of 9050A Angstrom, 40 or 80 times-per-second, and three photosensitive receivers. These beams are so narrow that they are only 1 in. (2.5 cm) wide 10 ft (3 m) from the source. Objects can, therefore, be located with a high degree of accuracy by discrete scanning. The upward projecting beam gives the user information about objects in the vicinity of the head, the forward beam detects objects in the travel path and immediate periphery, and the downward beam forewarns of downsteps (Fig. 32-11).

Using the Cranberg principle of optical triangulation, the device emits pulses of infrared light, which, if reflected from an object in the travel path, are detected by photodiodes located behind the receiving lens. The angle made by the diffusely reflected ray passing through a receiving lens is an indication of distance to object detected (Fig. 33-11).

The signal emitted by the down-directed channel is a low-pitched, rasping 200-Hz tone designed to alert the traveler of downsteps of 6 in. (15 cm) or greater which appear about 3 ft (0.9 m) in front of the cane tip or 6 ft (1.82 m) in front of the user.

Usually, an electronic travel aid sends out a beam of energy and receives echoes or reflections from objects detected, before displaying processed information to the user. The C5 *down* channel operates differently. As long as light pulses are received by the down-channel receiving optics, the output is silent. When a pulse is *not* received, the down-channel signal is activated and the user is warned of surface dropoff.

The forward channel has both tactile and auditory output signals. The auditory signal is a medium tone of 1600 Hz, and may be switched on or off. The tactile output of the C5 is a tiny, pin-like stimulator which vibrates against the index finger when an object is detected within the 5-ft to 12 ft (1.50-m to 3.60-m) range.

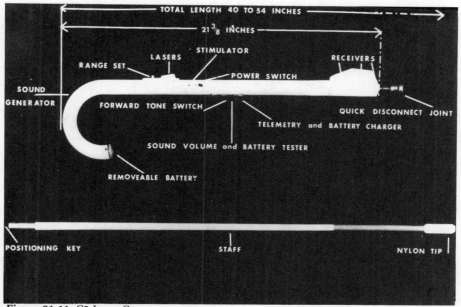

Figure 31-11. C5 Laser Cane.

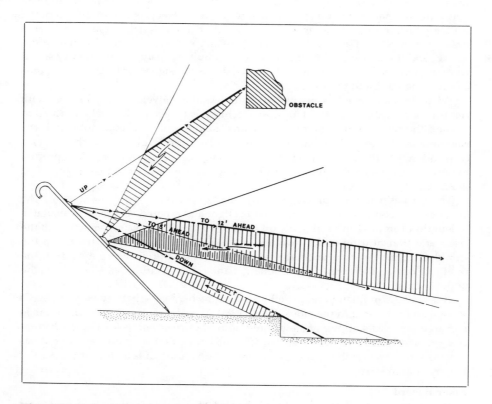

Figure 32-11. Laser Cane beam configurations.

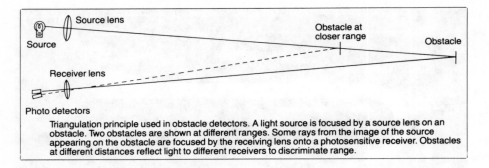

Triangulation principle used in obstacle detectors. A light source is focused by a source lens on an obstacle. Two obstacles are shown at different ranges. Some rays from the image of the source appearing on the obstacle are focused by the receiving lens onto a photosensitive receiver. Obstacles at different distances reflect light to different receivers to discriminate range.

Figure 33-11. Triangulation principle.

The forward beam will detect objects extending upward about 2 ft (0.60 m) from the walking surface. The forward channel has a range control which can be set to detect objects from a distance of 5 ft (1.50 m) to a maximum of 12 ft (3.60 m) from the cane tip. Range potential of electro-optical aids such as the C5 vary according to the size, shape, color, or angle of approach to the object. So when a maximum range is designated, it means that it was on the best possible target, a large and light-colored one.

The up-channel signal is a high-pitched tone of 2600 Hz activated by objects 30 in. (76 cm) in front of the cane tip and 6 ft (1.80 m) above it. In addition to detecting overhangs, the up channel will respond to objects which extend from the walking surface up to head level. The forward-channel signal would be activated first; then at 30 in. (76 cm) from cane-tip distance, the up-channel signal would sound, and the user would hear both signals simultaneously, if the auditory signal were on. Otherwise the user would receive the tactile signal for targets ahead plus an audiosignal if a high target appeared.

When in use, the C5 is pivoted laterally like the conventional long cane with certain modifications of the long-cane technique to get peripheral information beyond the cane tip or to monitor pedestrians, guidelines, or automobiles. If the electronic elements fail to function, the traveler is still able to use the C5 as a conventional, although somewhat heavier, long cane. The C5 weighs approximately 16 oz (0.45 kg) compared to the long cane which is approximately 8 oz (0.225 kg).

The C5 Laser Cane separates into two parts for easy carrying or storage. The lower section contains no electronics and is light and tapered. The cane is available in lengths of from 42 to 54 in. (106 to 137 cm) in 1-in. (2.54-cm) increments. All the lasers and transmitting optics, two miniature electromagnetic speakers, the tactile stimulators, the laser-pulse drive circuits, the sound-output volume control, the receiving optics, the printed circuit boards, and other electronics are housed in the upper section.

A 6-volt, 225-milliampere, nickel-cadmium rechargeable battery powers the C5 system and is located in the crook. The battery is easily replaced, takes 12 hours to recharge, and lasts approximately three hours between charges. A small battery charger is included with the cane. The C5 cane has no battery status control but has a battery test switch that generates a tone, the volume of which is indicative of battery charge status.

Laser Hazard

When laser canes were introduced, hazard of radiation exposure to users was raised. However, studies indicated that gallium arsenide (GaAs) lasers used in the C4 and C5 are of such low power that radiation danger is negligible (Epstein & Meyer, 1970; Sliney & Freasier, 1969; United States Air Force, 1970).

Limitations

It is the nature of electronic travel aids to have problems, and the laser cane is not excluded. It will not receive reflections from clear plate glass in windows and doors unless there is dirt on the glass or some object is within range behind the glass. However, it will detect door handles, frames, and kick plates. The beam will not pick up low objects, and will fail to inform of gradual slopes. Glossy and highly polished surfaces both risk oblique reflection of the beam with failure of the forward channel detection range and increase the possibility of mistakenly activating the down-channel signal. Heavy precipitation (particularly snow) causes the up and forward channel signals to go off constantly. Under these circumstances, it is best to shut off the electronics and use the cane in the conventional long-cane manner. Because the IR beam is very narrow, one must be certain to keep it pointed in the direction of travel.

Training

Training to use the laser cane is more complex than that for the Pathsounder, but less so than for the Sonicguide. For persons who are already proficient with the long cane, the Veterans Administration training course, four hours, five days a week, takes from three to five weeks to complete.

The teaching manual for the C5 Laser Cane (Farmer, Benjamin, Cooper, Ekstrom, & Whitehead, 1974) is VA oriented and is consistent with current ETA programs at the VA Blind Rehabilitation Centers.

At the Oakland Intermediate School District and Rehabilitation Institute in Pontiac, Michigan, several adults and youths were trained to use the C5 Laser Cane. They confirmed findings that those who used the Laser Cane traveled with more confidence than they did with long canes, that their pace was speeded appreciably, and that their self-image improved (Goldie, 1976). Experience here also showed that young people have less tolerance for breakdowns and downtime than older VA consumers, who continue to use the Laser Cane faithfully despite electronic and mechanical problems.

Some students were hearing impaired and had trouble with traffic alignment. However, they used the Laser Cane to shoreline buildings to establish parallel relationships with them and the traffic, and to maintain more direct travel courses. They also used the canes to monitor pedestrians and trail them across streets.

THE SONICGUIDE

The Sonicguide (Binaural Society Aid, BSA), was developed by Kay at the University of Canterbury, Christchurch, New Zealand, and is manufactured by Wormald International Sensory Aids Limited, Christchurch. Telesensory Systems, Inc. (TSI) handle assembly and distribution in the United States, Canada, and Brazil.

From its inception, the Sonicguide attracted international attention and study, and involved professionals from many and varied disciplines. The idea was conceived in 1959 but the technology for its instrumentation was not available at that time. Instead, Kay developed a sensory aid called the Torch (Kay, 1970).

The Torch

The Torch, a hand-held, ultrasonic environmental sensor with a one-channel or monaural system, explored the field of view with a wide sonic cone of approximately 30° on either side of the midline direction in which it was pointed (Fig.

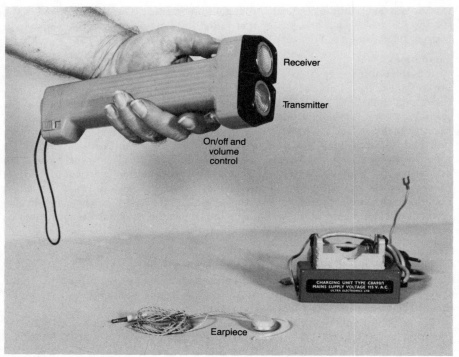

Receiver

Transmitter

On/off and
volume
control

CHARGING UNIT TYPE C8A90/1
MAINS SUPPLY VOLTAGE 115 V. A.C.
ULTRA ELECTRONICS LTD.

Earpiece

Figure 34-11. The Sonic Torch.

34-11). It weighed 9 oz (252 g) with all the electronics self-contained. It had two ranges, 7 ft (2.1 m) and 20 ft (6 m), and an auditory display delivered through an earpiece (Elliott, 1969).

The Torch has been evaluated in more countries than any other sensory aid, but was unsuccessful in the sensory aids market because it was introduced and used as a primary travel aid. In addition, it was not accepted on a universal scale by the blind population because it was hand-held.

The Binaural Sensory Aid (BSA)

By 1966, Kay had added another channel on the principle employed in the Torch for a two-channel (binaural), head-mounted sensory aid known as the Binaural Sensory Aid (BSA). In 1969, limited training and field testing procedures were possible, and Robert Pugh, an American mobility specialist, trained four sighted persons (under blindfold) to travel using the long cane and the BSA.

The Canterbury Team, consisting of Leslie Kay; Robert Pugh; mobility specialist Nancy Bell; electronics engineer, Derek Rowell; and a psychologist with additional training in audiology, William Keith, conducted a year-long evaluation for long cane travelers in New Zealand and dog guide users in Australia.

International Evaluation

An international evaluation of the BSA in the United States and Britain was formulated and was ready for implementation by early 1971, calling for formally trained specialists to teach the use of the BSA to blind travelers in both countries. In 1971, binaural sensory aid instructional courses for mobility specialists were held at Boston College and Western Michigan University. The four-week courses were attended by a total of 17 specialists.

The BSA underwent extensive training and evaluation, with many agencies from the United States, Britain, New Zealand, and Australia, participating. Not only was the device itself under scrutiny, but teacher training formats, teaching methods, teaching skills, length of effective training periods for teachers and trainees were also investigated. Questionnaires were sent to teachers and different ones to trainees (Airasian, 1973), and the response rate was 84 percent from the mobility specialists and 79 percent from the trainees. Survey results indicated that the BSA, with modifications, had potential for a certain segment of the blind population.

The Sonicguide Mk II

The Sonicguide exemplifies the analog system, collecting and displaying an abundance of environmental information to the user with the option of using all or whatever part of the messages one wishes to use, or is capable of using. As Russell suggests, the Sonicguide gives the text rather than the headlines delivered by such "go-no go" devices as the Pathsounder and Laser Cane. The aid was designed to give the blind user greater perception of the environment through the auditory sense. It supplies the user with three kinds of information, distance estimation, azimuth or directional appreciation, and interpretation of tonal characteristics which make object identification possible; the latter, however, only with much practice and experience.

The Sonicguide gives protection from above the head to about knee height. The sides of the body are more than adequately protected by the very wide sonic cone which exceeds 45° to the right and left. It does not, however, provide information about downsteps or very low objects in the travel path.

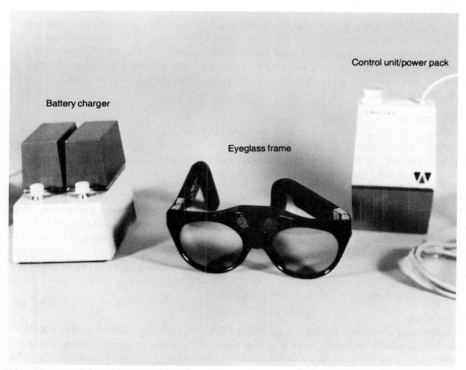

Figure 35-11. Sonicguide Mk II.

The Sonicguide Mk II is a secondary ETA to be used in conjunction with either a dog guide or long cane (Fig. 35-11). The electronics, three miniature, wide-band transducers (a central tiny ultrasonic transmitter located just above the bridge of the nose), and two small microphones (receivers) above and on each side of the loudspeaker (transmitter), are housed in a pair of spectacles and a control box. The auditory output is directed into the ears by means of ear tubes that do not obstruct ambient sound. Sounds coming from the right will be heard by the right ear sooner and will be slightly louder. Sounds coming from the left will be heard by the left ear sooner and will be slightly louder. Sounds coming from straight ahead will be heard in both ears simultaneously and will be equally loud (Fig. 36-11).

The Sonicguide signals enable the user to estimate distance by relating it to pitch. The transmitting transducer generates electrical signals that are converted into ultrasonic waves and pulsed out into the environment. It has a maximum range of 20 ft (6 m) with specular targets (large, smooth surfaces like walls or plate glass) and an effective range of 12 to 15 ft (3.6 to 4.5 m) with diffuse objects (smaller or rough surfaces like trees or foliage).

Object Identification by Signal Timbre

The Mk II enables perception of tonal characteristics that give information about the nature of the presenting surface, whether it is specular or diffuse, as well as its range, direction, and dimensions. If a user "looks" at a smooth, round aluminum post, the reflected echoes will have a single-frequency, pure-tone quality. However, a tree presents many branches and leaves with multiple frequency components. The echoes reflected from these surfaces will be scattered, presenting an electronic image of the totality of a tree, through signals of a scratchy, harsh quality.

Power

The power supply is housed in a small control box, not much larger than a deck of cards, with an on-off/volume control knob. The control box is connected to the left temple of the spectacle frame by a flexible cable. A battery charger supplied with the Sonicguide accommodates two rechargeable, nickel-cadmium batteries. A battery charge lasts about five hours, and a 14-hour recharge will restore a totally discharged battery.

Sonicguide for Children

The Sonicguide Training Aid for Children is a version of the Mk II with a smaller frame and adjustable temples. The aid was designed for use in concept development, and as an environmental training aid to enhance spatial awareness and sound localization skills in blind children (Telesensory Systems, Inc., 1977).

Limitations

In addition to the fact that the Sonicguide does not offer protection from dropoffs, there are other limitations. High winds can affect reception, and it may lose sensitivity in heavy rains or become inoperable in snowstorms because of constant echoes from snowflakes. There may also be ambient disturbances from neon signs, although they could be used as landmarks in areas frequented by a traveler. The Sonicguide output is auditory, and the signals quite possibly could be masked in certain very noisy situations.

Training

Because the Sonicguide is a complex ETA, the training period in the VA Blind Rehabilitation Centers is from four to six weeks, three to five hours a day. Training methods and formats may be found in the training manual written by the Canterbury Team (Kay, Bell, Keith, Pugh, & Rowell, 1971) and in articles by

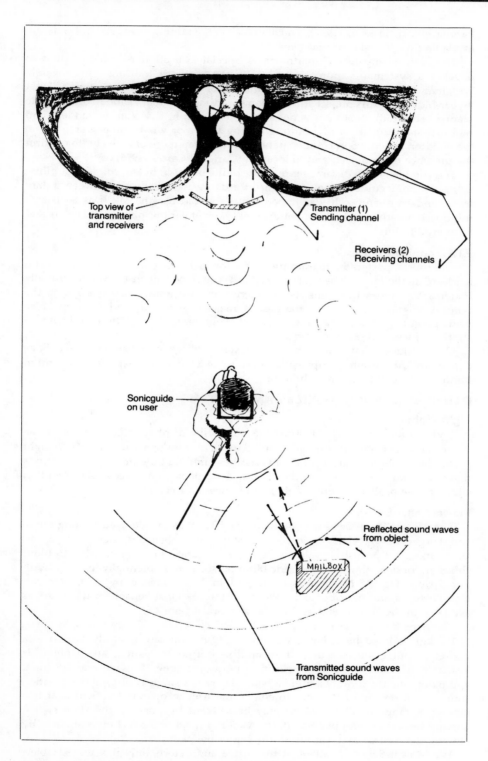

Figure 36-11. Sonicguide transmission and reception.

Farmer (1975), Jackson (1977), and Baird (1977). Training manuals and aids are available from Telesensory Systems, Inc.

The New Hampshire Department of Special Education received a grant to develop a systematic approach to low vision distance training with severely impaired children and adults through the use of the Sonicguide (Carter, 1975). A 9-year-old boy in this project still had some minimal residual vision in one eye. He scanned so rapidly that he was not able to use what little vision he had left, and had extreme difficult in pinpointing exactly where or what things were. Use of the children's model Sonicguide enabled him to scan more effectively, to confirm the presence of an object, and to locate it (Carter & Carter, 1976).

The youngster also became more aware of the use of light and color in mobility, using the Sonicguide to look for light in a doorway or contrast between a dark frame and an opening. It was hoped that he would use the Mk II as a distant-information-gathering tool, for better assessment of various objects and colors and to interpret blurs.

ETA Training Courses

A six-week postgraduate training course for specialists, in the use of ETAs and teaching methods, has been established at Western Michigan University initially under a VA contract. It consists of practical exposure and experience with the Lindsay Russell Pathsounder, the Laser Cane, and the Sonicguide, and includes principles of operation, teaching methods, program implementation, and demonstration of less well-known devices.

Other courses have been held at Boston College and San Francisco State University. At the latter, emphasis was on use of ETAs for concept development in blind and visually impaired children.

OTHER ELECTRONIC DEVICES AND SYSTEMS

Light Probes

Light probes are simple instruments consisting of photocells connected to an electronic circuit and in turn to transducers with one or more outputs. A light probe detects light sources and converts them into audible or vibratory outputs that vary with the intensity of the source. Attachments and accessories are often added to the probes to enhance their usefulness and versatility.

Mowat Sonar Sensor

The Mowat Sonar Sensor is a secondary ETA that can be used by dog guide and long cane travelers to locate bus-stop signs, benches, doorways, other landmarks, and pedestrians. It can be useful in concept development with blind children, for deaf blind and geriatric blind persons, and potentially for those with low vision (Fig. 37-11). It was developed in New Zealand by G. C. Mowat, manufactured and distributed by Wormald International Sensory Aids, and it is available in the United States, Canada, and Brazil from TSI.

The Sensor measures 6 in. x 2 in. x 1 in. (15 cm x 5 cm x 2.5 cm), weighs 6.5 oz (0.182 kg), is hand held, has a vibratory output, and can be easily carried in a pocket or purse until needed. If an audible output is desired, an earphone is available. The device emits an elliptical ultrasonic cone 15° wide and 30° high, approximating the form of a human body. There is a single control, three-position slide switch on top of the unit to enable the user to operate the Sensor at two ranges. A range of 13.2 ft (4 m) may be selected by pushing the slide switch forward from the center position (Off). A shorter range of 3.3 ft (1 m) is attained by moving the control backward from the center position.

The Mowat Sensor is silent in free space and detects only the nearest object within beam range. When an object is detected, the Sensor vibrates at a rate which

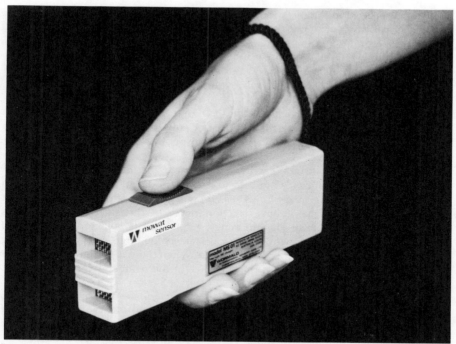

Figure 37-11. Mowat Sonar Sensor. (Courtesy of Telesensory Systems, Inc., Palo Alto, California.)

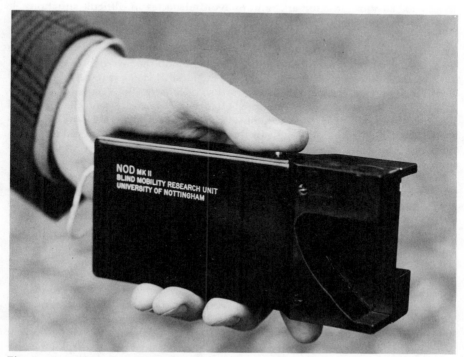

Figure 38-11. Nottingham Obstacle Detector. (Courtesy of Psychology Department, University of Nottingham, Nottingham, England.)

is inversely related to the distance from the object; at 13 ft (4 m) from a target, the aid vibrates at a rate of 10 pulses-per-second and increases to a vibratory rate of 40 pulses-per-second when the traveler advances to within 3.3 ft (1 m) of the target. The aid is powered by a rechargeable battery made in New Zealand but 9-v non-rechargeable transistor batteries can also be used.

The Nottingham Obstacle Detector

The Nottingham Obstacle Detector (NOD) is a small hand-held ultrasonic device that transmits pulses of high-frequency sound (40 kHz) in a narrow beam ahead of the user. Like the Mowat Sonar Sensor, it is useful in certain specific situations (Fig. 38-11).

The aid has eight outputs; each note (the notes of the major musical scale) corresponding to a small range of obstacle distance; 0-12 in. (0-30 cm) will give an output signal of one tone, 12-24 in. (30-60 cm) will give an output signal of another tone, and so on. The maximum detection range of the aid, 7 ft (2.10 m), is subdivided into eight 12-in. (30-cm) zones, each with its own individual signal tone. The signal tones go down the musical scale as the target is approached. The device is silent when no object is within range. When there is more than one object in the field of view, NOD signals the presence of the nearest object (Armstrong, 1974; Heyes, 1975).

The NOD has an on-off control, and a small loudspeaker to supply audio output. Provision is made for the use of an earphone with volume control if needed. The addition of an optional display, using tactile coding, is currently under consideration (J. D. Armstrong, personal communication, October 21, 1976).

A study indicated that users had no difficulty in learning the relationship between the major scale notes and the distance being represented. The aid is used mostly for location of landmarks and to avoid obstacles in difficult situations. It may also be useful in teaching concept development and spatial awareness.

The FOA Swedish Laser Cane

The Bionic Laser Cane inspired the work begun on the Swedish Laser Cane in 1972 by the Research Institute of the Swedish National Defense (FOA) (Benjamin, Benham, Bolgiano, & Meeks, 1967; Fornaeus, 1973; Fornaeus & Jansson, 1975).

The FOA Laser Cane has only one oblique, upward-directed channel. It is designed to be competitive in weight with the conventional long cane, approximately 8 oz (0.225 kg). Although in the development and evaluation stage and not yet in serial production, its cost is considerably less than the C5 Laser Cane with three channels.

The single up channel has only an auditory output, and the optics are adjusted to detect objects approximately 6 ft (182 cm) in front of the user. Objects extending upward from the ground may be detected by the up channel at a distance of 20-39 in. (50-97 cm).

The lighter weight and lower cost of the cane are achieved at a sacrifice of output. Justification for designing a one-channel information transfer capacity (ITC) device was that the consumers could not use a three-channel device efficiently. However, there has not been significant evidence in the American experience with the Bionic Laser Cane to support this belief. Consumers trained in the use of the Bionic Laser Cane have had little difficulty in processing, and utilizing three-channel information. The 16-oz (0.45-kg) weight of the Laser Cane has never been a factor because users are taught to neutralize the weight of the cane by bending the elbow and relaxing the wrist instead of employing the straight-arm conventional long-cane position. The battery in the crook also raises the center of gravity, giving a comfortable balance.

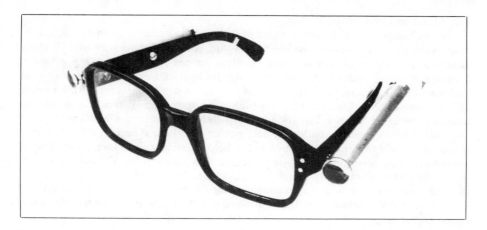

Figure 39-11. Mims Infrared Mobility Aid. (Courtesy of Forrest M. Mims III.)

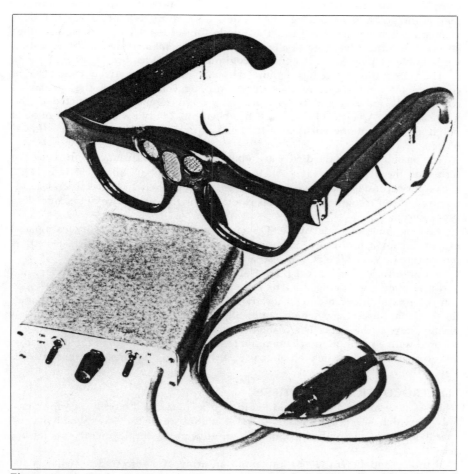

Figure 40-11. Single Object Sensor (Bui Device). (Courtesy of Department of Electrical Engineering, University of Canterbury, Christchurch, New Zealand.)

The Mims Infrared Mobility Aid

The operation of the Mims Infrared Mobility Aid is similar to the Laser Cane. The developmental versions of the Mims Aid consist of two narrow cylinders attached to temples of conventional eyeglass frames (Fig. 39-11). One cylinder contains a pulse-modulated, light-emitting diode (LED) optical transmitter that emits a train of 20-microsecond pulses of infrared radiation at a repetition rate of 120 Hz. The other cylinder contains a high-gain optical receiver and a miniature magnetic receiver. Both cylinders are completely self-contained and incorporate individual lens elements, batteries, and power switches. When an object illuminated by the infrared transmitter enters the field of view of a receiver, a signal tone is conveyed to one of the user's ears through a thin plastic tube. The tube does not block the external auditory canal (Mims, 1972a, 1972b, 1972c, 1974). No curb detection is provided so the aid should be used with a long cane or dog guide.

Farmer and Whitehead (1973) recommended redesign of this ETA to extend the range and incorporate a three-zone detection scheme.

The Single Object Sensor (SOS) Bui Device

For those who feel that the information displayed by the Mk II Sonicguide is too complex for effective use, there is a head-mounted aid with capabilities between the "go-no go" and the analog ETA. A new Canterbury Team is developing and evaluating a head-mounted aid, the Single Object Sensor or Bui Device (Fig. 40-11). It has the advantage of a limited environmental sensing capability with a very simple display (L. Kay, personal communication, October 22, 1976).

The SOS or Bui Device has binaural display with a comparatively wide beam of coverage (45°) for direction determination. The complexity of the display is considerably reduced and the sensing of the environment is restricted to the nearest object. A vertical beam of 25° has been provided to warn the user of head height objects, but one must move the head up or down to detect higher or lower objects.

The basic sounds of the device are repetitive clicks with distance being coded in terms of the repetition rate. At 16 ft (4.8 m) from an object, a rate of 30 clicks-per-second is heard, while at 6 in. (15 cm), the rate is 1000 clicks-per-second. Some character recognition of signals is retained in the Bui Device but is much less pronounced.

An experimental model of the SOS has been undergoing laboratory testing and evaluation for a few years. It has not, as yet, been extensively field-tested. A monaural version of the SOS is also available.

A Canterbury Child's Aid (Fig. 41-11) has been developed and standardized and a few are now being used in work with children in several countries. The components normally found in the frames of adult aids are placed in a durable, flexible, foam head band which can be adjusted to fit any head size by a snap-on elastic strap at the back. For cosmetic purposes, the ultrasonic transducers are covered with a nylon mono-filament material. The aid is designed for short range use so that a child can make better use of the sensing features (Strelow, Kay, & Kay, 1978).

ELECTROCORTICAL PROSTHESIS

ETAs now in use are designed to aid in orientation and mobility performance only. Research is in progress to try to develop a substitute for vision which may be useful not only for mobility, but also in education, employment, and leisure activities.

Brindley and Lewin (1968) implanted an array of 80 electrodes in the visual cortex of a newly blinded woman to demonstrate that electrical stimulation of the cortex could induce phosphenes (light spots or illusions of light).

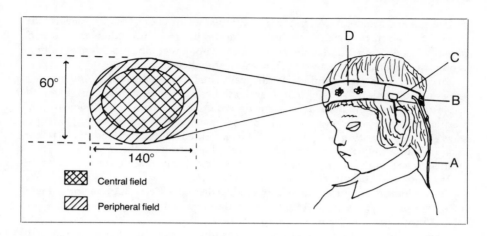

Figure 41-11. Canterbury Child's Aid.

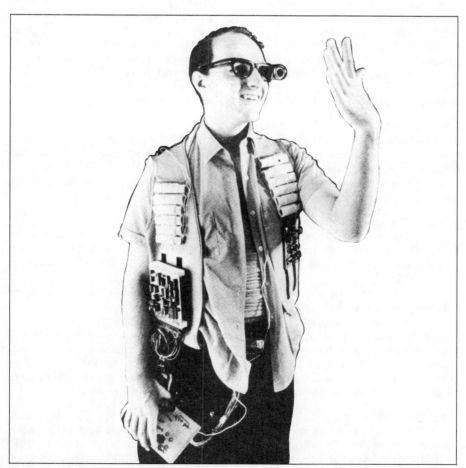

Figure 42-11. Tactile Vision Substitution System. (Courtesy of Smith-Kettlewell Institute of Visual Sciences, San Franciso, Calif.)

Dobelle and Mladejovsky, in 1973, positioned an array of 64 platinum electrodes in contact with the visual center of the brain and succeeded in inducing phosphenes in two blind subjects, one of whom was able to identify simple geometric patterns and letters of the braille alphabet.

Prospects for a successful electrocortical visual prosthesis that would result in some useful vision, satisfy moral and medical considerations, and meet the approval of the consumer and scientific community, seem remote for the immediate future because of the possible physiological risks (inducing epileptic seizures or overheating of brain tissues by electric currents) involved in electrocortical implantation: the erosion of implanted electrodes, the great number of electrodes and multiple leads required for sufficient information transfer, discomfort to user, and subminiaturization limitations.

Technological advances have provided at least partial solutions for some of these concerns. Platinum electrodes embedded in teflon have a slower erosion rate, subminiaturized cameras, components, and circuitry are now a reality, and the use of miniature computers to preprocess information might serve to reduce or bypass present hardware (Sterling, Bering, Pollack, & Vaughan, 1971; Hambrecht & Reswick, 1977).

A vision substitution system now under investigation consists of a lens and a subminiaturized camera that would be placed in an eye socket and attached to the eye muscles. A miniature computer in the temple of eyeglasses would convert light transmitted from the camera into electrical impulses, and send the impulses to an array of electrodes implanted against the visual cortex to induce phosphenes that would provide some degree of visual experience (Dobelle, 1977). Other investigators (Dawson, 1977) have proposed intervention and stimulation at other points along the visual pathway. So far, all are experimental.

Elektroftalm

The Elektroftalm is a portable, opto-electro-mechanical mobility aid that translates converted optical images formed on the photodetectors into mechanically stimulated tactile images displayed on the forehead of the user. Witold Starkiewicz has continued the work with the Elektroftalm in Poland and evaluation of the device is currently underway at the Pomeranian Medical Academy.

The Tactile Vision Substitution System

The Tactile Vision Substitution System (TVSS) is another experimental device designed at Smith-Kettlewell Institute of Visual Services to present two-dimensional patterned information to blind users through the skin of the abdomen (Fig. 42-11).

In the test procedures with the TVSS, a fairly complicated obstacle course was devised for tests using blind and blindfolded sighted subjects. They were able to discern a clear passageway through these obstacles, walking quickly and accurately and avoiding collision with the obstacles solely by means of information provided by the portable system (L. A. Scadden, personal communication, 1976).

Future development plans call for the design and construction of miniature mechanical stimulation matrices that will eliminate the use of existing cumbersome electrocutaneous displays (C. C. Collins, personal communication).

Impact on Mobility

The impact of ETAs on the rehabilitation of blind people has been widespread, and perhaps may have been a catalyst for the extensive introduction of mobility training programs. For example, the Sonic Torch has probably been more responsible for spreading orientation and mobility and long cane skills, particularly outside of the United States, than any other event.

Walter Thornton, an Englishman blinded during World War II, was taught to use the Torch by Kay, and said that it supplemented the cane and improved mobility performance in some travel situations (W. Thornton, personal communication, 1976). St. Dunstan's (an institution serving the war blinded in Great Britain) asked Thornton and others to assess the training system in the United States for possible use in Great Britain. As a result, American specialists went to England to train mobility specialists, to develop mobility programs at various agencies, and to establish a course to train future instructors.

In the past 10 years, 198 instructors have been trained and there are an estimated 5000 long cane travelers in Great Britain. The impact of ETAs was largely responsible for what has happened in Britain—it opened the door to a formal and professional approach to orientation and mobility with non-electronic aids.

The BSA also gave rise to the establishment of mobility programs and the introduction of long cane skills in New Zealand and Australia. When Kay arrived at the training and testing stage with the BSA, he brought Pugh and Bell from the United States to train blind (and sighted blindfolded) persons to use the aid in conjunction with the long cane. Up to this time there were no trained mobility instructors or instruction of any kind in the use of the long cane.

Imaginative and resourceful specialists in the United States are now using ETAs to enhance mobility performance and to enrich rehabilitative training for children, youths, and adults.

It is true that ETAs, like most electronic devices, are far from perfect, and they are expensive. Jackson (1977) discusses sources of funding for training programs and individual users. They do, however, offer advantages to many visually impaired people, addressing many special travel needs.

A mobility specialist may question the future of electronic travel aids and sensory systems. The fact is that the value and potential for supplementary use of ETAs by properly selected and trained blind and visually impaired persons has been established. It remains for the proper authorities to help make them more easily available, and for consumers and mobility specialists to use ingenuity and creativity in their use. Mobility instructors should play an active role in furthering refinement of the use of these devices.

Bibliography

Airasian, P. W. *Evaluation of the Binaural Sensory Aid*. Boston: Boston College, February 1973, 51.

American Foundation for the Blind. *Aids and Appliances for the Blind and Visually Impaired, 1977-78*. New York: Author, 1977-78.

American Foundation for the Blind. *International Guide to Aids and Appliances for Blind and Visually Impaired Persons*. New York: Author, 1977.

Armstrong, J. D. Mobility problems—a review of methods and aids. *Report on European Conference on Technical Aids for the Visually Handicapped*. Stockholm: March 1974, 64-73.

Bach-y-Rita, P., Collins, C. C., Sanders, F., White, B. & Scadden, L. Vision substitution by tactile image projection. *Nature*, 1969, **221;** 963-964.

Baird, A. S. Electronic aids: Can they help blind children? *Journal of Visual Impairment and Blindness*, March 1977, **71**(3), 97-101.

Ball, M. J. Mobility in perspective. *Blindness 1964—AAWB Annual*, 107-141.

Bauman, D. M., Gerstley, R., Neuman, L. A., & Ochsner, R. The collapsible cane project. New York: *American Foundation for the Blind Research Bulletin*, August 1963, 3, 1-12.

Benham, T. A. Evaluation and Development of a Guidance Device for the Blind. Paper given at AAAS, Dec. 28, 1953.

Benham, T. A. *Evaluation of the Signal Corps Sensory Aid for the Blind* AN/PVQ (XE-2), Washington, D.C.: Veterans Administration 1952 (Report of April 25, 1952, Contract No. V1001M-1900).

Benham, T. A. Guidance device for the blind. *Physiology Today*, 1954, **7**(12).

Benham, T. A., & Benjamin, J. M., Jr. Active energy radiating systems: An electronic travel aid. *Proceedings of the International Congress on Technology and Blindness*. New York: American Foundation for the Blind, 1963, **1**, 167-176.

Benjamin, J. M., Jr. A review of the Veterans Administration blind guidance project. *Bulletin of Prosthetic Research*, BPR 10-9 Spring 1968, 63-90.

Benjamin, J. M., Jr., Benham, T. A., Bolgiano, D. R., & Meeks, E.D., Jr. A laser cane for the blind. *Digest of the 7th International Conference on Medical and Biological Engineering*. Stockholm: 1967.

Benjamin, J. M., Jr. The Bionic Intruments C-4 Laser Cane. *Proceedings of the Conference on the Evaluation of Mobility Aids for the Blind*. Washington, D.C.: National Academy of Engineering, June 1970, 13-20.

Benjamin, J. M., Jr. The New C-5 Laser Cane for the Blind. *Proceedings of the 1973 Carnahan Conference on Electronic Prosthetics*, University of Kentucky Bulletin 104, November 1973, 77-82.

Bennett, L., & Murphy, E. F. Slipping cane and crutch tips: Part I—Static performance of current devices. *Bulletin of Prosthetic Research*, Fall 1977, BPR 10-28, 71-90.

Bionic Instruments, Inc. The Model G-5 Obstacle Detector, Contract No. V1005P-9217, July 1961—June 1963, December 1963.

Bionic Instruments, Inc. Users Manual, Veterans Administration Obstacle Detector. Model G-5, VA Contract Co. V1005P-9216, September 1962, 9.

Biophysical Electronics, Inc. Electronic obstacle and curb detectors for the blind, Summary Report on VA Contract No. V1001M-1900, January 1, 1953 to June 30, 1960, 199, September 1960 (Biophysical Electronics, Inc. was later reorganized as Bionic Instruments, Inc.).

Bliss, J. C. Sensory aids for the blind. *McGraw-Hill Yearbook of Science and Technology*. New York: McGraw-Hill, 1966, 357-360.

Brindley, G. S., & Lewin, W. S. The sensations produced by electrical stimulation of the visual cortex. *Journal of Physiology*. (London) 196, 479, 1968.

Carter, K. The sonic guide and distance vision training. *Optometric Weekly*, September 1975, 21-26.

Cicernia, E. F., & Hoberman, M. Crutch management drills. Reprinted from *Modern Medicine*, **26**(19), October 1958, 86-95.

Collins, C.C. Tactile sensory replacement. *Proceedings of the San Diego Biomedical Symposium*, 13, February 6-8, 1974, 12.

Collins, C. C. Extemporaneous comments on proprioceptive aids. *Workshops on Sensory Deficit & Sensory Aids*, San Francisco, Smith-Kettlewell Institute of Visual Sciences, Pacific Medical Center, March 23-25, 1977.

Collins, C. C., & Saunders, F. Tactile television: Electrocutaneous perception of pictorial images. *Neuroelectric Research*, D. Reynolds & A. Sjoberg (Eds), Kingsport, Tenn.: Kingsport Press, 1970, 55-64.

Cranberg, L. Sensory aids for the blind. *Electronics*, March 1946, 116.

Crouse, R. J. The long cane in Great Britain. *The New Outlook for the Blind*, January 1969, **63**(1), 20-22.

Dawson, W. W., & Radtke, N. D. The electrical stimulation of the retina by indwelling electrodes. *Investig. Ophthalm and Vis. Sc.*, 1977, **16**:249:252.

Deatherage, B. H. The evaluation of the Haverford-Bionic Instruments obstacle detector. *Proceedings of the Rotterdam Mobility Research Conference*, L. L. Clark (Ed.), New York: American Foundation for the Blind, May 1965, 201-233.

Deaver, C. C., & Brown, N. E. *The challenge of crutches*. New York Institute for the Crippled and Disabled, 1947, v.p. (Reprint: *Archives of Physical Medicine*, 6 parts, July 1945-November 1946).

Dobelle, W. H., Mladejovsky, M. G., & Girvin, J. P. Artificial vision for the blind: Electrical stimulation of visual cortex offers hope for a functional prosthesis. *Science*, 183:440-4, 1 February 1974.

Dobelle, W. H. Current status of research on providing sight to the blind by electrical stimulation of the brain. *Journal of Visual Impairment and Blindness*, September 1977, **71**(7), 290-297.

Dobelle, W. H., & Mladejovsky, M. G. Phosphenes produced by electrical stimulation of human occipital cortex and their application to the development of a prosthesis for the blind. *Journal of Physiology*, December 1974, **243**(2), 553-76.

Dobelle, W. H., & Mladejovsky, M.C. The directions for future research on sensory prostheses. *Transactions: American Society for Artificial Internal Organs*, 1974, 20 B:425-9.

Dupress, J. K. The requirements for successful travel by the blind. In L. L. Clark (Ed.),

Proceedings of the International Congress on Technology and Blindness, New York: American Foundation for the Blind, 1963, 1, 7-11.

Electronic vision. Newsweek, February 1974.

Elliott, P. H., & Roskilly, D. In E. Elliott (Ed.), *Sonic mobility aid.* London: St. Dunstan's International Manual, July 1969.

Epstein, R. A., & Meyer, R. G. *Output measurements for the Laser Cane.* Laser Laboratory, Children's Hospital Research Foundation, Medical Center, University of Cincinnati, January 1970.

Farmer, L. W., Benjamin, J. M., Jr., Cooper, D. C., Ekstrom, W. R., & Whitehead, J. J. *A teaching guide for the C-5 Laser Cane: An electronic mobility aid for the blind.* Kalamazoo: College of Education, Western Michigan University, 1975, 78.

Farmer, L. W., & Whitehead, J. J. *Preliminary investigation and assessment of the E-2 Seeing-Aid.* New York: Research Center for Prosthetics, Veterans Administration, August 1973.

Farmer, L. W. Travel in adverse weather using electronic mobility guidance devices. *The New Outlook for the Blind,* 1975, **69**(10), 433-439 & 451.

Fish, R. M., & Fish, R. C. An electronically generated audio display for the blind. *The New Outlook for the Blind,* September 1976, **70**(7), 295-298.

Fish, R. M. Visual substitution systems: Control and information processing considerations. *The New Outlook for the Blind,* September 1975, **69**(7), 300-304.

Fornaeus, L. *The Swedish Laser Cane for the blind.* FOA 2 rapport, C 2654-H5, Stockholm: Handikappinstitutet, February 1974.

Fornaeus, L., & Jansson, D. G. The Swedish Laser Cane—development and evaluation, *Report on European Conference on Technical Aids for the Visually Handicapped.* Stockholm: Handicappinstitutet, August 1974, 61-65.

Freiberger, H. *Notes from the conference on the VA-Bionic Instruments C-4 Laser Typhlocane.* Hines, Illinois VA Hospital, September 3, 1970, prepared by Research and Development, Prosthetic and Sensory Aids Service, Veterans Administration, New York: September 1970, 7.

Galton, L. New devices to help the blind and near-blind. *Parade Magazine,* Chicago Sunday Sun Times, April 1977, 18-21.

Goldie, D. *Some considerations on the use of the C-5 Laser Cane with school age children.* Paper presented at the Michigan Chapter of American Association of Workers for the Blind, October 11, 1976.

Goldie, D. Use of the C-5 Laser Cane by school age children. *The Journal of Visual Impairment and Blindness,* October 1977, **71**(8), 346-348.

Guarniero, G. Tactile vision: A personal view. *The Journal of Visual Impairment and Blindness,* March 1977, **71**(3), 125-130.

Hambrecht, F. T., & Reswick, J. B. (Eds.) *Functional electrical stimulation: Applications in neural prosthesis.* Biomed. Engng. and Instr. Series (3) 543 pages, 1977.

Heyes, A. D. The work of the Blind Mobility Research Unit, *Proceedings of the International Conference on Devices and Systems,* Philadelphia: Krusen Center for Research and Engineering, Temple University Health Sciences Center, April 1975, 160-165.

Illinois Visually Handicapped Institute. *The Conference on the Ultrasonic Spectacles for the Blind.* Chicago, Illinois: Author, June 1970.

Jackson, D. M. *Electronic Travel Aids in the Urban Environment.* Paper presented at the Conference on Orientation and Mobility in Urban Environment, sponsored by American Foundation for the Blind, New York, March 1977.

Jansson, G. *The detection of objects by the blind with the aid of a laser cane.* Report 172, Department of Psychology, University of Uppsala, Sweden, 1975.

Jansson, G., & Schenkman. *The effect of range of a laser cane on the detection of objects by the blind.* Report 211, Department of Psychology, University of Uppsala, Sweden, 1977.

Juurmaa, J. On the accuracy of obstacle detection by the blind—Part 2. *New Outlook for the Blind,* 1970, **64**, 104-118.

Kallman, H. E. Optar, a method of optical automatic ranging as applied to a guidance device for the blind. *Proceedings I.R.E.,* **42**, 1438-1446, 1954.

Kallman, H. E. Optar, a new system of optical ranging. *Electronics,* 1950, **23**(4), 102-105.

Kay, L. Active energy radiating systems: Ultrasonic guidance for the blind. *Proceedings of the International Congress on Technology and Blindness.* New York: American Foundation for the Blind, 1963, **1**, 137-156.

Kay, L. An aid to mobility for the blind—what progress in ten years? In P. W. Nye (Ed.), *Proceedings of the Conference on the Evaluation of Mobility Aids for the Blind.* Washington, D.C., National Academy of Engineering, November 1970, 20-28.

Kay, L. A sonar aid to enhance spatial perception of the blind: Engineering design and evaluation. *The Radio and Electronic Engineer,* November 1974, **44**(11), 605-627.

Kay, L. *Blind Aid, U.S. patent Specification No. 3,366,922.*

Kay, L. Sonar glasses for the blind, a progress report, New York: *American Foundation for the Blind Research Bulletin,* January 1973, 25, 25-58.

Kay, L. The Sonic Glasses evaluated. *The New Outlook for the Blind,* January 1973, **67**(1), 7-11.

Kay, L. Ultrasonic mobility aids for the blind. In L. L. Clark (Ed.) *Proceedings of the Rotterdam Mobility Research Conference.* New York: American Foundation for the Blind, May 1965, 9-16.

Kay, L., Bell, N. E., Keith, W. J., Pugh, R. W., & Rowell, D. *Lesson notes for training course on the Binaural Sensory Aid.* Chestnut Hill, Mass.: Boston College, April 21-May 7, 1971.

Kay, L., Bui, S. T., Brabyn, J. A., & Strelow, E. R. Single Object Sensor: A simplified binaural mobility aid. *Journal of Visual Impairment and Blindness,* May 1977, **71**(5), 210-213.

Keen, K. Coupling the output of the "Sonicguide" to the ear of the user. *The New Outlook for the Blind,* September 1976, **70**(7), 304-306.

Kurcz, E. Elektroftalm—a mobility aid with a tactile display. *Report on European Conference on Technical Aids for the Visually Handicapped,* Stockholm: March 1974, 67-73.

Laenger, C. J., Sr., Owen, T. E., Peters, W. R., & Suhler, S. A. *A proposal for a mobility aid for the blind.* San Antonio: Southwest Research Institute, April 1973.

Louchek Products, 870 South Gramercy Place, Los Angeles, California 90005: Author, 1976.

Malamazian, J. D. The first 15 years at Hines. *Blindness—1970—AAWB Annual,* Washington, D.C.: American Association of Workers for the Blind, 59-77.

Mallinson, G. G. Prosthesis for the blind—one billion dollars in ten years. *Blindness 1966—AAWB Annual,* Washington, D.C.: American Association of Workers for the Blind, 147-153.

Mann, R. W. Technology and human rehabilitation: Prostheses for sensory rehabilitation and/or sensory substitution. Reprinted from: *Advances in Biomedical Engineering.* New York: Academic Press, 1974.

Martin, H. L. *New type of cane for the blind (Wheeled Cane).* Alabama: George C. Marshall Space Flight Center/NASA. MFS-21120, October 1970.

Massachusetts Institute of Technology. Final report to Vocational Rehabilitation Administration, Department of Health, Education, and Welfare, Washington, D.C. From Sensory Aids Evaluation and Development Center, Cambridge, Mass.: Author, October 31, 1965.

Mims, F. M., III. An active infrared mobility aid for the blind. *Proceedings of the Electro-Optical Systems Design Conference,* 1972a, 14-18.

Mims, F. M., III. An infrared eyeglass mobility aid for the blind. *Proceedings of the Southwest IEEE Conference,* April 1972b.

Mims, F. M., III. Energy radiating mobility aids for the blind: Design considerations and a progress report on an eyeglass mounted infrared aid. *American Foundation for the Blind Research Bulletin,* April 1974, 27, 135-158.

Mims, F. M., III. Eyeglass mobility aid for the blind. *Journal of the American Optometric Association,* June 1972c, 673-676.

Mims, F. M., III. *LED circuits and projects.* Indianapolis: Howard W. Sams, Inc., 1973a, 138-153.

Mims, F. M., III. Sensory aids for blind persons. *The New Outlook for the Blind,* November 1973b, **67**(9), 407-414.

Miyagawa, S. H. My experiences with the Laser Cane. *The New Outlook for the Blind,* November 1974, **68**(9), 404-407.

Moricca, L. S., & Slocum, R. V. Pattern recognition on the forehead: An electronic scan system. *Journal of Visual Impairment and Blindness,* April 1977, **71**(4), 164-167.

Murphy, E. F. Some notes on canes and cane tips. *Bulletin of Prosthetics Research,* BPR 10-4, VA, Fall 1965, 65-76.

National Academy of Sciences, Advisory Panel for the Evaluation of the Laser Cane. *A preliminary evaluation of the Bionic Instruments—Veterans Administration C-4 Laser Cane.* Washington, D.C.: Subcommittee on Sensory Aids, Committee on Prosthetics Research and Development, Author, 1973.

National Academy of Sciences. The Conference on the Evaluation of Sensory Aids for the Visually Handicapped, Washington, D.C.: Author, 1972.

National Academy of Sciences. The Minutes of the Conference on the Evaluation of Electronic Mobility Devices for the Blind, Chicago: Illinois Visually Handicapped Institute, NAS/NRC, 1972, 33.

National Academy of Sciences. *Sensory aids for the blind.* Washington, D.C.: Author, Publication 1691, 1968.

National Research Council. The cane as a mobility aid for the blind. A report of a conference sponsored by the CPRD, Division of Engineering: Author, September 10-11, 1971, NAS 1972.

Newcomer, J. Sonicguide: Its use with public school blind children. *Journal of Visual Impairment and Blindness,* June 1977, **71**(6), 268-271.

Nye, P. W., & Bliss, J. C. Sensory aids for the blind: A challenging problem with lessons for The future. *Proceedings of the IEEE,* 1970, **58**(12), 1878-1898.

Preston Corporation, J. A. *Equipment for health care and rehabilitation,* Catalog 1095, New York: 1974.

Riley, L. H., Cohen, A. Y., Gunther, M. W., Weil, N. Evaluation of the Sonic Mobility Aid. *Bulletin of Prosthetic Research,* BPR 10-6, Fall 1966, 125-170.

Rowell, D. Auditory factors in the design of a binaural sensory aid for the blind. In *Proceedings of the Fourth Annual Meeting of the Biomedical Engineering Society.* Los Angeles, California (Session V), January 1973.

Rowell, D. The binaural sensory aid for the blind. In *Proceedings of the Conference on Engineering Devices in Rehabilitation, Boston.* Cambridge, Massachusetts: Massachusetts Institute of Technology, May 1974.

Rowell, D. *Lecture notes on the principles of the operation of the Binaural Sensory Aid.* Cambridge, Mass.: Massachusetts Institute of Technology, September 1974.

Rowell, D., Lawrence, P., & Perron, A. Volitional control for a scanning sensory aid for the blind. In *Proceedings of the Conference on Engineering Devices in Rehabilitation, Boston.* Cambridge, Massachusetts: Massachusetts Institute of Technology, May 1974.

Russell, L. *Operating instructions for E Model Pathsounders,* Cambridge, Mass.: Sensory Aids Evaluation and Development Center, M.I.T., June 1974.

Russell, L. *Operating instructions for SE Model Pathsounders,* Cambridge, Mass.: Sensory Aids Evaluation and Development Center, M.I.T., July 1975.

Russell, L. *Pathsounder instructor's handbook.* Cambridge, Mass.: Sensory Aids Evaluation and Development Center, M.I.T., January 1969.

Russell, L. Travel Pathsounder and evaluation. *Proceedings of the Conference on the Evaluation Sensory Devices for the Blind.* R. Dufton (Ed.), London: St. Dunstan's, 1966, 293-297.

Russell, L. Travel Pathsounder and evaluation. *Proceedings of the Conference on the Evaluation of Mobility Aids for the Blind,* Washington, D.C.: National Academy of Engineering, June 1970, 36-46.

Russell, L. Travel Pathsounder. In L. L. Clark (Ed.), *Proceedings of the Rotterdam Mobility Research Conference.* New York: American Foundation for the Blind, May 1965, 73-78.

Saunders, F. A. Electrocutaneous displays. *Proceedings of the Monterey Conference on Cutaneous Communication Systems and Devices,* (B.A. Geldard, Chairman), Monterey, California, 1973.

Scadden, L. A tactual substitute for sight, *New Scientist,* March 1969, 677-678.

Scadden, L. A. The tactile vision substitution system: Applications in education and employment. *The New Outlook for the Blind,* November 1974, **68**(9), 394-397.

Science for the Blind products brochure. 231 Rock Hill Road, Bala Cynwyd, Pa. 19004: Author.

Sliney, D. H., & Freasier, B. C. *Evaluation of a Laser Cane.* Radiation Protection Special Study No. 42-089-69170, U.S. Army Environmental Hygiene Agency, August 1969, 17.

Snider, A. J. New "eyes" for the blind. *Science Year: The World Science Annual,* Field Enterprises Educational Corporation, Chicago: 1976, 68-79.

Starkiewicz, W., & Kuliszewski, T. Active energy radiating systems: The 80-channel Elektroftalm. In L. L. Clark (Ed.) *Proceedings of the International Congress on Technology and Blindness,* Vol. I. New York: American Foundation for the Blind, 1963.

Sterling, T. D. Report on progress in the development of visual prostheses. *New Outlook for the Blind,* February 1970, **64**(2), 41-45.

Sterling, T. D., Bering, E. A., Jr., Pollack, S. V., & Vaughan, H. G., Jr. (Eds.). Visual prosthesis the interdisciplinary dialogue. *Proceedings of the Second Conference on Visual Prosthesis.* New York: Academic Press, 1971.

Strelow, E. R., Kay, N., & Kay, L. Binaural Sensory Aid: Case studies of its use by two children. *Journal of Visual Impairment and Blindness,* January 1978, **72**(1), 1-9.

Strelow, E. R., & Hodgson, R. M. The development of a spatial sensing system for blind children. *The New Outlook for the Blind,* January 1976, **70**(1), 22-24.

Suterko, S. Long cane training: Its advantages and problems. *Proceedings of the Conference for Mobility Trainers and Technologists.* Cambridge: Massachusetts Institute of Technology, December 1967.

Telesensory Systems, Inc. *Sonicguide, a mobility aid for the blind.* Palo Alto, Calif.: Author, 1977.

Thornton, W. The Binaural Sensor as a mobility aid. *New Outlook for the Blind,* December 1971, **65**(10), 324-326.

Thornton, W. Four years' use of the Binaural Sensory Aid. *New Outlook for the Blind,* January 1975, **69**(1), 7-10.

United States Air Force, School of Aerospace Medicine, Oculo-Thermal Branch, Radiobiology

Division, San Antonio: Letter, 23 July 170, to Research and Development Division, Prosthetics and Sensory Aids Service, Veterans Administration, New York.

Veterans Administration. *Model C-4 Laser Cane, User's Manual.* Produced by Bionic Instruments, Inc., Contract No. V5244P-675, Veterans Administration, Department of Medicine and Surgery, March 1969.

Veterans Administration. *Specifications for the long cane (Typhlocane).* Veterans Administration, Washington, D.C., April 1964. (Reprinted in the Long Cane Newsletter, Vol. 1(1):2-4, 1965; and in Proceedings of the Rotterdam Mobility Research Conference.) New York: American Foundation for the Blind, May, 1965, 243-251.

Zahl, P. A. (Ed.). *Blindness: Modern approaches to the unseen environment.* Princeton, New Jersey: Princeton University Press, 1950. (Reprint, New York: Hafner, 1962.)

11

Appendix A

Specifications for the Long Cane (Typhlocane) Veterans Administration

I. Purpose

These specifications were developed to provide a standard cane for use by persons who have a severe visual impairment or who are totally blind.

II. Definitions

A. *The Long Cane* is a cane specifically designed to serve as a mechanical object detector and environmental perceptor to facilitate physical orientation and self-dependent mobility for persons having severe visual impairment or blindness, (Fig. 43-11).

B. *The Shaft* refers to the main portion or "body" of the Long Cane and extends from the base of the crook to the tip end of the cane, (dimension B, Fig. 44-11).

C. *The Crook* refers to that portion of the upper end of the Long Cane which has been bent or curved to form an arc or "hook," (dimension C, Fig. 44-11).

D. *The Grip* refers to that portion of the Long Cane which has been adapted for grasping by covering with leather, plastic, rubber or other suitable material, (dimension A, Fig. 45-11).

E. *The Tip* refers to the element located at the lower end of the Long Cane and is that portion which normally contacts the floor or ground, (dimension B, Fig. 45-11 and Fig. 46-11).

F. *The Shaft End* refers to the lower end of the shaft into which the tip is fitted.

III. Types

A. The rigid one-piece shaft, or Long-Cane-type canes.

B. The multipiece shaft, or telescopic and folding-type Long Canes.

IV. Application

The following specifications are for the rigid one-piece Long Cane:

A. Materials

1. All metal parts of the Long Cane shall be fabricated from drawn aluminum tubing having the alloy formula 6061-T6. The chemical composition, mechanical properties and tolerances for this tubing shall

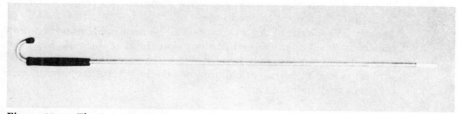

Figure 43-11. The Long Cane.

conform to G.S.A. Federal Specifications WWT-700/6B. Nominal dimensions of tubing shall be:

a. Outside diameter (OD) 0.500 in. (1.27 cm).

b. Wall thickness, 0.062 in. (0.157 cm).

c. Inside diameter (ID) 0.375 in. (0.95 cm).

2. The grip shall be a standard rubber golf club grip known as Grip-Rite, manufactured by the Fawick Flexi-Grip Company, Box 111-C, Akron 21, Ohio, or equal.

3. The tip shall be made of opaque white nylon rod, nylatron rod or equal.

4. The plastic cap closure for the open end of the crook shall be of suitable white plastic or rubber material.

B. Design

In general, the Long Cane shall be designed so as to include a crook, shaft, tip, and grip in accordance with the specifications outlined below.

1. The Crook. Beginning at a point approximately 3.75 in. (9.52 cm) from the unthreaded end of the initially straight shaft, the tubing shall be bent to form an arc of 180° on a 1-in. (2.54-cm) internal radius. The end of the crook shall extend tangentially to the arc and parallel to the shaft for a distance of approximately 0.50 in. (1.27 cm), dimension C, Fig. 44-11.

2. The Crook Cap. The open end of the crook tubing shall be fitted with a white plastic or rubber cap to cover any rough edges of the metal tubing. The cap shall be designed with walls of uniform thickness approximately 0.062-in. (0.157 cm) thick, with the covered or closed end having approximately twice the wall thickness, (detail 1, Fig. 45-11).

3. The Shaft. The shaft or body of the Long Cane shall be the straight section of the cane extending from the arc of the crook to the plastic tip, (dimension B, Fig. 44-11). The tip end of the shaft shall be threaded on the *in*side for a distance of 8 in. (20 cm). The threads will be 7/16-20 UNF threads matching those cut on the tip, (dimension D, Fig. 44-11).

4. The Tip. The tip shall be machined from opaque white nylon, nylatron, or equivalent. The tip shall have an overall length of 3.25 in. (8.25 cm) and have 7/16-20 UNF threads applied to one end for a length of 1.156 in. (3.13 cm). This shall be followed by an undercut of 0.093 in. (0.24 cm) in width and 0.046 in. (0.12 cm) in depth. The unthreaded end shall be ground with a ⅛-in. (0.32-cm) chamfer. The diameter of the tip shall be 0.50 in. (1.27 cm), (Fig. 46-11).

5. The Grip. The grip shall be fitted on the cane so as to extend downward on the shaft from a point 0.25 in. (1.1 cm) above the point at which the shaft begins to form the crook. The closed end of the golf grip shall be drilled or cut to provide an adequate hole to permit the application over the crook. The length of the grip shall be reduced to 8.5 in. (22 cm) beginning at the crook end. All material excess to the 8.5-in. (22-cm) length is to be removed from the end of the grip having the lesser diameter. The grip, cut to appropriate size will be applied to the cane so that the flat surface lies in the same plane as the crook and faces "outward" for a right-handed user.

6. Length. The length of the long cane shall be measured from the top of the crook to the extreme end of the nylon tip *after* the cane has been assembled. Generally, only two lengths will be required—48 in. and 54 in. (1.2 m and 1.37 m). For children or people of unusual height, some revisions may be necessary.

C. Weight

The complete and assembled cane including grip, crook, end closure, and

nylon tip weight:
1. For the 48-in. (1.2-m) cane—10 oz (180 g).
2. For the 54-in. (1.37-m) cane— 8 oz (230 g).
D. Accessories
1. Accessories for each completed cane shall include one package of Scotchlite Reflective Tape or coating containing one white adhesive 2 in. (5 cm) wide and 6 in. (15 cm) long for covering the shaft of the cane.
2. Each cane will be furnished with one tip as part of the completed cane, and two additional spare tips.

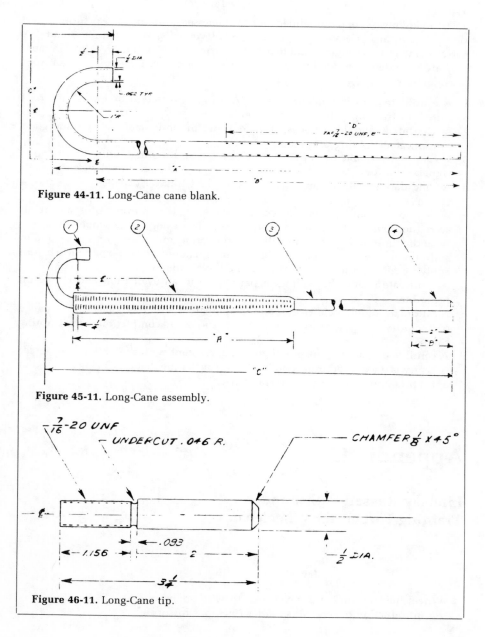

Figure 44-11. Long-Cane cane blank.

Figure 45-11. Long-Cane assembly.

Figure 46-11. Long-Cane tip.

Appendix B

Electronic Travel Aids Program for Blinded Veterans

The following general guidelines for candidate selection for the electronic travel aids program are offered to acquaint blinded veterans, their families, and VA personnel with this program and to assist referring agents who serve the veterans; they are intended as guidelines and do not necessarily exclude any veteran from consideration:

1. A candidate who is totally blind or with light projection or less seems best suited for training with the sensory aids.
2. A candidate should possess sufficient health and stamina to undergo a concentrated training program.
3. A candidate should be capable of perceiving and distinguishing the various signals (auditory, tactile, vibratory, or other) of the electronic devices.
4. A candidate should be an active, independent traveler capable of utilizing a sensory aid.
5. A candidate should have successfully completed a training program at an accredited blind rehabilitation center or agency or dog guide school.
6. A candidate should have completed an orientation and mobility program and in addition had a reasonable amount of independent travel experience before applying for training with the electronic travel aids.
7. A candidate should be willing to participate in an evaluation and follow-up procedure.
8. A candidate should be aware of and in agreement with the policy that issuance of a sensory device is contingent upon the successful completion of the training course.
9. A candidate should be aware of and in agreement with the policy that device issuance is on an indefinite loan basis until such time that it is no longer used or appropriate in meeting that veteran's needs.

Appendix C

Lindsay Russell Pathsounder Training Format for Wheelchairs

I. Wheelchair training and travel with the Pathsounder
   A. Introduction to the Pathsounder (includes history)

1. Review the Pathsounder Instructor's Handbook before initiating any training procedure.
B. Areas of usefulness
   1. Secondary ETA for long cane travelers.
   2. Travel aid for the multiply handicapped.
   3. Collision avoidance aid.
   4. Protection against collision with objects in vicinity of head.
   5. Early warning of in-path objects.
C. Practice putting on device
D. Checkout of coverage above and below the waist
E. To protect the hands, wear gloves and put curb feelers on wheels of chair (Fig. 47-11). Curb feelers may be purchased at auto part stores.
F. Precautions
   1. Work in very familiar areas.
   2. Avoid areas of travel with stairways.
G. Facings and wheelchair negotiations and maneuvers
   1. Do 90°, 180°, 45° facings, etc., incorporating compass directions awareness.
H. Trailing
   1. Trailing is done by propelling the wheelchair forward and reaching over and touching the guideline (wall) with the back of the hand after it has attained its most forward position; then return the hand to the wheel for the next and successive thrusts. If curb feelers are on the wheelchair, trailing may be achieved by maintaining contact with the guideline with the curb feelers.

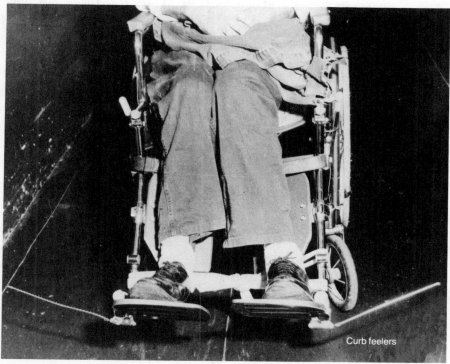

Figure 47-11. Curb feelers.

    2. The guideline may be contacted with each forward stroke, with every second or third stroke, or as often or infrequently as desired.

I. Free-lance practice
    1. Maneuver the wheelchair in the training room and in the corridors, practicing facings and moving about without trailing.
    2. Initially, the specialist may move about in front of the wheelchair to act as a guide and sound source.
    3. The Pathsounder may be placed on the front of the wheelchair (Fig. 48-11) for trainees who are semi-ambulatory and they can walk behind the wheelchair until they become tired. They can sit in the chair and rest and either resume their mobility in the wheelchair or get behind it again and push it along.

J. Detectability. Define, discuss, and give practice in experiencing and understanding the following concepts:
    1. Objects too small.
    2. Viewing wall frontally.
    3. Viewing wall obliquely.
    4. Oblique cylinder.
    5. Frontal cylinder.
    6. Corner view of square post.

K. Post drills
    1. Find the post (avoid making contact with chair).
      a. Ride up to the post after locating it with the Pathsounder beam, sonically line up with the post, and point directly to it.
    2. Circle right and circle left drills
      a. The wheelchair is placed in the center of circle of posts (or objects); all posts are equi-distant from the center of the circle. The trainee turns the chair and locates each post sonically around the circle to the right and points to each one. Repeat the drill but circle to the left.
      b. Repeat the above drill but alternate the posts around the circle in buzz (chestvibes/control unit for SE model) and beep (neckvibes/control unit) distances from the center.

L. Ride-by (discuss blind inside corners with trainee)

M. Corridor practice (define, discuss, and give practice in experiencing and understanding the following occurrences):
    1. Wall chatter.
    2. Stationary pedestrian.
    3. Double-check.
    4. Cut-across.
    5. Head-on collision.
    6. Backbouncing.
    7. Passer.

N. Familiarization of various areas in wheelchair

O. Elevator familiarization

P. Destination runs
    1. The regular O & M indoor travel routes may be used.

II. Training Format for Crutches and Walkers
    A. Introduction to the Pathsounder (includes history)
    B. Areas of usefulness
      1. Secondary ETA for long cane travelers.
      2. Useful as travel aid for the multiply handicapped.
      3. Collision avoidance aid among pedestrians.

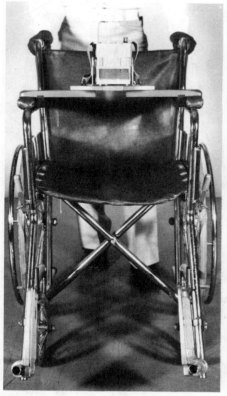

Figure 48-11. Pathsounder on wheelchair.

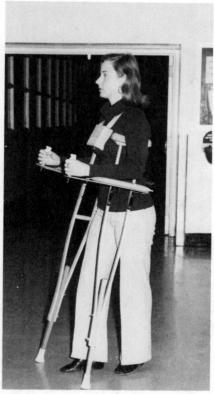

Figure 49-11. E Model Pathsounder in use with forearm trough crutches.

    4. Protection against collision with objects in vicinity of head.
    5. Early warning of in-path objects.
C. Practice putting on device
D. Checkout of coverage above and below the waist
E. Precautions
    1. Work in very familiar areas.
    2. Avoid areas of travel with stairways, initially.
F. Introduction to crutches
    1. Kinds of crutches
      a. Wooden and aluminum adjustable crutches.
      b. Aluminum Forearm or Canadian crutches.
      c. Trough Forearm crutches (Fig. 49-11).
G. Crutch gaits
    1. Four-point crutch gait (Fig. 50-11)
      a. This is the most basic of the crutch gaits, it insures that three points are always in constant with the surface, and it is a good gait to use in crowded areas because it requires very little space.
      b. It is a slow but safe gait.
      c. Order of crutch-foot movements
        (1) Advance right crutch forward
        (2) Advance left foot forward

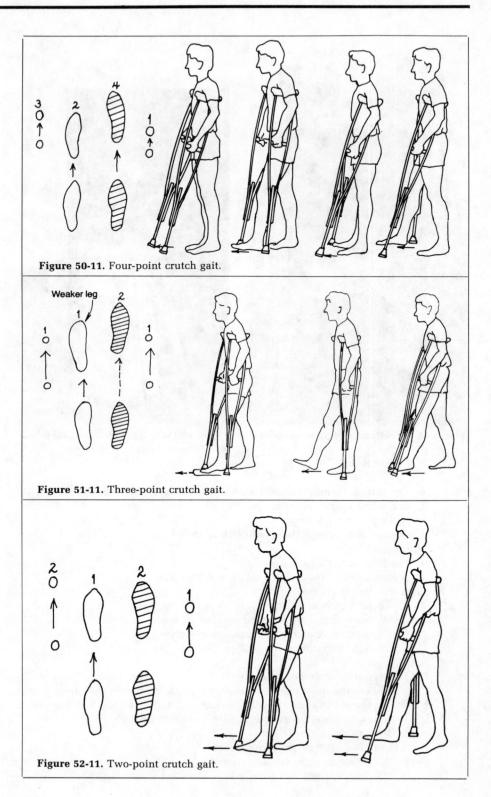

Figure 50-11. Four-point crutch gait.

Figure 51-11. Three-point crutch gait.

Figure 52-11. Two-point crutch gait.

        (3) Advance left crutch forward

        (4) Advance right foot forward

        (5) Repeat the sequence as necessary

  2. Three-point crutch gait (Fig. 51-11)

    a. This gait may be used when one has a weak lower limb which cannot support the body weight and a stronger lower limb which can support the body.

    b. Both crutches and the weak lower extremity are always on the surface at the same time.

    c. Order of crutch-foot movements

      (1) Advance both crutches and the weak lower extremity forward.

      (2) Advance the strong lower extremity forward.

      (3) Repeat the sequence as necessary.

  3. Two-point crutch gait (Fig. 52-11)

    a. This gait enables one to walk at a faster pace.

    b. It can be used by persons having good strength and control in the upper extremities and shoulders.

    c. There are only two points of contact on the surface simultaneously so better control of balance is required.

    d. Order of crutch-foot movements

      (1) Advance right crutch and left foot forward simultaneously.

      (2) Advance left crutch and right foot forward simultaneously.

      (3) Repeat the sequence as necessary.

H. Facings and crutch negotiation and maneuvers

  1. Do 90°, 180°, 45° facings, etc., to right and left, incorporating compass directions awareness.

  2. To turn, put one crutch off to one side and rear of the body. Move the other crutch across and in front of the body, pivot on feet, and turn body toward the crutches.

  3. The trainee might have to make small turns initially but with practice should be able to make a full quarter turn in one maneuver and a 180° turn in two movements.

I. Investigatory (clearance) crutch swing check before each forward step

  1. When moving crutch forward, swing crutch across the body (long cane style) to clear spot for next forward step. Do this gently so as not to bruise any pedestrians should contact be made.

J. Trailing

  1. Maintain contact with the guidelines with the crutch on that side away from the guideline by swinging it across the body. Again take care not to swing the crutch too hard and be mindful that the crutch will contact the guideline at a higher point than would the long cane.

K. Free lance (refer to #3 of wheelchair training format and adapt drills)

L. Introduction to walkers

  1. Kinds of walkers

    a. Standard walkers

    b. Walkerettes

    c. Folding walkerettes

    d. Push-button walkerettees

    e. Walk-A-Matic Reciprocal Motion Walker (Fig. 53-11)

    f. Walkerette with crutch attachments (Fig. 54-11)

M. Areas of usefulness

  1. Walkers may have to be used during early ambulation. One may have relatively good strength and power in the upper extremities but weak

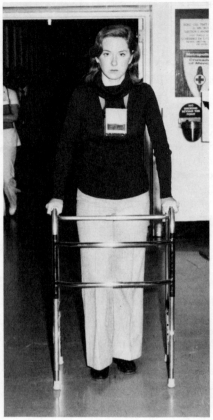

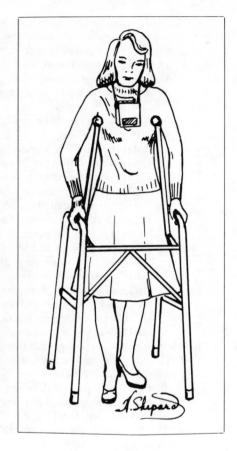

Figure 53-11. E Pathsounder used with Walk-A-Matic Reciprocal Motion Walker.

Figure 54-11. E Pathsounder used with Walkerette with crutch attachments.

lower extremities and poor balance and coordination.

2. The Walk-A-Matic Reciprocal Motion Walker offers a good, supportive and safe means of teaching a blind person early reciprocal gait training and the proper steps used in walking with the long cane.

3. A combination of the walker and Pathsounder may be used to give a person support and security and freedom from fear of making physical contact with objects which could result in injury.

N. Post drills (refer to wheelchair training format and adapt drills for crutches and walkers).

O. Corridor practice (refer to wheelchair training format and adapt for crutches and walkers).

   1. The trainee who may later travel with a support cane, long cane and Pathsounder, or two support canes and the pathsounder, before becoming fully ambulatory with just the use of the long cane and Pathsounder or the long cane alone.

P. Familiarization of various areas with crutches or walker.

Q. Elevator familiarization

R. Destination runs (use the regular O & M indoor travel routes).

Additional Handicaps

Topic 1. The Visually Impaired Amputee

A. James Enzinna

Mobility specialists may occasionally find themselves working with a client who is an amputee. A certain amount of specialized knowledge is required, including a good understanding of the proper application and functioning of prostheses, the use of crutches and wheelchairs, and the irregularities of gait peculiar to lower extremity amputees. In addition, there are considerations that relate directly to the teaching of mobility. It is with the latter that this section is concerned.

The approach to the design of a mobility program for a visually impaired amputee requires two basic considerations; which extremity, the arm or the leg, has been amputated, and where the amputation is located on the extremity. Mobility adaptations are different for a client with an arm (upper extremity) amputation than those for one with a leg (lower extremity) amputation. A client whose leg has been amputated below the knee or whose arm has been amputated below the elbow has much more strength in the amputated extremity than does a client whose amputation is above the knee or above the elbow.

THE UPPER-EXTREMITY AMPUTEE

In dealing with an upper-extremity amputation, the mobility specialist must first deal with three factors:

1. Whether the arm has been amputated above or below the elbow

2. Whether the amputation is on the client's dominant side

3. Whether the client uses a prosthetic arm.

While it is generally preferable for a client to use the long cane in the intact hand because more information can be "felt" that way, the client who has a prosthetic arm should be given the choice of using the long cane in the prosthesis or the hand. There are some whose upper-extremity amputation is on the dominant side or those who find it necessary to carry a briefcase or luggage regularly, who may prefer or even insist upon using the long cane with the prosthetic hook.

There are several disadvantages to using the long cane with the prosthetic arm. The client is less sensitive to information that comes from cane contact with various surfaces and textures such as a grassy surface, asphalt, or cement. When using the long cane in the prosthetic arm, the client's movement of the cane to

413

describe an arc must stem from the shoulder rather than the wrist. Movement from the shoulder is much more difficult to control than movement from the wrist, so many more hours of practice are required to develop a consistent arc when using the shoulder for movement of the cane.

The bilateral-hand amputee, of course, has no choice but to use the prosthesis to carry the long cane. Because this client's tactile sense is greatly diminished, the mobility specialist will have to find adaptations for grasping and using the long cane, and help the client to find ways to establish sensitive contact with sources of information. A bilateral-hand amputee who uses two prostheses loses "feel" completely. If one arm has been amputated below the elbow, a client may choose to use that arm for surface contact and use a prosthesis on the other arm. The Krukenberg operation is one solution to the problem of "feel" and grasp. It is a surgical operation that consists of splitting the forearm between the ulna and radius, mobilizing the radius which then moves independently away from, and against, the ulna. The Krukenberg operation is possible only when the client's forearm stump is at least one half the length of the forearm. The end result appears as two long fingers, which can be used in a forceps-like way to grasp things. By pronating and supinating the arm (as in turning the palm up and down), objects can be grasped in a pincer movement approaching that of normal human fingers. Enzinna described a complete orientation and mobility program for visually impaired bilateral-hand amputees in the *New Outlook for the Blind*, March 1975.

Adaptation of the long cane is necessary if the client is going to use it with the prosthetic arm. The adaptation consists of cutting off the crook of the cane and replacing it with a 6-in. (15-cm) plug tooled on the end with a groove to fit into the hook's grasping joint, and a rigid plastic loop for use with the Krukenberg (Figs. 1-12 and 2-12). Some adapted canes have been grooved to allow the "fingers" of the hook to grasp the cane and keep it firmly clasped, but providing this type of cane is technically difficult.

THE LOWER-EXTREMITY AMPUTEE

The lower-extremity amputee may walk on a prosthesis with the help of crutches or be in a wheelchair. Obviously, both the amount and the kind of mobility employed will determine the training method used. Some clients with prosthetic devices must, from time to time, resort to crutches or a wheelchair and so will need to be taught techniques for more than one means of travel.

The first consideration when beginning mobility lessons with a lower-extremity amputee who has a prosthetic leg is the location of the amputation. A below-the-knee (BK) amputee will have much more strength and stability than the

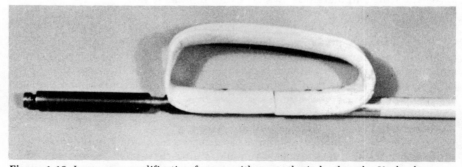

Figure 1-12. Long cane modification for use with a prosthetic hook and a Krukenberg.

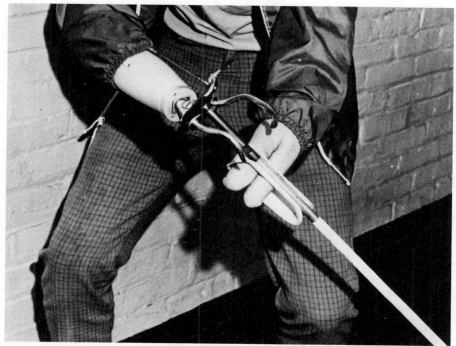

Figure 2-12. Fitting modified long cane into prosthetic hook using Krukenberg.

person with an above-the-knee (AK) amputation. The BK amputee is much more sensitive to gradients in the terrain, and is more capable of walking a direct line with less tendency to move laterally. The AK amputee will probably require a support walking cane to control lateral movements, which are a deterrent to direct line travel.

Use of a support walking cane along with a long cane creates problems. Because the client must put weight on the support cane, the area traveled by the support cane must be explored with the long cane. Therefore, the arc of the long cane must be slightly wider than normal in order to cover the entire area. The client must also be taught to move the long cane's tip close to the walking surface in order to detect surface discrepancies to avoid tripping. The touch-and-slide technique may be necessary. Here, when the tip makes contact with the surface, instead of tapping it, it slides over the surface lightly, describing an arc. Because of the shortened stride of the amputee, the cane arc explores the surface two steps ahead of the user, rather than the normal one step ahead. The mobility specialist must also spend considerable time helping the client to develop skill in interpreting textures and gradients.

Curbs and drop-offs require special techniques for the leg amputee. For the lower-extremity amputee, it is not usually possible to determine when to begin to cross the street, step off the curb, and continue the crossing. The lower-extremity amputee may have to step off the curb and then stop momentarily to regain balance before continuing the crossing. He should be taught to step down off the curb onto prosthetic leg in order to control his weight with the normal leg while shifting body weight onto the prosthetic leg.

When stepping up onto stairs or curbs, the lower-extremity amputee controls his shifting weight by stepping upward with the normal leg first. In other words, when ascending, the normal leg goes first; when descending, the prosthetic leg goes first.

Escalators

The mobility specialist should insist that lower-extremity amputee clients use handrails wherever they are available but *especially* when using an escalator. When using an escalator, the lower-extremity amputee should step onto the moving stairs with the normal leg to determine the surface, and off the escalator onto the prosthesis as soon as the normal leg determines the terminal point of the escalator. The railing and escalator steps level off, and movement ceases. Meanwhile, the prosthetic leg is in position to swing off the escalator and into the next step. While on the escalator, the client can hold the long cane in one of two ways, in a diagonal or crossbody fashion, or set in front of him on the moving stair to detect the terminal point of the escalator before it is reached. Either way, the client holds the cane at a diagonal to provide protection.

OTHER MOBILITY MEANS

It may be necessary for the client to use a wheelchair or crutches from time to time when the prosthetic leg needs repairs and adjustment, or there is tissue breakdown. Diabetic clients are sometimes subject to tissue breakdown and not able to use the prosthesis for a long time as the healing process is slow. When using crutches or a wheelchair, mobility is usually limited to indoors.

Crutches

The mobility specialist's first concern in instructing a client using crutches is to teach the location of stairways, particularly stairs going down, as it would be next to impossible to regain balance were he to overstep. When using crutches, the client cannot use a cane in front of him. Therefore, mobility must be limited to a controlled, indoor area. He will learn to move about by clearing his path of travel with one crutch, by making a sweeping movement in front of him. He will then proceed to swing-through onto his foot in a pendulum fashion while his arms support all of his weight. This is called a three-point, swing-through crutch gait (see Chapter 11, Fig. 51-11). He may need to utilize the crutch to trail the wall when attempting to locate a doorway or corridor. It is emphasized again that the client must be alert and familiar with the location of all stairways.

In ascending or descending stairs with crutches, the client must hold both crutches under one arm while using the handrail for support with the other arm. When descending the stairs in this manner, the crutches *precede* from the top of the stairs down each step; then the weight is lowered onto the crutches and down one step with use of the handrail to steady and support. To ascend the stairs, the weight is supported on the crutches as the intact leg moves up each step. The handrail is used for pulling the weight up and the crutches follow to the current level.

Wheelchair

When a client is confined to a wheelchair, mobility considerations are largely directed to avoidance of unnecessary contacts with a paralleling wall. To help avoid injury to the hands in this case, it may be advisable to modify the wheelchair by adding curb feelers, which are available at most automotive parts stores. The wheelchair footrests generally serve as forward bumpers. To locate particular doorways or corridors, manipulation of the wheelchair with one hand is necessary while trailing the wall with the other. The sphere of travel for a visually impaired client traveling in a wheelchair is very limited.

In conclusion, it must be understood that teaching mobility to the multiply handicapped client requires special additional knowledge of the application and functioning of prostheses, the use of crutches and wheelchairs, and the ability to recognize irregularity of gait as a sign of possible tissue breakdown. These concerns must be capably managed to promote complete and effective programs for these particular visually impaired, multiply handicapped clients.

Topic 2. The Visually Impaired Diabetic Client

A. James Enzinna

The orientation and mobility specialist working with a diabetic client has special concerns that are both unique and critical. For a better understanding of the client's behavior, it is worthwhile to know some of the basic physiology involved in diabetes. To accept the seriousness of the malady more readily, we need to realize that the increased incidence of diabetes mellitus makes it of greater concern to the medical profession and those people involved in the rehabilitation of blinded individuals. It is a fact that diabetic retinopathy is the leading cause of blindness in the United States today.

PHYSIOLOGY OF DIABETES

Basically, the physiology of diabetes is that the body is not able to metabolize carbohydrates due to the lack of a hormone called insulin, which is manufactured in the pancreas. Because the diabetic is not able to use sugars and starches properly, he is required to treat his condition by special diet, insulin injections, or other medications that may be taken orally to control the amount of sugar in the blood. *Diabetic retinopathy* occurs in the diabetic when tiny blood vessels in the retina break and cause small hemorrhages on or in the retina, resulting in loss of vision. A more severe form of retinopathy, *retinitis proliferans,* causes formation of scar tissue and retinal detachment, resulting in total loss of vision. The exact cause of retinopathy has not been determined. The significant fact is that the longer a person has diabetes, the more likely retinopathy will occur.

Another disease likely to occur in persons with diabetes is *chronic glaucoma,* a condition causing the pressure of the fluid in the eye to become too high, subsequently destroying the optic nerve. In this case, the loss of vision is gradual with peripheral vision being the first to deteriorate. If detected early, the condition can be treated and arrested. However, any loss of vision cannot be restored.

Emphasis must be placed on the importance of the mobility specialist's learning about his client's illness and about the subject of diabetes itself. *How to Live with Diabetes,* by H. Bolger and B. Seeman, published by W. W. Norton, is recommended reading.

Hypoglycemia

The early stages of the diabetic's participation in a mobility program are usually the most critical, and require close scrutiny on the part of the specialist. Increased activity requires a lowering of insulin intake. If the client remains on the insulin dosage he was accustomed to when less active, the results would probably be a reaction called *hypoglycemia.* The condition may reveal itself in one or many ways, the most likely being pronounced perspiration. The client may appear pale and may breathe rapidly. In more advanced stages of hypoglycemia the client may tremble and appear to lack coordination, and speech may be impaired temporarily. On the spot remedies for hypoglycemia are provided in the immediate consumption of sugar, preferably in a liquid form. Soft drinks are often easily available in an area away from home. Sugar and water are just as effective; as are fruit juices. At this time, the client may be temporarily disoriented and work may need to be postponed for several minutes and possibly for the entire session, depending on the severity of the setback. When it is possible to anticipate hypoglycemia, the client may carry candy. It is extremely important that the mobility specialist be in contact with the client's physician when this type of problem exists. The doctor will be interested in the necessity of making adjustments in the dosage of the client's insulin intake.

Ketosis

Other conditions may come to the surface that require the mobility specialist's attention, although they are less prevalent than hypoglycemia. A client may be affected by a ketosis condition that may lead to diabetic coma. One must be alert to recognize related symptoms. In *ketosis,* a client experiences excessive thirst and the skin may appear very flushed and dry. Deep, labored breathing and vomiting may take place, and the client may seem weak, drowsy, and lethargic. This condition can occur when a client neglects the insulin schedule and his diabetes goes untreated, or if he fails to follow the prescribed diet. The client must realize his responsibility if he is to contemplate active participation in a rehabilitation program of orientation and mobility.

Diabetic Neuropathy

The diabetic client may have related degrees of neurological affliction, and *diabetic neuropathy* may be evident. A client may complain of strange sensations in the extremities. A degree of numbness may be prevalent in the arms and legs. The mobility specialist must consider this condition in relation to the client's effectiveness in trying to gain travel information about changes in terrain, or in the lack of sensitivity to information perception that he should feel through the cane. This condition may necessitate special techniques such as the "touch-and-slide" to give him more information about the walking surface and its irregularities.

Emotional Symptoms

In some instances, unusual emotional behavior may occur as a result of abnormal blood sugar, which may have a temporary effect upon the client's personality. He may be unusually nervous and easily excited, or may appear very moody and even become hostile. It would be advisable for the mobility specialist to ease or avoid situations that could provoke any incidents whenever these symptoms appear. Again, a program adjustment may be in order.

AWARENESS AND OBSERVATION

It goes without saying, that the most significant requirements of a specialist working with a diabetic person are a thorough understanding of the health condition, learning the client's tendencies toward particular diabetic reactions, and coping with them. The specialist can obtain information about the client's medical history through the physician. It is extremely important to know the client's frequency of reaction if the history states such, and whether a particular pattern of incidence exists. Preventative measures are more effectively applied, if, indeed, such a tendency is apparent. The specialist may find the client's condition is controlled and stable, that he has been active, and that his physical endurance is good. The program plan for this client will be determined principally from this information. Physical capacity will be tested in a progressive manner to determine how extensive mobility lessons can be. The pursuit of a progressively extended program of mobility would be a safeguard in avoiding hypoglycemic conditions that are caused by sudden increase of physical activity. As the mobility program

418

gets underway, close scrutiny must be maintained to observe whether there is a need to readjust the client's intake of insulin.

A close rapport should be maintained with the client in order to be aware of any changes in his physical well-being. The client should communicate freely any changes in physical condition that may be pertinent. As the client gets further into the program and lessons are of a long and extended nature, the rigors of the program may require adjustment in insulin dosage. If he requires less insulin, it leads to the related consideration that once the insulin dosage has been lowered the client needs to be involved in some physical activity on those days or weekends when there is not a mobility lesson. He may choose to practice travel routes he has become familiar with, or have an exercise arrangement at home such as utilizing an exercycle or a calisthenics program.

The diabetic client is usually more physically capable early in the morning and early in the afternoon; periods following closely after breakfast and lunch. At these times, low blood sugar is less likely to present a problem. Close attention to this fact is important when scheduling all mobility appointments for diabetic clients. When scheduling is not possible in these time slots, one should schedule the client for periods as close to these hours as possible. To plan a late afternoon program for a diabetic client would be inviting difficulty.

Physical injury to any degree is to be avoided with the diabetic client. A seemingly slight bruise or bump might develop into serious complications. It must be remembered that a circulatory problem exists with the diabetic, and that bruises or cuts can become gangrenous sores, particularly in the lower extremities. It is not unusual to encounter a diabetic who has had a foot or leg amputation caused by a sore which did not heal and became gangrenous. One must be extremely alert to any slight change in the client's gait which would indicate an improperly fitting shoe, a blister, or an ingrown toenail.

In program planning, the mobility specialist should always be concerned with setting realistic goals for the client. This is particularly important when dealing with the diabetic. The specialist needs to make a judgment based on physical capacity as well as ability. He needs to be honest with the diabetic client in making clear any physical limitations that he feels are necessary. Often it is found that extended, lengthy patterns of travel are too taxing on the client's physical endurance. Therefore, the client may need to learn to plan shorter routes to destinations and the techniques for utilizing public conveyances. He needs to learn to pace himself in order to avoid exertion while traveling with the long cane. It is most critical that techniques offer the most protection at all times in order to avoid encounters with objects that could cause physical injury.

FAMILY

It is important to point out that any client's program is enhanced by the participation of an interested family member. The mobility specialist should encourage a wife, husband, or other family member to observe the client's performance periodically at a point when the client is well underway in his application of learned skills and techniques. It would then be possible to demonstrate the client's ability to travel independently. This matter is extremely important when there is reason for the specialist to suspect that the client is being overprotected by his family. It is necessary that the family see firsthand that the client is able to travel safely. In many cases, overprotective restrictions are placed on client's activities because family members are uninformed of the degree of independence a client has achieved in the mobility program. Such restrictions can easily destroy self-confidence and the effectiveness of all of the labors of the client as well as the mobility specialist.

Topic 3. Visually Impaired Older Persons

Richard L. Welsh*

Various attempts to establish the prevalence of blindness and visual impairment have resulted in widely differing statistics. Depending upon how visual impairment was defined and the methodology of the study, estimates of the number of visually impaired people in the United States range from 400,000 to 1.7 million (Hurlin, 1960; National Society for the Prevention of Blindness, 1966; Scott, 1969; and Goldish, 1972). In spite of the large differences in projections of the total number of visually impaired people, most studies agree on one demographic characteristic, that the majority of visually impaired people can be classified as older adults. Most studies indicate that as many as two-thirds of the visually impaired are 65 years of age or older.

This elderly sub-population of the visually impaired is not expected to decline in the near future. Worden (1976) cites statistical projections indicating that even larger percentages of the visually impaired population will be older in future years and that this will mean a growth in the absolute number of visually impaired people as well. This is explained, of course, by the increase in longevity of the population in general.

Despite strong evidence that older persons make up the majority of the visually impaired population, studies have demonstrated that these people receive a very small proportion of the rehabilitation services, especially orientation and mobility (Organization for Social and Technical Innovation, 1971). Several factors might explain this imbalance in services.

THE NEED AND THE PROBLEM

Most of the funds for establishment of formal orientation and mobility services have come from sources that do not address the needs of older persons. These services have been supported by federal and state programs oriented toward special education and vocational rehabilitation. The priorities of these programs are directed to those who are considered to be employable. More recently, some older persons have been rehabilitated through vocational rehabilitation programs as homemakers or to free other family members to seek employment, but for the most part, older persons have not been considered eligible for such services.

Many of the myths and stereotypes associated with old age have worked against the delivery of orientation and mobility services to this population. Rehabilitation professionals and many older people themselves have been influenced by cultural beliefs suggesting that old age is a time of hopelessness and that older people cannot be expected to benefit from rehabilitation. Many felt that the concomitant impairments that frequently accompany old age would make travel without vision or with reduced vision impossible. The higher incidence of hearing loss, balance problems, poor general health, memory loss, and other problems is generalized to all older persons and used to rationalize why mobility services would not be appropriate for this group.

THE RIGHT TO REHABILITATION

Recently, however, there has been a strengthening of the conviction that older

*The author acknowledges the ideas contributed to the chapter by Martin Yablonski, Guiding Eyes for the Blind, Yorktown Heights, N.Y.

visually impaired persons can benefit from and have a right to professional rehabilitation services, including mobility instruction. This has developed within the context of a general growth in awareness of the rights of the older members of society. This growth has been generated largely by the public education and lobbying activities of groups of older persons themselves, such as the American Association of Retired Persons, the National Senior Citizens Council, the Grey Panthers, and others. Older persons have worked for such changes as the elimination of mandatory retirement ages, the improvement of social security and medical benefits, improved housing opportunities, and other community services designed to help older persons cope with the demands of living. This increased awareness has been expressed formally in legislation and regulations such as the Older Americans Act, 1965, and the Rehabilitation Act, 1973, which address the particular needs of older visually impaired persons.

Stereotypes and Myths

Service to any client must be based on an assessment of the particular needs and assets of that individual. However, there are general characteristics of certain segments of the population that should receive special attention when an assessment is made for any individual member of that group. When a pre-service assessment is made of an older visually impaired person, attention must be given to the effect of cultural myths and stereotypes on the client and on the judgments of the professionals making the assessment. "Agism," which has been identified by Butler (1974) as a form of discrimination against older people simply because they are older, may affect the older person's own interest in mobility as well as the mobility specialist's judgment about the feasibility of such services. For many people, aging is associated with losses and dying and not with re-involvement and rehabilitation.

Among the particular myths Butler and Lewis (1973) have identified, which might affect the judgment of professionals and clients themselves about the suitability of services, are:

1. The myth of chronologic age which mistakenly relates advances in chronological age with the effects of aging

2. The myth of unproductivity which suggests that because a person is old he cannot contribute to society

3. The myth of disengagement which implies that older persons prefer being alone or associating only with their peers

4. The myth of inflexibility which suggests that older persons are resistant to change

5. The myth of senility which attributes normal emotional reactions of grief, anxiety, and depression to irreversible senility

6. The myth of serenity which implies that old age is a period of tranquility and few concerns.

As a result of these myths, older persons may refuse services or professionals may feel that a particular client would probably not want or benefit from instruction. Professionals must be able to recognize when and how these stereotypes affect their thinking and they must develop skills in helping older persons to make judgments independent of these myths.

Health

Older persons are more likely to have health problems that might affect the course and type of mobility instruction that can be provided. Birren (1959) has pointed out that the incidence of chronic disease rises in older persons, and that there is little likelihood that any person over 65 picked at random would be free from all diagnosable conditions. The mobility specialist must make a special effort to obtain an assessment of the older client's state of health and be ready to make whatever alterations in the mobility service are indicated by other conditions. Faye (1971) has discussed the most common diseases that cause visual loss in the elderly, including cataract, macular degeneration, glaucoma, and diabetes. It is important that the mobility specialist be familiar with these diseases and their effects, noting especially that most of the eye diseases leave the client with some useful vision, placing most older visually impaired persons in the low vision category.

Disease, or the aging process itself, may alter sensory and motor functioning in older clients. The mobility specialist must give special attention to the older person's potential for using other than visual channels to receive information necessary for independent travel. In other words, are the older person's auditory and haptic abilities also impaired? In addition, problems with motor control, coordination, and balance may increase the difficulty and danger of independent walking for the older visually impaired person. Many fear falling with the greater likelihood of broken bones at this age. The mobility specialist must construct an assessment process that provides information in these areas so that methods and expectations can be modified appropriately.

Psychosocial problems, including lack of motivation and lessened expectations of significant others to the extent that they are frequently characteristic of older clients, may affect training particularly for clients in the highest age ranges who live in nursing homes or other long-term care facilities. Snyder, Pyrek, and Smith (1976) demonstrated a positive relationship between vision and mental functioning and discussed the possibility that some patients may have been inappropriately labeled as mentally impaired as a result of unresolved vision needs. Held and Wartenburg (1961) discussed the emotionally paralyzing effects of vision loss on elderly clients and suggested that appropriate instruction can be instrumental in helping a client through such a stage. As Bledsoe (1958) pointed out, the mobility instructor might be perceived as the concrete affirmation of a person's permanent loss of vision, and so such instruction might be strongly resisted by someone not yet ready to make this admission.

The impact of the individual's family and significant others on one's willingness to consider and benefit from mobility instruction should also be determined. If the overwhelming message communicated by others is that the person cannot function independently, then this may have a very negative effect on instruction.

Environment

An additional area that should be considered and assessed before commencing mobility instruction with an older visually impaired person is the effect of life space and physical environment on mobility needs. The person who lives in an institution or in a semi-sheltered environment is usually in the highest age range and will have different needs than the person who is living independently in the community. Some institutional environments discourage independent travel especially when the person must use a long cane, because the cane is perceived as dangerous to the visually impaired person or other residents who may be tripped by it. As Allen (1977) pointed out, many city dwelling older persons, visually impaired or not, have rather limited mobility needs. Allen cited a study by Cantor (1975) suggesting that as older persons cease to work, have limited incomes, and grow frailer, they become increasingly neighborhood based and often neighborhood bound. The mobility instructor must distinguish between client needs that result from limitations brought on by the visual loss and the limitations that are the result of aging even for persons who do not have visual loss.

APPROACH TO INSTRUCTION

Certain adaptations of the usual approach to mobility instruction may be necessary for older persons in general while other modifications may be necessary for particular clients.

An andragogical approach should be used in teaching all adults as contrasted to the classical pedagogical approach. The concept of andragogy as presented by Ingalls (1973) capitalizes on the fact that adults realize they are capable of self-direction in their learning and that their own life experiences can contribute to it. In the andragogical process, the instructor is more a facilitator (helping the person to organize his own learning), than an authoritative teacher. The older person should be much more involved in the selection of the learning goals and in the evaluation of the results.

Using the andragogical approach, the sequence of instruction may have to be modified to accommodate the wishes or needs of the older person. When a client constructs a learning sequence that reflects his current needs and interests, the instructor may realize that certain preliminary skills are necessary before the plan can be accomplished. The instructor's responsibility is to present this information and to help the client to alter his plan to reflect the sequence deemed necessary. If the client objects, the instructor must be ready to modify his own preferred way of approaching the goals within the limits of what is safe and professionally responsible.

When compared to typical pedagogical methods, the andragogical approach seems to produce a more positive change in the adult's self-concept as a result of the atmosphere of shared communication and mutual respect. The application of this approach to the teaching of orientation and mobility to older visually impaired persons was described by Allen, Griffith, and Yablonski (1976).

Another difference frequently found in teaching mobility to older adults is the limit to the ultimate goals. This may result from the limited interests, needs and desires of the older client or it may reflect the effect of other impairments and limitations on ability. This is sometimes difficult for the mobility specialist to accept because it is not as interesting and challenging as the more advanced travel some clients are capable of achieving. However, there is a challenge in helping older clients find ways to meet their limited needs despite other restrictions and impairments.

The mobility specialist should be careful not to misinterpret the initial expression of limited goals. In some cases, this may be a most appropriate response given the older person's fear or expectation of failure, or his embarrassment at needing this kind of special service. It is another effect of cultural stereotyping. However, as the client begins to experience success, perception of interests and goals may also change, necessitating a flexible program structure and attitude on the part of the instructor.

Special Considerations

The health and medical problems of many older clients may necessitate modifications in mobility training. Certain disease processes such as those involving the cardio-pulmonary system may make it difficult for the client to endure stress or pressure for very long. For some clients, lessons of much shorter duration than usual will have to be constructed, or short rest periods included. Long routes, excessive work on stairs, or exposure to cold and wind may be contraindicated.

Some clients may have additional mobility problems as a result of medication they are taking. Its effect may make the client less aware of certain information that needs to be processed to complete a travel route. A medication may also cause light-headedness and susceptibility to falling. Those who suffer from diabetes may experience difficulty in balancing insulin and sugar intake. (See Enzinna, this chapter.)

Gait and balance problems occur frequently among older clients and require additional thought and planning. If an individual must use a walker, crutches, or a support cane to maintain balance, the mobility specialist will have to develop a method of using such devices either with the long cane or instead of it for information gathering purposes. In Chapter 11, Farmer discusses some of these devices and how they may be used by the visually impaired person. Gait and balance problems also account for the reluctance of some dog guide agencies to accept older persons as clients.

The need for medical care as a result of other health problems may interrupt the flow of mobility instruction for a period of time or bring a halt to the rehabilitation program altogether. The mobility specialist must be prepared for this possibility when working with older persons.

Sensory Limitations

Among the modifications in the mobility program necessitated by sensory limitations, the effect of presbycusis may be the most common and the most problematic. *Presbycusis* (see Wiener Chapter 6) is a gradual loss of hearing beginning in the upper frequencies, and thought to be associated with age. Since many of the auditory cues in the environment, especially those associated with the use of reflected sound, are in the upper frequencies, presbycusis affects the mobility of persons with reduced vision. Once the disease progresses to the point of affecting the speech ranges, it may also interfere with communication between the instructor and the client. The instructor may have to encourage the client to depend less on auditory cues and more on tactile information in the environment. More patience when communicating with certain clients, remembering to double check reception of verbal communication, may also be needed.

Birren (1959) concluded from his review of the research on reaction time and motor coordination among the elderly that there was relatively little change of speed or accuracy in simple tests of reaction time. However, in complicated tasks requiring coordination of what a person perceives with what he does, aging results in greater changes in speed and accuracy. Because of changes in sensory and motor functioning, the instructor may have to help the client over-learn certain basic tasks and functions to insure safe performance.

In discussing sensory-motor coordination, Birren (1959) noted that the older person performing motor tasks seems to need continuous reassurance or new information as he proceeds, which he obtains through repeated visual examination of the stimulus and of his own performance. According to Birren, "The perceptual and conceptual models of the world seem to diminish, and certainly form less easily with age, so that this steady information reinforcement becomes essential" (Birren, 1959, p. 271). If so, the client with no means of visual reinforcement will probably require additional feedback and information from the instructor when learning motor tasks. Paskin (1977) presented useful samples of sensory training activities used with older visually impaired clients.

Motivation

Some older clients have emotional problems and a lack of motivation that make participation in mobility training unlikely. They cannot be motivated by the reasoning that is so useful with children and younger adults—that mobility training is necessary preparation for later aspects of life. Instead, the source of motivation must be found within the mobility learning situation. For example, if the relationship between the instructor and the client can be trusting and rewarding in itself, it may be sufficient to motivate client participation in the program.

Because the client is a genuine partner in the learning situation and participates in its planning, the andragogical approach may be another source of motivation. Of course, some kind of interest is necessary at the outset to get the client involved in the planning. The andragogical approach stresses beginning where the client is, and focusing on real problems and needs that he perceives. A less personal, more abstract approach may further alienate someone whose motivation is marginal at the outset.

While the client may not be motivated by the usual approach of preparing for some future life tasks, it may help to present mobility instruction as an aid in preventing further deterioration and alleviating some of the losses already being experienced. If the client is feeling increasing isolation as a result of losing friends to death and relocation, the ability to travel independently may facilitate maintaining contact with others. Skills in independent functioning may also be favorably perceived by the client as a means of remaining in the community, forestalling placement in a long-term care facility. For individuals living in an institution, helping the client realize how mobility instruction can help him become a little more independent in this setting, making him less dependent on others to fulfill his basic needs, may be enough.

ATTITUDES OF THE MOBILITY SPECIALIST

The success of mobility instruction with older visually impaired persons depends as much on the instructor's attitude as on his skills. Working with these clients can be sufficiently different for the mobility specialist that attention should be given to its emotional impact.

Initially, the instructor must be able to recognize and deal with the effects that cultural stereotypes and myths have on his own and the client's attitude. He has to be able to evaluate each client objectively in spite of the strong inclination to anticipate many complications in addition to the visual impairment. Even though statistical studies have demonstrated that combinations of impairments are more likely in older persons, each individual must be assessed separately and his program planned individually. That is the client's right and the instructor's obligation. Some clients are free of the complications that frequently accompany visual loss among the elderly.

Whenever the mobility specialist does encounter a client whose visual loss is accompanied by other impairments, he might have a sense of hopelessness and futility. He may despair of being able to have an impact on the individual's ability to function more independently. This attitude, if it persists, can be the most serious impairment that the client has to overcome. The mobility specialist must discipline himself to focus on abilities and potential as a necessary step toward helping the client reach that potential. This skill, for the mobility specialist, relates to his ability to draw satisfaction from the actual gains of individual clients, even though they may be small in comparison to those of clients not burdened with the complications of advanced years or other impairments. The focus must be on helping the client reach goals that make the most sense for him and not on those most meaningful for the instructor.

The instructor must be able to relinquish a strong authoritative role in his relationship with the client, and allow the older client, indeed every adult client, full partnership in the decision making and lesson planning that takes place. This can be difficult for mobility specialists who have taught in more traditional educational settings before working with adults. The extent to which the mobility specialist can create this type of relationship may relate directly to the client's motivation to continue instruction.

The mobility specialist must be very knowledgeable about human functioning in order to devise alternative methods of receiving and processing information for individuals whose usual channels are blocked by impairments. Thus, the specialist working with older persons must be very knowledgeable and resourceful in drawing on a wide body of information to cope with the needs of older visually impaired persons.

Finally, the mobility specialist working with visually impaired older persons must be unequivocally convinced of the worth of working with this group. This kind of commitment is necessary to counteract the strong cultural tendencies in the opposite direction that he will encounter in others, including his clients.

FINANCIAL SUPPORT

One of the reasons for the lack of mobility services for older visually impaired persons has been the difficulty of finding appropriate sources of financial support. A number of possibilities, however, do exist, at least in spirit, in some legislation, and the challenge is to convert this legislative intent into services.

Some older persons can receive mobility and other rehabilitation services through state and federal vocational rehabilitation programs, especially if they are between the ages of 55 and 65. These individuals might still be justified under a vocational plan. Others benefit from vocational rehabilitation funds when they are rehabilitated as "homemakers." This category is being used more frequently than in the past, as recognition that individuals can contribute to the family's economy by taking care of the home or by freeing others to assume paid employment.

A second source of possible support for mobility services is the Older Americans Act of 1965 and recent amendments. The special needs of older blind persons are mentioned in this legislation, and there is the intent of providing some funds for services for them. In spite of this, not many programs have been developed using this source of support.

The Rehabilitation Act of 1973 also mentioned the possibility of research and innovative projects for older blind persons. The legislation encouraged the use of vocational rehabilitation funds for this population as one of the types of severely disabled groups that were the special focus of the 1973 act and its later amendments.

More recently, Title XX of the Social Security Act directed federal funds toward certain populations at risk and with particular goals in mind. One such goal was to prevent the institutionalization of individuals who, with a reasonable amount of assistance, could be helped to continue to live in the community. The regulations implementing this legislation referred to older visually impaired persons among others as a target group that could benefit from such services. This legislation has generated a number of special projects for older blind clients at various agencies around the country. However, the competition for Title XX funds is intense, and many more projects have been proposed than have been funded.

Finally, the prospect of some type of national health insurance seems to offer still another possibility for the funding of mobility services for older visually impaired persons. A precedent exists in the support that is provided for physical therapy and speech therapy under current Medicare and Medicaid provisions. For many older visually impaired persons, mobility services can help to restore health and to prevent further medical deterioration.

This premise is based upon the accumulating evidence that seems to indicate a connection between inactivity and further deterioration of various body systems in older persons. (Bonner, 1969; Brunner, 1970; Hein and Ryan, 1960; and Shock,

1967). The older person who becomes visually impaired frequently becomes sedentary as a result of the inability to move about independently. In some care facilities, visually impaired persons have even been confined to bed, supposedly for their own safety. The cumulative effect of lack of activity on a person whose original impairment was just loss of vision can seriously affect cardio-pulmonary systems too. The services of a mobility specialist if they result in helping a person to remain mobile and active may help to prevent the onset of other health problems and the deterioration of other systems.

REALITY ORIENTATION

Similarly, increasing attention is being given to the effects of reality orientation activities and to their possible role in delaying senile deterioration (Barnes, 1974; Richman, 1969; and Taulbee and Folsom, 1968). The core of reality orientation is to keep older persons interacting with their environments in a concrete way and to maintain their sensory contacts with the surrounding world. These theories and experimental programs have possible implications for visually impaired older persons who have lost a main contact with the environment with loss of vision. If the theory related to "reality orientation" is correct, such individuals could benefit from any efforts to help them relate positively to their surroundings. This implies another possible role for orientation and mobility services for older visually impaired persons. Mobility instruction is a practical way to help individuals to relate to their environments and to help persons prone to senile deterioration to stay in contact with their surroundings for a longer period of time.

If mobility services can be demonstrated as helping to prevent the onset of circulatory and respiratory problems by keeping a person mobile and active or to stave off senile deterioration or other emotional reactions by helping an individual stay in contact with the environment, such services can be shown to relate to maintaining the overall health of visually impaired older persons. As a result, other sources of funds might be available through the channels that support health-related services.

CONCLUSION

If the orientation and mobility profession is to keep its commitment to serve visually impaired persons in the community as implied in the profession's Code of Ethics (Wiener, Welsh, Hill, La Duke, Mills, & Mundy, 1973), an effort must be made to contact and effectively serve the largest segment of the visually impaired population, the elderly. Effective service to this group will require that mobility specialists increase their knowledge about the various effects of aging and age-related diseases, the modifications in mobility instruction that are implied by this knowledge, and the various ways to generate increased support in the culture for making such services available to those who need them.

Bibliography

Allen, W. *The elderly visually impaired traveler in the urban environment.* Paper presented at the Conference on Orientation and Mobility in the Urban Environment, New York City, March 1977.

Allen, W., Griffith, A. & Yablonski, M. Realistic orientation and mobility for the elderly blind person. *The Long Cane Newsletter,* 1976 (Winter).

Barnes, J. A. Effects of reality orientation classroom on memory loss, confusion, and disorientation in geriatric patients. *The Gerontologist,* 1974 (April) 138-141.

Birren, J. E. *Handbook of aging and the individual.* Chicago: University of Chicago Press, 1959.

Bledsoe, C. W. Rehabilitation of the blind geriatric patient. *Geriatrics,* 1958 (February), 91-96.

Bonner, C. D. Rehabilitation instead of bed rest. *Geriatrics,* 1969, **24,** 109-114.

Brunner, D. *Physical activity and aging.* Baltimore: University Park Press, 1970.

Butler, R. N. Successful aging and the role of the life review. *Journal of the American Geriatric Society*, 1974, **22** (12) 529-535.

Butler, R. N. & Lewis, M. *Aging and mental health* St. Louis: C. V. Mosby Co., 1973.

Cantor, M. H. *The formal and informal social support system of older New Yorkers*. Paper presented at the symposium: The city a viable environment for the elderly? Jerusalem, Israel, 1975, 3-4.

Carney, J. An orientation and mobility program for the geriatric blinded adult. *The New Outlook for the Blind*, 1970, **64,** 286-287.

Faye, E. Visual function in geriatric eye disease. *The New Outlook for the Blind*, 1971, **65,** 204-209.

Goldish, L. H. The severely visually impaired population as a market for sensory aids and services: Part one. *The New Outlook for the Blind*, 1972, **66,** 183-190.

Hein, F. & Ryan, A. The contributions of physical activity to physical health. *Research Quarterly*, 1960, **31,** 263-285.

Held, M. & Wartenburg, S. Blind people—fifty and over. *The New Outlook for the Blind*, 1961, **55,** 165-168.

Hubbard, J. A program of orientation and mobility for the aged blind in the community. *The New Outlook for the Blind*, 1969, **63,** 211-213.

Hurlin, R. G. Estimated prevalence of blindness in the United States and in individual states, 1960. *The Sight Saving Review*, 1962, **32,** 2-10.

Ingalls, J. D. *A trainer's guide to andragogy*. Waltham, Mass.: Data Educational Inc., 1973.

National Society for the Prevention of Blindness. *Estimated statistics on blindness and visual problems*. New York: Author, 1966.

Organization for Social and Technical Innovation. *Blindness and service to the blind in the United States*. Cambridge, Mass.: OSTI Press, 1971.

Paskin, N. *Sensory development*. New York: New York Infirmary/Center for Independent Living, 1977.

Richman, L. Sensory training for geriatric patients. *The American Journal of Occupational Therapy*, 1969, **23**(3), 2-6.

Scott, R. *The making of blind men*. New York: The Russell Sage Foundation, 1969.

Shaw, J. A. Mobility and the aging process. *The New Beacon*, 1970, 315-317.

Shock, N. Physical activity and the rate of aging. *Canadian Medical Association Journal*, 1967, **96,** 836-840.

Snyder, L. H., Pyrek, J., & Smith, K. C. Vision and mental function of the elderly. *The Gerontologist*, 1976, **16,** 491-495.

Taulbee, L. R. & Folsom, J. C. Reality orientation for geriatric patients. *Hospital and Community Psychiatry*, 1968, 135-138.

Wiener, W., Welsh, R., Hill, E., LaDuke, R., Mills, R., & Mundy, G. A code of ethics for orientation and mobility specialists. *Blindness*, 1973, 6-16.

Worden, H. W. Aging and blindness. *The New Outlook for the Blind*, 1976, **70,** 433-437.

Topic 4. Visually Impaired Children

Robert J. Mills

Before World War II, visually impaired children were educated primarily in residential schools. The prevalent attitude among the general public seemed to be that blind persons could not take even limited responsibility for their own safety. Society as a whole did not seem to consider the individual and his strengths and assets, but rather focused on the stereotyped weaknesses and limitations imposed by blindness and attributed them to all blind persons. As a result, there was no

12

systematic approach to independent travel being offered that would enable a child to be as independent as an adult. Some children taught themselves to travel and shared their techniques with their peers. Others were taught by low vision students or by alumni who were sometimes added to the faculty as physical educators.

Following World War II, successfully rehabilitated blinded veterans and self-emancipated blind adults were having a positive impact on society's attitudes toward the blind. In addition, the parents of blind children pushed local educational programs into providing services for their children. Attention began to turn toward preparing blind children for integration into society (Lowenfeld, 1973; 1975).

At first, some educators attended summer workshops in orientation and mobility conducted by mobility specialists on leave from the Veterans Administration. As university based programs began to appear, public and residential schools began to employ mobility specialists as part of the regular staff. These early instructors experienced difficulty in trying to apply techniques developed initially for adventitiously blinded veterans to congenitally blind children.

SPECIAL NEEDS OF CHILDREN

Some of the problems encountered by these instructors included the difficulty of expecting a child who had always lacked the integrating sense of sight to use his other senses to substitute for lost vision. Second, children could not be expected to have correct and meaningful concepts and an understanding of the spatial organization of the environment that sight usually provided incidentally as the individual developed. Third, the instructors had to remember that their students were still children or adolescents, not mature veterans. Finally, the problem that these students experienced was learning to live, not learning how to return to living in a way closely resembling a way they had lived before blindness.

The School Years

Research and demonstration projects funded by United States Office of Education during the 1960s produced evidence that children could benefit from formal orientation and mobility instruction during their school years.

Costello and Gockman (1966) indicated that the mobility skills used in the Veterans Administration Program did not need to be revised for children. However, it was also pointed out that orientation skills and knowledge needed to be developed further, primarily because blind children lack experiences with their environment. Children have a greater need for orientation materials that can be classified as educative rather than rehabilitative.

The project done by the Detroit Metropolitan Society for the Blind (1963) concluded that blind children and teenagers could be taught to overcome problems that limit their ability to move freely in the environment. It was also noted that public schools provide many opportunities to develop mobility. By illustrating the rewards of independent travel, the public school environment helps children to regard mobility as a useful skill—not as an isolated subject.

The acceptance of university trained professionals as the providers of formal orientation and mobility instruction for children became evident as the Office of Education initiated additional university programs to train specialists to serve children. The rapid move of mobility specialists to positions in educational settings was documented by studies done in the early 1970s.

Blasch and Wurzberger (1971) reported that while 49 percent of graduates with a master's degree were employed in rehabilitation agencies, and 8 percent in hospitals, 18 percent were employed in residential schools and 25 percent in public school systems. This suggested that more than 40 percent of mobility specialists were working with children. Welsh and Blasch (1974) reported that 45 percent of the mobility specialists work with school age individuals, individuals in residential schools for the blind, residential schools for other handicaps, and public school systems. This would suggest that 55 percent of the mobility specialists, those working in rehabilitation agencies, production training workshops, and hospitals, are primarily working with adults. However, some of the mobility specialists working in the rehabilitation agencies reported that they spend some of their time working with children, usually through a contractual arrangement with a school district. This is verified by the fact that responses to the survey indicated that 28 percent of all the agencies provide some services for children, infancy to age six; 57 percent provide some services for young persons age 7 to 14; and 73 percent serve adolescents age 15 to 18 in some capacity. From this, Welsh and Blasch concluded that more than 50 percent of the mobility specialists are involved in delivering services to school age persons who, according to the American Foundation for the Blind (1973), represent only 10 percent of the blind population.

When to Begin

Teaching orientation and mobility skills to visually impaired children does differ in certain respects from teaching adults. One area of difference relates to the concern about the appropriate time to begin mobility instruction. Generally, it is important to relate the expectations of visually impaired children to the stages of development of non-impaired children at the same age. It is not reasonable to expect or to encourage visually impaired children to function without vision at developmental levels beyond the stages usually achieved by non-impaired children of the same age. On the other hand, if efforts to help visually impaired children move independently are delayed beyond the normal ages when such skills appear in the non-impaired population, this delay in itself may have the effect of compounding the handicap and creating new problems.

Ideally, mobility specialists should be involved with visually impaired children and their parents while the child is still an infant and throughout the preschool years. The focus of such involvement is to encourage and provide assistance to the child and parents to help the child to achieve expected stages of normal development as closely as possible given the visual impairment.

Preschool

Recently in a few pilot projects, itinerant teachers of visually impaired children have been working with parents, infants, toddlers and preschoolers in their homes. Other programs are being offered by rehabilitation centers for day care preschoolers who are visually impaired. While such programs exist and ideally will increase, most mobility specialists can expect that the children with whom they are about to begin instruction have not had the benefit of formal and effective efforts to help them maintain a developmental pace that is as close to normal as possible. For this reason, it is necessary to assess the level of psychomotor development of each child considered for mobility instruction so that training can begin at the level of development most appropriate for that child.

ASSESSMENT

Cratty and Sams (1968) and Lord (1970) have developed instruments that are useful in checking out some of the basic psychomotor skills of visually impaired children. The Cratty instrument, *Body Image of Blind Children*, is designed to assess the child's ability to identify body planes and body parts, and to demonstrate various body movements—laterality and directionality. Lord's instrument, *Orientation and Mobility Scale Short Form*, assesses the child's ability to make turns and to use polar centric directions, to execute certain movements in space, and to demonstrate various self-care skills. Other more general instruments have been developed by Frostig and Maslow (1977), Roach and Kephart (1966), and others.

As a result of the assessment, it might be discovered that remedial or supplementary activities are needed to improve on or make up for deficient development or the lack of experience related to the impairment. While some children may require remedial activity, almost all children would seem to benefit from structured opportunities to strengthen or further develop their psychomotor abilities. As an example of the kind of program that might be developed, students at the Ohio State School for the Blind are periodically screened by orientation and mobility specialists and/or other staff to assess their level of psychomotor development. Based on these screenings, prescriptions for each student are written by the mobility specialist that call for instruction and learning activities in any or all of the following areas: 1.) tactile perception, 2.) vestibular perception, 3.) proprioception, 4.) auditory skills, 5.) low vision perception, 6.) olfactory perception, 7.) kinesthetic perception, 8.) body awareness, 9.) spatial relations, 10.) distance, time, and speed estimation, 11.) laterality and directionality judgments, 12.) movement and motor planning, 13.) orientation skills, 14.) concept development, 15.) expansion of experiences, 16.) use of polar centric directions, 17.) maintaining an awareness of turns and a sense of balance during purposeful activity, 18.) learning to be responsible for their own safety during movement.

Information related to various components of psychomotor development and the normal stages of growth and how they are interrupted by visual loss is presented by Hart in Chapter 2.

Concept Development

Before formal mobility instruction is begun, it is also necessary to assess the level of concept development of each child. As mentioned above, and as discussed by Hill and Blasch (Chapter 9), development without vision leads to deficiencies in the range and variety of concepts that are attained by visually impaired children. Efficient mobility instruction is not possible if the child is lacking basic concepts, especially spatial and environmental concepts. Examples of some of the deficiencies that children might experience in this area are represented by the following:

1. A child may not understand the concept of a hall and how a hall is used to travel from one room to another

2. A child may lack an accurate concept of a square or a rectangle and therefore have difficulty understanding street patterns or intersections

3. A child lacking an accurate concept of a "room" may think that a large room has more walls than a smaller room.

Some of the instruments for assessing concept development presented by Hill and Blasch should be administered before formal mobility instruction is attempted. When deficiencies are noted, time must be spent in helping the child to develop the necessary concepts. Although this has frequently been the responsibility of the mobility specialist in the past, it does not have to be. It can be done as part of the child's learning in other classes, or it can be provided through specially trained and supervised aides. The mobility specialist should, however, be closely involved with this aspect of the total program to help make these activities as relevant as possible for later mobility needs.

The activities for concept development suggested by Hill and Blasch (Chapter 9) may be of assistance in this part of the program.

There are various recorded materials that have been helpful in the areas indicated:

Educational Activities, Inc.
Freeport, L. I., New York 11520

> *The Development of Body Awareness and Position in Space.* LP 605, used for developing body awareness and position in space.
> *Developing the Perceptual—Motor Abilities of Primary Level Children.* LP 606-7, helps to develop balance, agility, and movement.
> *Relaxation Training.* AR 655, focuses on body image and control of all muscle groups.
> *Pre-Tumbling Skills for Impulse Control.* AR 656, body control movement through relaxation, falling, turning and falling, simple rolls.
> *Dynamic Balance Activities.* AR 657.
> *Dynamic Balance Activities, Balance Beam.* AR 658.
> *Basic Concepts through Dance (Body Image).* EALP 601.
> *Basic Concepts through Dance (Position in Space).* EALP 603.
> *Auditory Perception.* Eight Record Kit, Unit One. AKR 113.

Classroom Materials Co.
93 Myrtle Drive
Great Neck, New York 11021

> *Developing Body Space Perception Motor Skills Album 1.* CM 1056, develops early motor skills and concept of body image.
> *Developing Body Space Perception Motor Skills Album 2.* CM 1058, develops large muscle coordination, space perception, laterality, directionality, coordination, eye/hand movement.
> *Developing Body Space Perception Motor Skills Album 3.* CM 1079, focuses on body parts; planes; laterality to self, objects, and other people, above and below.
> *Listening Skills for Pre-Readers.* CM 1065, includes indoor and outdoor sounds, discrimination, identification in sequence (2 or 3), simultaneous sounds.

Educational Recordings of America, Inc.
Beardsly Station; P.O. Box 6062
Bridgeport, Connecticut 06606

> *Rhythms for Physical Fitness.* Primary, intermediate and junior-senior grades isometrics

Kimbo Educational Records
Box 246
Deal, New Jersey 07723

> *Developing Everyday Skills.* LP 7016, LP 7017, LP 7018, LP 7019, LP 7020, LP 7021, series of songs combines action movements, educational learning, concepts and physical movements.
> *Exercise is Kid Stuff.* LP 2070, posture conditioning and body coordination.
> *Rhythmic Activities and Physical Fitness.* LP 1077.
> *Jazz U.S.A.* LP 2040, jazz exercises and coordinating body movement.
> *U.S.A. on the March.* LP 2030, formal exercises, Volume 3.

Golden Records
250 W. 57th Street
New York, New York 10019

> *What Can The Difference Be.* LP 271, songs about opposites, differences and opposites in size, shape, directions and textures.
> *Songs and Games of Physical Fitness for Boys and Girls.* LP 114, postural exercises.

Columbia Recording
Follett Publishing Co.
Chicago, Illinois

> *The Horn That Wanted To Know.* 3499, listen and hear program.

432

Integrated Play/Learning

Some equipment used by physical therapists and occupational therapists may be useful in psychomotor development and concept development programs for visually impaired children. Equipment such as walkers, balance beams, vestibular training barrels, etc. might best be used with the assistance and consultation of therapists who are most familiar with the applicability of these aids. Some commercially produced games and puzzles lend themselves well to tasks that help the visually impaired child to keep pace with normal development. They might include different types of felt boards to help children learn body parts, types of clothing, geometric forms, and various other shapes and concepts. Many of them can be obtained through the American Printing House for the Blind and are described in their catalog.

More frequently, the mobility specialist or teacher of the visually impaired child will find that the most useful aids can be made from common materials and supplies such as dowel sticks, peg boards, pieces of carpeting, sand paper, etc. Different sized balls, jump ropes and other toys can be useful in encouraging children to develop their sensory skills and discrimination abilities. Bells, whistles, clickers, and other noise makers can also help to stimulate the child and to encourage movement as well as sensory awareness.

Low vision children can benefit from exercises using various art supplies, jigsaw puzzles, flash cards, playing cards, slides and slide projectors, mazes, and a wide range of other materials.

The Ohio State School for the Blind has attempted to integrate a number of psychomotor and conceptual training tasks in a practical learning situation through the use of a simulated grocery store. Using containers in which the real products had been purchased, a grocery store was set up in a large area of the school and the children were oriented to the layout and operation of a typical store. The arrangement of aisles and other parts of the store was explained and its logical pattern discussed. The children then became involved in learning how to select various products in the store by the identification of the different packages and cans. The activity provided the child with some easily transferable skills in size and weight discrimination, in haptic exploration and identification of various shapes, in the discrimination of a variety of textures that are characteristic of different products, in color identification and recognition of the visual symbols of certain labels, and to a certain degree the development and use of olfactory discrimination abilities.

INITIATION OF INSTRUCTION

Once the student's level of psychomotor development has been assessed and any needed remedial efforts have begun, and the level of concept development has been determined and improved if necessary, it is possible to consider the initiation of orientation and mobility instruction. The mobility specialist recognizes that orientation and mobility education, like other school subjects, cannot be crammed into a few weeks or even one year of the student's academic experience. It should begin when the child enters school at whatever level is appropriate, and be available as needed as he grows and proceeds toward commencement. Educators do not wait until a student is a senior to begin teaching language arts. Part of every year the child is in school is devoted to language arts. Orientation and mobility education must also be ongoing during the child's school life to culminate in independence.

One way to begin mobility instruction for children is to expose young students to the concept of how they may travel when older. Sighted children at this age know that they will drive a car when they are older. But few young visually impaired children have parents who are also visually impaired and able to provide an example of travel without vision. Older students who are independent travelers may serve as useful models for younger children, talking to them, explaining sensory training and the cane, and relating some of their own travel experiences. It may also help to adapt several canes to the appropriate length for the children and, after demonstration, allow them to employ some basic skills to move across the room using the cane as a bumper and as an extension of the haptic sensing system.

Beyond this type of exposure, the needs of a particular child and his ability to take responsibility for his own safety should determine when he enters formal mobility instruction. Several years ago, some of the elementary students at the Montreal Association for the Blind were integrated into a nearby neighborhood school. They learned to use a cane and to cross streets to go to school; an experience approximating the experience of sighted children attending the same school with regard to residential travel.

Very young children can be exposed to formal instruction and many can master the fundamentals of the long cane. Often, however, these students will have to relearn long cane skills when older if their need for them initially is limited to travel in their home areas and on quiet streets in residential neighborhoods. Relearning these skills when older, and applying them to more complex urban and suburban situations should be easier because of the early exposure. Such formal mobility instruction with young children must be given only with the approval of parents, and the students must be mature enough to take responsibility for their own safety in the limited situations in which they are to travel.

In deciding when to offer formal mobility instruction, it is important to realize that children need to keep pace with their peers. There should be a recognized need for the use of the skill on some regular basis. The mobility specialist, the parents, and the child must agree to this regular use and practice if the educational process is to be most effective and the child is to grow and mature along with his peers.

While mobility instruction should be available as needed by the individual student throughout his academic experience, certain general patterns may appear and the length and frequency of lessons may vary at different points in the process. For primary level students, formal mobility instruction should be offered on a daily basis and should last a minimum of 30 minutes but should not exceed 50 minutes because of the attention span of this age group. For elementary level students (4th, 5th, 6th grade), depending on the child, mobility instruction may expand the child's area of travel beyond the immediate neighborhood and include street crossings plus a review of all previous skills necessary to travel in a residential area. Instruction should still be on a daily basis and should last from 40 to 80 minutes to provide sufficient time for reinforcement and to insure an interval of practice necessary for proficiency.

As day school students enter junior high, their needs will generally change as they leave their neighborhoods to attend centralized schools. They probably will not be able to walk to school by themselves or with friends as they did in elementary school. They will need orientation to the new school and they will have to learn how to locate the school bus at both ends of the trip. The student may require special understanding at this time of puberty and adolescence. Orientation and mobility may be the furthest thing from the student's mind. The instructor must be patient, understanding, and accepting. When the instructor tries to understand the student's world vicariously, he is more likely to be able to help the student cope with his normal growth and to acquire needed skills. At this stage, instruction will typically expand the world of the child beyond the confines of the home residential area or the campus of the residential school to nearby small or medium business areas and shopping centers.

Lessons for junior high school students should last a minimum of 50 minutes and be offered on a daily basis. If this is not possible, lessons might be offered a minimum of three times a week, but the lesson time should be extended to insure an interval of practice commensurate with the student's ability to learn.

In senior high school, if it is at all possible, all formal orientation and mobility instruction should be completed, preferably before grade 11. The instruction should further expand the world of the student to the entire city including the downtown area and the use of public transportation.

Generally speaking, orientation and mobility lessons should be conducted at different times of the day throughout the week. This will require the student to practice using his orientation skills in varying situations with the sun in different positions, with traffic flow varying from morning rush hour to mid-morning to early afternoon and to evening rush hour, with stores opened and closed, when bus stops are crowded, and when there are many pedestrians or few.

Providing mobility instruction to children may require special abilities, characteristics, and attitudes of the mobility specialist. With very young children, the mobility specialist may have to be able to set aside some of his adult mannerisms and language to be able to relate to the child more effectively. He may have to enter the world of the child and be able to do a lot of teaching through games and other high-reward activities. As mentioned above, the instructor of adolescents may need special patience and understanding of the turmoil and uncertainty that accompanies the age.

COUNSELING

Students in mobility training may need to be counseled individually and in small groups about their handicap, and they may need some suggestions for developing an outgoing attitude in meeting, making, and maintaining friends. They should also be advised what to expect of sighted people when confronted with their blindness.

In addition to individual counseling, students can profit immensely from group counseling sessions while receiving orientation and mobility instruction. Group meetings should be conducted weekly by a qualified psychologist. Groups should be composed of students in various phases of orientation and mobility instruction, allowing the students an opportunity to express themselves in a permissive setting and to share experiences with peers about channeling emotions, fear, anxiety, embarrassment, and frustration resulting from dealing with the public or the environment while traveling. Students need support and a heterogenous grouping allows more experienced travelers to share with the novice the ways in which they dealt with similar situations when they were learning.

The same psychologist may be instrumental in counseling parents of youngsters who strongly resist the idea of their child traveling independently. The psychologist should observe lessons over a period of time to insure understanding of the problems the students encounter. The mobility specialist should also meet with the psychologist weekly before the group meeting, to relate progress, problems and unusual happenings on lessons of the past week.

When working with children, the mobility specialist should not accept sloppy, inappropriate techniques but strive to help the child to develop perfect techniques. Adults may be allowed to experiment with modifications in developing their own set of techniques but children must be helped to develop the skill that the mobility specialist knows is best, and which affords the maximum warning and protection.

ORIENTATION SKILLS

The orientation and mobility specialist must not take for granted that a visually impaired student who is supposedly ready for training already has all of the necessary information about himself and the environment. Cane techniques are essential, but so too are orientation skills. When working with children, the orientation and mobility specialist may have to spend two-thirds to three-fourths of his time on orientation and teaching the student to develop a method of structuring space. The following questions may help the student to be aware of the essential points of information needed to remain oriented in an environment:

1. What block am I within?

2. What is the street pattern in this area?

3. What is the name of the street I am walking along?

4. In what direction am I traveling?

5. What side of the street am I on?

6. How is the traffic flowing; on which side, and in which direction?

7. What are the names of the parallel and perpendicular streets in this area?

MOTIVATION AND REWARD

The use of special motivation and reward systems is usually necessary when working with children. With younger children, the teaching of concepts, psychomotor skills, and mobility techniques in the context of games may provide the necessary motivation and stimulation to learn. Some students, particularly the multiply handicapped, may need extrinsic concrete rewards, such as food or tokens, to hold their attention and stimulate their learning. For many students, the approval of the instructor or of other significant adults may be the most effective reinforcer. Still others like adults are motivated by a desire to master the skills involved because they realize how important they are for accomplishing other desirable goals.

The Pass System

For students in residential schools, a pass system may represent a motivational device while also functioning as a regular part of a program designed to help use the skills learned. Considered a privilege, a pass, earned by students who have completed various phases of formal mobility instruction has worked well at various residential schools. A system which allows a child to travel independently off campus during free time, also allows the child to grow and mature while practicing and maintaining the skills mastered. The pass is a tangible symbol of achievement and personal privilege.

An annual evaluation of a student's travel ability should be made by the mobility specialist before the pass is re-issued each year. It should be done routinely, and may require considerable understanding on the part of the faculty and administration as some disruption of class attendance will occur during evaluations. As the administration is responsible for children on or off campus, cooperation is usually easily obtained, and the policy of annual evaluations can be instituted as school policy.

As an example of the success of such a pass system, the number of students leaving the campus of the Ohio State School for the Blind has steadily climbed since the system was initiated in 1965. The holders of unlimited passes may be gone for extended periods of time during the day for such things as a shopping trip downtown, to a movie for three or four hours, or other non-school activities.

An effective pass system also requires the cooperation of houseparents or other staff members. Such staff members should be supplied with a list of students who have demonstrated their ability to travel safely off campus, and a method of consulting mobility staff if there is any doubt regarding the information on the student's pass or the ability to do what is proposed. Houseparents and/or other staff should verify the possession of a pass by a student at time of departure from campus and should enforce restrictions indicated on the pass. A record should be kept whenever a student leaves campus and the name of a companion if any. In addition to recording time of departure and expected return the reports indicate the frequency with which the student uses previously learned skills, and the number of times the student traveled alone. Such records may motivate travel where awards are given to successful travelers each year.

FAMILY INVOLVEMENT

Any mobility program designed to help students to learn how to travel must also give special attention to the involvement of parents and family members. The mobility specialist and/or psychologist must counsel parents from the beginning about realistic abilities of a child and help them to cope with their feelings about the child's independence. From the time the child begins to receive service from the school, the orientation and mobility specialist must insure that information and help to the parents and other family members is available. When a student is capable of teaching a sighted member of his family how to be an effective sighted guide, the beginnings of understanding on the part of the student and the parents will be evident.

THE SCHOOL SETTING

The type of school setting in which mobility instruction takes place may affect the quality of services and the type of modifications that are necessary. The educational setting presents many opportunities for the specialist to share his knowledge about the child as well as his own skills with administrators, teachers, houseparents, and other professionals. There is also the opportunity to gain meaningful insights about the child from colleagues who have observed and/or worked with the child. The school setting may also have roadblocks to providing a sufficient quantity of instruction at intervals which are most beneficial to the child.

Scheduling

The first and most difficult of all roadblocks is the "schedule" and the attitude that once it was established it could not be changed. The second most common roadblock is the lack of insight into innovative and positive approaches by the specialist himself to understanding administrative problems and becoming involved in working out mutual solutions. Another roadblock may be the attitude of teachers toward interruption in class when a student leaves for or returns from a mobility lesson. Still another problem may be the student's attitude toward mobility instruction whenever he experiences difficulty making up classwork missed during the mobility lesson.

School Administration

The quality of the mobility instruction offered is not entirely dependent on the mobility specialist's ability, but many times is determined by the attitude of the administrator of the educational setting. The mobility specialist should be informed about the policy of administration with regard to the provision of orientation and mobility instruction before accepting a mobility position in a particular educational setting. It is important to be clear about the priority that mobility instruction receives in that setting. Is it given status as a regular class? Are sufficient and appropriate blocks of time available? Are sufficient funds and other resources available? Can the schedule be modified as needed to meet legitimate needs of the mobility program? The mobility specialist needs a firm commitment from the administrator regarding budget, availability of low vision services and equipment, and the amount of clerical and other support services available for the preparation of records and reports.

The mobility specialist must also be responsible for working with other staff, both teachers and houseparents (in residential settings), to assist them in understanding and supporting the goals of the mobility program. This is necessary so that all members of the staff may communicate consistent expectations to the child concerning independent travel throughout the building and beyond.

Progress

In a relatively short period of time, the applicability of formal instruction in orientation and mobility to the needs of visually impaired children has been firmly established. Present day programs are not yet as effective as they could be, nor do all children who need this instruction currently receive it. It is expected that the effect of recent federal legislation to insure the right of all handicapped children to the most appropriate education will further expand the role of orientation and mobility instruction in educational programs for visually impaired children.

Bibliography

American Foundation for the Blind. *Facts about blindness*. New York: Author, 1973.

Blasch, B. & Wurzburger, B. Mobility instruction: A professional challenge. *Long Cane News*, 1971, **IV**(3), 1-5.

Costello, H. J. & Gockman, R. *Ability training for junior and senior high school students*. VRA Project RD-1082-S. Chicago Project Summary, Catholic Charities Archdiocese of Chicago, 1966.

Cratty, B. & Sams, T. *The body image of blind children*. New York: American Foundation for the Blind, 1968.

Frostig, M. & Maslow, P. *Learning problems in the classroom*. New York: Grune & Stratton, 1973.

Lord, F. E. *Short form of orientation and mobility skills for young blind children*. United States Office of Education, Project 6-24641, 1970.

Lowenfeld, B. *The changing status of the blind: From separation to integration*. Springfield, Ill.: Charles C Thomas, 1975.

Lowenfeld, B. *The visually handicapped child in school*. New York: John Day Company, 1973.

Metropolitan Society for the Blind. *Education program to maximize independent mobility of blind children in public schools at elementary, junior, and high school levels*. VRA Project 1228, Detroit: Author, 1963.

Roach E., & Kephart, N. *Purdue perceptual-motor survey*. Columbus, Ohio: Charles E. Merrill, 1966.

Welsh, R. L. & Blasch, B. B. Manpower needs in orientation and mobility, *The New Outlook for the Blind*, 1974, **68**, 433-443.

Topic 5. Deaf-Blind Persons

Dennis A. Lolli

The deaf-blind client presents a unique challenge to the mobility specialist. However, as with any challenge, the endeavor demands careful examination and an organized approach. The term *deaf-blind* does not necessarily mean that a

TABLE 1-12

Characteristics of Clients Served at Helen Keller National Center Headquarters from 6-24-69 to 12-31-75

Characteristics	Number of Clients	Per- centage
Male	68	61.3
Female	43	38.7
Visual acuity (better eye with best correction)		
Total blindness	19	17.1
Light perception	16	14.4
Better than light perception and up to and including 5/200	19	17.1
Better than 5/200 and up to and including 20/200	24	21.6
Better than 20/200, all with limitations in the visual fields so severe as to place them within the classification of "blind"	33	29.8
Primary cause of blindness		
Retinitis pigmentosa	57*	51.4
Optic atrophy	11	9.9
Glaucoma	8	7.2
Congenital cataract	11	9.9
Cataract	3	2.7
Macular degeneration	3	2.7
Phthisis bulbi	4	3.6
Corneal scars	3	2.7
Retrolental fibroplasia	2	1.8
Albinism	1	0.9
Chorioretinopathy	1	0.9
Retinal degeneration	2	1.8
Diabetic retinopathy	2	1.8
Anophthalmos	1	0.9
Bilateral retinoblastoma	1	0.9
High myopia	1	0.9

*All but 5 of these (46.8%) were congenitally deaf.

Auditory functionality
(Results of speech discrimination testing—
Stimulus: CID W-22 or Haskins Kindergarten PB Word Lists
Loudness Level: Most comfortable loudness level for speech)
Test results on better ear; optimal test conditions

Discrimination score		
81-100%	0	0.0
61- 80%	3	2.7
41- 60%	2	1.8
21- 40%	5	4.5
0- 20%	101	91.0
Congenitally deaf	80	72.1
Quality of speech		
Normal	15	13.5
Defective, but understandable	22	19.8
Occasional words can be understood	21	18.9
No understandable speech	53	47.8

TABLE 2-12
Seven State Subsample of AFB Sample of Deaf-Blind Children:
Conditions in Addition to Deaf-Blindness

Persons Reported (N = 130)	Number	Percentage
No conditions additional to deaf-blindness	59	45.4
With conditions additional	71	54.6
Additional conditions reported (N = 215)*		
Mental retardation	73	34.0
Speech problems	62	29.0
Brain damage	27	12.5
Cerebral palsy	10	4.6
Orthodontic defects	9	4.1
Cosmetic defects	7	3.2
Cleft palate	5	2.3
Emotional conditions	5	2.3
Other conditions**	17	8.0
Total	215	100.0

*Total conditions exceed number of persons as several had more than one additional condition.
**Includes abnormal skull, heart conditions, short arm or leg, dwarfism, quadraplegic, anemia, paralysis, diabetes, and allergies.

person has no useful vision and/or hearing. In fact, data indicate that only a small percentage of persons referred to as deaf-blind are totally blind (no light perception) and profoundly deaf. The 1976 Annual Report of The Helen Keller National Center for Deaf-Blind Youths and Adults, (Table 1-12) presents a detailed analysis of the characteristics of clients served at the center. An indication of the involvement of additional handicapping conditions within the deaf-blind population can be gained from Table 2-12 (Graham, 1970, p. 9).

The deaf-blind population, therefore, is not a homogeneous group which fits nicely into preconstructed categories. There are variations in time, degree, and mode of occurrence of the disabilities that may suggest ways to understand the client's orientation and mobility needs, goals, and limitations. Initially, the mobility specialist must determine:

1. Whether the client is adventitiously or congenitally deaf-blind

2. Whether he is a victim of a syndrome with additional handicapping conditions

3. Whether the client is totally or partially deaf and/or blind.

It is from these considerations that the picture of the client begins to form.

Chart the Handicap
For example, it is useful to the orientation and mobility specialist to know whether a client has visual memory upon which to build, whether there may be related handicapping conditions to consider, and whether there may be useful auditory and/or visual potentials to encourage. One way to keep track of the possible handicapping combinations is to record them in a chart. The first line in the chart would indicate whether or not the impairment was congenital. The second line would indicate whether or not the impairment was related to a syndrome. The third line would indicate whether the impairment resulted in total blindness or deafness.

440

	Deaf	Blind
Congenital	✓	
Syndrome		✓
Total	✓	

The example indicates someone who was born totally deaf with no additional handicaps and later lost most of his vision in a manner unrelated to the deafness but as part of a syndrome such as diabetes. The etiology of the deaf-blindness will probably indicate what resources to consult in order to gain an understanding of its nature. For example, with retinitis pigmentosa, one is fairly certain of the progressively worsening nature of the eye condition and of night vision problems.

From the three mentioned considerations and sometimes in addition to them, the concept of a primary handicap may arise. This is not to say, however, that in every deaf-blind person there is an identifiable primary handicap. A primary handicap could be considered to be the handicap which appears to have had the major effect on the client's past learning experiences. If, after systematic investigation, it seems that a client is unable to understand certain geometric shapes fully and is, therefore, having difficulty with familiarizations, one might infer that the problem is vision-based. When the same client appears to have additional vision-based difficulties, one may further infer that for this particular deaf-blind person, vision appears to be a handicap with a greater learning impact than hearing, therefore a primary handicap. However, this is an untested concept that may be helpful in some situations but may not be applicable in others.

It can be seen, therefore, that it is useful to know the ordering of the handicap as well as its etiology. Also, there may be cases when either or both handicaps are degenerative in nature, such as a blind client who may be in the process of losing hearing or vice versa. In some cases, such as the one described above, it may be necessary to provide that training which is immediately needed or acceptable to the client and supplement it with additional instruction at a later date when the client is better adjusted to the sensory loss.

COMMUNICATION WITH CLIENT

A major concern for the mobility specialist is how to communicate with the client. There are some deaf-blind persons with whom one may speak in an almost normal manner; raising the voice or slowing the rate of speech may be adequate compensation. Much of the deaf-blind population, however, uses a manual method of communication, such as signing and/or fingerspelling. In rare cases, the services of an interpreter may be available, but when working regularly with deaf-blind persons, it is advisable to take the time to learn some fingerspelling. When greater ease and fluency in communicating with the deaf-blind client is necessary, signing is an invaluable skill for the mobility specialist to possess. Commonly used methods of communication are:

1. One-hand manual alphabet—placing manually-formed letters lightly in the deaf-blind person's hand, pausing between words. Usually, this method is used with totally deaf and blind individuals.

2. Sign language—using symbolic hand and arm movements representative of words. The client should have some residual vision.

3. Todoma Method—placing the thumb and index finger of the client on the lips and throat of the speaker, allowing speech, motion and vibrations to be interpreted. Usually, this method is used with totally deaf and blind persons.

4. Also, in cases where there is enough residual vision, communication can occur

by notewriting. This is an especially important ability for deaf-blind persons who can use it as it gives them the ability to converse with the general public when needed.

RELATED CONSIDERATIONS

Once it becomes possible to communicate with the client, the mobility specialist must attend to other considerations. Complete medical, educational, psychological, and social records should be reviewed, particularly the hearing and vision reports. In addition, care should be given to avoid overlooking other factors such as physical endurance, haptic considerations, and speech therapy.

Physical Endurance

It is especially necessary not to overlook clients who have cardiovascular limitations because of age or congenital syndrome. Lessons should be planned with rest or break sessions, and strenuous sessions should be avoided on hot days.

Haptic Considerations

Usually, the haptic sensing system is the major near sense that the deaf-blind person has on which to rely, although this may not be true for the client with neuropathies. There should be a sensitivity on the part of the mobility specialist to incorporate, whenever possible, the haptic sense into lessons and thereby encourage the development and continued use of this sense.

In initial instruction, care should be given to avoid training sessions on carpeted surfaces as they minimize the general vibrations and feedback that the client receives from his environment and can also discourage the client from developing the haptic sensing system. The specialist should later structure training to introduce the difference between carpeted and non-carpeted surfaces. Additional important information about the haptic sense is provided in Chapters 4 and 5.

Speech Therapy

Some clients may have a speech pattern that is difficult to understand. In many instances it can be improved through the work of a speech therapist. This can have a positive effect on the traveler's self-concept, especially if it enables him to use speech in dealing with the public as opposed to other communication systems.

TRAVEL AIDS

Once in training, there are a number of aids and program modifications that will enable the deaf-blind client to have more meaningful instruction. The haptic sense is the major remaining sense for totally deaf and blind clients. The mobility specialist should capitalize on it by using as many tactile models and maps as are available or as are needed.

The long cane is generally used as the main travel aid for deaf-blind clients. For many low vision deaf clients, the cane may be useful for identification purposes.

An electronic device which has been found useful to some totally deaf-blind clients is the E Model Pathsounder, (Russell, 1974), equipped with a chest and neck unit that vibrates when the user is a certain distance from an object. (See Chapter 11.) The chest unit is activated at 6 ft (182 cm) from an object, and the neck unit at 30 in. (76 mm).

The role of dog guides as a travel aid is somewhat uncertain and varies with different dog training agencies. Those agencies that do not work with deaf-blind persons cite the following as concerns:

1. The candidate should be able to hear vehicle traffic well enough to determine its proximity and direction in relation to where he is standing.

2. Since instruction in the use of the dog is given orally and in classroom settings,

the client may not be able to hear the lectures.

3. The deaf-blind client should be able to hear a spoken voice from a distance so the instructor can communicate from a distance.

In this last instance, it is very important that the instructor be able to be at a distance from the dog and new master so that the dog begins to relate to its new master. In those cases when dog training had been provided, it appeared that clients had a degree of residual hearing or vision or both. Guiding Eyes for the Blind trained one totally deaf and blind client who had previous dog guide experience before losing her hearing. It appears that some pedestrian aid would still be needed in such an instance when the dog user arrived at street crossings.

Street Crossings

Clients who are totally deaf and blind are not able to cross streets independently with safety. Obviously, if there is sufficient useful vision the low vision, profoundly deaf person can be taught to cross streets. With this combination of handicaps, however, the mobility specialist should emphasize the importance of the client being visually alert to the possibility of traffic turning in front of the line of travel. It is also important to discover whether the client is able to detect the proximity of traffic through vibrations felt from the pavement through the feet.

Traffic light systems that emit sounds in conjunction with walk signs can provide a supplemental system to reinforce the walk-cycle detection. The low vision, profoundly deaf client can feel vibrations in the traffic light pole that correspond to the bell-ringing during a walk cycle, and serve to "verify" detection of the walk cycle. These auditory systems are not widespread, however, and should only be used as a support to other methods of traffic flow analysis. In addition, even when they do exist at an intersection, the poles that contain the vibrating mechanism only exist at one or two of the intersection corners. Such an aid is most useful when a client is being familiarized to only one route and it contains this type of traffic control. Additional information regarding the effects of hearing loss upon street crossings is presented in Chapter 8.

COMMUNICATING WITH THE PUBLIC

If a client's self-concept permits, the hearing aid should be clearly visible so that the public is aware of a hearing disability in advance. This can avoid embarrassing situations for everyone involved. It is also wise to discuss with the client some attitudes that the public has regarding hearing aids, such as that the person is hard of hearing and must be shouted at, or that the hearing problem is corrected and there is no need to alter the volume of speech.

Another explanation that can be given to the client to reduce the possibility of an embarrassing situation is that the manual alphabet and/or signing are not generally known by the public who will probably not know how to respond when approached by someone using one of those methods of communicating. Also, the client who has nonintelligible speech should be helped to realize that an unexpected voice tone may startle the typical person on the street. In both of these instances, if the client is able to write notes, he will be better served by that method of communicating.

For various reasons, note cards with braille index codes may be useful in establishing communication. Introductory messages on the cards could be:

1. I am blind and have poor hearing. Could you please help me (to be filled in with appropriate need). Thank you.

2. I am deaf and do not see well. Could you please help me . . . etc.

3. I am deaf and blind. Could you please help me . . . etc.

An example of an appropriate need might be "Could you please help me to cross Maple Street" or "to board the Harvard Square bus." It is advisable that the client catalogue the cards and that they be retained in the client's hand when in use. The reason for retaining the card is to reduce the possibility of the public thinking that the client is making a request for a contribution or handout.

Another method sometimes used to identify a deaf-blind person, a deaf-low vision person, or a blind person with a hearing problem, is the wearing of a large button on outer garments with the appropriate message. However, the client may not feel comfortable with this arrangement. Some common reservations have been that the handicap is being "advertised," that the public may not take the message seriously and consider it a "joke" button, and that it is a bother to change it to each piece of outerwear or to have enough buttons.

Sidewalk Travel

The client with severe hearing limitations can travel more safely by making some simple adjustments in sidewalk travel. For example, if a deaf client is walking along a residential sidewalk and approaching a driveway, he is, theoretically, in more danger than a hearing client unless he notices the driveway and visually scans it and the parallel street for possible turning or exiting traffic. Often, in these instances, the client is helped by the visibility of the cane for identification as a handicapped traveller. The visually handicapped client who is unable to see a vehicle has an even greater dependence on the cane to serve as an identifier to a driver. It is important that the deaf-blind traveler discover the locations of driveways, parking lots, and the like and become completely familiar with them so as to proceed with extra caution in these areas.

Physical proximity is needed between client and mobility specialist for communication. It is wise to be within quick reach of the client as observations cannot be effectively called out from behind. This is especially true in the beginning phases of instruction when both parties are becoming familiar with one another's communication skills and it is an easy time for discrepancies to occur.

Nonverbal Clients

Many rubella and other multiply impaired deaf-blind clients may have limited receptive and/or expressive language. This greatly infringes on the mobility specialist's reliance on verbal feedback, which usually supplements the client's physical demonstration. Thus, the specialist may be in a situation where physical demonstration of a travel ability must substitute for verbal feedback. In this instance, it is wise to select the setting based on the objective of the lesson. For example, in attempting to assess a client's skill in scanning for traffic before crossing streets, the client might be asked to mail a letter at a mailbox, with which he is familiar, two blocks away. This will allow the mobility specialist an opportunity to observe the client at a task which cannot be verbally described to him. It is important, however, that the skill remain as the focal point, rather than the completion of the task.

In making suggestions for correcting unsafe behavior in a client, the method of skill imitation can be used, providing the client has sufficient vision. That is, the mobility specialist should play the role of the person about to cross a street and demonstrate the sequence and/or behavior which the client needs to emulate. Depending upon the functioning level of the client, demonstrations can contain gestures, physical exaggerations and/or a mime-like approach. It is important, however, that a critical attitude be maintained by the mobility specialist toward the consistency, reliability, adaptability, and overall quality of the client's assimilation of the skill. The specialist must be careful not to oversimplify or generalize.

There are, of course, as many modifications as there are clients and specialists. Therefore, any attempt to present a total picture of orientation and mobility for deaf-blind persons will be incomplete. A strong first step is for the mobility specialist to contact those agencies, services, and personnel who have background and experience with this type of client. It is through this type of careful and organized approach that the deaf-blind client is assured of receiving appropriate and meaningful instruction.

Bibliography

Chess, S., Korn, D.J., & Fernandez, P. B. *Psychiatric disorders of children with congenital rubella*. New York: Brunner/Mazel Pub., 1972.

Efron, M. & DuBoff, B. R. *A vision guide for teachers of deaf-blind children*. Raleigh: North Carolina Department of Public Instruction, 1975.

Ficociello, C. *Total approach to educating deaf-blind children*. Paper presented at the Deaf-Blind Child Determining a Direction Workshop, Seattle, May, 1975.

Gallaway, A. *Orientation and mobility readiness skills for the pre-school deaf-blind child*. Proceedings of a Special Institute Conference for Teachers of Deaf-Blind Children, Berkeley, California, June, 1970.

Graham, M. *The deaf-blind: Some studies and suggestions for a national program*. New York: American Foundation for the Blind, 1970.

Guldager, V. *Body image and the severely handicapped rubella child*. Watertown, Mass.: Perkins School for the Blind, 1970.

Hammer, E. K. *What we know about deaf-blind children and early development*. Paper presented at the 50th Annual Convention, Council for Exceptional Children, Washington, D.C., March, 1972.

Kinney, R. *Independent living without sight and hearing*. Arlington Heights, Ill.: The Gray Dove, 1972.

Lin-Fu, J. *Rubella*. Washington, D.C.: Department of Health Education and Welfare, 1970.

Montagu, A. *Touching: The human significance of skin*. New York: Columbia University Press, 1971.

O'Brien, R. *Alive . . . aware . . . a person*. Rockville, Maryland, Montgomery County Public Schools, 1976.

O'Rourke, T.J. *A basic course in manual communication*. Silver Springs, Md.: National Association of the Deaf, 1970.

Quarterman, F. *Instruction in physical orientation and mobility for deaf-blind persons*. Paper presented at the workshop for Paraprofessionals Working with Deaf-Blind Children, Chicago, sponsored by the Midwest Regional Center for Services to Deaf-Blind Children, Lansing, Michigan, 1974.

Russell, L. *Pathsounder instructor's handbook for E-model Pathsounders*, Cambridge, Massachusetts Institute of Technology, 1974.

Sherrick, C. E. *1980 is now*. Los Angeles, Calif.: John Tracy Clinic, 1974.

Topic 6. The Visually Handicapped Person with Cerebral Palsy

Sandra J. McCloskey Gamble

Cerebral palsy can be defined as a difficulty with movement caused by a benign lesion in the brain and occurring before the second year of life (Mohr, 1975). To understand cerebral palsy, one must first understand normal movement. Muscles work in patterns and with groups of muscles. The brain responds to the intention to move using these groups in a series of movements, not using the contraction of a single muscle. Because of brain damage, these patterns are abnormal and uncoordinated in a cerebral palsied person. To accomplish a certain task, the cerebral palsied person must compensate with abnormal movements and must expend extra energy. Since by definition cerebral palsy occurs early in a child's development, all of his movements are affected by learning with abnormal patterns (Finnie, 1975).

CLASSIFICATION

There are two basic methods of classifying cerebral palsy: one by the type of movement disorder, and the other by the area of the body that is involved. The movement disorder classification includes spasticity, athetosis, ataxia, and hypotonicity. *Spasticity* is an increase in muscle tone resulting in limited movements. *Athetosis* is characterized by frequent uncontrolled movements with wide patterns of motion. *Ataxia* is a lack of balance and smooth motor patterns. *Hypotonicity* or floppy is defined by a marked decrease in muscle tone (Bobath & Bobath, 1973). Each of these types of cerebral palsy represents distinct characteristics, but they are rarely seen in their true form. For example, a child may have spastic extremities and a floppy or hypotonic trunk. Therefore his arms and legs are stiff and have few motions while his trunk has little or no ability to maintain an upright position for sitting or standing. To complicate the categories of cerebral palsy further, there is a wide range of severity of each type. Some persons have such marked motor difficulty that they cannot control their heads or have any purposeful movements of their arms and legs. Others are able to ambulate only with crutches for short distances. More mildly involved persons may have observable gait or coordination deviations, but functionally they can carry out most tasks.

The second type of cerebral palsy, referring to the areas of the body involved, includes quadriplegia or double hemiplegia, diplegia or paraplegia, and hemiplegia. Quadriplegia or double hemiplegia refers to disturbances in the four extremities, the head, and the trunk. Diplegia or paraplegia means that most of the involvement is in the legs. Hemiplegia means that one side of the body is affected. Most people use terms from both classifications to describe motor involvement in a cerebral palsied person. For instance, spastic diplegia means that the person has increased muscle tone in his lower extremities. Athetoid quadriplegia means that the person has wide uncontrolled movements affecting all four extremities (Bobath & Bobath, 1973).

Cerebral palsy, except in very rare cases, is not a progressive disorder. The main lesion in the brain causing the motor disturbances does not change. A person may, however, develop contractures or bony abnormalities because of persistent movement patterns during growth. On the other hand, functional and motor capabilities may improve through proper treatment and through normal maturation.

Other disturbances often accompany the motor abnormalities that characterize cerebral palsy. These include deficits in perception (visual, auditory, haptic, and proprioceptive), integration of perceptual motor tasks, speech, cognitive abilities, social and psychological adjustment, and general life experiences (Bobath & Bobath, 1973). This rather involved definition indicates that cerebral palsy is a comprehensive term describing a person who has some difficulty with movement due to brain damage at a very young age. Also it points out that very often the motor deficit is accompanied by other abnormalities and that there is a wide range of characteristics and a wide range of involvement within each of the characteristics.

12

TEAM EVALUATION—MANAGEMENT

Such a complicated involvement requires thorough evaluation by a team consisting of a mobility specialist, a physical therapist, an occupational therapist, a speech therapist, a psychologist, an eye specialist, a social worker, a vocational counselor, a teacher (if the client is a child in school), the client, and the family. Information should also be shared with the client's managing physician. Each of these disciplines has unique capabilities to promote better growth and development for the client. For a good team approach to work, each member must know what the professional and personal qualifications are for fellow team members to prevent overlapping of effort and to utilize each member's capabilities more fully.

The team first conducts separate and unique evaluations of the client and then meets to discuss the evaluations and to set realistic and objective goals. The client and his family must be an active part of the goal setting. A team leader should be appointed for each client. It is the team leader's responsibility to see that the suggestions of the team are carried out and to schedule any future meetings about that client. An effective team approach requires ongoing evaluations of the client and constant formal and informal communication among the team members, not only to provide a better program for the client, but also to establish a good learning experience for team members.

The mobility specialist must define his role with each client and use the evaluation tools at his disposal for his part in the team evaluation. The evaluative tools should include concept testing, functional vision evaluations, observations of the client's present mobility status, and a discussion with the client about his objectives for a mobility program. This should give the mobility specialist specific information for the team meeting.

In addition, the mobility specialist should ask questions of other team members about ambulatory status, endurance, balance, perceptual motor problems, adaptive devices needed (especially for ambulation), communication skills, cognitive development, hearing, residual vision, and social history. Although much of this information can be gathered on a trial and error basis or by rough screening techniques, it can be obtained more accurately from other professionals. Using this procedure enables the mobility specialist to concentrate in areas where he is most skilled. Many members of the team have input that would affect the mobility program, but they do not know exactly what information the mobility specialist needs. Good communication is necessary to enable the team approach to work effectively. A mobility specialist will sometimes have to work without benefits of an organized team, but he can still formulate questions and seek information from other sources by using formal consultations or informal information gathering techniques.

Goals

The mobility goals set up by the team (or by the mobility specialist with input from other professionals) can cover a wide range depending on the capabilities of the client. Some may achieve maximum independent travel only in familiar, barrier-free, indoor settings. Others may become fully independent travelers. In a particular instance, one client reached his potential of independent travel in a wheelchair with a Pathsounder in a residential building specifically designed for handicapped people. The client had cerebral palsy defined as spastic paraplegia, was totally blind, and had very limited experience with any independent travel. Over half the time used for mobility lessons was devoted to practicing routes in the building where he planned to live. If he were to move to a new building, a significant amount of time would be required to teach route travel in the new setting. Another client, also totally blind with spastic paraplegia, had reached a

447

level of independent travel in a small business area. She walked without any assistive devices, but had difficulty with travel in unfamiliar areas. Her delayed reaction time often caused her to fall when she came to a curb unexpectedly. She also had trouble in slippery conditions because of poor balance. In addition to the long cane, she was given an orthopedic cane to use when traveling in unfamiliar areas and during slippery conditions.

Developmental Help

In addition to a regular mobility program, a blind child with cerebral palsy needs special developmental help. A mobility specialist working with children should be familiar with normal motor development, the age ranges for each developmental step, and the quality of normal movements, in order to understand motor problems and to keep demands realistic. For instance, according to Gesell (1940), a child learns to ascend stairs independently and with alternating feet at the age of three years. A child cannot descend a long stairway unsupported and with alternating feet until he is five years old. A child who has not mastered these tasks should be taught first to ascend stairs. It is unrealistic to demand the mastery of both skills at the same time.

Sound Localization Skills

Children or adults who have to use their hands for support on crutches or to propel a wheelchair cannot gather much haptic information when traveling, so they must rely more heavily on sound clues. A client whose reaction time is slower may need more familiarization and specific information about his environment. This would enable him to anticipate stairs or obstacles and to travel more slowly in danger areas. The mobility specialist can assist in assuring safety of movement for a multiply handicapped person by teaching sound localization skills or the use of hearing for indoor travel.

Gross Motor Skills

The mobility specialist should institute work with physical therapists, occupational therapists, and physical education personnel to establish a gross motor program. Children who have had limited movement experiences benefit greatly from this type of program that gives them safe, creative, and pleasant opportunities to move more freely within their environment. A gross motor program for children with cerebral palsy must be designed for the type of movement that is best for each individual client. A spastic child needs slow rhythmical movement, because fast movement increases spasticity of muscle tone and decreases the ability to produce good quality movements. An athetoid child is generally able to move better when standing or sitting than when lying down. Each child's unique movement needs should be evaluated in setting up individual goals. A movement program demands a one-to-one individualized program to establish a favorable atmosphere for success. The approach can also be used with adults and adolescents, but the benefits are greatest for preschool and primary-school-aged children. At this age, positive experiences with gross motor movements can lay a firm foundation for good mobility skills.

CONCEPT DEVELOPMENT

Concept development takes on added importance with the cerebral palsied client, as the capacity for sensory intake may be damaged as well as the ability to integrate the sensory information on a cortical level. It is important for the team to set goals in keeping with the client's perceptual motor capabilities. It is unrealistic to ask a person who shows signs of tactile defensiveness to develop concepts tactually without advance preparation. Ayers (1964, p. 8) defines a tactile defensive person as one who has "feelings of discomfort and a desire to escape a situation where certain types of tactile stimuli are experienced." There is an imbalance between their protective system and their discriminating system when reacting to tactile stimuli, with the protective system predominating. Tactile defensiveness is a malfunction in sensory integration. An example would be a negative response to the map of an intersection being drawn on the back of a person's hand. The response could take the form of a grimace, increased motor activity, negative verbal remarks, or inattention. In each instance, ability to learn or process information is decreased at the moment of negative response. Ayers notes that the response is less severe when the person touches an object as opposed to his being touched or when he can anticipate the stimulus. If a client shows consistent difficulty in processing sensory information, further testing and evaluation by the physician or the occupational therapist is indicated.

The mobility specialist has a unique opportunity to offer new experiences and concepts as building blocks for future travel programs. This can be done in individual mobility lessons or by the mobility specialist acting as a consultant to teachers and other rehabilitative personnel on concepts to be taught. A mobility specialist might work on developing a better body image as an objective during mobility class. At the same time the mobility specialist could suggest related activities to the classroom teacher, using the skills learned in mobility class for visiting stores or for indoor travel.

When working with multiply handicapped people, it is imperative to define the role of each discipline, especially in relation to concept materials. Duplication of effort is unfortunate, but unavoidable, because these clients need help in so many areas.

AN INDIVIDUALIZED PROGRAM

Each multiply handicapped client has such differing problems and also unique capabilities that an individualized program is necessary. There are practical suggestions that can be helpful in dealing with architectual barriers, inclement weather, stress factors, reaction time for processing information, veering problems, timing for crossing streets, modification of cane skills, effects of speech problems, experience lessons, and splinter skills.

Architectural Barriers

In indoor and outdoor travel the most obvious difficulty occurs with architectural barriers—stairs, curbs, narrow doorways, revolving doors. Each poses different ambulation problems to different clients. Those with balance problems or with slow reactions should be familiar with an area in order to anticipate drop-offs, or else slow their walking pace in an unfamiliar area. Clients who have difficulty ascending or descending a curb should practice the skill in a variety of situations with different height curbs so that they will know what they can handle and where they will need assistance. Clients who are interested should also be informed of various organizations, public and private, working to reduce architectural barriers so that they can provide information regarding their own needs.

Weather

Slippery conditions, such as rain, snow, or ice, can make travel hazardous to clients with even mild balance problems. These conditions require more energy and endurance from the client. The client may have to resort to additional support for travel. If a client usually travels with crutches, a wheelchair may be needed in slippery conditions. A person who usually walks independently may need an orthopedic cane for support.

Stress

Stress factors create a more subtle obstacle for traveling. Fatigue, increased noise and confusion, and emotional upsets are the most common stress factors. Stress can precipitate abnormal motor problems not seen in more comfortable situations. For example, under stress a person with spastic diplegia might exhibit an increase in muscle tone, which could narrow the base of support, make balance more unstable, and a fall more likely.

Reaction Time

As mentioned before, reaction time may be slow for multiply handicapped clients causing them to take longer to process information about their environment before responding to it. This could cause them to trip over curbs or run into objects even though they have received feedback about their placement. Several techniques can be applied here. A longer cane can be used to increase the time between touching an object and running into it. Thorough familiarization with an area is indicated so that objects or drop-offs can be anticipated and reaction time shortened. A client can be encouraged to slow down in unfamiliar areas so that he has more time to respond to new information. If he has good control over his gait and can change it, the center of gravity should be shifted backwards so that weight is over the heels instead of the the balls of the feet. This enables the client to stop more quickly and prevent falls, especially at drop-offs.

Veering

Veering is common with multiply handicapped persons because ambulation and coordination problems make it difficult enough to walk a straight line even without a visual handicap. A visually handicapped person with cerebral palsy has a double reason for veering. Two approaches can be used: stress auditory skills so that the client can line up with traffic patterns or use a solid building line to give a straight line clue; consistent feedback for self awareness of movement is helpful so that the client can fully understand his tendency to veer and the direction of the veer he usually takes. If the client has a consistent problem, he can build in a correction in potentially confusing areas, such as street crossings.

Crossing Time

Crossing streets with or without a light puts a time limit on completing the task. The most common length of a traffic light cycle is 30 seconds. If, after practice, a client's gait is so slow that he cannot complete the crossing in 30 seconds, he should solicit aid to complete the crossing safely.

Cane Skills

A fair amount of motor planning and coordination is required to learn the touch cane technique successfully. Some clients may have to use a modification of the touch technique, such as sliding the cane along the ground when moving it from side to side to give a tactual clue about the placement of the cane tip. The mobility specialist may also have to make exceptions to his expectations of hand placement and wrist motion. It is more important for the client to have good coverage with the cane than to have perfect technique. Remember that stress, both emotional and physical, can cause a cerebral palsied client to exhibit increased motor disturbances. A client, therefore, could have difficulty with the touch cane technique under certain circumstances. There should be varied opportunities in traveling to evaluate any potential problems.

Speech Problems

Speech problems can cause difficulties in interacting with the public. The first step is for the client and the mobility specialist to know the client's capabilities and limitations. In many cases, practice through role playing and lessons graded in difficulty can increase the client's capabilities. Severe speech problems may necessitate carrying written requests to solicit aid.

Experience Lessons

Persons who are multiply handicapped often have had little opportunity to experience a variety of travel experiences. During the mobility program, every client should have the opportunity to visit a variety of stores and public buildings. For some it may mean that the mobility specialist acts as a sighted guide or pushes the client in a wheelchair. The client may never expect to travel independently in these buildings, but just going through them is a valuable experience. The client can be given the responsibility of making a purchase or asking for information, even if he is not traveling independently. All of these experiences help to alleviate the experiential deprivation and the verbal unreality common in multiply handicapped clients. It is also important that parents, families, or other personnel working with clients be taught the safest and smoothest means of transporting them, so that these experiences can be continued after the mobility program is completed.

Splinter Skills

With adolescents and adults it is often necessary to teach splinter skills rather than to adhere to a strict developmental sequence. "A splinter skill is very much like a motor skill; it is specific for a particular behavioral response" (Roach & Kephart, 1966). Therefore that skill is learned for only that particular situation and cannot be carried over to other similar situations, such as climbing steps using a technique that cannot be carried over to stepping up on a curb. This also relates to learning route travel instead of learning independent travel skills. When it is necessary, it is imperative to have mobility actually taught in the client's home, work, and recreational areas. Then the client does not have to make the transition from the lesson to his home area. Again, good evaluation is necessary so that the right decision is made to teach the splinter skill rather than teaching all the steps leading to that skill.

OTHER CLIENTS

These suggestions for adapting a mobility program for a visually impaired person with cerebral palsy may also be applied to clients with other movement disorders. They include those who have had strokes, head trauma or brain tumors causing neuromuscular problems, spina bifida or myelomeningocele, multiple sclerosis, and accidents requiring a period of time on crutches or in a wheelchair. In all cases the first step is an understanding of the client's abilities with input from a variety of personnel. Evaluation, goal planning, and team approach are all necessary for good programs.

CHALLENGE

Working with cerebral palsied persons is an exciting field in need of innovative thinking, documentation of programs, and an ongoing team approach. The mobility specialist needs to define his role more specifically as very little work has been done in mobility, especially with clients at a very low developmental level. Evaluative tools need to be developed and standardized. Also, successes and failures of present programs need to be documented so that better programs can be developed. Since the number of multiply handicapped clients involved in programs for the visually handicapped is increasing, attention needs to be given to innovative programs now. A challenge exists for mobility specialists to develop good programs for cerebral palsied clients with a visual handicap.

Bibliography

Ayers, J. *Sensory integration and learning disorders.* Western Psychological Services, 1972.

Ayers, J. Tactile functions. *The American Journal of Occupational Therapy,* 1964, **1**(XVII), 6-11.

Barsch, R. *Achieving perceptual motor efficiency: A space oriented approach to learning.* Seattle: Special Child Publications, 1967. 2 vols.

Bobath, K. The neuropathology of cerebral palsy and its importance in treatment and diagnosis. *Cerebral Palsy Bulletin,* 1959, **1**(8), 13-33.

Bobath, K., & Bobath, B. *Neurodevelopmental Training Course Syllabus.* (Unpublished.) 1973.

Bobath, K., & Bobath, B. The facilitation of normal postural reactions and movements in the treatment of cerebral palsy. *Physiotherapy,* August, 1964.

Cratty, B., & Sams, T. *The body image of blind children.* New York: American Foundation for the Blind, 1968.

Finnie, N. *Handling the young cerebral palsied child at home.* New York: E. P. Dutton & Co., 1975.

Gesell, A. *First five years of life: A guide to the study of the preschool child.* New York: Harper, 1940.

Illingworth, R. S. *The development of the infant and young child.* (5th ed.) Baltimore: Williams and Wilkins, 1972.

Illinois Department of Children and Family Services. *Orientation and mobility for the visually handicapped: A guide for parents.* Author.

Kephart, N. C. *The slow learner in the classroom.* Columbus: Charles E. Merrill Books, Inc., 1960.

Los Angeles County Schools. *East San Gabriel Valley School educational program for multi-handicapped children.* (1st ed.) Los Angeles: Author, 1972.

McGraw, M., & Lydon, W. *Concept development.* New York: American Foundation for the Blind, 1972.

Mohr, J. Neurodevelopmental treatment. Course presented at the Home for Crippled Children, Pittsburgh, July, 1975.

Roach, E., & Kephart, N. *The Purdue perceptual motor survey.* Columbus: Charles E. Merrill Publishing Co., 1966.

Scrutton, D. R. Some thoughts underlying the treatment of hypertonic cerebral palsy. *Physiotherapy,* 1967, 53.

Topic 7. The Mentally Retarded Visually Impaired Person

Nancy W. Bryant and Wayne A. Jansen

Increased integration into the school and the community makes it essential that visually impaired, mentally retarded persons be adequately prepared for and skilled in moving through the environment during the course of their daily activities. Educational and living alternatives that are less restrictive than in the past may cause a student to be faced with requirements for independent mobility that are beyond his capacity. The mentally retarded, visually impaired person may experience great difficulty in learning skills that will enable him to better cope with his environment. The ramifications of etiology and severity of mental retardation and how these factors interact with visual impairment are complex and often difficult to understand. Mental retardation not only may complicate, delay, and/or diminish the acquisition of orientation and mobility skills, but its presence will challenge an instructor's creativity in devising suitable teaching techniques for the special client.

The sometimes complex adaptations needed to simplify concepts which must be incorporated by the student of limited ability cannot be found in a compendium. The mobility specialist will find little in the literature and will most often have to depend on resourcefulness. Each client is different and should be treated as such. This section will attempt to present educational principles drawn from the fields of visual impairment and mental retardation that can be related to the development of programs of orientation and mobility for the visually impaired mentally retarded person.

PLANNING

The first step in the design and implementation of an orientation and mobility program for the mentally retarded is the instructor's planning. Although the steps are not significantly different than those required for any good training program, careful advance review of an individual's attributes can pave the way for success while avoiding frustration and failure for both student and instructor.

There are two considerations that must be taken into account:

1. Mental retardation is a condition that exists in as many variations and forms as does visual impairment. The interaction of the degree of visual loss and the degree of mental retardation is obviously of primary importance. The mildly retarded, partially seeing adult presents an entirely different training challenge from a severely retarded, blind child. The degree or extent of each disability must be considered separately as well as in relationship to each other when goals are established and the training sequence planned.

2. Neither the difficulty nor the effectiveness of the training is necessarily related to the severity of the handicaps either individually or in combination. Every individual can profit from instruction that is realistically designed, creatively implemented and periodically evaluated for its effectiveness.

With this in mind the following outline is offered as a guide for acquiring and assimilating information relevant to the design of a training program for the retarded student:

PHYSICAL CHARACTERISTICS
Visual Acuity and Efficiency

Visual acuities obtained in conventional ways by professionals who have limited experience with the retarded may be inaccurate. A true picture of the student's visual efficiency may only come as the result of observation. As the derived visual acuity may be affected by mental retardation, the individual's potential for visual efficiency may also be diminished for concept development and/or the inability to reason, draw conclusions, and report these conclusions may result in what appears to be poor use of residual vision. An alert instructor should be able to separate these strongly interactive factors through close observation over a period of time.

Other Handicaps

The presence of one or more impairments in an individual increases the probability that other impairments will also be present. The interaction of additional problems which may affect the student's ability to profit from mobility training must be taken into account.

Chronological/Developmental Age Disparity

The mentally retarded individual will not be able to perform at a developmental level commensurate with his chronological age. General estimates of this disparity can be obtained from psychological tests, developmental histories, and behavioral observations. This disparity will affect the nature, time, and length of instructional units presented to the student.

General Health

Although the student's health is always an integral part of the planning process, it is of particular importance with a mentally retarded individual. He/she is more susceptible to both chronic and acute diseases. Some of an individual's particular susceptibilities (i.e., elevated blood pressure, upper respiratory infections, allergies, etc.) will influence the nature and course of the training program.

MENTAL CHARACTERISTICS

Intellectual Level and Etiology

Certain causes of mental retardation may have specific behavioral characteristics. For example: Down's Syndrome clients are usually trainable (30 to 50 IQ), placid, and manageable. Certain kinds of brain damage are associated with hyperactivity, distractibility, and perseveration. The general intellectual abilities of a student will influence the level of instruction but the behavioral characteristics will also affect the program's nature. A relatively able student who is mildly mentally retarded may only profit from short lessons covering one concept repeated numerous times due to distractibility, inattentiveness, or other behavioral characteristics.

Learning History

The knowledge of a client's general response to training/education may assist the specialist. It is also possible that a mentally retarded student may appear totally unskilled in mobility only to have the record reveal his "graduation" from a program in another setting. It would be important to know the nature of the former program and the student's response to it in order to revive, retrain, and retain those skills necessary to his successful travel. One of the salient characteristics of a retarded client are deficits in the area of retention and/or the inability to apply previously learned skills to new settings (transfer of training).

Socialization/Interaction Style

Most mentally retarded students are aware of their deficiencies, at least in general. Their lack of confidence in trying to learn new skills could result in the failure of a perfectly designed program. The relationship between the instructor and client is often the key to its success. Previous history could influence the way in which initial contacts with the client are made.

Motivation

Many mentally retarded persons have impaired motivation, particularly toward tasks that represent "school-like learning," due to past history of failure. Because orientation and mobility may be perceived as offering new freedom, it is important to know if the client can understand the value of such training. It may also be important to project just how long the student can work toward a long-range goal of increased freedom. Mentally retarded clients may be easily discouraged by early failure. This will influence the amount of work and number of concepts presented in any given lesson. Motivational level will also influence the pace of instruction.

Fear and Anxiety Level

An unfortunate or unplanned event could cause major setbacks in the progress of the retarded client. However, because of the retarded client's inability to reason effectively or seek cause and effect relationships, fears are not easily allayed. Retarded clients may also suspect supernatural intervention (God never really meant for me to travel with a cane!). More than the usual assurances may be necessary.

Self-Concept, Self-Worth

As with normal clients, the mentally retarded person who has a healthy regard for himself will more likely be motivated to acquire new skills which will give him greater access to the world about him. Though not the primary goal of the mobility specialist, he can reinforce the client's positive feelings of self-worth through success in training. Attention to success is even more important to the retarded person whose self-concept has often suffered many indignities by the time he is considered for mobility training.

ENVIRONMENTAL DEMANDS
As Perceived by Client's Advocate

The characteristics of both the present and future setting where the student will spend the majority of time (i.e., home, school, community, etc.) will influence the skills a retarded client needs. If the retarded individual can only achieve a certain level, it is logical that his most important needs take priority over skills that may be of little long-term value. These needs should be ranked with the input of parents or caretakers, teachers, and vocational/rehabilitation counselors.

As Perceived by Client

The client can provide valuable information for selection of skills to be learned. The client's life-style including recreational skills and preferences must be taken into account.

SPECIAL FEATURES
Realistic Tempo

Beginning lessons should be well organized and closely supervised to provide a realistic tempo while maintaining the retarded student's interest. The student's performance is often best the first few times a skill is attempted. The practice periods should be short with frequent changes of activity to avoid frustration brought on by failure to maintain the desired level of performance. Certain skills should be practiced frequently to establish them well. These practice periods should be spaced so as to maintain interest and enthusiasm. New activities should be introduced early in a period because the student is likely to fatigue as the hour progresses. Pacing throughout the period should be varied unless the client requires a very rigid schedule to profit from instruction. As the student progresses, mobility sessions can be lengthened in accord with mental and physical development.

Activities

The selection of activities for the retarded student should be based on the individual's background, needs, interests, and abilities. The lessons should meet the student's immediate and long range practical mobility needs. The student's mental age is an important factor in the selection of activities. Verbal directions should be few, simple, and at a level easily understood by the student. Educational level must also be considered. A student cannot be expected to read even simple directions if they are beyond his capability. To a greater extent than for normal students, repetition and review are essential components of any lesson. Familiar sites and activities for training should be used in the beginning. The mentally retarded individual will be better able to relate to the requirements of known situations. As training progresses, coping with the unfamiliar can be programmed into lessons. Activities must be continually evaluated and modified to find those most suitable for a particular student in a particular situation.

Instructor-Student Relationships

When a student is learning mobility skills and concepts, praise and encouragement are indispensable for achievement and progress. Even if the student's efforts do not result in successful performance, the effort that is expended can contribute to his mental and physical development when handled positively. Demonstration and participation by the instructor are crucial for the retarded learner. Physically moving the student's body through the movements desired is often effective in bringing about results. Patience is not only required of the instructor, but is an important goal for the student. When he is patient with himself he will be happy and progress at a reasonable and satisfying rate.

In order for the student to lead a happy life, he needs to be given the opportunity to know himself and to develop the ability to think for himself. He needs a feeling of worthiness and competence in both physical and mental tasks. The mobility specialist has an opportunity to provide these experiences and foster personal growth of his retarded student. A good relationship between instructor and student will enhance skill acquisition for independence as well as interpersonal skills with other individuals and as a member of a group. Mentally retarded students may misinterpret or exaggerate the traits of parents and teachers, such as kindness, anger, confidence, etc. As models, we must be sensitively aware of our effect on mentally retarded students for not only what we teach but *how* we react may remain with the student for many years hence.

Expectations

Deficient transfer of training capability is a characteristic of the mentally retarded learner. In the beginning the student will show little transfer of skill from one activity to another. However, once a skill is well learned, the mentally retarded person has a usable tool for problem solving, and will be able to integrate skills over a long period of time, if the instructor perseveres. Many times the student will reach a plateau before moving on to achieve another skill. Regression in a particular skill is also common because of insufficient practice or poor understanding of the ask. Instruction must be slow, deliberate, progressive, and concrete. Expectations must be realistic but always provide a goal toward which a student must strive. The mobility specialist is the key to coordinating expectations for successful gains by the student.

SPECIAL CONSIDERATIONS
Confidence Levels

It is particularly important to be aware of a mentally retarded client's level of confidence. A student who lacks confidence needs a setting where he will learn to feel good about himself and his ability to be mobile. This may take time and so a setting should be chosen where he will be comfortable and have a good beginning. The specialist will want to encourage the student toward a realistic attitude to travel, recognizing strengths as well as weaknesses. Overconfidence may cause the student to experience more failure than necessary. The instructor will also want to assist the student in being very realistic about his long-term capabilities for mobility in the community. A realistic appraisal of one's own abilities is an important aspect of safe travel.

Emotional Instability

Emotional instability along with an intellectual and visual handicap may be the most severe problem for both student and mobility specialist to overcome. A student's extreme shyness, impulsiveness, aggressiveness, or other neurotic or psychotic behavior, interferes with teaching or learning of mobility. The behavior often conflicts with the goals of mobility as well as creating barriers between the client and the world . . . including the instructor. Emotional instability may require the specialist to spend a great deal of time counseling. However, other professional help should be sought if the training program is seriously affected.

Variable Learning Styles

Some mentally retarded students require a firm, regimented structure for learning where others need flexibility and a relaxed atmosphere. Some students can memorize sequences; some must be reminded of each step. Some can perform in a particular fashion one day and not on the next. In working with the retarded, expectations must be flexible: expect the unexpected both within the same and between various clients. Learning styles will become evident with experience with a particular client but the variability encountered will test the specialist's initiative, ingenuity, and resourcefulness. The ultimate goal of training for any student is the acquisition of sufficient skills for structuring his own life-style within the limits imposed by his visual and mental deficits. Awareness of the client's learning style will enhance this process.

Concept Development

The mentally retarded student will require more repetition and patterning when learning concepts. Small segments gradually expanded to form a broader, more general constellation of concepts will have practical and lasting value to the student. It is important to review the student's level of concept development prior to training. We cannot expect the retarded student to draw logical conclusions unless trained to do so. The building block approach will allow the student to progress from the unknown and often feared to the known usable skill which he may call upon out of need as the situation presents itself. Success will reinforce the student's problem solving behavior and develop the confidence needed to exercise it. The student will usually reach learning plateaus where very little progress is made. This time may be needed for the purpose of assimilating material learned to that point. When a plateau is recognized, practice and review of previous successes may be helpful for this time can be fraught with frustration for both the student and the instructor. Following a plateau, a new direction or conceptual series can allow enthusiasm to blossom once again.

Hearing Impairment

The presence of a hearing impairment can cause many additional problems. Directions should be given slowly, clearly, and repeated when necessary to make sure the student knows what is expected of him. Repeated failure may come from the inability to hear or understand, or both. The instructor should seek interpretation of the effects of a hearing loss from an audiologist so functional hearing levels can be targeted in the same way that lessons are planned to accommodate intellectual deficits. If sign language or finger spelling is used, the specialist should make sure he is signing in a fashion known to the client. One of the biggest problems that may arise is hearing only part of a direction. It is, therefore, important to repeat that direction several times and possibly provide a demonstration before asking the student to perform. Misunderstandings that arise from missing, or misinterpreting messages can also cause affective problems which have an effect on the relationships between student and teacher.

Low Vision

Partial vision presents special problems. The student may have enough vision to compare himself with sighted peers but may fall short of his expectations. He may equate visual ability with self-worth. It is essential that the student learn what his abilities are and how to use them most effectively. When he can separate his own self-worth from his visual disability, he will be free to explore and select satisfactory answers that are within his intellectual reach to problems of mobility caused by visual limitations. Specific impairments such as color-deficient vision, restricted field, and retinal detachment cause the same problems they do with normal clients. Additionally, impaired intellectual function may limit the client's problem solving ability needed to cope with these conditions. As with impaired hearing, the interpretation by an expert in low vision will augment the specialist's observations of the client.

Multiple Disabilities

The presence of a number of handicaps in addition to deficits in intelligence and vision complicate the training program even further but should not necessarily exclude an individual from mobility instruction. The multiply handicapped person may be in need of this training far more than his less severely handicapped peers. Seek the knowledge of experts' opinions to interpret the nature of the disabilities present. Priorities then need to be established because gains may be limited. It is important that the effort expended by both teacher and client be directed toward achievable goals that will improve the quality of life of a multiply handicapped person. Successful mobility training of the multiply handicapped, as with training in other skills, seems to be directly related to the creativity and perseverance of the instructor. There is no cookbook, but there are ways to maximize an individual's strengths while minimizing weaknesses.

Student Reactions to Mobility Training

The following reactions to mobility are commonly encountered by the specialist working with the retarded student:

1. The student may become angry with himself, others, or his environment. Anger may present itself in many forms: withdrawal, absenteeism, open hostility, or tantrums. The mentally retarded student may not only have an impaired understanding of events, but may lack sufficient impulse control to deal with frustration, etc.

2. The student may give up. He may invent a fantasy world where there are no demands on him and where he does not have to perform, especially in areas requiring mobility.

3. The student may appear entirely disinterested and uninspired to learn travel techniques, preferring to let others take the responsibility for getting him from place to place. Hard work is seen as neither desirable nor rewarding. The retarded client is less able to delay gratification and, therefore, has difficulty seeing the value of working for independence in the future. Being dependent also has its rewards.

4. The student may talk incessantly about everything but the task at hand. If he is talking, he doesn't have to listen or think about what he is doing! The mentally retarded student is easily distracted and may have difficulty focusing on a task.

5. The student may treat the instructor as a parent, seeking approval beyond what is usually expected of teachers. Such a student has difficulty assuming responsibility for his own behavior and may attempt to create a symbiotic relationship in this one-to-one situation.

Problems with students arise for many different reasons. Very often, however, unrealistic expectations underlie them. The training program must be realistically designed and appropriately paced for each individual student. As the ultimate goal is for the student to think for himself, he must be aware of his own strengths and weaknesses and be able to participate in decisions about pacing his progress. This can be orchestrated by the specialist through intimate knowledge of the client and sensitive interpretation of his needs. Flexibility, adaptability, determination, and stability are uncharacteristic traits for the mentally retarded learner but still must be stressed as important goals during training and in life.

Bibliography

Addison, M., & Luckey, R. *The profoundly retarded: A new challenge for public education.* Arlington, Texas: 1974.

American Foundation for the Blind. *Proceedings of the regional institute on the blind child who functions on a retarded level.* New York: Author, 1969.

Boe, E.N., & Zubrycki, T.H. Dog guide training for the mentally handicapped: An interagency approach. *New Outlook for the Blind,* 1976, **70**(8), 326-328.

Danler, T., Jeanblanc, A., & Nichols, G.W. *Mobility training program for visually impaired, mentally retarded, institutionalized individuals.* Dixon, Illinois: Dixon Developmental Center, 1977.

Ellis, N.R. *Handbook of mental deficiency.* New York: McGraw-Hill, 1963.

Harley, R., Merbler, J., & Wood, T. Programmed instruction in orientation and mobility for multiply impaired blind children. *New Outlook for the Blind,* 1975, **69**(9), 418-423.

Harley, R. & Wood T. *The development of a program in orientation and mobility for multiply handicapped blind children.* Nashville, Tenn.: Peabody College, 1974.

Hill, E., & Ponder, P. *Orientation and mobility techniques: A guide for the practitioner.* New York: American Foundation for the Blind, 1976.

Jordan, T.E. *The mentally retarded.* Columbus, Ohio: Charles E. Merrill, 1972.

McDade, P.R. The importance of motor development and mobility skills for the institutionalized blind mentally retarded. *New Outlook for the Blind,* 1969, **63**(10), 312.

McDade, P.R. Orientation and mobility problems for the blind mentally retarded. *Long Cane News,* 1968, **2**(6), 12-15.

McClinchey, M.A., & Mitala, R.F. Using environmental design to teach ward layout to severely and profoundly retarded blind persons: A proposal. *New Outlook for the Blind,* 1975, **69**(4), 168-171.

Schultz, P.J. *Mobility and independence for the visually handicapped: Psychological dynamics of the teaching process.* Van Nuys, Ca.: Muse-Ed Company, 1977.

Snow, C.C. *A sequential approach to the mobility training of educable and trainable blind mentally retarded.* Arkansas Children's Colony-Conway Unit (unpublished document).

Uslan, M.M. Teaching basic ward layout to the severely retarded blind: An auditory approach. *New Outlook for the Blind,* 1976, **70**(9), 401-402.

Training for Persons With Functional Mobility Limitations

Bruce B. Blasch and Richard L. Welsh

There has been a tendency to disregard the mobility problems of other handicapped groups based, perhaps, on the assumption that these individuals are able to teach themselves how to travel. Because many handicapped individuals go to hospitals and clinics and receive physical and/or occupational therapy and instruction in the use of various prosthetic devices, this assumption is reinforced. In addition, many handicapped individuals are independently mobile. We see them on the streets and in public places. This situation is not unlike that of a visually impaired person prior to formal mobility programs. Some had been able to teach themselves how to travel through the community and some still do.

THE NEED FOR MOBILITY TRAINING

Many visually impaired individuals, however, for a variety of reasons are unable to achieve this goal on their own. Formal or systematic mobility services have been developed to guarantee each individual the opportunity to learn how to travel to the fullest extent of his abilities. Without a formal educational system, some individuals (handicapped and nonhandicapped) would still learn about the world and how to interact with it. However, a society must take steps to assure that *each* member will have this opportunity and that the acquisition of knowledge is not left to chance. Similarly, it is important not to assume that every handicapped person will develop independent travel skill without structured intervention. It must be emphasized, however, that just because a person has a handicap or is old he will not necessarily need mobility training.

The opportunity for formalized orientation and mobility instruction must be provided for all handicapped and elderly persons who need such assistance. This is necessary if we are going to be consistent with policies to integrate such people into the mainstream of our society more readily. Making policies, changing the environment, and developing new equipment is not enough. Appropriate learning experiences must be provided when needed.

Many programs developed to assist persons with certain mobility limitations to learn how to use prosthetic devices or other equipment such as wheelchairs to assist in locomotion, or to learn or relearn the use of muscles needed for walking have not systematically addressed the many subtle factors involved in independent travel. Programs for mentally retarded persons have sometimes helped such persons to develop the concepts needed for moving independently through the community, but most of these efforts have not been directed at the entire process of independent travel nor considered the needs of the total individual.

Among the skills of independent travel that might concern the mobility specialist regardless of the disability of a particular client are:

1. Orientation skills such as map reading and route planning

2. Valid concepts of the environment

3. Social competencies such as asking questions, getting directions, asking for help when needed, politely refusing assistance when not needed, and dealing with other aspects of a stigmatized identity

4. Related skills such as handling money, telling time, estimating distances, and reading signs and schedules

5. Movement skills, and knowing the capabilities and limitations of such skills

6. Skills in using whatever prosthetic devices might be necessary

7. Skill in using whatever types of transportation systems might be available

8. The ability to generalize these skills to as many environmental situations as possible.

Background Methods

Early methods for systematically teaching orientation and mobility to the visually impaired focused primarily on compensating for the visual loss. Most of the early instruction was provided by individuals with corrective therapy, physical therapy, or physical education backgrounds. Instruction focused on the physical aspects of ambulation and on devices, such as the cane, dog guides, and electronic aids, that could be used to obtain information from the environment. At first, emphasis was on the physical skills needed to use the long cane to scan, and to use a dog guide. Persons with corrective and physical therapy backgrounds were originally selected for the Hines Veterans Administration mobility program for blinded veterans because they had worked with other handicapped individuals to increase their physical mobility and ambulation.

As systematic orientation and mobility instruction for the visually impaired began to expand beyond the Veterans Administration and to serve populations with additional and in many cases more complicated mobility problems (for example, congenitally blind persons, older blind persons, and persons with developmental handicaps in addition to blindness), it became apparent that the initial approach to instruction, emphasis on the physical skills, was not sufficient. Problems such as poor concept development, family overprotectiveness, inadequate motivation, and mental retardation affected the teaching and learning process. Mobility specialists began to realize that many of the problems of independent travel without vision were not always the most obvious and expected ones. With many clients, much of the instructional time was spent on overcoming the effects of negative expectations of family members, learning to think logically to solve orientation problems, and to cope with the reaction of others on the street, problems which only became apparent as the instructor and client became involved in the total process of learning to travel. A more complete understanding of the mobility process also grew from efforts to serve low vision clients more appropriately. Many low vision clients did not need a long cane or a dog guide, but they did need to learn to use residual vision, to plan routes, to deal with people and develop confidence about travel.

Awareness

As the total process of orientation and mobility instruction, including the significance of the less obvious factors, became more apparent, awareness of the travel problems of persons who were not visually impaired but who had functional mobility limitations resulting from other impairments, grew. As a result, formalized mobility instruction for persons with other impairments was suggested (Welsh, 1972; Laus, 1974 and 1977; Welsh & Blasch, 1974).

462

Obvious limitations to a person's mobility include impairments such as: sensory loss; loss of limbs as in amputation; loss of limb functioning as in diseases of the neuromuscular system; muscle, bone, or joint disorders; cognitive and perceptual deficits such as in mental retardation; some of the effects of aging; and height and size disorders.

A number of subtle factors not due to physical or intellectual limitations, which limit a person's ability to travel independently, also became apparent through systematic instruction of visually impaired persons:

1. Lack of travel experience, which in itself can be a strong deterrent to independent travel

2. The effects of overprotection and experiential deprivation, including insufficient knowledge about and understanding of the environment

3. Fear and anxiety related to traveling alone

4. Lack of confidence in one's travel and orientation abilities

5. Communication problems

6. Difficulties with problem solving and decision making

7. Lack of endurance and stamina related to age, medical problems, or insufficient opportunities to develop the necessary endurance

8. Stigmatizing or embarrassing aspects of visible disabilities or atypical behaviors

9. The reactions of others

10. The fears and expectations of family members.

While mobility specialists working with visually impaired persons have come to appreciate the many dimensions of travel problems, professionals working with persons with other primary limitations have not always recognized similar problems in their clients (Welsh, 1972; Laus, 1977).

Physical therapists provide instruction and assistance in basic mobility for persons who have lost the functioning of their legs or have certain neuromuscular problems. This therapy is usually provided in the clinic only and does not deal with the total travel situation. It does not generally cover orientation, strategies for soliciting assistance when needed, and learning to cope with the stigmatizing nature of the disability in public.

Educators and rehabilitators of hearing impaired persons may teach the client how to communicate in situations when aid is needed, but they do not usually provide opportunities for supervised experiences in travel situations nor do they deal with the reaction of a deaf client to orientation problems and dangers when they occur.

Teachers of mentally retarded persons teach their students to recognize bus and street signs and may take them on group trips (Tobias, 1963; Tobias & Cortazzo, 1963; Tobias, 1965; Tobias & Gorelick, 1968; Cortazzo & Sansone, 1969) but they do not help them to become confident with strategies for coping with disorientation and other problems while traveling alone.

Elderly persons may be able to use a special transportation system to get from their homes to the business district. However, they are unable to go from one store to another within the business district because it means crossing a very wide and busy street that they fear they could not negotiate safely.

THE REAL ENVIRONMENT

Methods used by mobility specialists working with the visually impaired to help clients overcome some of the factors which limit mobility in subtle ways are also applicable when dealing with similar problems among clients with different primary mobility limitations (Welsh, 1972; Laus, 1977). The methods that apply to work with all handicapped groups are: use of the real environment, individualized instruction, lessons of graduated difficulty and responsibility, and the synthesis of specific travel skills.

Mobility specialists have discovered that instruction can be adequately provided only in real environments similar to those in which the client will travel later. While training in simulated and protected environments may be necessary for beginning instruction, it is not sufficient for the development of all needed skills. Real environments are qualitatively different from the hallways of institutions and hospitals. In real environments there is a bombardment of stimuli and a variety of competing concerns such as existing dangers, the reactions of passersby, the possibility of getting lost, and the preoccupation with the actual business of the trip. The only method that has proven to be the best way to prepare for such situations is practice in the real environment.

Individualized Instruction

Training in independent travel also requires individualized instruction. Because of the variety of components that are involved it is unlikely that any two clients will be able to proceed at the same rate. Attempting to train two clients at one time will result in danger for the clients or inefficient training. Because part of the focus of mobility instruction must be on individual problem solving, training with another person deprives one or the other of the clients of the opportunity to learn to make decisions on his own and to bear their consequences, which he will have to do when he travels independently. Individualized instruction also enables the mobility specialist to structure the situation to reflect the level of complexity that is most needed by a particular client at that time in training.

Graduated Lessons

Another important teaching strategy in mobility training is the need for *lessons of graduated difficulty and responsibility*. Various components have to be broken out of the total mobility task and presented sequentially. It is important to develop certain basic skills before the client can be expected to deal with other people in travel situations. For example, the client should be able to handle less congested areas of travel before proceeding to more complicated areas. A client should also develop confidence in his own travel abilities before he works on the skills of soliciting and using assistance. While the particular sequence or approach may differ somewhat for individual clients, and the approach used for persons with different disabilities may be found to vary from that which has been most helpful for the visually impaired, mobility specialists should be expert in planning sequenced lessons of graduated difficulty and responsibility. Such skill is necessary for work with persons with all types of mobility limitations particularly as it relates to the development of the person's self-confidence in his travel abilities and the overcoming of any fears and anxieties that may exist.

Synthesis of Skills

Another common factor that has emerged in mobility training of the visually impaired is that the whole of independent travel is greater than the sum of its parts. No matter how expertly the client performs the various subskills in isolation, the various components frequently do not come together as smoothly as expected. Unless the client gets an opportunity to put it all together in practice situations with an instructor available for feedback and assistance, it is likely that the person will not be able to learn to travel to his full potential, at least not as soon as he might with such assistance.

Responsibility

Finally, one of the most important elements of mobility training that has application to services for persons with various mobility limitations is the designation of mobility instruction as the primary responsibility of one or more full-time staff members of an agency or program. Where mobility instruction of some sort is offered in programs for persons with limitations other than visual impairment, it is usually done by someone whose main responsibility lies elsewhere and who provides travel instruction only when time permits or when the need is so obvious and pressing that other duties must be put aside. Giving specific staff members responsibility for mobility instruction is an important step in the recognition and development of this service as an essential part of the program. The presence of mobility specialists in a program also indicates that someone in the organization, as a professional responsibility, will focus attention on this area and on the literature to learn how to improve the service. A designated person is able to devote his full attention to this service without the distractions of other responsibilities.

EVALUATING MOBILITY FUNCTIONING

Efforts to address mobility deficiencies in persons with all types of mobility limitations should begin with a reliable and valid assessment of the individual's characteristics and the environmental characteristics which relate to mobility functioning. The individual's characteristics can be grouped as psychomotor abilities, cognitive skills, and emotional or psychological factors. The characteristics of the environment can be considered as physical-architectural-situational factors and social factors.

The psychomotor abilities category can be subdivided into body awareness, posture and gait, sensory-perceptual abilities, perceptual-motor coordination, and other psychomotor characteristics.

Body Awareness

Frostig (1970) has differentiated the more general term, body awareness, into three components—body schema, body concepts, and body image. *Body schema* refers to the individual's awareness of the location of the various parts of the body at any particular moment and in general. It is a type of proprioceptive awareness that is always available to the person though often not consciously. *Body concept* refers to the cognitive awareness of the names of the various body parts and the verbal description of their relationship to one another. *Body image* embraces the full range of an individual's emotional reactions to his body.

Instruction of visually impaired children has led to the realization that these children frequently have difficulty developing an accurate awareness of all the body parts, their names and functions and how they relate to each other (Cratty & Sams, 1968; Kephart, Kephart, & Schwartz, 1974). In addition, many children as well as adults experience a negative emotional reaction toward their own bodies whenever they have serious impairments (Goffman, 1963; Wright, 1960). Mobility specialists have become aware of the effect that these deficiencies produce on an individual's ability and willingness to travel independently. Clients express a reluctance to be seen in public or to have their visible impairments readily apparent. Some clients try to cover eye defects with dark glasses; others refuse to use a cane or other equipment which draws additional attention to their impairments.

Children who are retarded, or who have certain learning disabilities or physical impairments, particularly when they are congenital, will probably experience difficulty in developing adequate body awareness. Deficiencies in both body concepts and body schema can make it difficult for the child to learn to use his body for physical activities, including travel. Other problems have been noted in amputees. For example, when an individual loses a limb he frequently continues to experience sensations from the stump which create the feeling that the limb is still functional. This illusion is referred to as the "phantom limb" (Reddoch, 1941; Haber, 1955; Haber, 1956; Simmel, 1956).

Improvement in physical skills, including independent movement through the environment, seems to result in an improved body image, that is, the emotional reaction that the individual has toward his own body. This applies to congenitally impaired persons as well as to adventitiously disabled individuals.

A wide variety of learning activities have been developed to assist people to improve or develop their awareness of their body parts and how they function. Such activities are also used for nonhandicapped children at certain times in their education. As Mills pointed out in Chapter 12, many of the learning activities for nonhandicapped children such as games like "Simon Says" and dances like "Hokey-Pokey," can be easily adapted for persons with other impairments.

As visually impaired persons do, persons with other impairments may have to be helped to develop or improve body awareness early in any remedial or training effort which is directed toward travel or other physical skills. Body awareness is the fundamental support of any skilled or purposeful use of the body or its parts.

Posture and Gait

Directly or indirectly, many impairments, both congenital and adventitious, result in deficiencies in posture and/or gait. Some physical and neurological impairments involve the skeletal and neuromuscular components of the body that are responsible for a person's ability to stand upright and to ambulate with an erect posture. Other impairments affect posture and gait indirectly through the difficulties a person has in perceiving correct posture and making changes in his own stance in relation to the vertical, or as a result of the reluctance of parents and teachers to expect and reinforce correct posture in children with handicaps. In some cases distinctive postures and gaits result from institutionalization while in others one individual's abnormal gait may be modeled by the other clients (Haring & Schiefelbush, 1967). Some temporary conditions such as broken bones result in permanent posture and/or gait problems.

Poor posture and gait can make movement through the environment impossible, inefficient, or uncomfortable. Some posture and gait deficiencies make movement more precarious since they impair the reflexes through which the individual draws back from danger. Others make reactions slower and movements less precise (Aust, Chapter 3). Posture and gait problems may deter movement as a result of the stigmatization that results from the impairment or from the correction of the impairment such as braces and walkers. Some people hesitate to move freely in public if they feel that they will draw extra attention to themselves as a result of their manner of locomotion.

Sometimes posture and gait problems can be remedied through physical therapy or direct instruction. When this is effective, the person can move freely and the deficiency is no longer visible or influencing the locomotion. In other instances, the best physical therapy will not completely remediate the problem nor make it invisible.

The person may need assistance in learning to cope with the stigmatization, the posture and gait deficiency, or in planning his movement through the environment in order to neutralize the problems that remain.

466

Perceptual Abilities

Safe and purposeful movement through the environment requires that the traveler take in, interpret, and react to information about the environment through which he is moving. Movement can take place without this, but it will neither be oriented nor necessarily safe. Many people have difficulty with independent travel because their systems for receiving and interpreting both external and internal information are deficient. In some cases a handicapping condition (for example, hemiplegia or unilateral poliomyelitis paralysis) also affects other sensory perceptions such as the perception of the vertical or the horizontal (Werner & Wapner, 1952; Lorenze & Cancro, 1962; DeCencio, Leshner, & Voron, 1970).

Deficiencies in the information processing systems may be caused by impairments of the sense organs themselves as in visual and hearing impairments, or they may be caused by problems in the perceptual mechanisms through which the person makes sense out of the sensations picked up and delivered by the sense organs. Perceptual difficulties of this type are characteristic of certain learning disabilities and neurological impairments and some kinds of mental retardation. In some instances, this type of perceptual difficulty is unavoidable and apparently nonremediable. In others, these problems can be remedied through systematic and appropriate learning experiences.

Lack of the usual sensory inputs may necessitate the use of special equipment such as a long cane, a hearing aid, a low vision aid, or special techniques to pick up the information necessary for safe and oriented movement. In other situations the person may have to learn how to depend on another type of information in the environment which is helpful when the other is not available (i.e., auditory information rather than visual). In some cases the individual, because of a particular handicapping condition, may have to learn to attend to certain otherwise extraneous and unimportant environmental cues and information, for example, visual displays for mentally retarded persons or sound cues for visually impaired persons.

Perceptual-Motor Coordination

Some individuals have an impaired ability to direct their movement based upon the sensory information they receive. The problem does not exist in the receptive mechanisms but rather in the person's ability to produce accurate movements based upon the information received. This can cause difficulties in locomotion as well as in driving a vehicle (Bardoch, 1971). Some individuals because of a lack of or a distortion of sensory input may need a very structured and systematic presentation of stimuli to facilitate perceptual motor coordination.

Some of these deficiencies can be remediated through training and learning activities. Congenitally impaired persons frequently need opportunities to practice some of the perceptual/motor coordinated activities in order to develop independent travel skills.

The mobility specialist should make a systematic evaluation of the individual's level of psychomotor development (see Hart, Chapter 2). This is especially important for congenitally impaired children. The results of this evaluation are used to design an individualized sequential curriculum. The mobility specialist must identify the movement behaviors relevant for mobility and the individual's level of maturation and proficiency of specific movement behaviors to structure a movement program focusing on independent travel, tailored to the individual's needs, and encompassing the appropriate levels of behavior as presented by Harrow (1972).

COGNITIVE ABILITIES

The second category of individual characteristics that must be assessed is cognitive abilities, which are subdivided into concept development, orientation skills, and problem solving abilities.

Spatial and Environmental Concepts

The skill of independent travel requires a person to have clear and functional concepts of three-dimensional space of areas, and shapes, and of the constructs in the environment such as streets, intersections, and the layout of neighborhoods and buildings (Hill & Blasch, Chapter 9).

Many disabilities impair an individual's ability to develop these concepts, or distort such concepts either because of limited intake of sensory information about characteristics of the environment, or because of perceptual or cognitive problems that make it difficult to synthesize the information perceived into usable concepts.

All travelers must be able to form and retain these concepts and to use them to facilitate efficient travel. To the extent that an individual has difficulty in forming and using concepts about space and the environment, he will be more limited in the variety of places to which he can travel and in the variety of ways he may get to the same objective.

Some impairments do not affect an individual's ability to develop concepts directly, but restrictions placed on the person as a result of the impairments, for example, the parents' reluctance to allow a child to explore the environment freely, prevents the natural interaction with the environment that results in the development of spatial and environmental concepts.

Orientation Skills

Independent travel requires that the individual be able to establish his orientation in relation to the environment and to maintain it as he moves through the environment. The individual must understand the environment well enough to plan and execute routes, and reverse and alternate routes as necessary. His ability to remember must be sufficient to allow him to keep track of which parts of the routes he has already traveled and which still lie ahead. Related to these skills is the ability to read maps or other representations of the environment as aids in planning a route or understanding an area.

Problem Solving

Deficiencies in the ability to solve problems that arise during travel or difficulty in making necessary decisions which affect safe and efficient travel are related to the deficiencies in concepts that some people have and to the orientation process. Some individuals cannot reorient themselves when they are lost or effectively choose an alternate route when necessary because they do not have complete concepts about a particular area or about grid patterns of city streets or other configurations. Some individuals who do possess the necessary concepts cannot use them efficiently because of anxiety or other emotional problems or a lack of confidence in their own ability to solve a problem or to orient themselves when lost. Since the ability to solve such problems is essential, an inability to do so seriously impedes independent travel.

Some impairments, especially those which affect cognitive functioning directly, obviously affect a person's reasoning powers and therefore his problem solving abilities. For others, difficulties with reasoning and problem solving are related more to their lack of opportunity to be responsible for themselves, a pattern of social interaction in which the person with the impairment is never allowed to make decisions and suffer the consequences of wrong ones. Without such experiences, a problem solving skill does not generally develop (Hughes, Smith, & Benitz, 1977).

EMOTIONAL-PSYCHOLOGICAL FACTORS

A third group of individual characteristics which must be assessed by the mobility specialist are *emotional or psychological factors.* For many handicapped persons, there is a complex interaction between independent travel and psychological factors. For example, the lack of independent travel may lead to increased dependency, isolation, hopelessness, and a poor self-concept, and all of these reactions themselves represent obstacles that must be overcome to get a handicapped person moving. On the other hand, success in independent travel tasks, even at the beginning levels, can bring about an improved self-concept, a greater sense of independence, and improved motivation for other tasks (Welsh, Chapter 8).

Efforts to help people with mobility limitations to learn to move independently must take psychological factors into account. Structured learning experiences must not only be directed toward the motor, sensory, and orientation skills that are necessary, but also toward elimination of emotional obstacles and development of a positive psychological attitude toward independent travel. It does no good to help a person improve his ability to ambulate or to use hearing more effectively unless the individual has enough confidence in himself to use the skills and the ability to overcome fears and other negative feelings about independent travel.

The individual's characteristics interact with characteristics of the environment in ways which determine the level of mobility functioning that the individual can master. The environment can be divided into two categories, the social and the physical.

SOCIAL AND FAMILY FACTORS

Like most other human activities, independent travel is a social act both affected by and dependent on others. This is especially true for persons with impairments who must deal with the reactions of others on the street and the reactions of family members.

Many persons must learn to cope with the fact that they are stigmatized by their impairment and frequently by the techniques and devices that they use to overcome some of their limitations. This stigma must be confronted directly when the person begins to travel independently. Previously, the person with an impairment may have spent most of his time with sympathetic family members, friends, or professionals. Any ventures into the community were usually with an escort who served as a buffer in interactions and absorbed or avoided most of the negative effects of confrontations.

This problem is complicated by the fact that many impairments make interaction more necessary than for other pedestrians since the person with a mobility limitation may need assistance in a number of situations. Many such persons curtail their travels greatly or entirely because of difficulties in coping with offers of help, expressions of curiosity, and expressions of sympathy. Efforts to help people with impairments put the client in situations in which interacting with the public is necessary and unavoidable and then help him develop strategies for interacting effectively and minimizing the negative aspects of such exchanges.

Other social components which cause mobility limitations for persons with impairments are the fears and low expectations of members of their families. Family members often dread exposing the person with the impairment to the dangerous and embarrassing aspects of travel and do not always appreciate the importance of mobility to adjustment. Some persons with impairments, after receiving training in travel and in the use of special mobility equipment, are prevented from using this training by family attitudes and restrictions.

The fears of family members are real and understandable. Efforts to help people learn to travel include taking responsibility for bringing families to an understanding and acceptance of its importance for people with impairments. Specific observations or group activities may be needed to help family members overcome their anxieties and learn how best to contribute to and support the client's effort to travel independently. At the other extreme, some families have unrealistic expectations and place handicapped individuals in situations beyond their abilities. This usually increases anxiety and reinforces a negative attitude toward independent travel.

ENVIRONMENTAL FACTORS

The remainder of the environment can be subdivided into physical, architectural, and situational factors.

The physical structure of the environment itself seriously affects the ability of people to travel through it. Each of us has limits in terms of the types of terrain we can traverse, but persons with certain impairments experience serious limitations with ordinary environments which have been constructed with the able-bodied traveler in mind (Morgan, 1976). Some impairments can never be remediated enough to enable the person to travel over or through certain parts of the environment such as turnstiles and stairs. Other persons will travel more efficiently and safely if the lighting or directional signs are improved.

When the physical environment must be changed to facilitate the travel of persons with certain limitations, community planning and/or social action may be necessary to promote reconstruction or modification. Even when such modifications are made, it may still be necessary to assist the person with the impairment to develop confidence in moving through the reconstructed or modified area.

The assessment of the mobility potential of an individual with an impairment must consider how the individual's limitations interact with the variety of physical, architectural, and situational factors suggested by the following list:

I. Buildings
   A. Public
      1. Entrances, doors, doorways, doorhandles
      2. Stairs, ramps, and handrails
      3. Hallways, corridors, and aisles
      4. Floors and floor coverings
      5. Toilet facilities
      6. Furniture
      7. Elevators and escalators
      8. Telephone locations
      9. Drinking fountains
    10. Suspended objects and projections
    11. Display islands
    12. Signage, e.g., raised numbers
    13. Concessions and vending machines
    14. Coatracks and cloakrooms
   B. Commercial
      1. Counters and aisles
      2. Seating
      3. Cafeteria lines, ordering and utensils
      4. Box office
      5. Turnstiles
   C. Residential
      1. Furnishings
      2. Shower and tub

3. Kitchen counters, cupboards, appliances
4. Controls (light and heat)

II. Street Traffic and Street Furniture
  A. Residential
    1. Curbs, curb cuts, curb ramps, and gutters
    2. Crosswalks
    3. Traffic signals
    4. Signage
    5. Sidewalks
    6. Driveways
    7. Manhole covers and gratings
    8. Mailboxes, fire hydrants, trash receptacles
    9. Overhanging branches, shrubbery, and fences
    10. Public telephones
    11. Drinking fountains
  B. Small business and shopping
    1. Parking, passenger loading zones
    2. Barricades
    3. Outdoor steps and stairs
    4. Projections, control boxes and poles
    5. Parking meters
    6. Vending machines
    7. Furniture
    8. Landscaping, outdoor planters, and ornamental structures
  C. Metropolitan
    1. Street widths
    2. Crowd congestion
    3. Masking noises
    4. Safety islands
    5. Open excavation sites
  D. Manufacturing/industrial
    1. Entrances
    2. Gates
    3. Platforms, loading docks
    4. Industrial machines and equipment

III. Transportation
  A. Bus/trolley
    1. Steps
    2. Railings
    3. Seating
    4. Crowd congestion
    5. Fare
  B. Subways/elevated trains
    1. Turnstiles
    2. Platforms
  C. Airplanes and trains
    1. Terminals
    2. Stations
    3. Airports
  D. Cars, taxis, and vans

IV. Recreation
  A. Public parks; monuments, historic sites, and trails

     1. Width of walkways
     2. Surface of walkways
     3. Access to swimming facilities
     4. Recreation equipment
     5. Access to information and directions
  B. Amusement parks
  C. Athletic centers and facilities

V. Climatic factors
  A. Weather
  B. Pollution

Situational Factors

In some situations, persons with impairments experience new or exaggerated travel difficulties as a result of changes in traffic laws and regulations. For example, laws permitting a right turn on a red light have serious implications for the ability of some persons to cross streets safely.

Many impairments make driving impossible. Others do not, but require special equipment or training. Hand controls and special mirrors may make driving possible for orthopedically impaired or deaf persons. Persons with certain neurological impairments may have difficulty with particular aspects of driving a car, such as coordinating vision and steering (Hofkosh, 1970), especially where visual perception has been affected. Congenitally impaired persons without community experience may take a long time to learn how to establish their orientation in the community and how to make decisions under pressure while driving. The inability to drive is very difficult for some persons to accept. Driving has considerable importance in this society and many feel that the inability to do so limits their participation in the society and seriously affects their own identity (Maye, 1976). This can lead to denial and to risk-taking that endangers the individual as well as others on the road. Counseling or other interventions may be needed to assist the person in coming to terms with the inability to drive.

More disabled persons than non-disabled depend on public transportation, yet the use of public transportation is difficult or impossible for some people as a result of their physical, sensory, or cognitive impairments. For some, training in the use of special equipment or techniques makes the use of public transportation possible. This frequently includes the need to depend on bus drivers, motormen, or conductors. For others, modification of public transportation vehicles or facilities is required. To secure these modifications, increased lobbying or community efforts may be needed.

MOBILITY LIMITATIONS

Reviewing a representative list of disabling conditions and causes of such conditions, such as that which follows, produces many examples of how certain physical, cognitive, and/or psychological conditions interacting with environmental factors result in mobility limitations.

I. Sensory disorders
  A. Blindness
  B. Low vision
  C. Deafness
  D. Hard of hearing
  E. Vestibular and kinesthetic dysfunction

II. Circulatory disorders
  A. Arteriosclerosis

B. Heart disease

III. Orthopedic disorders
   A. Amputations
   B. Arthritis
   C. Muscular dystrophy

IV. Disorders of the central nervous system
   A. Stroke
      1. Spasticity
      2. Rigidity
      3. Hemiplegia
   B. Neoplasma—tumors
   C. Epilepsy
   D. Cerebral palsy
      1. Spasticity
      2. Athetosis
      3. Ataxia
      4. Tremor and rigidity
      5. Mixed types
   E. Multiple sclerosis
   F. Parkinson's disease
   G. Spinal cord dysfunction
      1. Paraplegia
      2. Quadriplegia
   H. Spina bifida

V. Respiratory disorders
   A. Emphysema
   B. Asthma and allergies

VI. Cognitive and perceptual disorders
   A. Learning disabilities
   B. Mentally retarded, educable
   C. Mentally retarded, trainable
   D. Mentally retarded, profoundly
   E. Mentally ill and emotionally disturbed

VII. Geriatric (general conditions in addition to other disabling conditions.)

VIII. Endocrine disorders
   A. Obesity
   B. Body disproportion
   C. Diabetes
   D. Body structural disorders
      1. Gigantism
      2. Dwarfism

IX. Communicative disorders
   A. Articulation
   B. Retarded speech development
   C. Aphasia

Deaf persons usually have no difficulty walking safely or appropriately, but have serious problems interacting with strangers when the need arises. Some deaf

473

people have had little experience traveling alone because of family overprotection and so may have little confidence in their ability to travel independently. They may also be more vulnerable to dangers in the environment because they cannot hear warning sounds.

The person who has lost the use of his lower limbs through amputation or disease may have been taught how to use a wheelchair, crutches, or a prosthesis, and still have travel problems. If he fears falling or losing his balance in public, he may depend on others for assistance. He may lack appropriate or effective strategies for soliciting assistance whenever he must move through an inaccessible area. He may fear that he cannot cross wide streets quickly enough to safely reach the opposite side before traffic begins. He may shudder at the thought that others may look at him with pity and curiosity.

The mentally retarded person may, like the hearing impaired person, experience communication problems and, like the congenitally blind person, lack certain basic concepts about the environment (Laus, 1977). He is likely to be unable to understand the general layout of the environment sufficiently to solve orientation problems and to take alternative routes. He may be stigmatized by certain visible aspects of his retardation or by inappropriate behavior in public. Many mentally retarded persons also have basic posture and gait deficiencies and lack basic safety information. All of these difficulties can create interaction problems for the person and make his family strongly resist his traveling alone.

A person who has recently been discharged from a hospital for the mentally ill can have travel difficulties too. He may lack confidence in his ability to handle the complexity and the confusion of large city environments. He may have developed what has been referred to as an "institutional gait" which may stigmatize him on the street (Haring & Schiefelbusch, 1967). He may exhibit inappropriate behaviors which cause interaction problems with others. Orientation problems and crossing busy streets can cause stress and discourage travel. The person who has been institutionalized for a long time will not know how the community has changed or the location of community resources especially if he is discharged to a new neighborhood. The new environment may be strange and frightening, the exact opposite of the secure institution he has left. He may have difficulty planning trips and allowing sufficient time to get to appointments or may allow too much time and arrive inappropriately early for job interviews or work.

Individuals with certain learning disabilities also have travel problems. Some are unable to sort out the complex stimuli of the urban environment and become disoriented, particularly if they are away from a frequently traveled route. They may be unable to read street signs and store names and have to develop other strategies for remaining oriented and for locating objectives. Some persons with learning disabilities are unable to use the numbering systems in large buildings and thus have orientation difficulties. They may have coordination deficiencies that make driving difficult or impossible.

Elderly persons have a number of mobility problems associated with the diseases and disabilities that frequently accompany old age. They may be unable to drive or to walk long distances and have difficulty on stairs and inclines. They may fear falling and the complications that come with injury, and they may fear that they cannot cross wide streets quickly enough to guarantee their safety. Some older persons have their mobility limited by their environment, where they feel vulnerable to attacks and muggings. Others are embarrassed to pass through their old neighborhoods in a manner which advertises their disabilities and limitations.

FURTHER TRAINING NEEDED

While some of the elements of training individuals with other mobility limitations are similar to those employed by the mobility specialist teaching the visually impaired, there are a number of things that mobility specialists have to learn if they are going to become effective in the delivery of such training.

Mobility specialists have to learn more about the other disabilities, including how they originate, their characteristic effects, and how they are treated. Information would also be needed about the remaining skills available for the client to use and adapt.

In addition to knowing about the disabling conditions, the mobility specialist would have to become especially knowledgeable about the strategies for coping with those conditions. For example, for mentally retarded clients the appropriate structuring of learning activities to compensate for the reduced learning abilities must be known. When dealing with clients who have lost the functions of their lower limbs, the mobility specialist must be knowledgeable about the proper use of crutches, wheelchairs, braces, and prosthetic devices. It is important to emphasize that the mobility specialist should not be the person teaching such techniques originally. This should be done by the physical therapist. However, the mobility specialist will have opportunities to observe the client's use of these procedures during the training in independent travel, so he should be in a position to remind the client of techniques that are being performed sloppily or ineffectively and be able to tell when the follow-up services of the physical therapist are needed.

When working with deaf clients, the mobility specialist must be able to communicate with them and will need to understand the operation of hearing aids. For clients with learning disabilities, the mobility specialist must know what is involved in each condition and understand how to limit the distracting aspects of certain learning situations and structure other learning activities to facilitate the growth of the client. For clients with psychiatric problems, the mobility specialist will have to be able to recognize the symptoms of recurring pathologies and provide appropriate support as well as know when to involve other professionals.

The mobility specialist should also have the ability to interact effectively with other professionals who have information and knowledge about various disabilities. The mobility specialist would not enter the situation to deal directly with the main effects of the other disabilities, but rather to deal with the problems of independent travel as these are affected by the disability. It is not necessary that the mobility specialist become as knowledgeable about the conditions as the physical therapist, the teacher of the mentally retarded, or the deaf educator are in their own areas. Instead he should become skillful at working in collaboration with those who have expertise in specific areas.

The need to train mobility specialists to work with a variety of impairments becomes increasingly apparent considering the increasing number of multiply handicapped individuals. If the mobility specialist is going to offer training in mobility to the multiply handicapped and other disability groups he must gain additional knowledge and competencies.

This concept of mobility training represents the profession's response to the needs of disabled individuals at a time when society is becoming more aware of the importance of the right to independent mobility.

Bibliography

Bardoch, J. L. Psychological factors in the handicapped driver. *Arch. of Physical Medicine and Rehabilitation*. July, 1971.

Cortazzo, A. C., & Sansone, R. Travel training. *Teaching Exceptional Children*, 1969, **3**, 67-82.

Cratty, B., & Sams, T. *Body-image of blind children*. New York: American Foundation for the Blind, 1968.

De Cencio, D. V., Leshner, M., & Voron, D. Verticality perception and ambulation in hemiplegia. *Arch. of Physical Medicine and Rehabilitation.* February, 1970.

Frostig, M. *Movement education: Theory and practice.* Chicago: Follett Educational Corporation, 1970.

Goffman, E. *Stigma: Notes on the management of spoiled identity.* Englewood Cliffs, N.J.: Prentice-Hall, Inc., 1963.

Haber, W. B. Effects of loss of limb or sensory functions. *Journal of Psychology,* 155, **40,** 115-123.

Haber, W. B. Observations on phantom limb phenomena. *Arch. Neurol. Psychiat.,* American Medical Association, 1956, **75,** 624-636.

Haring, N. G., & Schiefelbusch, R. L. *Method in special education.* New York: McGraw-Hill Book Co., 1967.

Harrow, A. *A taxonomy of the psychomotor domain.* New York: David McKay, 1972.

Hofkosh, J. Teaching disabled individuals to drive—A symposium. *Psychological Aspects of Disability,* March 1970, **17**(3), 8-15.

Hughes, M. C., Smith, R. B., & Benitz, F. Travel training for exceptional children. *Teaching Exceptional Children,* Summer, 1977, **1**(4), 90-91.

Kephart, J. G., Kephart, C. P., & Schwartz, G. C. A journey into the world of the blind child. *Exceptional Children.* March, 1974.

Laus, M. D. Orientation and mobility instruction for the sighted trainable mentally retarded. *Education and Training of the Mentally Retarded,* April, 1974, 20-72.

Laus, M. D. *Travel instructions for the handicapped.* Springfield, Ill.: Charles C Thomas, Publisher, 1977.

Lorenze, E. J., & Cancro, R. Dysfunction in visual perception with hemiplegia: Its relation to activities of daily living. *Arch. of Physical Medicine and Rehabilitation.* October, 1962.

Maye, J. (Chm.) Report of the first day, Panel IV. Panel presented at a workshop in Washington, D.C. *Personal Licensed Vehicles for the Disabled.* Moss Rehabilitation Hospital, Philadelphia, Pennsylvania. June, 1976.

Morgan, M. Beyond disability: A broader definition of architectural barriers. *American Institute of Architects Journal.* May, 1976.

Reddoch, G. Phantom limbs and body shape. *Brain,* 1941, **69,** 197-222.

Simmel, M. L. On phantom limbs. *Arch. Neurol. Psychiat.,* 1956, **75,** 637-697.

Tobias, J. Teaching trainables on travel. *Digest of the Mentally Retarded,* 1965, **3,** 166-172.

Tobias, J. *Training for independent living.* New York: Association for Help of Retarded Children, 1963.

Tobias, J., & Cortazzo, A. C. Training severely retarded adults for greater independence in community living. *The Training School Bulletin,* 1963, **60,** 23-27.

Tobias, J., & Gorelick, J. Teaching trainables to travel. *Digest of the Mentally Retarded,* 1968, **3,** 175-181.

Welsh, R. L. Cognitive and psychosocial aspects of mobility training. *Blindness,* 1972, 99-109.

Welsh, R. L. & Blasch, B. B. Manpower needs in orientation and mobility. *The New Outlook for the Blind,* 1974, **68,** 433-43.

Werner, H., & Wapner, S. Experiments on sensory-tonic field of theory of perception: IV. Effect of initial position of a rod on apparent verticality. *Journal of Experimental Psychology,* January, 1952, **43,** 68-74.

Wright, B. *Physical disability: A psychological approach.* New York: Harper and Row, 1960.

Environmental Modifications

Kent Tyler Wardell

Efforts to assist visually impaired persons to travel independently must consider the effect of the environment on safe and efficient movement. The manner in which the environment is constructed can facilitate or impede travel by persons with disabilities. While this fact has been generally recognized in regard to persons who are confined to wheelchairs or who experience other types of ambulation problems, it is only now beginning to be considered in regard to visually impaired persons.

Mobility specialists can be proud of the progress that has been made in helping persons to adapt their travel skills to the environment as it exists. Yet it is obvious that not all dangers have been eliminated. Some of these could be prevented through relatively simple and inexpensive modifications. Others could be eliminated by more careful and knowledgeable planning for future construction. Travel by visually impaired persons might even be made more convenient and efficient through other modifications in the environment. This chapter will present some suggestions for how this might be done, and will analyze some of the issues involved. The discussion will consider how the mobility specialist should be involved in planning and proposing such modifications and how these concepts interact with the current philosophy and practice of orientation and mobility instruction.

Consideration of environmental modifications for visually impaired travelers has been motivated in part by the success with which these ideas have been pursued on behalf of persons who are wheelchair bound or whose travel is limited by other physical impairments. The central theme of their effort was accessibility to buildings by the elimination of barriers that prevented free movement of the wheelchair such as stairs, curbs, and narrow doors.

ESTABLISHMENT OF STANDARDS

The first national effort to solve the problem of architectural barriers came about in 1959 through the combined efforts of the President's Committee on Employment of the Handicapped, the National Society for Crippled Children and Adults, and the American Standards Association. The University of Illinois received a grant for research on the problem of architectural barriers and for recommendations of standards to eliminate them. In 1961, the *Standards Making Buildings Accessible and Usable by the Physically Handicapped,* American National Standards Institute (ANSI), were adopted by the American Standards Association. They formed the basis for revised building codes and for legislation. Some of the principles involved included the following:

1. At least one entrance to a building had to be freely accessible from the ground level

2. Ramps instead of stairs had to be provided at a minimum of one location into a building

3. Doorways had to have at least 32 inches of clear space to accommodate a wheelchair

4. Restrooms had to have the necessary space to accommodate a wheelchair

5. Safe parking access had to be provided.

While these initial standards provided a positive impact, they were deficient in one respect: they did not apply to private residences and to apartments.

Architectural Barriers Act

In 1965, Congress authorized the creation of the United States Commission on Architectural Barriers to Rehabilitation of the Handicapped to study the scope of architectural barriers and suggest ways to eliminate them in future construction. Their final report was a key factor in the passage of the Architectural Barriers Act of 1968. The intent of this legislation was to assure that all buildings constructed in full or in part with federal funds would be accessible to physically handicapped persons. It also led to the adoption by the Department of Health, Education, and Welfare of the ANSI standards to assure accessibility in buildings constructed or remodeled with federal funds.

The Rehabilitation Act of 1973 created the Architectural and Transportation Barriers Compliance Board to monitor federally supported construction in order to insure compliance with the accessibility standards. The Board was given the power to conduct investigations, hold public hearings, issue orders to comply with the accessibility standards and withhold the funds for construction if necessary. In 1976, Congress again acted on this issue as part of the Tax Reform Act that grants tax deductions to businessmen who eliminate barriers to the handicapped, including the deaf and the blind.

Other indicators of success for this movement included the 1969 adoption of the international symbol of accessibility which is used to identify facilities that are totally accessible to the physically handicapped. Also in 1974 the major groups interested in this topic formed a coalition to promote a barrier-free environment. Called the National Center for a Barrier-Free Environment, membership is open to all persons who are interested in this goal.

Recently, a grant was awarded to Syracuse University to revise and update the original "ANSI" standards. Such a revision was called for by the U.S. Department of Housing and Urban Development, and it is expected that the revisions will include private residences under the standards.

In spite of this success, many individual battles still had to be fought at the local level and with private industry. Lawsuits and intensive lobbying have been used to promote barrier-free hotels, airports, shopping centers, restaurants, and public transportation. Those who have advocated such changes have demonstrated that the cost of such modifications is not significant in a new building. The cost of removing barriers from an existing structure can be expensive but new tax incentives add to the desirability of undertaking such changes. It has also been pointed out that money spent on these changes is not spent unjustly. These modifications would benefit the 7.6 million people with heart conditions, the 1.1 million with leg braces, and the 20 million people over age 65.

The movement for a barrier-free environment for those in wheelchairs has been generally successful. Extensive literature has been amassed on the topic. Familiarization with it will provide a good learning experience for those concerned with the effect of the environment on the independent travel of visually impaired persons. A number of these references are listed at the end of this chapter. In addition, the ANSI standards which are being revised will make reference to the needs of visually impaired persons. Such a combined effort is necessary to assure compatibility among the standards that have been suggested to meet the needs of different handicapped persons.

FOR THE VISUALLY IMPAIRED

A variety of special environmental modifications for visually impaired persons have been suggested over the years. However, concern has only recently been expressed about this issue by orientation and mobility specialists. Although agreement is not yet available about what modifications are necessary and feasible, some clarification of the issue is offered by the distinction between an obstacle and a hazard.

Obstacle

An *obstacle* is defined as an architectural or environmental obstruction in the path of travel that *can* be detected and negotiated with standard long cane techniques, such as trash cans on the sidewalk, a child's wagon in the travel path, parking meters, etc. Figure 1-14 shows cars protruding onto a sidewalk, presenting an obstacle to the long cane traveler but not a hazard. The arc coverage of the long cane, when used properly, would contact the cars and warn of their presence. The traveler could experience cane contact with a number of the cars and be forced to

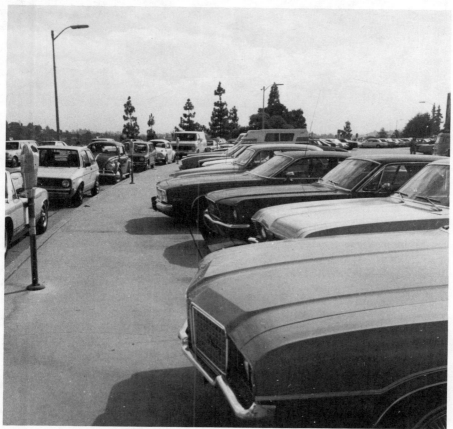

Figure 1-14. Travel obstacles.

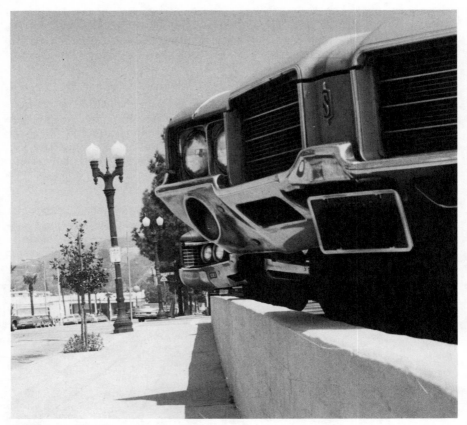

Figure 2-14. Travel hazards.

make appropriate adjustments in his line of travel. The problem of the cars overlapping the sidewalk could be eliminated if cement parking stoppers were installed to block the tires. But, for our purposes, the cars here do not represent a travel hazard.

Hazard

A *travel hazard* is defined as an architectural or environmental obstruction in the path of travel that *cannot* be detected and negotiated with standard long cane techniques, such as metal support cables for utility poles, some public telephones, some stairs and escalators, some store windows, incorrect placement of railings on stairs, irregular intersections with offset corners, and curb ramps designed with only the wheelchair in mind. Figure 2-14 represents a travel hazard. The parking lot is elevated above the sidewalk level. The lack of parking stoppers permits the cars to overhang the sidewalk. The arc coverage of the cane would not detect this situation, resulting in a hazard. The possibility of physical injury is very great.

There are a wide variety of hazards located at face and chest height. The advances made in new guidance devices employing laser beams and reflected sound waves will help neutralize these problems. However, only a small number of these devices are presently in use, and they may never be used by a majority of visually impaired people.

A dog guide can be an effective deterrent to this type of hazard. The dog's proficiency at this task depends upon the master's enforcement of the dog's original training standards. But most visually impaired travelers do not use a dog guide. Estimates place the number of dog guide users at less than five percent of the blind population.

PROS AND CONS

The issue begins to take shape. The environment could be modified to foster safe and convenient movement for the visually impaired. The dilemma is: should these modifications be made, and if so, to what degree?

Various considerations influence one's response to this question. Several factors influencing *affirmative* responses are:

1. The feeling that modifications made for the visually impaired would benefit others. The hazards faced by the visually impaired may also be hazards to the sighted person at night or in areas of poor lighting. Many children and adults simply do not watch where they are walking. The elimination of hazards for the visually impaired would make a safer environment for all pedestrians.

2. The feeling that visually impaired people are being victimized. They are forced to function in a visually oriented travel environment. Visually impaired travelers are a minority, but are entitled to equal rights with the sighted majority. One of these rights is the ability to move freely and safely in a travel environment designed to meet the needs of *all* people.

3. The feeling that different travelers have different needs. Architectural and environmental modifications should provide valuable assistance to those need-ing this assistance and yet could be ignored by those visually impaired travelers who do not require the modifications. For example, some travelers would detect a smooth curb ramp while others might need a distinctive texture on the ramp to facilitate haptic identification through the feet or cane. Some travelers could see the number buttons in a self service elevator while others might benefit from braille symbols and/or raised Arabic numerals.

4. The feeling that modifications should be expanded beyond *just* the elimination of travel hazards. Modifications should be made whenever they would make independent travel more comfortable and convenient for the visually impaired. Examples of this thinking are reflected in the proposals for audible traffic signals and brailled buttons in the self service elevators.

Other considerations that influence negative responses against architectural and environmental modifications are:

1. The feeling that modifications made for the visually impaired are counter-productive since they call unwanted attention to these individuals and thus set them apart from the mainstream of society.

2. The feeling that it is unrealistic and unnecessary to expect the sighted majority to cater to the needs of the visually impaired.

3. The feeling that all pedestrians are exposed to some dangers. All of these dangers cannot be eliminated and should also be accepted as part of everyday life by the visually impaired.

4. The feeling that sighted assistance can be an alternative to modifications. One can solicit temporary sighted assistance if the environment becomes too difficult or dangerous for independent travel. The visually impaired person assumes a dependent mode of travel for the time needed to deal with the problem, then resumes independent travel.

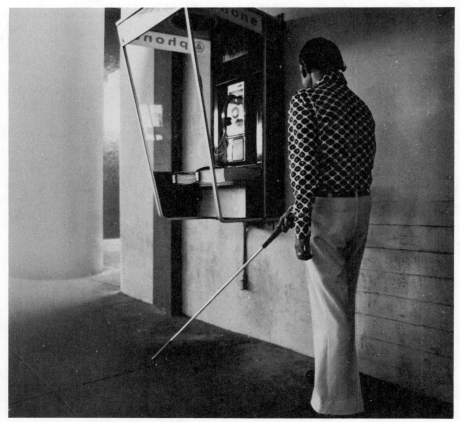

Figure 3-14. A telephone booth as a travel hazard.

5. The feeling that the cost of the modifications would be prohibitive; the expense is not justified because of the small numbers of visually impaired pedestrians.

SPECIFIC PROPOSALS

The extreme value positions represented above are most likely to be elicited by the general question of whether the environment should be modified to meet the needs of the visually impaired traveler. However, a consideration of some of the specific proposals for modifications usually results in greater unanimity. The following pages will review some of the travel hazards for the visually impaired and some of the modifications that have been suggested for the elimination of these hazards. There will also be a discussion of the importance of compatibility of modifications made for one group with the needs of other disability groups. Other discussions will relate to proposed modifications for added convenience of travel as opposed to modifications made strictly for safety of travel. Included also will be a discussion of special "nature trails" for the visually impaired. Finally, material will be presented that can guide the mobility specialist in his efforts to influence the community's decisions about the implementation of modifications for visually impaired travelers.

Public Telephones

Placement of public telephones can cause a travel hazard (Fig. 3-14). The

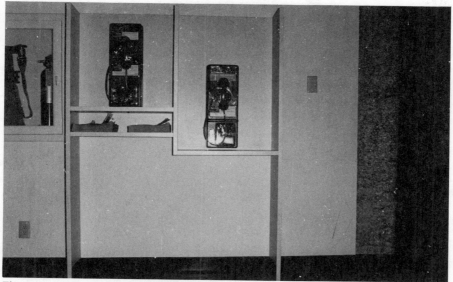

Figure 4-14. Hazard-free telephone mounting.

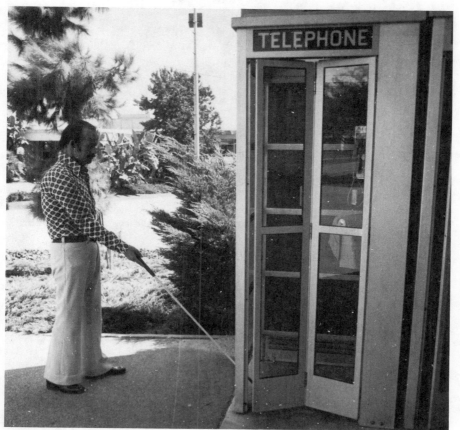

Figure 5-14. Telephone booth that is not a travel hazard.

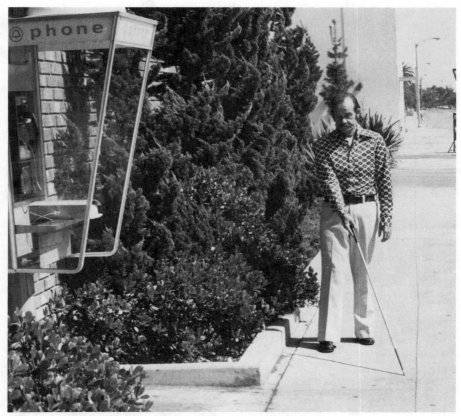

Figure 6-14. Wall-mounted telephone offset from normal line of traffic.

telephone is wall-mounted at approximately chest height. The side panels of the enclosure project outward from the wall but do not extend to ground level. The cane could go under the enclosure. If any cane contact is made, it would be high on the shaft or at the grip. This would provide very little time to stop. The possibility of injury is increased if the person is trailing the wall to locate a specific doorway. The cane would go under the enclosure, and not provide the necessary warning because there is nothing present to contact.

One solution is to provide the cane with something to contact. The side panels should be extended to within 12 in. (30.5 cm) of the ground or extend all the way to the ground. The panels should be the same width from top to bottom in order to prevent the top from projecting outward. The interior width between the two side panels should be constructed to allow adequate space for those in wheelchairs. Figure 4-14 illustrates this type of telephone situation.

The telephone booth in Fig. 5-14 does not present a travel hazard. The cane contacts the enclosure and provides warning of an obstacle.

A more desirable solution would be the elimination of the hazard through better building design. The telephone could be recessed into the interior walls. This telephone alcove could be designed to reflect the needs of the visually impaired traveler as well as a person in a wheelchair. Figure 6-14 shows a solution for the telephone located outdoors. The wall-mounted telephone is offset from the normal line of pedestrian traffic.

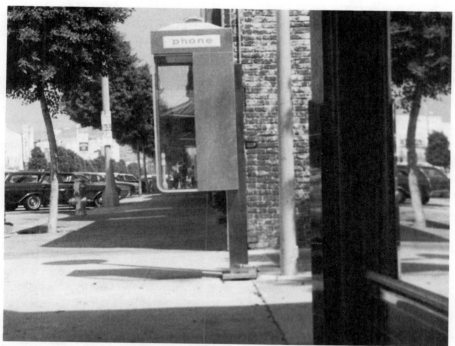

Figure 7-14. Pole-mounted phone as travel hazard.

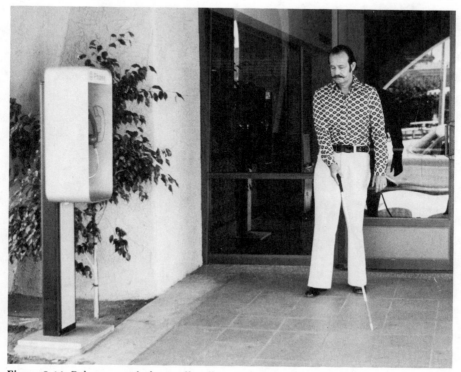

Figure 8-14. Pole-mounted phone off walkway out of line of traffic.

Another style of telephone is the pole-mounted variety. Here again, the cane may go under the telephone enclosure. The placement of the pole-mounted telephone in Fig. 7-14 could not be worse. It is placed directly in the path of travel, presenting a hazard to the visually impaired traveler as well as the sighted public.

Figure 8-14 shows a different style of pole-mounted telephone. It does not have the large box-like enclosure that can become a hazard. This telephone is correctly positioned just off the walkway and out of the pedestrian line of travel.

Guy Wires

Guy wires are metal cables used to support utility poles. Placement of these wires can result in a travel hazard (Fig. 9-14). The angular position of the guy wire creates the hazard. This person's head would make contact with the wire before his cane could provide the warning to stop.

Figure 10-14 shows a better placement of the guy wire. The angular placement of the wire is gone. The wire is now perpendicular to the ground and the cane will provide adequate warning. The utility pole and the wire may remain obstacles to travel but they are no longer dangerous hazards. Figure 11-14 shows a different placement with the guy wire strung to the side of the walk.

In the ideal situation, there would be no guy wires near the sidewalk at all. If they must be present, the placements in Figs. 10-14 and 11-14 are recommended. In those rare cases where the angular wire must be maintained, a protective covering or padding should be applied to the abrasive surface of the wire.

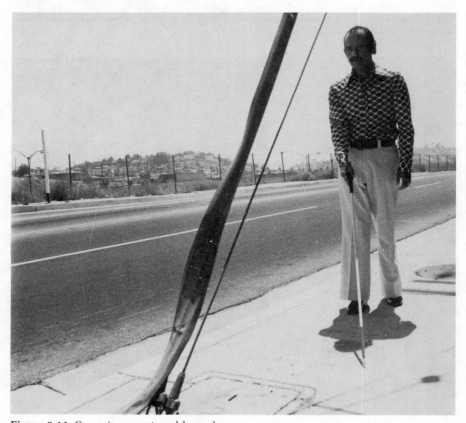

Figure 9-14. Guy wires as a travel hazard.

14

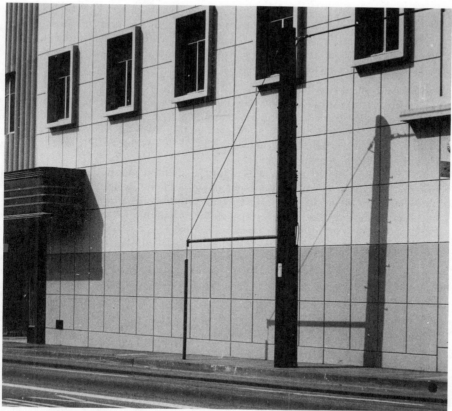

Figure 10-14. Safer placement of guy wires.

Wall Fixtures

Protruding objects attached to the wall and not extending to the floor create a travel hazard. The placement of fixtures recessed into the wall should be stressed. The wall-mounted ashtrays in Fig. 12-14 are an example. The original design of the building should have specified ashtrays recessed into the wall. This would have been less costly than having the fixtures placed in the wall after the building was completed. In this example, a solution would be to remove the wall-mounted ashtrays and replace them with the floor-standing variety.

"In the wall placement" should also apply to other types of wall fixtures such as fire extinguishers, drinking fountains, telephones, etc. This principle also applies to the exterior walls when the public walkway is very near the building line.

Stairs and Escalators

Under certain circumstances, stairs and escalators can become a travel hazard at face height. In Fig. 13-14, the traveler had veered slightly to the left of his intended line of travel. The hazard occurred when the underside of the staircase was open and there was nothing for the cane to contact.

Unfortunately, this type of hazard also occurs indoors. Figure 14-14 illustrates a dangerous open area under stairs. The traveler approaching the stairs from the side could strike his face and chest on the overhang of the ascending staircase. An area of this kind, both indoors and outdoors, should be enclosed with wood paneling or other type of building material. Another solution would be to box in the dangerous area with a solid line of decorative planters or shrubbery, or a small wall.

The escalator in Fig. 15-14, was in a two-story shopping center and posed the same potential danger. It is another example of an area that should be enclosed, so that the cane has something to contact.

Planters and Shrubbery

Planters and shrubbery can be used to neutralize some travel hazards by filling the open space beneath stairs and escalators. However, a poor choice of planter or shrubbery can create new hazards. Most planters used on commercial property are large circular or boxlike structures. They rest on the floor surface and are approximately four feet in height.

The planter in Fig. 16-14 was chosen for the visual appeal of its unusual design. No thought was given to the potential dangers of the design. The flaring sides could cause problems for the cane traveler. Another disturbing fact is that the sharp corners are at face level for any children walking or running through the shopping center without paying proper attention.

Good judgment should also be used in the choice of plants and shrubs. This is particularly important when they are to be used near a door or walkway. Figure 17-14 depicts such a hazard in a semi-business location. The long, narrow leaves of the plant are ridged, and the end of the leaf has a needle-like point. The dangers

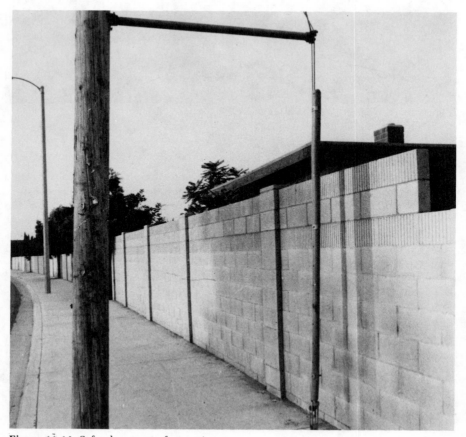

Figure 11-14. Safe placement of guy wires.

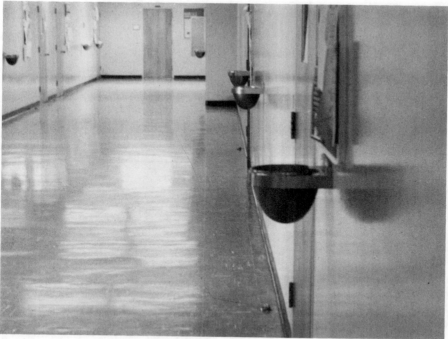

Figure 12-14. Wall-mounted ashtrays as travel hazards.

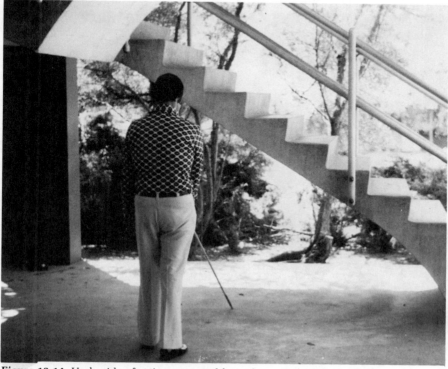

Figure 13-14. Underside of stairs as a travel hazard.

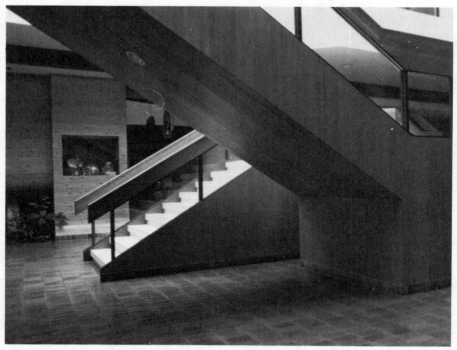

Figure 14-14. Underside of indoor stairs as a travel hazard.

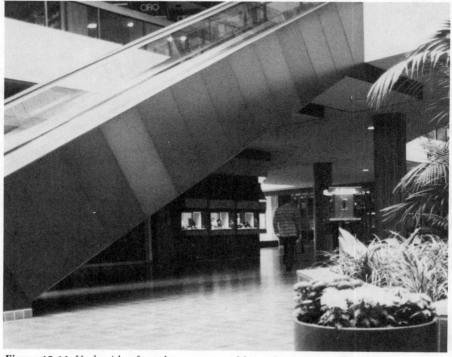

Figure 15-14. Underside of escalator as a travel hazard.

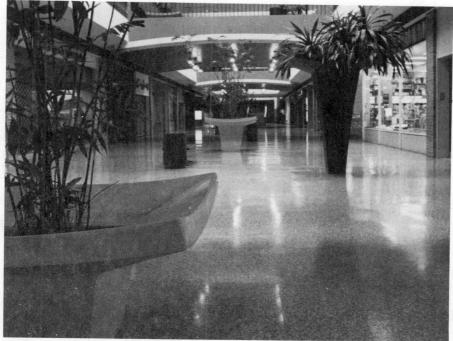

Figure 16-14. Planter as a travel hazard.

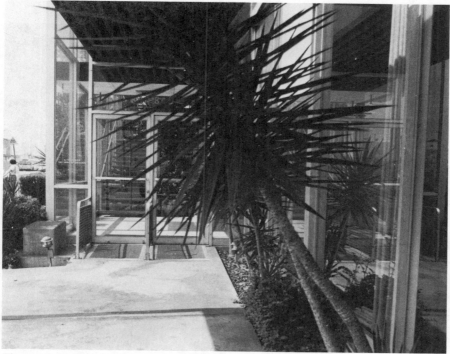

Figure 17-14. Plant leaves as a travel hazard.

are obvious. The same type of shrub presents a hazard situation on a residential sidewalk (Fig. 18-14).

The varieties of dangerous plants differ according to geographical area, and most areas have several varieties that should not be used in areas of pedestrian travel.

Proper trimming of shrubbery is also important. Shrubbery overhanging the sidewalk at face level is one of the most common travel hazards. Most communities have ordinances requiring that shrubbery around sidewalks be well trimmed. Complaints to city officials about specific violations will get results.

Street Signs

The placement of street signs can create a travel hazard. The law in many localities states that the bottom of a sign must be at least seven feet from ground level, but there are far too many violations of this law. There are times when the cane will contact the pole supporting the sign and give adequate warning. Unfortunately, there are other times when a sign extends outward too far for the pole to be contacted. The low sign nearest the traveler in Fig. 19-14 may cause a bump or bruise. The position of the second sign could cause a facial laceration as the edges of most signs are knife sharp. These hazards can be eliminated. Signs placed at dangerous heights and angles should be reported to city officials.

Display Windows

Some display windows are unrecognized hazards. Once again, the problem is an object without much ground level support. Figure 20-14 illustrates a potential danger. In this example the traveler does get some warning. However, the contact is very high on the cane shaft giving little warning time. The traveler's momentum might carry him forward to the point of bumping his head on the window. Some

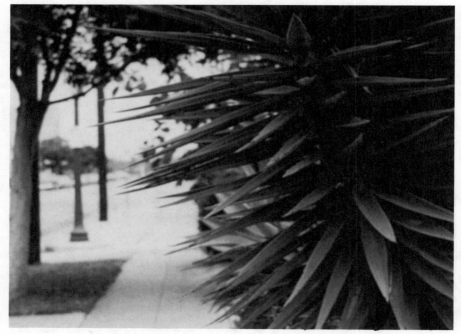

Figure 18-14. Overhanging shrubbery as a travel hazard.

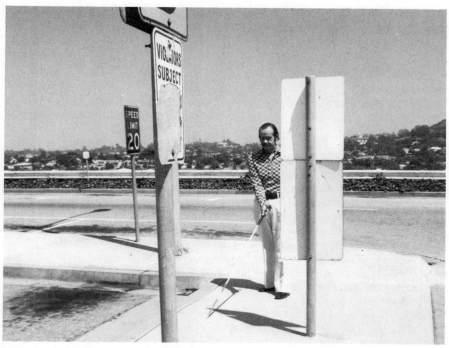

Figure 19-14. Street signs as travel hazards.

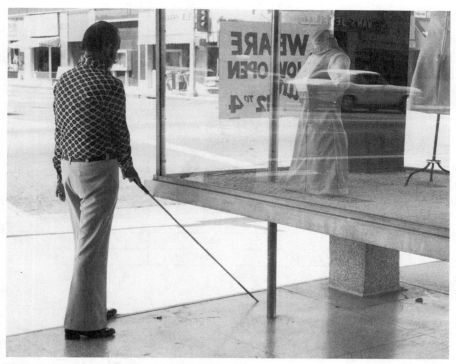

Figure 20-14. Display window as a travel hazard.

display windows are elevated even higher from the ground, and no warning of their presence would be received from the cane.

The solution is simple. Give the cane something to contact. If the base of the display window cannot be enclosed with wood or masonry, the techniques of filling such spaces with planters discussed earlier would apply.

Stair Handrails

The benefits of handrails are obvious, but their placement is also important. The handrails on the exterior stairs of a post office were positioned as shown in Fig. 21-14.

In the following set of circumstances, these handrails could become a travel hazard. The traveler has been told that he can locate the entrance to the post office by trailing the wall on his left. He does this and his cane indicates the stairs. He turns left and places the cane in his left hand and grips the railing with his right hand. Note that the handrail is attached to the face of the building and the door is actually on the other side of the handrail. Without vision or appropriate auditory clues, the traveler may sidestep in search of the door. If he sidesteps without first checking with his cane, he could fall off the edge of the stairs with resulting injury.

When informed of the potential hazard the post office altered the handrails as shown in Fig. 22-14. Additional railing to block the dangerous portion of the stairs was added to handrails already in place. All pedestrian traffic is now safely directed to the door.

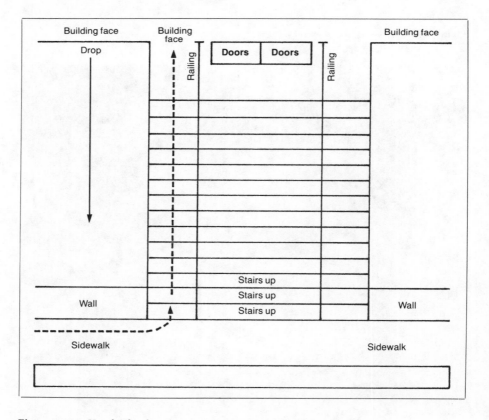

Figure 21-14. Handrails placed so as to lead to a travel hazard.

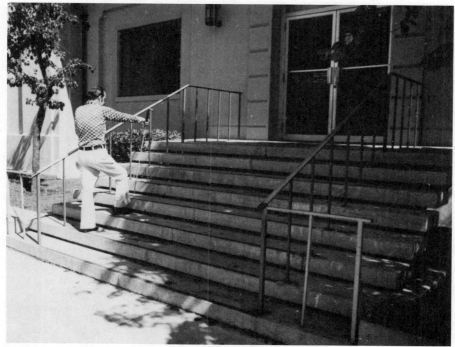

Figure 22-14. Handrails placed so as to provide safe access.

Handrails on interior stairs also deserve comment. Many people such as the elderly blind, those with leg braces, or with balance problems depend upon handrails for necessary support. Therefore, it is recommended that the handrails be continuous around the landing area and be placed on both sides of the stairs. This would make an uninterrupted handrail from one floor to the next floor. It is also recommended that the handrails extend completely to the end of the flight of stairs, and not end prematurely two or three steps from the end. In fact, the handrail should begin 12-18 in. (30-45 cm) before the first step and continue 12-18 in. (30-45 cm) beyond the last step.

The handrail should also be of contrasting color to the walls of the staircase. This would make them easier to locate by people with low vision.

Some propose that the railings in large buildings be equipped with plastic, wood, or metal plates to indicate floor numbers. The plates could use raised Arabic numerals, color contrasted for the low vision person, and braille symbols for the totally blind. This modification would make travel more comfortable or convenient but does not involve the elimination of a travel hazard.

IRREGULAR INTERSECTIONS

Many visually impaired students learn to cross regular intersections (two streets crossing at right angles) in a safe and independent fashion. This typical intersection is found almost everywhere.

Unfortunately, there are other types of intersections atypical in design. The two streets may not cross at right angles. The corners of the intersection may be offset, necessitating a line of travel at an angle from the traffic flow. Figures 23-14 and 24-14 depict irregular intersections.

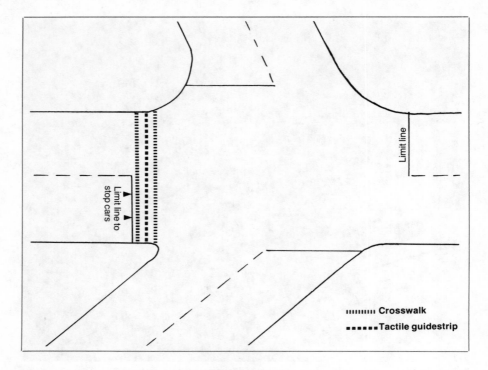

Figure 23-14. Tactual guidestrip in atypical intersection.

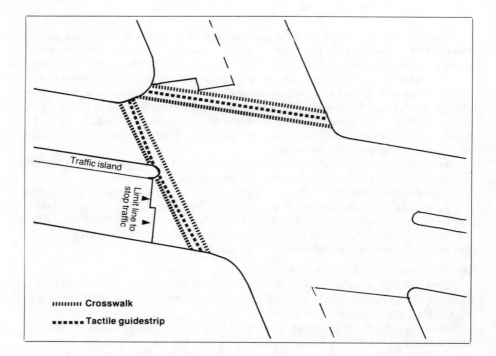

Figure 24-14. Tactual guidestrip in atypical intersection.

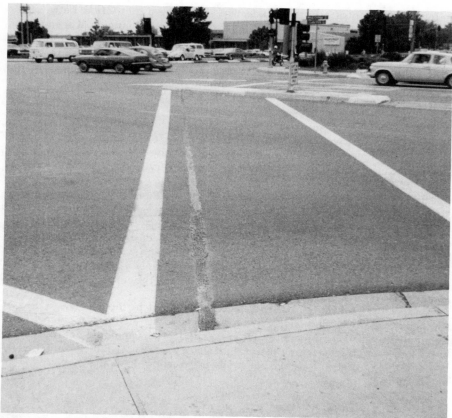

Figure 25-14. Tactual guidestrip.

Irregular intersections often require the visually impaired traveler to seek sighted assistance. In fact, orientation and mobility training stresses when and how to use sighted assistance. However, the problems caused by irregular intersections are compounded if they are located in areas of very little pedestrian traffic. It is particularly annoying if these intersections cannot be avoided by using a convenient alternate route. The irregular intersection may be located on the best route to a rehabilitation center, school, or place of employment.

Tactual Guidestrips

A tactual guidestrip (Elias, 1974) may provide a solution. It gives the traveler a safe guide to follow across an irregular intersection. A tactual guidestrip is a raised line of 0.25 in. (0.6 cm) thick epoxy cement with 0.25 in. (0.6 cm) pea gravel pressed into it. The guidestrip is 2 in. (5 cm) wide and is followed with the cane as the traveler crosses the intersection. A tactual guidestrip is pictured in Fig. 25-14.

The visually impaired traveler can be aided in locating the guidestrip by the placement of a tactual indicator on the curb face (Fig. 26-14). The traveler locates the curb using the touch technique or the touch and slide technique. He then pivots the cane into a diagonal position and moves the cane laterally across the curb face. The cane locates the tactual indicator and the guidestrip is in the street directly below and out from this point. The touch and drag technique can be used to parallel the guidestrip across the difficult intersection.

497

Implementation of a tactual guidestrip should be a joint effort between the mobility specialist, the blind traveler, and the appropriate municipal agency. The blind traveler may express a concern regarding difficult crossing conditions at a particular intersection. The mobility specialist evaluates the intersection to determine if the standard crossing techniques apply, or can be safely modified to fit the peculiarities of the intersection. He should also determine how much pedestrian assistance is available and how practical a tactual guidestrip would be at that intersection.

If the use of a tactual guidestrip is decided upon, the mobility specialist and the blind traveler must work together to arrive at its best placement. The city traffic engineer, or other appropriate official becomes involved at this point to evaluate structural considerations, secure financing, and supervise the actual construction of the guidestrip.

The tactual guidestrip presents no problems to others. It is not confusing to drivers because it is not painted white and actually looks as though the street had been patched. The guidestrip is not harmful to car or bicycle tires. It is placed near one of the crosswalk lines and will not trip sighted pedestrians as it is parallel to their line of travel, nor will it hinder the movement of a wheelchair.

It should be stressed that the tactual guidestrip is only a directional aid. It will not insure a safe crossing if the traveler does not leave the curb at the proper time, and exercise normal safety precautions while crossing.

Most of the guidestrips currently used are located in the San Diego area of Southern California. They are used on a limited basis at irregular intersections frequented by visually impaired travelers. Experience has pointed out the danger of the general public viewing the guidestrip as a panacea. The mistaken rationale is that if the guidestrip is beneficial at one intersection, it should be placed at all intersections.

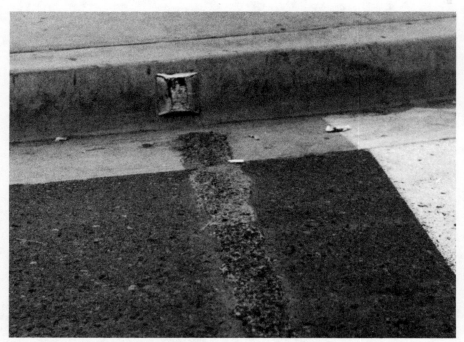

Figure 26-14. Tactual indicator for guidestrip.

Little is known about the effect of winter weather conditions on guidestrips. At present they are used in Southern California, and have not been tested in the harsh snow climates of the midwest and eastern states. The effects of severe temperature change, rock salt, and snow removal equipment are not known. Test projects are recommended so that communities can determine the adaptability of the tactual guidestrip to local conditions and climates.

THE LOW VISION PERSON AND ENVIRONMENTAL MODIFICATIONS

Many environmental modifications discussed thus far relate to the low vision person as well as the blind traveler. However, several additional concerns are relevant for low vision persons not using long canes. In reality, this is quite a large portion of the visually impaired population.

Step-down Situations

Because of poor depth perception characteristic of many visual impairments, a major concern of the low vision traveler is the step-down situation. When the color of the sidewalk blends with the color of the down-step, a misleading impression of a level sidewalk may be perceived. This situation may also be found in a long hallway where a few steps lead down to a lower level of the same hallway. The colors blend and a long level hallway is perceived.

One solution is the use of materials of different color and texture preceding the edge of the step-down area. Figure 27-14 shows a potentially dangerous situation that has been improved through the use of color contrast.

Color contrast has additional uses. The edge of each step, in a flight of stairs, should be identified by color contrast. A contrasting color should also be used on a landing to help to identify the end of the stairs and minimize the possibility of those jarring extra steps taken when an individual thinks that the stairs continue. A point made earlier applies here too—the desirability of the handrail contrasting in color with the walls of the stairwell.

Figure 28-14 shows a portion of an indoor shopping center. The walkway changes elevation at this point and the stairs have been contrasted in color to enhance recognition of this change. A ramp has been constructed in the center of the stairs. It is refreshing to see the ramp incorporated as part of the original building design and not added later as an unattractive afterthought.

Stairs, up or down, should not be built in close proximity to entrance and exit doors. A person with low vision may experience poor eye adaptation to the sudden change in light intensity as he enters or exits a building. Poor eye adaptation could cause a person to fall at stairs near a door. The light intensity in this area of the building should be regulated to help facilitate eye adaptation. It would be desirable to use transitional lighting in building areas near entrance and exit doors.

The problems are not over when a low vision person is safely out of a building. The sidewalk from a building may lead to a step-down situation at a parking lot or public sidewalk. The gray cement of the walk from the building may blend with the gray coloration of the parking lot or public sidewalk, and the step-down may not be recognized by the low vision person. The solution is to employ materials of differing color and texture just preceding the step-down. The edge of each step should be painted a contrasting color.

More Use of Color Contrast

The use of color contrast could be expanded to solve problems faced by the low vision traveler in the monochromatic environment characteristic of large institutions and government buildings. Floor tile should contrast in color with the sides of the hall. Doors and door frames should be lighter or darker than surrounding

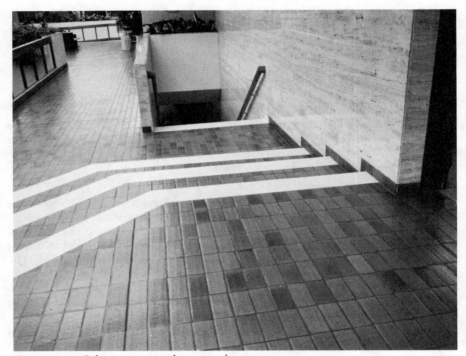

Figure 27-14. Color contrast to show step-down.

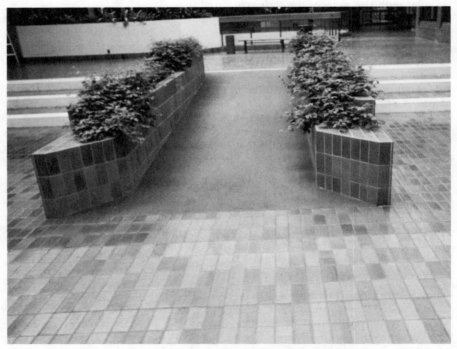

Figure 28-14. Color coded stairs for recognition of floor elevation change.

wall surfaces. If the floor tile is light in color, dark tile can be used in front of major offices, or classrooms to facilitate visual location and door counting. The contrasting tile should be the width of the door and extend 3 to 4 ft (90 to 120 cm) from the door into the normal sized hallway.

The effects of glare such as light streaming through large expanses of plate glass and reflecting off floor and wall surfaces add to the difficulty of safe movement. Several approaches could be taken to make these areas more hospitable to the low vision traveler. Coatings can be applied to the glass to soften the light intensity. Nonreflective floor surfaces can be used. When choosing the type of wall coating to be used near large areas of glass, the problem of potential glare should be considered.

In addition to glare, large expanses of glass create problems for the low vision person. Doors are often camouflaged in this wall of glass. Exit doors should be clearly visible to everyone using the building by making the door frames and if possible the doors contrast with the wall color. A contrasting colored floor tile in front of these doors would also provide needed visual clues.

Large areas of plate glass are a potential hazard to *anyone* using a building. It should be standard practice to apply a decorative design or decal at face level on the glass. The contrast in color provided by this visual clue can prevent dangerous physical contact with the glass.

Color Contrasted Signs

Informative signs often blend into the color of the walls and are not seen by the low vision person. Even when the signs are seen, the print size is often too small to be read. Signs throughout buildings should have large letters. A letter height of at least 2 in. (5.1 cm) is recommended, in a Helvetica semi-bold print style.

Room number and signs should be easy to locate and read as a low vision traveler moves down a hall. Room numbers attached to an office or classroom door are not easily visible when the door is propped open, and numbers located above the door may be difficult to read, therefore signs and room numbers should be on the wall on the right, left or both sides of the door frame at a height of 5 ft (150 cm) from the floor surface. Some propose that they should be raised letters or numerals for tactual identification. A standardized position and height would facilitate the location of the tactual information by blind travelers.

The colors of a sign should contrast in two ways: the color of the letters should contrast boldly with the background of the sign and these two colors should also contrast with the surrounding wall surface. Creative use of artificial light can also be used to call attention to signs such as illuminating them from behind, the way exit signs are commonly lit in a theater.

THE COMPATIBILITY FACTOR

It was mentioned earlier that most of the present activity in the field of architectural and environmental modifications centers around the needs of those in wheelchairs. In most cases, their needs are compatible with the independent functioning of the visually impaired. However, problems can arise if proper precautions are not exercised. One area of particular concern is curb ramps.

Curb Ramping

The implementation of curb ramping is an example of modifications designed primarily for one segment of the population having both positive and negative ramifications for other segments of the population. Persons in wheelchairs find curbs a major impediment to independent travel. Properly constructed curb ramps have proven to be a desirable solution to this problem. Curb ramps have also proven useful to elderly pedestrians, to individuals in leg braces or on crutches,

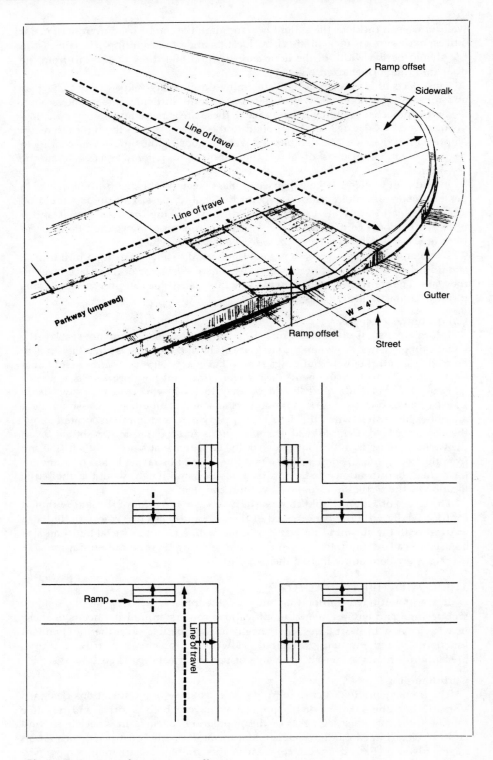

Figure 29-14. Ramp location one, offset.

and even to mothers pushing baby carriages.

Curb ramps have various implications for blind travelers using the long cane. Traditionally these travelers have used one or more of the following methods to locate the end of a block: employing touch and slide technique to increase the chances of the cane tip sliding over the edge of the curb, listening to perpendicular and parallel traffic, and using time-distance estimation and landmarks in familiar neighborhoods to anticipate the end of the block.

The major clue in curb location is the recognition of the change in elevation between sidewalk and street. The ramp replaces this pronounced change in elevation with a gradual one. The concern is that a blind traveler could descend the ramp and enter the street without realizing his mistake.

Two solutions have been proposed to minimize the chances of this occurrence. The first calls for texturing the ramp. It should differ, to a marked degree, from the regular sidewalk surface. The texture should be very pronounced and easily distinguishable under a nylon or metal cane tip. The texturing should not, however, impede the movement of a wheelchair. It fact, proper texturing can provide a non-slip surface on the ramp which is helpful to the wheelchair traveler. The type of texturing differs from community to community. Some have elected to swirl a very coarse pattern into the wet cement with a wood float or broom finish. Others have inscribed lines in the wet cement forming a ribbed pattern that is perpendicular to the pedestrian line of travel. The important element is that the texture of the ramp be easily distinguished from the texture of the sidewalk.

A second solution is the incorporation of a small lip at the point where the ramp meets the street. This lip provides at least a minimal drop in elevation under the cane tip. It may not be distinguishable to some blind pedestrians, but it does provide important help to others. This lip should be compatible with the needs of those in a wheelchair. A ½ in. (1.27 cm) maximum lip has been proposed by some as a compromise. They feel that the ½ in. (1.27 cm) lip can be recognized by the cane traveler and will not seriously impede the wheelchair if it is beveled at a 45° angle. It is important to note that the lip does not replace the texturing techniques described earlier. The dual clues of texture and elevation change are used to maximize the traveler's ability to distinguish the end of the sidewalk and the beginning of the street. Some propose making the ramps a distinctive color to help the low vision person locate the ramp.

A very important factor for visually impaired persons in the use of curb ramps is consistency of placement. The ramps should be in the same location at all intersections within the community. Several options are available. In some cases, the ramp can serve as an indicator of good crossing alignment. In other cases, the ramp is in the wrong crossing position. Consistency is the key factor. The ramps must be located in the same position at all intersections. The blind traveler learns to use the ramps or to avoid the ramps. There are five possible locations for ramps. *Location One:* The ramp here is offset from the normal line of travel (Fig. 29-14). It would seem that this position would minimize the chances of a blind traveler finding himself on the ramp. Here, the desired line of travel would bring the traveler to the regular curb. The ramp would be slightly to his right or further from his parallel traffic.

Some travelers may wish to use the ramp as an indicator of a good crossing position. The ramp projects a line of travel within the crosswalk lines and provides a crossing position permitting the luxury of some veer without being in the intersection.

Opponents of this ramping style point out that two ramps are necessary at each corner, and that the cost would be double that of the single-ramp system in Location Two. Another objection is that much "street hardware" such as fire

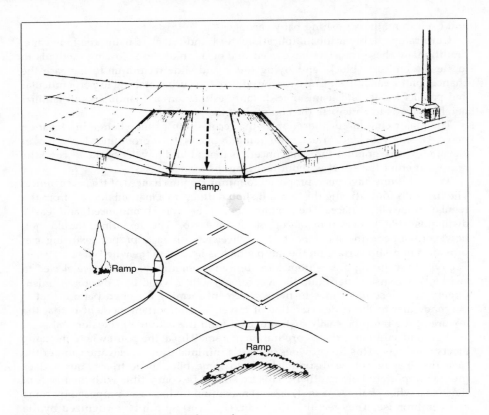

Ramp

Ramp

Ramp

Figure 30-14. Ramp location two, diagonal.

hydrants, street signs, utility poles, switch boxes, police telephones, etc., is located in the desired ramp position.

Location Two. The ramp here is positioned diagonally toward the center of the intersection (Fig. 30-14). In this situation a blind traveler would be taught not to cross from the ramp position. If a traveler found himself on the ramp, he would move from the ramp on this corner to the right and line up as usual facing north. He could also move to the left of the ramp and line up to face directly west. Proponents of this ramping system cite the cost economy of the one-ramp system over the two-ramp system. They also point out that this portion of the corner is usually free of street hardware, therefore the ramps could be placed in the same position at all corners.

There are also negative aspects to the diagonal ramp system. Some blind travelers unfamiliar with the diagonal position may line up with the ramp. This would project a line of travel directly into the middle of the intersection.

The diagonal ramp also prolongs the length of time a person in a wheelchair is in the street. When crossing, he must come down the ramp, make a turn around the corner and then cross. When he reaches the far side he must again turn around the corner to locate his ramp. This movement around the corner is done in the street. It necessitates altering the crosswalk lines to include the area around the face of the corner in the crosswalk area.

Location Three: Here there are two ramps-per-corner directly in the line of travel and facing in cardinal directions (Fig. 31-14). In this case, the visually impaired

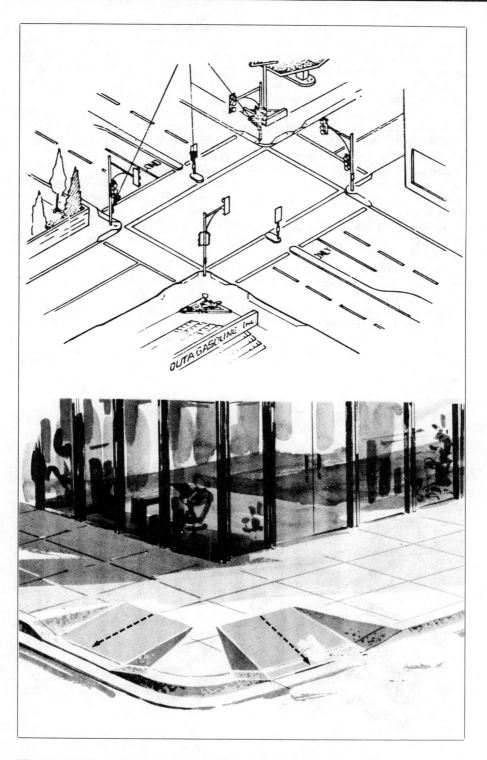

Figure 31-14. Ramp location three, two ramps-per-corner in pedestrian line of travel.

person can be taught to seek the ramp. A centered position in the ramp helps assure a good crossing position and projects a straight line of travel to the opposite corner. The negative aspects of this system would again be the cost factor and the possibility of not being able to place the ramps consistently in this position on all corners. The traveler would have to deal with a ramp at every corner as opposed to Location One where the ramps were offset from the line of travel.

Location Four.   In this instance the entire corner is flush with the street surface and serves as a ramp (Fig. 32-14). This type of construction is commonly called a blended curb. The cane traveler would use touch and slide technique to attempt to distinguish the textural change from the cement surface of the sidewalk to the coarse texture of the blacktop street. Occasionally, added help is provided by the cane tip sticking in the expansion joint formed at the junction of these two surfaces. The traveler would, of course, also use traffic sounds and other clues mentioned earlier.

However, blended curbs are difficult for many travelers to distinguish. The difficulty is increased because the sidewalk has a very minimal slope downward toward the street.

Texturing becomes even more important. It is recommended that at least the last four feet of sidewalk be textured to indicate the blending of street and sidewalk. The texture used should be different from the sidewalk texture and also differ from the street texture. It is important that the traveler recognize the sequence of the different textures. He should feel the texture of the transition area just before the street, then recognize the texture of the street.

Location Five.   The ramp here is built as an extension of the curb into the street (Fig. 33-14). This is the least desirable of the possible ramp constructions. It is inexpensive to construct, but the disadvantages outweigh this. It is hazardous to

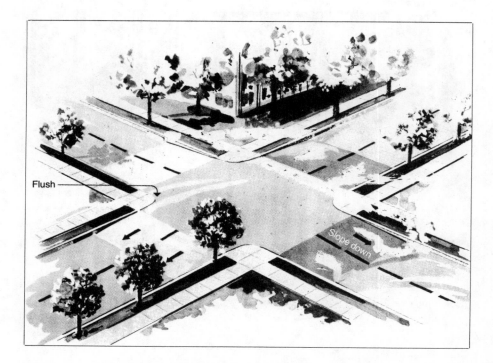

Figure 32-14. Street built up to level of sidewalk, no ramp.

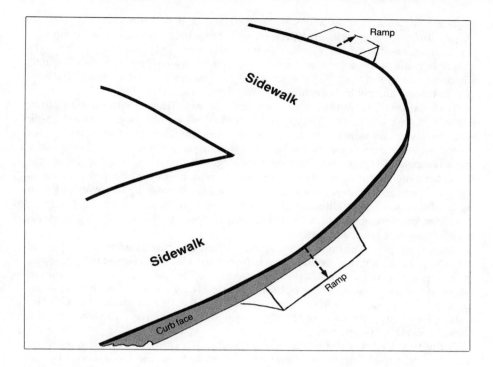

Figure 33-14. Ramp as extension of curb.

those in wheelchairs, as the wheelchair can easily tilt off the side of this ramp causing a serious fall. Those not in wheelchairs can also trip off the side of the ramp. The positioning of the ramp also creates drainage problems, as it interrupts water as it attempts to flow along the curb line forcing the water into the intersection.*

Curb ramps needed by those in wheelchairs can be made compatible with the independent functioning of the visually impaired, if proper precautions are taken to insure that the ramp surface is tactually distinct and that the ramps are consistently placed in the same location at each corner. Mobility specialists can then teach the traveler to avoid the ramps or to seek the ramp location to help to insure a straight street crossing.

MODIFICATIONS FOR CONVENIENCE

One purpose of architectural and environmental modifications is to eliminate travel hazards. A second purpose is to modify the environment for the improved convenience of the visually impaired traveler.

People's opinions differ on this issue. Some say that convenience is not a legitimate justification for architectural and environmental modifications. Others take the opposite position. Several situations are relevant to this discussion.

Self Service Elevators

Self service elevators do not qualify as a major travel hazard, but they do qualify as a major inconvenience to the visually impaired traveler, particularly when he

---

*The focus here has been from the point of view of the cane traveler. It has not attempted to deal with design criteria of ramp construction such as gradient of slope, width of ramp, etc. A source for this information is: A.P.W.A. Guidelines for Design & Construction of Ramps for the Physically Handicapped, American Public Works Association, 1313 East 60th Street, Chicago, Illinois 60637.

finds himself in a location where sighted assistance is not available.

The difficulty with self service elevators is their inconsistency. The position of the buttons outside of the elevator is not consistent. They may be on the right side or left side of the door. They may be high on the wall or low on the wall, and to the consternation of those in wheelchairs, they may be too high to reach. But, the real problems are the buttons on the inside of the elevator.

The location of the interior buttons is not standard. They may be on the right or left side of the elevator cab. They may be on the front wall of the cab or on the side walls. In some elevators the interior button panels are wisely placed on both sides of the elevator cab but may be out of reach from a wheelchair. The visually impaired person is faced with inconsistency again when he attempts to figure out the arrangement of buttons. The odd numbers may be in a row on either side of the panel, or the numbers may progress in sequential order up one row and then up the other row. The bottom button in the row may be basement, or it may be first floor, or even be second floor. There are additional problems in buildings with mezzanines and sub-basements.

Even the types of buttons differ. Some buttons are raised and must be pushed into the panel. They usually stay recessed until the elevator stops at that floor and then pop out to their original position. Some buttons are flush with the button panel and must be pushed. The button lights up giving a visual clue that is useless for the blind person. Perhaps the worst style is the heat sensitive button. The button panel may be unintentionally activated as the visually impaired person tactually explores the button panel.

If the traveler finds the proper button and presses it, the elevator moves. He does his best to estimate the direction and distance of the movement. This is difficult. Many travelers cannot be absolutely sure they are on the proper floor when the elevator stops. Perhaps two buttons were inadvertently pressed as the panel of buttons was explored, or perhaps the elevator stopped because someone on that floor pushed the exterior call button.

Several solutions are possible. One solution, of course, is to seek sighted assistance. There are many times when others are taking the same elevator and their assistance can be obtained. However, some suggest that self service elevators require modification for better reflection of the needs of the visually impaired traveler. They propose two additional solutions. The first is that brailled symbols and/or raised Arabic numbers be placed in standardized positions on the button panels, and on both sides of the exterior door casing. This modification would provide the visually impaired traveler with the convenience of checking the floor number for himself. When the door opens he reaches out of the elevator to the exterior door casing. The floor information appears at a standardized height on the casing.

Legislation can be used to mandate consistency. California, and possibly other states, have passed such a law. Section 4455.5 of the California Government Code relating to the access of public facilities by handicapped persons states,

All new elevators in public buildings or facilities after the operative date of this Section shall have braille symbols and marked Arabic numerals corresponding to the numerals on the elevator buttons embossed immediately to the right thereof.

All new door casings on all elevator floors after the operative date of this Section shall have the number of the floor on which the casing is located embossed in braille symbols and marked Arabic numerals on both sides at a height of approximately 42 inches from the floor.

Elevator Marking Standards

Standards for elevator markings were developed by Eugene Lozano, Jr. and the California Alliance of Blind Students:

1. Raised Arabic numerals and braille symbols corresponding to the numerals on the elevator buttons shall be provided immediately to the left thereof. Braille symbols shall be placed to the left of the corresponding raised Arabic numerals.

2. Buttons and switches shall be positioned to a maximum height of 55 in. (140 cm), minimum height of 35 in. (90 cm) above cab floor.

3. Type style to be known as RA-101.
   a. Arabic characters shall be a minimum of 0.625 in. (1.59 cm) high with a stroke width of 8 percent to 12 percent of the character height.
   b. Characters shall be raised a minimum of 0.030 in. (0.08 cm) and a maximum of 0.050 in. (0.13 cm) above the background.
   c. Cab control other than floor buttons shall be designated by raised symbols, refer to RA-101.
   d. Braille dots shall be on a 0.1-in. (0.25-cm) center in each cell with space between the cells 0.2 in. (0.5 cm). Dots shall be raised to a minimum of 0.025 in. (0.064 cm) above the background.

4. All door casings on all elevator floors shall have the number of the floor on which the casing is located, designated by raised Arabic numerals and braille symbols on both sides at a height of 60 in. (152 cm) above the floor. Braille symbols shall be placed directly to the left of corresponding raised Arabic numerals.

5. Type style to be known as RA-101.
   a. Arabic characters shall be a minimum of 1 in. (2.5 cm) high, maximum of 1.25 in. (3.18 cm) high with a stroke width of 8 percent to 12 percent of the character height.
   b. Characters shall be raised a minimum of 0.030 in. (0.08 cm) with a maximum of 0.040 in. (0.10 cm) above the background.
   c. Characters shall be white on a black background.
   d. Braille dots shall be on a 0.1-in. (0.25-cm) center in each cell with space between the cells 0.2 in. (0.5 cm). Dots shall be raised to a minimum of 0.025 in. (0.064 cm) above the background.

A second solution is to increase the use of spoken information in the elevator. The same technology used in the talking calculator could also be incorporated in the elevator buttons. The button panel would give immediate audio feedback stating what button has been pushed. A recorded message could state the floor number as the door opens to prevent someone exiting on the wrong floor. Many do not realize that this audio floor information could also be helpful to those in wheelchairs. It frequently happens that there is no room to turn a wheelchair in a crowded elevator. The person must ride facing the back of the elevator and therefore cannot see the visual floor indicator at the front. The audible information would let him know exactly when to back out of the elevator car. It eliminates the necessity of seeking this information from fellow passengers in the elevator.

TELEPHONE AND HALLWAY MARKING STANDARDS

Lozano and the California Alliance of Blind Students have also proposed standards for braille markings on pay telephones and hallway doors:

Pay Telephones

1. Raised Arabic numerals and braille symbols shall correspond to the phone number and area code and shall be provided immediately below the dial with the area code 0.25 in. (0.64 cm) above the phone number. Braille symbols shall be placed directly beneath the corresponding raised Arabic numerals with a

space of 0.25 in. (0.64 cm) between the horizontal lines of braille and Arabic symbols.

2. Type style to be known as RA-101.
   a. Arabic characters shall be a minimum of 0.625 in. (1.59 cm) high with a stroke width of 8 percent to 12 percent of the character height.
   b. Characters shall be raised a minimum of 0.030 in. (0.08 cm) and a maximum of 0.040 in. (0.10 cm) above the background.
   c. Characters shall be white on a black background.
   d. Braille dots shall be on a 0.1-in. (0.25-cm) center in each cell with space between the cells 0.2 in. (0.5 cm). Dots shall be raised to a minimum of 0.025 in. (0.64 cm) above the background.

Outside and Hallway Door Marking Standards

1. Raised Arabic numerals and braille symbols corresponding to the specific rooms shall be provided on the door jamb, on the same side as the door knob occurs at a height of 60 in. (152 cm).

2. In the case of double doors, the braille markings shall be on the extreme left and right sides of those door frames, whether it is one set or more of double doors. The braille markings shall have the name of the building and its address.

3. The arrangement of the name of the building and its address on the panels shall have the raised Arabic symbols for the name and address on two horizontal lines 0.25 in. (0.64 cm) apart and the braille symbols for the name and address also 0.25 in. (0.64 cm) apart directly below the raised Arabic with 0.50 in. (1.27 cm) between the last line of raised Arabic and the first line of braille.

4. In addition to the raised international symbol for handicapped accessibility on restroom doors, there should also be braille and Arabic symbols signifying men's and women's restrooms.

5. Braille symbols shall be placed directly to the left of the corresponding raised Arabic numerals with all symbols in Grade II Braille, at a height of 60 in. (152 cm).

6. Type style to be known as RA-101.
   a. Arabic characters shall be a minimum of 1 in. (2.5 cm) to a maximum of 1.25 in. (3.18 cm) high with a stroke width of 8 percent to 12 percent of the character height.
   b. Characters shall be raised a minimum of 0.030 in. (0.076 cm) and a maximum of 0.040 in. (0.010 cm) above the background.

7. Whether the raised Arabic numeral is either 1 in. (2.5 cm) or 1.25 in. (3.18 cm) high on the jamb panel, the numeral should have a minimum of a 0.50-in. (1.27-cm) border from the top, bottom, and right side of the last numeral on the right to the edge of the panel plate, as well as a 0.50-in. (1.27-cm) minimum between the first braille cell and the left edge of the first raised Arabic numeral.

8. Characters shall be white on a black background.

9. Braille dots shall be on a 0.1-in. (0.25-cm) center in each cell with space between the cells 0.2 in. (0.5 cm). Dots shall be raised to a minimum of 0.025 in. (0.64 cm) above the background.

The Information Center

Many sighted people seek out a building directory in the lobby of a large office complex or shopping center, visited for the first time. There is usually an alphabetical listing of offices or stores and perhaps a floor diagram depicting their location.

This type of helpful information could also be made available to the visually impaired traveler. An information center could be required in large buildings not containing a staffed reception desk. However, the information center is of no use if it cannot be found. Its location would have to be standardized. Perhaps it could be a certain distance within the building and to the right of each main entrance. It could provide large print and brailled directories of the offices or stores within the building. Diagrams of the floor plan would be displayed in a large print format with contrasting colors and also in tactual format for the blind traveler. A telephone extension with a direct line to an information source within the building could also be provided.

TRAFFIC AND PEDESTRIAN CONTROL

The scope of environmental modifications has been broadened by some to encompass control of vehicular and pedestrian traffic. Attention centers upon independent street crossings at intersections controlled by traffic lights. Proper interpretation of auditory information is a major factor in a safe street crossing for the visually impaired traveler. He is taught to "read" intelligently the auditory patterns formed by the parallel and perpendicular traffic. The traveler begins his crossing in conjunction with the surge of parallel traffic. However, there are times when this important information is either not present or not reliable. There are also times when the proper auditory information is present but the traveler hesitates because he doubts his interpretation of the auditory cues.

Three options are available in these troublesome situations:

1. Attempt the street crossing even though you are unsure that you are crossing at the proper time.

2. Delay the crossing and seek sighted assistance.

3. Delay the crossing and wait for more traffic to flow through the intersection. This provides more auditory information to use in determining the proper time to cross.

Auditory Traffic Signals

Some propose the use of auditory signals at traffic light intersections. An immediate consideration is what the extent of use will be within a community. They can be installed city-wide or installed at selected or particularly troublesome intersections. There are advantages and disadvantages to both of these options as seen a little later in the listing of advantages and disadvantages.

Another immediate consideration faced by a community is the type of system to be used. There are two general classifications, constant information systems or demand activated systems.

The *constant information system* provides auditory and/or tactual information every time the traffic light changes from red to green. The system functions constantly regardless of pedestrian need. The *demand activated system* functions only when activated by a pedestrian. Generally this activation occurs when a button is pushed on a control box mounted on the corner. However, Japan has experimented with a pocket size activation device. It is issued to visually impaired pedestrians and used when needed to activate the audible signals.

Three specific sensory patterns are possible in either a constant information system or in a demand activated system. One pattern is a *one-sound pattern* commonly called a scatter-light crossing or a scramble crossing. The traffic light functions normally for the parallel and perpendicular traffic flow but no pedestrian movement takes place until the light turns red in all four directions. An auditory signal is given and pedestrians cross in all four directions. Diagonal crossings are also permitted in some cities.

A second sensory pattern is a *two-sound pattern*, where pedestrians cross, as usual, with the flow of traffic parallel to their crossing position. One auditory signal such as a bell signifies the proper time to cross in north-south directions and a buzzer signifies an east-west crossing. Some cities use a monotone for one direction and a beeping tone for the other direction. A recorded speech system has even been attempted.

A third sensory pattern is a *combined auditory-tactile pattern*. Much of the work on these systems centers in Japan and Sweden. The Japanese system uses touch-posts on each corner of an intersection. The visually impaired or deaf blind person locates the tactile indicator and assumes a waiting position with his hand on the post. A distinctive audio-tactile pattern is presented at the proper crossing time.

Proponents of auditory traffic signals and combined auditory-tactile systems give the following advantages:

1. The information from the auditory or auditory-tactile systems can be used in conjunction with the usual system employing the sound of traffic surge. This dual cueing will remove much of the stress involved in crossing a major intersection.

2. In situations with little or no traffic, the system will provide a safe reference for the proper crossing time.

3. The system will help to facilitate safe crossings for the sighted pedestrian. Many sighted pedestrians miss the visual walk signal due to inattentiveness or visual distractions. The auditory signal combined with the walk sign would give dual cueing to the sighted pedestrian.

4. Demand-activated systems keep noise annoyance to a minimum, lessening discomfort to those living and working near intersections with audible signals.

5. Cost is minimized if the systems are used at selected or troublesome intersections instead of installation city-wide.

Opponents to these systems point to the following disadvantages:

1. The devices are susceptible to mechanical failure and vandalism.

2. Confusing auditory overlap may be heard when the auditory information at one intersection is confused with auditory information coming from another nearby intersection.

3. If speakers are centralized above the intersection, the auditory signal must be loud enough to be heard on all four corners. A signal of this intensity can mask the sound of the traffic surge thus destroying the possible double cueing benefits.

4. Another location for the speakers could be on the corner rather than above the intersection. The speaker box could be at shoulder level and of course constructed in such a way as not to form a travel hazard. The traveler stands near the box and listens for the signal to cross. However, this may require two boxes per corner. Auditory overlap may occur and the potential for vandalism is increased when the equipment is located near sidewalk level.

5. Proper education of all pedestrians and drivers is critical. They must know what the auditory signals mean. In a two-sound pattern, they must be oriented. They must know exactly what direction they are facing and the exact sound that signifies a safe crossing time in that direction.

6. The location of the push button in a demand-activated system can be a problem. The location could be standardized at a certain height and in a certain location at each corner of an intersection. However, the problems of a demand-activated system are compounded if they are installed at intersections scattered throughout a community as opposed to city-wide installation. The visually impaired person may need the auditory assistance but not know it is available to him at that particular intersection.

7. City-wide installation of constant information systems creates a noise problem for those living and working near the intersections.

8. City-wide installation is also expensive.

9. Travelers that could benefit from an audio-tactile system may be too self-conscious to use it. They may not wish to stand at the corner with their hand on a device waiting for the proper tactual signal.

Further information on Auditory Traffic Signals is available from:

Traconex, Inc.
336 Martin Ave.
Santa Clara, Calif. 95050

Nagoya Electric Works Co., LTD
1-36, Yokobori-cho, Nakagawa-ku
Nagoya 454, Japan

Dansk signal Industria A/S
175. DK-2650 Hvidovre
Denmark

Traffic Safety Research Center for the Blind
8-26 1 Chome, Minamigata,
Okayama, Japan

Right-Turns-On-Red

Another aspect of traffic and pedestrian control is the policy of permitting traffic to make a right turn even if the traffic light is red. This legalization of right-turn-on-red has been slowly growing since its inception in California in the late 1930s. The last decade has witnessed a dramatic increase in its use.

The basic objective of the system is the reduction of vehicular congestion and delay at intersections. A right-turn-on-red is permitted if the driver is in the proper lane, makes a complete stop before turning, and yields the right-of-way to pedestrians and vehicular traffic. Most states west of the Mississippi River permit this unless a sign specifically warns that it is not permitted at that particular intersection. States east of the Mississippi have mixed policies. In some states a right-turn-on-red is permitted only when a sign indicates this permission, and in other states right-turn-on-red is permitted at all times unless a sign specifically denies this permission. Only a small handful of states remain without some provision for right-turns-on-red. The system *is* a benefit to drivers and does accomplish its objective of reducing the delay at intersections.

The system does not, however, benefit pedestrians, particularly visually impaired pedestrians. It introduces two new elements of danger that would not be present without right-turn-on-red. The first is a false indication of a traffic surge as depicted in Fig. 34-14. The car to the traveler's left has accelerated to begin a right-turn-on-red. This could cause the visually impaired traveler to interpret this as the beginning of traffic flow in the parallel street and to begin his crossing at the wrong time. If the car comes to a quick stop and the traveler gets back on the curb, no great harm is done. However, the driver could come to a quick stop and the traveler could continue the crossing. He still thinks he has left the corner with the surge and the car was attempting to make a normal right turn on the green light. It is true that the proficient cane traveler would not be misled by this situation. He has been taught to begin his crossing with the parallel traffic surge of many cars, not just one. And even if he made the incorrect start, the flow of the perpendicular traffic should alert him to his error. However, all visually impaired travelers are not proficient travelers. The potential is present for this type of error.

A second element of danger is pictured in Fig. 35-14. The visually impaired traveler is crossing at the proper time to the southwest corner. The driver facing east wishes to make a right-turn-on-red and proceed south. He has been impatiently waiting for a break in the line of traffic going south. He sees a chance to make the turn and quickly accelerates. His attention has been on the traffic and not on the pedestrians who also have the right-of-way. He may turn quickly in

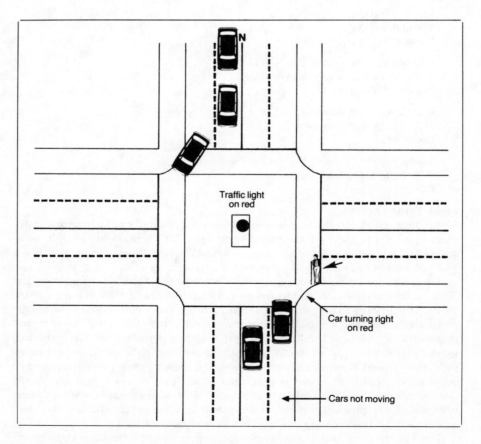

Figure 34-14. Turn-on-red hazard; false indication of traffic surge.

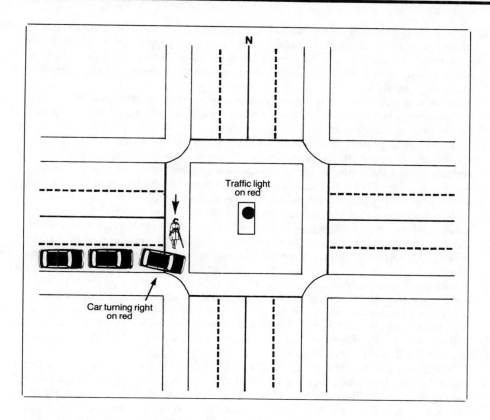

Figure 35-14. Pedestrian hazard; turn-right-on-red driver.

front of the pedestrian or may stop where he is. His stop is frequently in the crosswalk. This happens when the driver inches slowly into the beginnings of his turn before he actually has the chance to make the full turn. He finds himself stuck in the crosswalk. The cars behind him block his attempts to back up and the pedestrians must maneuver around the car in the crosswalk.

Mobility specialists as a profession should study the actual effects of the right-turn-on-red legislation and determine whether the needs of visually impaired travelers will be best met through efforts to modify or repeal these changes. In the meantime clients in mobility training should understand the dangers involved in this situation and the methods for coping with it.

NATURE TRAILS

Man's communal relationship with nature is probably as old as time itself. Nature's visual display is unsurpassed. However, the pleasures of nature transcend the visual spectrum. Nature is alive with the added dimensions of sounds, textures, and smells which have always been enjoyed by large numbers of blind individuals.

Proponents of modified nature trails attempt to promote greater interaction with nature. They point out that interesting objects found at random in nature can be organized into one trail or garden and then displayed in an environment that will encourage the best nonvisual interaction. The nature trail or scent garden greatly conserves the time and energy that would be required to find similar items at random in nature. These proponents also state that the educational experience provided at these trails and gardens can be a springboard for more in-depth exploration in the wilds. A further point often raised states that this organized environment for the blind can avoid the "do not touch" aspects of many museums and public exhibits.

Some of these trails are designed specifically for visually impaired people and are sometimes restricted to only these individuals. However, this does not seem to be the case in most instances.

The general philosophy of most existing nature trails seems to be that they should be as enjoyable as possible for *all* those who wish to use them. The construction of the trail should not deny access to those restricted to a wheelchair. Nor should the esthetic and educational elements of the trail be limited to a visual presentation. The trail should reflect the needs of all people.

It would seem that the sighted guide could solve the "special" needs of the non-visual participant. The guide could read the descriptive brochure describing the trail and could lead the way from display to display. The guide could also assist in the exploration of points of interest and could read the descriptive plaques at the displays.

However, the sighted guide does not seem to be a popular approach. Many people involved with the design and construction of nature trails feel that personal contact with nature revolves around an intimate one-to-one relationship. Therefore, the person should travel on his own. He should set his own pace and linger at will along the trail. They feel the self-guiding trail provides the opportunity for independent, meaningful, discovery.

The existing nature trails vary greatly in length. The Tribble Fort Reservoir Self Guided Trail in the Utah National Forest of Provo, Utah is 200 feet in length while the Handicapped Children's Nature Study Center in Davenport, Iowa has a 4,000 foot nature trail. Some trails are paved to facilitate ease of travel in a wheelchair, as is the La Pasada Enchantada Trail in Lincoln National Forest near Cloudcroft, New Mexico.

For many years the trails followed the same design. Guide rails of hemp rope, nylon rope, steel wire, or covered wire were strung from post to post along the full length of the trail. Some of these posts have brailled plaques or raised relief maps attached to describe points of interest along the route. The wisdom of this design is being questioned and some changes are being made. Recent years have seen some trails replacing the brailled plaques with brailled guidebooks. The initial expense is lower and the frequent vandalism of the brailled plaques has been eliminated.

The use of auditory devices is increasing in popularity. On some trails, such as the Shady Rest Nature Trail in the Inyo National Forest, Mammoth Lakes, California, a push button tape system describes the display at each of the eleven stops along the trail. Some trails, such as the Roaring Fork Nature Trail near Aspen, Colorado, provide battery powered tape recorders. A cassette tape describes the 22 exhibit stations along this 1/4 mile (0.4 km) trail.

Increasing thought is being given to the elimination of guide rails in favor of auditory maps. The cane traveler could check out a small tape recorder at the beginning of the trail. The cassette message would describe the points of interest along the trail and provide the necessary orientation information to reach the display points. Mobility specialists should be consulted to examine the trail for useful landmarks and sensory clues, and to write the script for the orientation aspects of the cassette tape.

Generally, the design of most trails reflects little knowledge or understanding of standard cane techniques. It would seem that a more natural environment could be maintained if the trails were designed to promote the use of independent cane skills. Guide rails could be eliminated in favor of cane techniques such as touch technique, touch and drag, or shorelining. Those individuals not proficient in cane skills would have arrived at the trail with a sighted guide and would continue to use that guide over the length of the trail. Some suggest that the surface of the trail could be modified to provide landmarks for the display areas. The dirt trail could incorporate a four foot strip of gravel or flat walking stones fitted closely together. This pronounced texture change would be perpendicular to the line of pedestrian travel. It would notify the traveler of a point of interest. It would be described in the brailled guidebook or on the cassette tape. The paved trails should use a texture very different from that of the trail. For example, a trail paved with asphalt could incorporate a 4-ft (120-cm) strip of cement embedded with pea gravel or raised aggregate. The texture should be easily recognized through the cane; however, it should not impede the movement of a wheelchair. These strips could be designed to contrast in color to the regular walking surface and thus provide a visual clue to a low vision person. Some thinking along these lines must have gone into the planning of Trout Pond Recreation Area, in the Apalachicola National Forest of western Florida. Plastic plates were sunk into the paved trail. They are raised slightly above ground level and form a tactual guideline that can be followed with a cane. A white line was also painted as a guideline for low vision persons.

The Touch and See Nature Trail at the National Arboretum in Washington, D.C. incorporated a gravel band to serve as tactual limit around the meadow. Cane travelers are informed that they may wander throughout the meadow but not go beyond the safe area bordered by the gravel band. The potentially dangerous marsh area is beyond this point. The meadow is one portion of the 1,640-ft (492-m) nature trail.

As might be expected, the concept of a self-guided nature trail has not gone unchallenged. Those against the idea are quick to point out that once again artificial environments are being created to set blind people apart. They usually go on to say that these artificial nature trails often serve as a poor substitute for meaningful experiences in the real world. These artificial environments are static and not really what nature is all about. Other questions are sometimes raised. Are some "Braille Trails" created for the sake of public relations or as promotional gimmicks for a fund-raising program?

A pivotal point in formulating a personal opinion on this topic seems to hinge upon the question of how much modification, if any, is necessary for the visually impaired person. Other questions need to be pondered. Are these modifications made solely for the visually impaired person? Would these adaptations also enhance the enjoyment of the trail for sighted visitors? Would the modifications cause special attention to be focused upon the blind person using the trail? Are the "sniffing" boxes (with odors of local plants) on a Virginia trail there for everyone or just the blind? Are the mounted animals on an Arizona trail there for everyone or because someone thought the blind visitor would need them?

ADVOCACY PROCEDURES

Blind and low vision persons have long been the forgotten minority in architectural and environmental concerns. It is time for a change. The voices of mobility specialists and visually impaired people speaking in concert can effect necessary changes.

Local

On a local level a united approach will expedite solutions to specific problems. The procedure would be to identify the problem, determine if standard techniques apply or can be modified to apply, develop workable solutions, and cooperate with local officials to implement the solutions. The most desirable course of action is to eliminate travel hazards before they are incorporated into community planning. This means greater involvement with local planning committees. One effective approach is active participation on the Mayor's Committee on the Handicapped and other such groups. There should be representation on these committees when decisions are being made. This means greater involvement by blind individuals, low vision persons, and mobility specialists. This representation works in two ways; it can be used to promote architectural and environmental modifications or to defeat modifications that are not desirable or compatible with the needs of the visually impaired.

National

Activity is also needed on a national level. Much public education work needs to be done. Educational films, filmstrips, and printed materials need to be made for national distribution. These materials should stress the travel capabilities of visually impaired people and the architectural and environmental concerns that affect their independent travel. Many travel hazards could be eliminated if the general public was aware of what a travel hazard really was.

Cooperative efforts could be explored with established national organizations such as the National Center for Barrier Free Environment, 8401 Connecticut Avenue, Washington, D.C. 20015. Greater participation is needed at the national and local levels. The blind and low vision person need not be the forgotten minority in architectural and environmental concerns.

Some moves are being made in this direction. The Orientation and Mobility Interest Group (Interest Group Nine) of the American Association of Workers for the Blind has established a standing committee on architectural and environmental concerns. Local organizations such as The California Association of Orientation and Mobility Specialists and New York State Association of Orientation and Mobility Specialists have committees working on public education and the elimination of travel hazards in their community.

Professional Education

The message should be brought to architects and building contractors. It needs to be heard by architectural and engineering students. New and expanded courses on this topic need to be added to the professional training programs of architects, engineers, and others related to construction and community development. If the root of the problem is lack of understanding, the time has come for an educational awakening. A safe, functional building takes precedence over the visual effect of unusual non-functional design. There is no need for confusing floor plans, sunken pools in a lobby, glass doors hidden in large expanses of wall glass, and dangerous overhangs. A safe building, functional for all who wish to use it, comes first.

Research

The area of architectural and environmental modifications would provide a fertile field for research studies. Important information could be gained in a large number of areas, for example, improved use of light. It might be feasible to develop special light patterns to warn low vision persons of danger. Perhaps variations of light intensity or colored light could be used as orientation aids in a building. Studies could be made to recommend the best color contrast to use in step-down situations and perhaps patterns of color that could be more easily seen by low vision people. The type and design of building entrances and exits could be studied for incorporation of transitional lighting that would help eye adaptation.

Other topic areas also deserve the attention of the researcher. It would seem that increased functional use of color and texture could be incorporated into the walking surface of large buildings, shopping centers, and transportation depots, to assist orientation. Research could tell us if a universal warning texture could be developed. This texture could be used around existing hazards that could not be removed. It could also be used to mark the edge of subway platforms, the point where the blended curb meets the street, and on the slope of curb ramps. The use of acoustics as an orientation aid in building design is virtually unexplored territory. The same could be said for the use of thermal, haptic, and kinesthetic landmarks as part of building design. We also need to know more about right-turn-on-red and its affect on the accident rate for the visually impaired pedestrian.

SUMMARY

An orientation and mobility course of instruction teaches a wide variety of techniques that will help visually impaired people move safely through the environment. But all dangers are not eliminated. Several factors account for this: not all travelers are equally proficient with the skills; some travelers are safe in one travel environment and not in others; the standard long cane does not provide protection for the upper parts of the body.

Many types of architectural and environmental modifications could be made. However, opinions differ on these modifications. Opinions on the merits of the modification are often based upon some of the following factors: the number of persons that could benefit, the amount of sighted assistance available, the amount of attention it could attract, the cost factor, the increased safety it would provide, the increased amount of travel convenience it would provide.

A travel hazard is defined as a dangerous element in the travel environment that cannot be safely and independently negotiated with standard or modified cane techniques. There are many hazards at face and chest height such as public telephones, guy wires, wall fixtures, stairs, shrubbery, street signs, and display windows.

There are other situations that could be travel hazards such as the incorrect placement of handrails, and irregular intersections. The correct positioning of handrails was discussed and tactual guidestrips were discussed as a possible modification for irregular intersections.

The low vision traveler has special concerns. Color contrast and new lighting techniques could be used to a greater degree. This is particularly true at step-down situations.

Modifications made for the benefit of one group must be compatible with the needs of others. Curb ramps are primarily designed for those in wheelchairs but they can be made compatible with the needs of the visually impaired if proper attention is given to consistency of placement, texturing, and a small bevelled lip at the end of the ramp.

The elimination of a travel hazard is one reason for making architectural and environmental modifications. A second reason is added travel convenience. Self service elevators could be modified to provide tactual and/or auditory information. Nature trails can be modified but these modifications should be for the benefit of all those using the trails, not just the visually impaired.

Traffic control problems were discussed. Auditory traffic signals have advantages and disadvantages. The increasing use of right-turn-on-red adds new elements of danger to independent street crossings.

Mobility specialists and visually impaired people are urged to take a more active and united role in advocacy procedures. Active participation can be used to promote architectural and environmental modifications or to defeat modifications that are not desirable or not compatible with the needs of the visually impaired traveler.

Bibliography

Abeson, A., & Blacklow, J. *Environmental design: New relevance for special education.* Arlington, Virginia: Council for Exceptional Children, 1971.

American Society of Landscape Architects Foundation. *Barrier free site design.* Washington, D.C.: U. S. Government Printing Office, 1975.

American Standards Association, Inc. *American standard specifications for making buildings and facilities accessible to, and usable by, the physically handicapped.* Chicago: National Society for Crippled Children and Adults, 1961.

Armco Student Design Program. *Designing to accommodate the handicapped: 1974 Armco student design program.* Middletown, Ohio: Armco Steel Corporation, nd.

Austin, R. L., & Hayes, G. A. *Playgrounds and playspaces for the handicapped.* Manhattan, Kansas: Theraplan, 1975.

Australia. *Australian standard code of recommended practice: Design for access by handicapped persons, Part I. Public buildings and facilities.* North Sydney, New South Wales: Standards Association of America, 1968.

Baker, M., Fischetti, M. A., Williams, L. A., & Young, E. M. *State and local efforts to eliminate architectural barriers to the handicapped.* Washington, D.C.: United States Department of Urban Studies, 1967.

Bayes, K., & Francklin, S. (Eds.) *Designing for the handicapped.* London: George Godwin, 1971.

Berenson, B. *Environmental design for mental retardation.* Washington, D.C.: United States Public Health Service, 1968.

Berla, E. P. Behavioral strategies and problems in scanning and interpreting tactual displays. *The New Outlook for the Blind,* 1972, **66,** 277-286.

Bernardo, J. R. Architecture for blind persons. *The New Outlook for the Blind,* 1970, **64**(8), 262-265.

Birch, J. W., & Johnstone, B. K. *Designing schools and schooling for the handicapped.* Springfield, Illinois: Charles C Thomas, 1975.

Blasch, B. B., Welsh, R. L., & Davidson, T. Auditory maps: An orientation aid for visually handicapped persons. *The New Outlook for the Blind,* 1973, **67**(4), 145-158.

Boe, Eric N. *Architectural hazards encountered by visually handicapped travelers.* New York: New York State Association of O & M Specialists.

Braf, P. G. *The physical environment and the visually impaired: The planning and adaptation of buildings and other of physical environment for visually impaired people.* Bromma, Sweden: ICTA Info. Center 1974.

Brett, J. J. Pathways for the blind. *The Conservationist,* 1971, **25**(6), 13-16.

Brody, W. Sound and space. *Journal of the American Institute of Architects,* 1964

Byrne, S. A design for a mobile audio-tactile exhibition for blind and sighted school-age children. *The New Outlook for the Blind,* 1974, **68**(6), 252-259.

Canada. *Building standards for the handicapped.* Ottawa: National Research Council, 1965.

Caniff, C. E. Architectural barriers—a personal problem. *Rehabilitation Literature,* 1962, **23,** 13-14.

Case, M. *Recreation for blind adults: Organized programs in specialized settings.* Springfield, Illinois: Charles C Thomas, 1966.

Chapanis, A. Relationships between age, visual acuity, and color vision. *Human Biology,* 1950, **22,** 1-31.

Chapman, R. H. *Approach to design—The functional space and utility programme.* Albany, New York: New York State Department of Hygiene, 1966.

Chermayeff, I. et al. *The design necessity.* Cambridge, Massachusetts: The MIT Press, 1973.

Cluff, A. W., & Cluff, P. J. Design for the elderly. *The Canadian Architect,* 1970, 34-40.

Collins, J. The braille trail. *Trends,* 1968, **5**(2), 1-3.

Committee on Barrier Free Design. *A survey of state laws to remove barriers.* Washington, D.C.: The President's Committee on Employment of the Handicapped, 1973.

Committee for Barrier Free Design. *The right to be abroad in the land: Human dignity revisited.* West Bloomfield, Michigan: Michigan Rehabilitation Association, nd.

Crouch, C. D. Lighting needs for older eyes. *Journal of American Geriatrics Society,* 1967, **15,** 685-688.

Cull, J., & Hardy, R. E. *Considerations in rehabilitation facility development.* Springfield, Illiois: Charles C Thomas, 1975.

Dattner, R. *Recreation design for play.* Cambridge, Massachusetts: MIT Press, 1974.

Department of Community Affairs. *Construction guidelines on housing for the elderly.* Boston: Department of Community Affairs, 1972.

Dethlefs, T. Modifications for handicapped persons in outdoor recreation. *Therapeutic Recreation Journal,* 1971.

Division of Vocational Rehabilitation. *Check list and graphic illustrations for designing facilities* which are accessible to the useable by the physically handicapped. Charleston, West Virginia: Division of Vocational Rehabilitation, nd.

Division of Vocational Rehabilitation. *14 Ways to make buildings and facilities accessible to the handicapped.* Charleston, West Virginia: Division of Vocational Rehabilitation, nd.

Dreyfuss, H. *The measure of man.* New York: Whitney Library of Design, 1968.

Droege, R. F. Giving handicaps the heave-ho: Braille trails and lion tales. *1972 Yearbook of Agriculture,* 1972, 268-272.

Eastman, E. E., & Blix, S. The importance of community recreation programs for visually handicapped people. *The New Outlook for the Blind,* 1971, **65**(5), 144-148.

Edinburgh, University of. Department of Urban Design and Regional Planning. *Planning for disabled people in the urban environment.* London: Central Council for the Disabled, 1969.

Education Committee of the President's Committee on Employment of the Handicapped. *Accessibility of junior colleges for the handicapped: A survey by the Education Committee of the President's Committee on Employment of the Handicapped.* Washington, D.C.: United States Government Printing Office, 1972.

Educational Facilities Laboratories. *One out of ten: School planning for the handicapped.* Educational Facilities Laboratories, 1974.

Elevator World. *The world of elevator consultants: Elevator worlds annual study.* Mobile, Alabama: Elevator World, 1974

Elias, H. A tactile guidestrip for blind pedestrians. *The New Outlook for the Blind,* 1974, **68**(7), 322-323.

Felleman, C. Integration of blind children in a recreational setting. *The New Outlook for the Blind,* 1961, **54**(7), 252-258.

Fishman, P. L. *Adaptive housing for the handicapped.* Boston: Tufts New England Medical Center, 1971.

Fokus Society. *Principles of the Fokus housing units for the severely disabled.* Stockholm, Sweden: Fokus Society, 1968.(Re-edited 1969.)

Gangnes, A. G. *New environments for retarded people.* Washington, D.C.: United States Government Printing Office, nd.

Garvey, J. M. Touch and see nature trail. *Science and Children,* 1968, **6**(2), 20-22.

Garvey, J. M. Touch and see. *Parks and Recreation,* 1969, **4**(11), 20-22.

General Accounting Office. *Report to the Congress by the Comptroller General of the United States: Further action needed to make all public buildings accessible to the physically handicapped.* Washington, D.C.: General Accounting Office, 1975.

Gerontological Society. *Housing and environment for the aged. Selected general bibliography.* Washington, D.C.

Gilbert, J. G. Age changes in color matching. *Journal of Gerontology,* 1957, **12,** 210-215.

Goldsmith, S. *Designing for the disabled.* New York: McGraw-Hill, 1967.

Goldsmith, S. The signposting of arrangements for disabled people in buildings. *Rehabilitation,* 1968.

Graham, R. Safety features in school housing for handicapped children. *Exceptional Children,* 1961, **27**(7), 361-364.

Great Britain Council for Codes of Practice British Standards Institution. *Access for the disabled to buildings.* London: British Standards House, 1967.

Hammerman, S., & Duncan, B. (Eds.) Barrier free design: Report of a United Nations expert group meeting. *International Rehabilitation Review,* 1975, **26**(1), 1-36.

Health and Education Resources, Inc. *Proceedings of National Conference on Housing and Handicapped.* Bethesda, Maryland: Health and Education Resources, 1974.

Helsel, E. D. Architectural planning for the mentally retarded to remove barriers and facilitate programming. Compl. by Elsie O. Heisel and Lemar J. Clevenger. *Mental Retardation Abstracts,* 1967.

Henning, D. N. Consideration of the physically disabled. *Canadian Building Digest,* 1971.

Henning, D. N. *Annotated bibliography on buildings for disabled persons.* Ottawa: Division of Building Research, National Research Council of Canada, 1971.

Henning, D. N. *A checklist for buildings used by the handicapped.* Technical Paper No. 289. Ottawa: Division of Building Research, National Research Council of Canada, 1972.

Hilleary, J. E. *Buildings for all to use.* Chicago: National Society for Crippled Children and Adults.

Jeffrey, D. A. A living environment for the physically disabled. *Rehabilitation Literature,* 1973, **34,** 98-103.

Kidwell, A. M. & Greer, P. S. The environmental perceptions of blind persons and their haptic representation. *The New Outlook for the Blind,* 1972, **66,** 256-276.

Kiernat, J. M. Promoting community awareness of architectural barriers. *American Journal of Occupational Therapy,* 1972, **26**(1), 10-12.

Kirk, L. *Accent on access.* McLean, Virginia: American Society of Landscape Architects Foundation, 1975.

Klement, S. *The elimination of architectural barriers to the disabled.* Toronto, Ontario, Canada: Canadian Rehabilitation Council for the Disabled, 1969.

Kliment, S. A. *Into the mainstream: A syllabus for a barrier-free environment.* Washington, D.C.: Rehabilitation Services Administration, 1975.

Knorr, J. *A United States guide to nature centers for the visually handicapped.* Madison, Wisconsin: The Center for Environmental Communications and Educational Studies, University of Wisconsin, 1973.

Koncelik, J. A. *Gerontology project group: Research in environmental analysis and design for the aging.* Ithaca, New York: College of Human Ecology, Cornell University.

Kuhn, H. S.—Taffen, Jr. Color discrimination in industry. *Archives of Ophthalmology,* 1942, **28,** 851-859.

Lander, R. *The goal is: Mobility!* Washington, D.C.: Social and Rehabilitation Service, United States Department of Health, Education, and Welfare, 1970.

Lassen, P. *Barrier free design: A selected bibliography.* Washington, D.C.: Paralyzed Veterans of America, 1974.

Lewis, R. B. A self guiding nature trail for the blind. *Bureau of Outdoor Recreation: Technical Assistance Bulletin.* Washington, D.C.: United States Government Printing Office, 1967.

Ludtke, R. H., & Shefelman, T.W. Environmental designs. *Proceedings of the Regional Institute on the Blind Child Who Functions on the Retarded Level,* 1969, 33-39.

Mace, R. I. *An illustrated handbook of the handicapped section of the North Carolina State Building Code.* Prepared for the Governor's Study Committee on Architectural Barriers and the North Carolina Department of Insurance, 1974.

Mallow, J. To see-without seeing: A nature trail for the blind. *The Maryland Conservationist,* 1973.

May, E. E., Waggoner, N. R., & Hotte, E. B. *Independent living for the handicapped and the elderly.* Boston: Houghton Mifflin, 1974.

McGlinchet, M. A., & Mitala, R. F. Using environmental design to teach ward layout to severely and profoundly retarded blind persons: A proposal. *The New Outlook for the Blind,* 1975, **69**(4), 168-171.

McNab, A. Designing for the elderly. *Official Architecture and Planning,* 1968, 641-643.

Montan, K. Environmental problems of the handicaps: In the foreground. *Social Medicine,* 1965.

Morris, R. H. A play environment for blind children: Design and evaluation. *The New Outlook for the Blind,* 1974, **68**(7), 408-415.

Morrison, J. *Guidelines for community residences constructed under Chapter 812 housing for elderly and handicapped.* Preliminary draft prepared for the Department of Community Affairs, Boston, Massachusetts.

National Center for Barrier Free Environment. *Report Newsletter.* Washington, D.C.: National Center for Barrier Free Environment.

National Research Council of Canada. *Building standards for the handicapped.* Ottawa, Canada: Associate Committee on the National Building Code, 1965.

National Research Council of Canada. *Building standards for the handicapped: Supplement No. 5 to the National Building Code of Canada.* Ottawa, Canada: Associate Committee on the National Building Code, 1975.

National Steel Products Company. *Body mechanics manual for the guidance of architects, hospital administrators, doctors, nurses, and therapists in the placement and use of reach grab bars for patient maneuverability and support.* Los Angeles: The Company, 1962.

Nellisi, I. *Planning buildings for the handicapped.* London: Crosby Lockwood, 1970.

Netherland Society for Rehabilitation. *Architectural facilities for the disabled.* The Hague, The Netherlands: The Netherlands Society for Rehabilitation, 1973.

New Mexico Department of Education. *Removing architectural barriers: An illustrated handbook of Chapter 41 of the 1973 New Mexico Uniform Building Code.* Santa Fe, New Mexico: Division of Vocational Rehabilitation, New Mexico Department of Education, 1975.

New Mexico Division of Vocational Rehabilitation. *Removing architectural barriers: An illustrated handbook of Chapter 41 of the 1973 New Mexico Uniform Building Code.* Sante Fe, New Mexico: New Mexico Division of Vocational Rehabilitation, 1975.

New York Department of Conservation, State Council of Parks and Outdoor Recreation. *Outdoor recreation for the physically handicapped.* Albany, New York: 1965.

New York State University Construction Fund. *Interim guide: Performance criteria on spatial organization for the physically handicapped.* Albany, New York: 1965.

New York State University Construction Fund. *Making facilities accessible to the physically handicapped.* Albany, New York: 1967.

Nichols, P. J. R. Door handles for the disabled: An assessment of their suitability. *Annals of Physical Medicine*, 1966.

Norley, D. *Design as a non-verbal language.* Washington, D.C.: President's Committee on Mental Retardation, 1973.

North Carolina Rehabilitation Association. *North Carolina State Building Code for the handicapped.* Charlotte, North Carolina: North Carolina Rehabilitation Association.

Nugent, T. J. Design of buildings to permit their use by the physically handicapped. *New Building Research.* Washington, D.C.: Building Research Institute, 1960.

O'Boyle, Robert L., Associates, Inc. *Site design for the handicapped.* Kalamazoo, Michigan: Robert L. O'Boyle Associates, nd.

Olin, H. B. Barrier-free environment. *Directors Digest*, 1975, **34**, 9-10.

Osman, M. E. Barrier-free architecture: Yesterday's special design becomes tomorrow's standard. *AIA Journal*, 1975, **63**.

Pantona, R. Architectural barriers for the handicaps. *Rehabilitation Literature*, 1967.

Pastalan, L. A. The simulation of age-related sensory losses: A new approach to the study of environmental barriers. *The New Outlook for the Blind*, 1974, **68**(8), 356-361.

Penny, M. F. *Bibliography on architecture of mental health facilities.* Washington, D.C.: Department of Health, Education and Welfare, 1964.

Phillips, M. H. Residential schools for the visually handicapped. *American Institute of Architects Journal*, 1962.

Potomac Valley Architecture. *Barrier free rapid transit.* Washington, D.C.: The President's Committee on Employment of the Handicapped, 1969.

President's Committee on Employment of the Handicapped. *Highway rest area facilities—designed for handicapped travelers.* Washington, D.C.

President's Committee on Employment of the Handicapped. *Making colleges and universities accessible to handicapped persons.* Washington, D.C.

President's Committee on Employment of the Handicapped. *A survey of state laws to remove barriers.* Washington, D.C., 1973.

Raschko, B. Physiological and behavioral characteristics of the elderly: A basis for design criteria for interior space and furnishings. *Rehabilitation Literature*, 1974, **35**(1), 10-15.

Rehabilitation Institute of Chicago. *Access Chicago: Architect's and designer's handbook of barrier-free design.* Chicago, Illinois: Access Chicago, Rehabilitation Institute of Chicago, nd.

Rehabilitation International. *Barrier free design—report of a United Nations expert meeting on architectural barriers and disabled people.* New York: Rehabilitation International, 1975.

Research Center, College of Architecture and Environmental Design. *Environmental criteria: MR preschool day care facilities.* College Station, Texas: Texas A&M University, nd.

Resnick, R. Recreation: A gateway to the seeing world. *The New Outlook for the Blind*, 1971, **65**(9), 291-296.

Rusalem, H. et al. Architectural barriers to the participation of disabled persons in community recreation activities. *Journal of Chronic Disease*, 1965, **18**, 161-166.

Rutberg, J. Orientation and mobility in the urban environment: A form of future shock. *The New Outlook for the Blind*, 1976, **70**(3), 89-93.

Salmon, C. F., & Salmon, F. C. The blind: Space needs for rehabilitation. *American Institute of Architects Journal*, 1965, **43**, 69-72.

Salmon, C. F., & Salmon, F. C. Architectural barriers and the blind. *Blindness Annual*, 1968, 27-30.

Salmon, F. C., & Ryan, A. *A report on barriers to the disabled.* Stillwater, Oklahoma: Oklahoma State University, 1974.

Salmon, F. C., & Salmon, C. F. *Sheltered workshops: An architectural guide.* Stillwater, Oklahoma: Oklahoma State University, 1966.

Schoenbohm, W. B. *Planning and operating facilities for crippled children.* Springfield, Illinois: Charles C Thomas, 1962.

Schoenbohm, W. B. Some special considerations in planning for crippled children. *Rehabilitation and Physical Medicine*, 1964, XIX.

Schwartz, Jonathan R. Survey of nature trails for the visually impaired. *The Journal of Visual Impairment and Blindness*, 1977, **71**(2), 54-61.

Shaw, J. A. Architectural barriers: A medical problem. *American Journal of Occupational Therapy*, 1971, **25**(1), 13-15.

Spinelli, A. Successful trails for the blind. *Environmental Education*, 1972, **3**(4).

State University Construction Fund. *Architectural checklist: Making colleges and universities accessible to handicapped students.* Washington, D.C.: President's Committee on Employment of the Handicapped.

Tica, P. L., & Shaw, J. A. *Barrier free design: Accessibility for the handicapped.* New York:

Institute for Research and Development in Occupational Education, 1974.

Tiffin, J., & Kuhn, H. S. Color discrimination in industry. *Archives of Ophthalmology*, 1942, **28,** 851-859.

Toll, D. Should museums serve the visually handicapped. *The New Outlook for the Blind*, 1975, **69**(10), 461-463.

United States Bureau of Outdoor Recreation. *Outdoor recreation for the physically handicapped*. Washington, D.C.: United States Bureau of Outdoor Recreation.

United States Congress, Senate. *A barrier-free environment for the elderly and the handicapped*. Hearings Before the Special Committee on Aging, 92nd Congress, 1st Session, October 18-20, 1971. United States Government Printing Office.

United States Department of Forest Service. *Developing the self-guiding trail in the national forests*. Washington, D.C. United States Department of Forest Service, 1968.

United States Department of Health, Education & Welfare. *Design of facilities for the mentally retarded*. Washington, D.C.

United States Department of Health, Education & Welfare. *Design for all Americans*. Washington, D.C.: National Commission on Architectural Barriers to Rehabilitation of the Handicapped, 1967.

United States Department of Health, Education & Welfare. *Standards for construction and equipment of facilities for persons with developmental disabilities*. Washington, D.C.: Rehabilitation Services Administration, Department of Health, Education, and Welfare, 1970.

United States Department of Health, Education & Welfare. *First report of the architectural and transportation barriers compliance board to the Congress of the United States*. Washington, D.C.: United States Department of Health, Education and Welfare, 1974.

United States Department of Housing & Urban Development. *Housing for the physically impaired, a guide for planning and design*. Washington, D.C.: United States Government Printing Office.

United States Department of Housing & Urban Development. *The building environment for the elderly and the handicapped: A bibliography*. Washington, D.C.: United States Government Printing Office.

United States Department of Housing & Urban Development. *Barrier free site design*. Washington, D.C.: United States Government Printing Office, 1975.

United States Department of the Interior. *Outdoor recreation space standards*. Washington, D.C.: United States Government Printing Office.

United States Department of the Interior. *Outdoor recreation planning for the handicapped*. Washington, D.C.: United States Government Printing Office, 1967.

United States Department of the Interior. *National park guide for the handicapped*. Washington, D.C.: United States Government Printing Office, 1971.

United States Department of Transportation. *Travel barriers*. Washington, D.C.: United States Government Printing Office, 1970.

United States Government Printing Office. *National park guide for the handicapped*. Washington, D.C.: United States Government Printing Office.

United States Government Printing Office. *Design for all Americans*. Washington, D.C.: United States Government Printing Office.

United States Government Printing Office. *Housing for the physically impaired: A guide for planning and design*. Washington, D.C.: United States Government Printing Office, 1968.

United States Government Printing Office. *Travel barriers*. Washington, D.C.: United States Government Printing Office, 1970.

United States Government Printing Office. *A barrier-free environment for the elderly and the handicapped, hearings before the Special Committee on Aging*, 92nd Congress, 1st Session, October 18-20, 1971. Washington, D.C.: United States Government Printing Office.

United States National Park Service. Nature trail for the senses. *Trends for the Handicapped*, 27-30.

United States Rehabilitation Services Administration. *Design for all Americans*. Washington, D.C.: United States Government Printing Office.

United States Rehabilitation Services Administration. *The goal is mobility*. Washington, D.C.: United States Government Printing Office.

United States Vocational Rehabilitation Administration. *Inaccessible buildings: A special report on architectural barriers*. National Commission on Architectural Barriers to Rehabilitation of the Handicapped, 1967.

Vermilga, H. P. *Building and facility standards for the physically handicapped time saver standards*. J. H. Callender, Ed. (4th ed.). New York: McGraw-Hill, 1966.

Virginia Polytechnic Institute and State University. *Design for the disabled*. Blacksburg, Virginia: College of Architecture and Urban Studies, Virginia Polytechnic Institute and State University.

14

Walz, T., Willenbring, G., & deMoll, L. Environmental designs. *Journal of the National Association of Social Workers*, 1974, **19**(1), 38-46.

Wheeler, E. T. Architectural considerations in planning for community mental health centers. *American Journal Public Health*, 1964.

Willenberg, E. P. A conceptual structure for safety education of the handicapped. *Exceptional Children*, 1961, **27**(6), 301-306.

Williams, R. A. L. *Barrier-free design graphics*. Detroit: League for the Handicapped-Goodwill Industries, 1975.

Worsley, J. C. *Check list and graphic illustrations*. San Francisco: California Council, The American Institute of Architects, nd.

Educational Aspects

Robert O. LaDuke and Richard L. Welsh

Mobility specialists are responsible for assisting visually impaired persons to move as independently as possible through the environment. Many visually impaired persons will be helped to change this aspect of their behavior through a teaching/learning process. Mobility specialists should be prepared to program effective teaching and learning sequences for a wide variety of visually impaired persons.

Early efforts to help people learn to travel were successful because they embodied a number of effective teaching principles. A common sense methodology consisting of an analysis of tasks and a logical sequencing of learning experiences characterized the early training. Because many of the original instructors came from professions that related to movement efficiency, such as corrective therapy, they had a very practical focus, concerned mainly with observable behaviors. They stressed the most efficient techniques to accomplish a task and the effective use of sensory systems other than vision. As graduate training programs for mobility specialists were initiated, curricula were developed which tended to reflect those elements which had been viewed as effective in the early programs. The similarity among clients allowed the use of fairly standard sequences and approaches.

With the availability of graduate mobility specialists, services were opened to a wider range of visually impaired persons. Many of these individuals had congenital visual losses as well as behavioral and mental deficits which interfered with learning. Many were elderly and experienced other impairments. Thus, rather than teaching young, physically active, and generally highly motivated war veterans how to substitute information received through other senses to regain travel skills, mobility specialists found themselves concerned more with basic problems such as how individuals interpreted the sensory information received, how concepts were developed, how to effect behavior change, and, in general, how to organize a learning program responsive to the individual needs of each visually impaired person.

It has become apparent that while changes in curricula and methodologies will continue, a solid background in principles of teaching and learning is of central importance to the mobility specialist so that adaptations in programming can be made to meet the needs of each individual.

THEORIES OF LEARNING

The world, be it the physical or social world, presents itself to us in a highly complex manner. The operation of the law of gravity is not immediately seen by the naive observer in such diverse events as two boys playing baseball, an orange falling from a tree, and the flight of a kite. Each of these events is complex and appears to be quite different from the others. But the science of physics has demonstrated that the basic principle of gravity is operating in each case.

In the social world there frequently seems to be little rationale behind a person's choice of clothes, his mate, his occupation, and his living environment. Yet there may be certain motivational laws operating through these activities and each behavior may be as clearly related to the others as the behavior of the baseball is to the kite and the orange.

The aim of every teacher, regardless of the setting, is to facilitate change in behavior in some desired direction. However, because of the complexity of human behavior, our understanding of how to initiate and maintain behavior change in a systematic way is not clear.

A number of theories that are systematic interpretations of an area of knowledge have been developed to explain human behavior and human learning. They generally serve two purposes.

1. They can suggest an approach to analyzing, discussing and doing research in a specific area.

2. They enable a large amount of knowledge about a specific area to be summarized so that predictions can be made when the theory is applied to a variety of situations.

Even though a variety of learning theories have been proposed, two general approaches have set the tone for much of the current research and discussion regarding learning.

Behavioral Theory

Man's interest in learning has a long history. Even though philosophers spent a great deal of time considering such topics as how we think, feel, and learn, psychologists feel that the establishment of a research laboratory by Wilhelm Wundt in Germany in 1879 was the point in history where experimental research into learning was firmly established (Hill, 1963). Wundt, like philosophers before him, was primarily interested in what has been called conscious experience. Basically, his interest was in the area of sensation and how thoughts, feelings, and recollections of past experiences could be experimentally demonstrated to relate to sensations. This approach to the study of learning became commonplace in Europe and America. However, Americans in particular never totally accepted it. A number of Americans were interested in observable behavior, what people did, as well as what they felt or thought. American researchers wanted to be able to obtain accurate measurements of human activity rather than rely on an individual's interpretation of sensory events.

John Watson is generally credited with popularizing a movement known as behaviorism. Watson's (1913) article, "Psychology as the Behaviorist Views It," was one of the first popular statements charging that one could not study consciousness objectively. He felt that only observable behavior could be measured objectively and, in fact, rejected attempts to explain concepts such as motivation, which were considered to be based on instincts. In Watson's time, sociability was attributed to the instinct of gregariousness, fighting to an instinct called pugnacity, and so on.

Watson felt that if we explain behavior as inherited in some way, we would do very little scientifically to broaden our knowledge of how learning takes place or how we might affect the way individuals function and operate in our environment.

Stimulus-Response Theory

Watson regarded all learning as a type of classical conditioning, a concept previously studied from the physiological standpoint by Pavlov in Russia. It was known that a certain stimulus produced a specific response. Pavlov demonstrated that a specific response could be elicited by new stimulus if the latter was paired with the original stimulus.

A dog guide in training is conditioned to respond to the Swiss word "pfui" as a result of the trainer having paired this word with a painful leash correction. In the terminology of stimulus-response theory, the force on the front of the dog's throat is the unconditioned stimulus (UC) which elicits the unconditioned response (UR) of pain. The word "pfui" would be considered a conditioned stimulus (CS) which would result in compliance which is the conditioned response (CR).

In a similar way, some clients come to feel comfortable and secure traveling independently as a result of the traveling being paired with the trusting relationship that the client shares with the mobility specialist. The relationship with the instructor is the unconditioned stimulus which elicits comfort and security in the client. Traveling independently may become a conditioned stimulus that also comes to elicit comfort and security.

In order to learn new responses Watson theorized that a process of serial combinations of simple responses was necessary. This was very difficult to demonstrate when studying the learning of complex behaviors. Miller (1962) discussed this theory in detail.

Hill (1963) felt that the main contribution of Watson was that his efforts to popularize a more thorough study of observable behavior were widely accepted.

Skinnerian Behavior Theory

Skinner's (1953) position was that reflexes, conditioned or otherwise, were primarily concerned with the internal physiology of the person. However, mobility specialists were most interested in behavior emitted by the individual that had some effect on the surrounding environment. Skinner maintained that this behavior referred to as operant behavior was different from that discussed by Watson. Operant behavior is defined by Skinner as behavior that operates on the external world or environment. It differs from the stimulus response of respondent behavior in that it is emitted by the individual rather than elicited by some stimulus. The operant response of reaching for food is not simply elicited by the sight of food, but may also depend upon other variables such as the individual's state of hunger, social situations, and many other stimulus conditions.

The learning of operant behavior is also known as conditioning but is different from the classical conditioning of reflexes. If an operant behavior occurs and is followed by a reinforcer, its probability of occurring again increases. Operant conditioning is a method of shaping or managing behavior. The unique feature of operant conditioning, at least from the Skinnerian standpoint, is the lack of concern regarding the stimulus which caused the operant behavior. Instead, Skinner focuses on understanding and controlling the reward or punishment that comes after the behavior and either strengthens it or extinguishes it.

The mobility specialist who rewards his young students with candy or food for finding a particular objective or the specialist who praises a client for maintaining his hand in the center is attempting operant conditioning, although not in its purest sense since the behavior which is being reinforced did not appear spontaneously but as the result of explanation or prompting from the instructor.

Skinner insists on talking only about behavior and its external determinants, and does not speculate about any mediating thought processes. Some of the specific procedures and principles of operant conditioning will be discussed and applied to orientation and mobility instruction later in this chapter.

Some of the confusion in the theoretical literature and in the understanding of psychologists is explained by Diggory (1972) who feels that behaviorism as a term is used by various people in three different ways:

1. Behaviorism as a label for traditional learning or stimulus response theory

2. Behaviorism as a label for Skinnerian theory

3. Behaviorism as a method of objectivity common to all learning theories including cognitive theories.

Cognitive Theory

Cognitive theorists stress the importance of the underlying causes of behavior, or the thought process that enables an individual to learn complex behaviors.

Like the behaviorist movement of Watson, cognitive interpretations of learning were an outgrowth of the European emphasis on studies of consciousness. Whereas Watson stressed the importance of studying observable behavior rather than conscious thought, cognitive theorists led by Max Wertheimer became concerned, not with the study of conscious thought, but rather with efforts to break conscious thoughts into units such as sensations and ideas. Wertheimer (1945) proposed that what should be done was to study consciousness as it appears in wholes rather than break it down into parts. Wertheimer used the German word Gestalt which means form, pattern, or configuration. The phenomenon of apparent movement is an excellent example. Everyone has seen advertising signs that appear to move or to have moving figures. This is accomplished when lights in one position are turned off and others turned on. There is an illusion of apparent movement. Wertheimer felt that this was an excellent example of the futility of studying the parts which make up the whole. The parts are separate lights going on and off but the whole perceived by the observer gives the impression of movement. Because of this concern with the whole pattern, the movement that Wertheimer started came to be known as Gestalt psychology.

In contrast to a Skinnerian behaviorist the Gestalt psychologist would seek to know how an individual has learned to perceive a situation rather than to focus solely on what the individual has learned to do. The assumption of the cognitive theorist is that the way a learner thinks about a situation will affect the type and amount of learning that takes place.

Gestalt psychologists have done a great deal of research into problem solving behavior (Kohler, 1925 and Koffka, 1935), and systems of predicting motivated behavior by describing the totality of facts which might determine behavior (Lewin, 1936).

Eclectic Approaches

Readers of the various theories of human learning are often dismayed by the seeming contradictions between theorists who are trying to understand and explain the same phenomenon, human learning. However, no theory yet proposed seems capable of explaining *all* of the various behaviors considered as learning. Each theory contributes somewhat to our understanding of the total range of learning phenomena, but the theorist becomes more involved in developing and articulating a coherent theory and loses sight of the totality of the behaviors he is trying to describe.

An integration of concepts from various theories appears in discussions of teaching strategies; especially those expressed by practitioners and teachers. Certainly there are examples of learning theorists who have developed and expressed teaching strategies consistent with their theories of learning. However, discussions of strategies that come from teachers themselves are eclectic and seem to draw concepts from seemingly contradictory learning theories to the extent that these concepts add to their effectiveness as teachers.

A good example of the eclectic integration of different concepts into a teaching strategy is the currently popular use of "behavioral objectives." Many aspects of this approach, including the title, its focus on concrete observable behaviors, and the breakdown of learning goals into a hierarchy of discrete steps suggest its origins in behavioral learning theories. On the other hand, the emphasis that is given to the value of involving the learner in the development of a plan for learning and the motivational aspects of the learner being able to see clearly the whole picture of what is to be learned and to be able to appreciate the progress that is being made, clearly draws upon some of the concepts of cognitive theories.

The teacher/practitioner, in his concern for finding out and using whatever works, seems more free than the learning theorists to pick and choose those concepts that will contribute to his effectiveness regardless of the seemingly conflicting origins of the ideas.

The mobility specialist as a practitioner shares this concern for discovering the teaching methods and strategies that will enable his client or student to reach the agreed-upon goals. Certainly it is helpful if the practitioner has read and understood the works of learning theorists, but the practitioner's purpose is not to prove or disprove a particular theory but to aid the client to reach desirable goals.

The teaching methods and strategies used by mobility specialists seem to incorporate ideas from different theories of learning, yet some consistency in these approaches seems to be emerging.

DEVELOPING THE CURRICULUM

Prior to the design of specific teaching plans for particular clients, the mobility specialist must develop a curriculum that is a general blueprint from which he will work with most clients. The particular assessment of the needs of each client will lead to the design of the teaching plan for that individual. However, the development of a general catalogue of skills that make possible independent travel and the methods for helping clients to develop these abilities is an essential part of providing effective mobility training.

Such a curriculum is usually based upon a logical analysis of the components of the tasks to be learned. This analysis is supplemented over time by input from consumers of the services who feed back to the curriculum needs that may have been overlooked or that only emerge in the peculiar circumstances in which certain clients find themselves. Curriculum designers should consult the literature and other professionals for additional ideas about curriculum content. Ideally, the contents of curricula should be submitted for empirical review using a research methodology to test the assumptions concerning the need for particular skills or the analysis of the critical subskills or prerequisites. None of the orientation and mobility curricula which have been developed have been researched in this way.

Orientation and mobility specialists have generally relied on the traditional notebooks of mobility techniques as the basis for the curricula developed for specific agency or school programs. These techniques have included skills in using a sighted guide; indoor protective and orientation techniques; cane skills; techniques for traveling in outdoor areas, and crossing streets; techniques for travel in business areas, and using public transportation; and special techniques for situations such as using elevators, escalators, revolving doors, soliciting aid from sighted pedestrians, etc. These techniques have been organized and taught in a sequence that roughly approximates a hierarchy of skills for the person who has not traveled previously without vision, although such a hierarchical assumption has never been verified empirically.

Usually the written techniques have also included suggestions for teaching methodology and for altering the techniques to meet the needs of special clients.

The mobility specialist has also had to develop lesson plans in a particular agency and nearby neighborhoods that would offer the opportunity to teach the variety of skills involved in the curriculum.

A comprehensive presentation of these techniques was published for the first time by Hill and Ponder (1976). More recently, Allen, Griffith, and Shaw (1977) published a similar list of techniques written in the format of behavioral objectives. Both of these curriculum guides share the same deficiency that has characterized the individualized technique notebooks. They are very thorough in the area of cane skills and in the movement skills that go into independent travel without vision, but they treat only minimally the skills of orientation, decision making, and interacting with the public that are also important areas in independent travel. Weisgerber and Hall (1975), as part of the research project supported by the Veterans Administration, attempted to isolate some of the skills and behaviors related to orientation, decision making, and other sensory and perceptual factors. Even though the latter material was not as thorough and comprehensive as it will have to become, it is significant as an effort to delineate orientation and other components of the mobility process that have not previously been dealt with in sufficient detail.

Prerequisite Skills

A comprehensive orientation and mobility curriculum should also contain units that would only be needed by some clients who are deficient in certain prerequisite skills. Programs serving children will need a unit directed toward remediating and/or enhancing the psychomotor development of visually impaired children whose development has been or may become delayed. The material presented by Hart (Chapter 2) indicates some of the skills and abilities that would have to be included in such a unit.

As Hill pointed out (Chapter 9), another unit may be needed to focus on the concept development of congenitally visually impaired clients. Similarly, units may be needed for training in the areas of low vision, audition, proprioception, haptic perception, or in the area of posture and gait training. In some settings, other specialists such as occupational therapists, physical therapists, audiologists, and classroom teachers may be available to take responsibility for some of these prerequisite areas. Where they are not, it usually falls to the mobility specialist to provide needed learning experiences if the client is to benefit as completely as possible from mobility training.

Many mobility specialists have not developed separate units to provide learning experiences in these prerequisite areas. Some attempt to provide the needed learning opportunities within the basic mobility lessons where the primary aim may be the learning of mobility techniques, but certain concepts or perceptual skills have to be developed in order to be effective with the technique. Some mobility specialists may feel that the training of perceptual skills in the actual situations where they are needed is more effective than practice in artificial situations with the hope of transfer to the real situation. Of course, the effectiveness of the methodology probably relates to the seriousness of the learner's deficiency.

In writing a curriculum, it is important that the skills and abilities be described in as much detail as possible to improve communication among those who read the curriculum and to add to the effectiveness of the instructor in planning and implementing individual lessons. Orientation and mobility instruction, by its nature has always contained a level of concrete specificity that exceeds other types of teaching and human service. However, Yeadon (1977) has suggested that mobility instruction could be made more effective through the use of behavioral objectives.

According to Yeadon, a properly written behavioral objective would begin with a verb that defines an observable "terminal behavior," one that will be accepted as evidence that the learner has accomplished the objective. Yeadon also discussed the advantages of this system, some of which will be presented here in other sections. Allen, Griffith, and Shaw (1977) have presented many of the traditional mobility techniques in the "behavioral objective" style.

The most difficult parts of the curriculum to write in specific detail are those that relate to less concrete and more variable skills and abilities needed for independent travel. Part of the mobility instruction process must focus on helping the client to develop sound judgment in a variety of quite different situations. Can the client be helped to function at a realistic level of risk taking? Can the client be helped to stay calm and make good decisions under the stress of being disoriented? Can the client learn to control his emotional reaction when approached by a helper who assists in a patronizing way? Can the client learn to be an effective problem solver? While each of these behaviors can be defined behaviorally, it is difficult to define which behaviors can be considered to demonstrate sound judgment.

The curriculum that is written must reflect a variety of levels of acceptable performance within it. Given the range of clients served, no one standard of successful mobility can be expected. The curriculum should be structured in such a way that individuals of varying levels of ability can be given learning experiences that are most appropriate for them in view of both their abilities and their aspirations.

THE TEACHING/LEARNING PROCESS

The fact that a general curriculum should be written first should not suggest that the client must be made to fit his needs to what the mobility specialist prefers to teach, in the order in which he prefers to teach it. Instead the curriculum should be viewed as the catalogue of possible skills and abilities and corresponding teaching methodologies from which the mobility specialist and client are likely to draw in establishing a particular mobility training plan.

The basic process of establishing the plan springs from John Dewey's (1933) description of an effective problem solving method based on his analysis of the human thought process. Dewey referred to five phases of reflective thinking:

1. Recognizing the difficulty

2. Defining or specifying the difficulty

3. Raising suggestions for possible solutions and rationally exploring the suggestions, which includes data collection

4. Selecting an optimal solution from among many proposals

5. Carrying out the solution.

Dewey's method of rational problem solving has been used extensively in education and in other human services. Recently, theorists have added the dimensions of evaluating the effectiveness of the attempted solutions and feeding the results of the evaluations back into the problem solving process in a type of feedback loop. Such a procedure seems particularly applicable for situations in which a professional is working with a client to help the client solve a particular problem. Dewey's basic process is also the foundation on which recent efforts to mount a systematic approach to andragogy, the science of teaching adults, are based (Ingalls, 1973).

Applying Dewey's method of problem solving to teaching, especially teaching orientation and mobility skills to adults, necessitates that the problems be thought of as the person's inability to travel independently. While the mobility specialist will usually hear of this "problem" first through some third party, such as the referral source or the rehabilitation administrator who assigns the case, it is important that the specialist hear the client's own view of the problem at the very first opportunity. Generally the problem will be remedied best as a result of the client learning a set of new skills that will enable him to travel independently. Occasionally, however, it may be that the desire to have the client take mobility instruction resides more with the client's counselor, spouse, or parent than with the client. This is quite a different problem, and one which will probably not be ameliorated by instruction.

A preliminary meeting between the mobility specialist and the client can provide the specialist an opportunity to hear from the client why he has come for instruction and what he hopes to accomplish. The specialist can share with the client what mobility instruction involves and the kinds of things that some clients have been able to accomplish as a result of instruction. It is important for the client to be able to express his goals and expectations from the instruction. Although it is likely that a client's initial goals will change in the direction of accomplishing either more or less than originally hoped, it is essential that both the mobility specialist and the client have some mutual understanding about the purpose of their work together. For both parties, the preliminary contact can be an opportunity to begin develop the trust and rapport that will be helpful as instruction progreses.

ASSESSMENT

The outcome of a preliminary meeting between client and mobility specialist should be an agreement to participate in mutual assessment of the client's background and potential for independent travel for the purpose of planning an appropriate sequence in instruction.

It is important to distinguish between two terms, *assessment* and *evaluation*, that are used differently among professionals and in the literature. Both terms refer to a process of making a judgment about an individual or situation based on information that has been collected. For the purpose of this discussion, *assessment* is used to indicate the data collection and decision making that goes on prior to the instruction for the purpose of deciding whether or not instruction should be provided and for planning the most appropriate type of lesson sequence. On the other hand, *evaluation* will be used to refer to the analysis and judgment that will be made about parts of the instructional process that have already taken place. The problem solving approach calls for evaluations to be made frequently throughout the instructional process to consider how it is proceeding and, if necessary, to make modifications in the program. The term *evaluation* will also be used to refer to the summative review of what the client has accomplished at the end of the instruction for the purpose of writing a formal report of the client's success and abilities in orientation and mobility. *Evaluation* will also be used to denote efforts to analyze the mobility instruction program itself and to judge its effectiveness.

Agency Oriented

It is also important to distinguish between two very different purposes for doing an assessment before offering mobility instruction. These purposes relate to the circumstances under which the instruction is being given and funded. It was fairly common recently, and may still be in some parts of the country, for an agency to be swamped with more requests for mobility instruction than it could possibly handle with the mobility staff available. There was also, at one time, some pressure to demonstrate the potential of mobility instruction quickly and dramatically so that additional support for this service could be obtained. In both of these situations, readiness assessments were done to decide which would be the "best" clients to enroll in mobility instruction. In some situations, best meant those clients who could be finished up, and, it was hoped, placed in employment quickly. It was important for the agency to be able to point to these successes in fund raising efforts. In other situations "best" merely meant those who could be served most quickly to allow the total number of clients served to increase more rapidly. As a result of some of these policies, less severely impaired clients were served first and more adequately than were the more severely impaired. Patton (1970) reported on efforts to analyze demographic data of successful and unsuccessful clients in mobility instruction and develop profiles based on demographic information about those clients who would be most likely to succeed in mobility training in the least amount of time. Other reports on developing instruments for "readiness assessment" seemed oriented to this same purpose. While this type of decision may still have to be made in some agencies at certain times, this is a matter of administrative policy that should be made on more equitable bases than a person's relative ability to benefit. In order to prevent those who most need services from being kept off the mobility schedules, mobility specialists should work with administrators to develop policies which Crouse in Chapter 16 described as "screening in" clients instead of screening them out.

Client Oriented

The second purpose for an assessment is based on the assumption that almost all visually impaired clients will be able to benefit from instruction in some way. The mobility specialist uses the assessment process not to eliminate some clients from training, but to determine both the client's actual needs as well as the type of learning program that will best meet those needs. The assessment process should begin first with the client's own perception of his needs and his goals for the mobility experience. The client can also be helpful in discussing his past travel experiences both with and without vision where applicable. The mobility specialist should attempt to understand the client's perception of the cause and course of his visual impairment. Is the client's understanding accurate? Does he expect that his vision will improve? Does his expectation in this regard agree with the prognosis of the vision specialists?

The interview with the client can also provide the mobility specialist with some insight into some of the psychosocial aspects of the client's life. It is important to understand how the client will react to the stigmatizing aspects of traveling in public. Is the client supported by significant members of his family in this endeavor? Do these others have unrealistic expectations for the client? Are they overly protective?

It is possible in this early interview to begin to understand what motivates the client. What rewards or reinforcers will work with this individual? Is he the kind of person who will work to master the skills for the sake of his own sense of competence, or will he be motivated most by praise from others? The best understanding of this aspect of the client, however, will usually come with time as the relationship between the client and the mobility specialist develops.

Medical, Visual, Audiological Assessment

Supplementary sources of information should be consulted with the client's permission during the fact gathering part of the assessment process. Information will be needed on the client's medical condition. Are there health problems which will necessitate modifications? Is the client taking medication of any kind? Is there a likelihood of emergency procedures being needed at some time during the training such as with epilepsy or diabetes?

Current ophthalmological and optometric information should be reviewed. How did the client function during the clinical vision evaluation? Is the condition stable? Might the client benefit from low vision aids? In a similar way, audiological information should be reviewed. Are there hearing losses? Of what magnitude and in which frequencies? Will amplification help?

In situations where medical, visual, and audiological information is lacking, the mobility specialist should make every effort to have such evaluations done and available. Proceeding without this type of background information is not conducive to the most efficient instruction.

There are other types of preliminary or background information that the mobility specialist might gather for certain clients when initial information or previous experience suggests it is necessary. He may request or perform an assessment of the individual's psychomotor development. If certain basic skills and reflexes have not matured or developed, instruction may be ineffective until remediation of some sort is attempted. The mobility specialist may observe a need for a thorough examination of the client's concept development, especially in the area of spatial and environmental concepts. There may also be a need for a posture and gait evaluation done by a physical therapist or by an orthopedic surgeon, if available. In some situations, the mobility specialist may have to do an approximation of these evaluations himself. There may be a need for some type of psychological examination in situations where the mobility specialist is worried about the client's ability to tolerate the stress and the frustrations of the training.

Mobility specialists, as a result of their experience with actual performance and functioning of clients and because of their emphasis on such practical matters, have learned that the results of clinical and isolated examinations in many of the areas discussed above do not necessarily describe the abilities of the client. Sometimes when clients are given an opportunity to demonstrate their skills and abilities in actual travel situations, they may do better or worse than the preliminary tests had led the mobility specialist to expect. This may be because of the validity and reliability of the examination procedures in the different areas, or perhaps because of the difficulty of understanding the complex reality of the whole person in particular situations. A client may do worse than anticipated as a result of the fear and anxiety that the real situation generates, or may do worse in the clinical testing situation where he is less sure of what is expected of him and where he feels the pressure to perform. On the other hand, the client may perform more adequately in the actual travel situation as a result of the motivational properties of accomplishing a particular task. Awareness of this phenomenon has grown particularly in relation to the visual functioning of low vision persons.

Initial Assessment

As a result of the discrepancy that is sometimes found between clinical findings and actual performance, mobility specialists usually include performance runs or functional evaluations as part of the fact gathering and assessment. Clients are put into travel situations and given an opportunity to demonstrate their abilities. Mobility specialists observe this functioning and attempt to evaluate both the overall abilities and some of the components that go into the skills being performed.

It has been common practice in orientation and mobility to treat the first 5 to 10 hours of instruction as an evaluation or assessment period. Usually the client is taken through the first few lessons with the mobility specialist making inferences from this performance about future instructional needs. This is necessary in those settings where the hours of instruction must be projected so that authorizations can be written by the agency funding the service.

Gathering information about a client's abilities does not usually extend to the kind of advance skills that come later in the program, such as crossing streets and dealing with people. It would be impractical to put many clients into advance travel situations where they do not have the skills to cope with them. People with low vision or with previous training or travel experience are frequently evaluated in a range of situations in which they have sufficient vision and travel experience to maintain their safety, and where the purpose of the assessment is to learn more about how the client uses his vision or his techniques under those conditions. Allen, Griffith, and Shaw (1977) have published a sample rating form and an appendix in their orientation and mobility manual.

While this informal type of functional mobility assessment may serve instructors well in planning lessons and a total program, it is generally felt to be insufficient for purposes of research. Armstrong (1972) and Weisgerber and Hall (1975) developed more formalized assessment instruments in connection with their respective research projects. While the instruments developed were limited in scope to the skills and abilities being researched, and were not intended for use as an assessment instrument in lesson planning, they did represent attempts to develop standardized and more specific instruments for functional mobility assessments.

Feedback

An important element of rational problem solving in a teaching/learning situation is that the process is continually monitored and evaluated, and that pertinent information gathered by the monitoring to improve the system is fed back at the appropriate stage. For example, the initial assessment may suggest that the client has sufficient vision to travel independently but needs additional travel experiences. As the lessons progress, however, it becomes clear that extra work is needed to help the client to learn to use vision effectively. This realization then leads to a slight reworking of the assessment and of the program that was built on that assessment.

After the initial fact gathering, and before beginning actual instruction, the mobility specialist should meet again with the client to share the implications of what has been learned in relation to the program that is to be planned. The client should understand as clearly as possible the components of the mobility program and the techniques and procedures that will be used to help him meet his goals. Yeadon (1977) suggested that a curriculum written as a behavioral objective makes for clearer communication about the curriculum between mobility specialist and client. The client is able to see the entire structure and the hierarchy of skills that, in some cases, serve as prerequisites for other skills.

Decision Sharing

Through this conference, the mobility specialist and client can make mutual decisions about the content of the mobility program and the methods to be used in achieving particular goals. This step in the process is crucial because the client has a right to participate in decision making about his own program. This kind of involvement in the planning of the program may have a favorable impact on the client's commitment to and motivation in the program.

Sharing planning decisions with the client in such an open process is not without its difficulties. While the instructor has an obligation to share with the client his own assessment of the client's ability and potential as well as his own judgment about the most appropriate content of the program, the client may insist on planning a program that does not agree with the instructor's best judgment. Depending on the seriousness of the disagreement, the mobility specialist may be faced with a choice that will have to be resolved in a manner consistent with his own ethical judgment. The client may want a program that the instructor feels might endanger the client or at least eventually discourage him from continuing training. The client may design a program that represents inefficient use of instructional opportunity or monies if state sponsored. Sometimes these conflicts can be resolved by proceeding in the manner that the client prefers and, by so doing, illustrate the problems of that method as the program progresses. In other situations the mobility specialist may have to terminate service to the client and, if possible, refer him to another mobility specialist. In this type of situation, the specialist should be certain that his judgment is sound and that the wishes of the client cannot be accommodated. Consultation with other specialists and supervisors is important in this event.

Sharing planning decisions with clients may also be difficult in situations where the sponsoring or funding agency imposes a firm, arbitrary limit to the number of instruction hours. This may be difficult to reconcile with a client when talking about actual mobility needs and the length of time needed to meet them adequately. However, clients may also become more aware of the problem of arbitrary limits to services and possibly become effective advocates on their own behalf or in union with other clients to change these policies.

The selection of goals for the training may have to deal with such difficult decisions as to whether or not the client will be able to travel independently at all or will be restricted to sighted guide travel only. Will the client be able to become a totally independent traveler in all situations, or will he have to limit his travel to familiar routes? In a few situations it may be possible to predict such outcomes early, but more frequently such realities only become clear gradually during the period of instruction. In situations where the potential of the client is unclear, the mobility specialist must not raise expectations unrealistically, but at the same time avoid taking away the client's motivation to try. In other words, the assessment process should result in a tentative plan viewed as changeable by all parties involved.

It is common practice for the assessment process to lead to a tentative written evaluation or a contract between the client and mobility specialist that outlines the findings of the assessment and the plan for meeting the needs of the client.

IMPLEMENTING THE PLAN

Once an assessment has been made, the mobility specialist and the client move into the central part of the teaching/learning process—the implementation of the plan. The written curriculum will provide a general structure for instruction in those areas that the client and specialist have included in the plan. The specialist should also have other resources available to implement the plan, especially appropriate neighborhoods and other training areas to provide the necessary range of real travel situations.

Motivation and Reinforcement

Attention should be given to the client's motivation for participating in the training and to appropriate reinforcers to maintain motivation and achieve success. Just as the different theories of learning present differing concepts about the nature and source of motivation and reinforcement, individuals are motivated differently. For some, especially children or severely mentally retarded clients, the most appropriate reinforcer may be a reward such as food, tokens, or privileges. Others may be motivated best by the instructor's attention and praise or by the approval of significant family members. There are those who are reinforced by the sense of competence or mastery that comes with success in training. The instructor's role may be to articulate these accomplishments for them so that they can fully appreciate them. Other clients may be motivated by the understanding that success in learning to travel provides access to other rewards such as the possibility of employment or increased social opportunities. Welsh (Chapter 8) presents a discussion of the variety of types of motivation that relate to the orientation and mobility situations.

Observation of clients during preliminary stages of program planning might suggest the most potent reinforcers. Behaviorists who rely on the Premac principle in selecting reinforcers hold that those behaviors occurring most frequently in the natural situation can be used to encourage behaviors which appear less frequently. In other words, if a child enjoys playing on the playground, and the preference is clearly demonstrated when he is free to choose from a number of activities, time for playing on the playground can be used as a reinforcer to reward a less natural but desirable activity such as using protective techniques when moving independently.

Adults can usually be relied upon to be more open about those activities which they enjoy and find rewarding. The mobility specialist may observe that some clients appreciate recognition from the specialist for skills accomplished. Others are rewarded by having members of their family observe lessons to see what has been acomplished. Some may dislike open praise and recognition from the instructor, preferring a simple, matter-of-fact statement of accomplishments as verification of their own judgment about their success.

Hall's (1975) list of potential reinforcers for children in public and residential schools included:

Privileges of activities—extra or longer recess, acting as group leader, going to the library, listening to records, individual conferences on progress, field trips, having parents observe, running errands

Social—verbal praise, posting student's picture, praise from the principal or other school officials, being voted most improved student in mobility

Token—badges to be worn for the day signifying staff to give positive attention, special certificate for work completed, points, notes to parents.

Schedule of Reinforcements

A frequent role for the mobility specialist is to control the distribution of reinforcers in a manner that will lead to the greatest amount of learning for the client. This is particularly true when the instructor is using an operant conditioning model. Behaviorists have identified six different "schedules of reinforcement" and the differential effect of each on learning:

1. Continuous reinforcement where every response is reinforced, and the rate of response is very high.

2. Extinction where no response is reinforced and the rate of response diminishes rapidly.

3. Fixed ratio schedule where a certain number of nonreinforced responses must be emitted for every reinforced response. For example, eight nonreinforced to one reinforced (8:1 ratio). The rate of response for this schedule is generally high and steady.

4. Fixed interval schedule where reinforcement is given only after a chosen time interval has elapsed. For example, one reinforcement ten seconds after the last reinforcement. The rate of response is generally low immediately after the reinforcement and gradually increases until the next reinforcement occurs.

5. Variable ratio schedule where the ratio of nonreinforced to reinforced responses, rather than being fixed, is changed after each reinforcement. For

example, 5:1, 18:1, 10:1, etc. The schedule may vary about an average ratio. The rate of response is high and steady and the response is highly resistant to extinction.

6. Variable interval schedule where the time interval between reinforcements is changed after each reinforcement. The schedule may vary about an average time interval. The rate of response for this schedule tends to be high and steady and the response is highly resistant to extinction.

The mobility specialist may need to use a formal operant conditioning procedure when working with low functioning, multiply handicapped clients (Webster, 1977), or when working with general clients on particular aspects of cane techniques or sensory training. In these situations a clear knowledge and purposeful use of the appropriate schedules of reinforcement is essential. In other situations when the mobility specialist is administering reinforcers for successful performance, it is important to be aware of what has been learned about response to schedules of reinforcement even when a formal operant conditioning procedure is not being used.

Interaction

The relationship with the mobility specialist could be a rewarding experience for some clients, so that interacting with the specialist might be a positive reinforcer. Frequently, however, the instructor only initiates interaction when the client's performance needs correction. According to operant theory, the reinforcement represented by this kind of interaction immediately after a client's mistake may encourage incorrect behavior. To be consistent with operant theory, if the instructor interacts with the client immediately following an undesired behavior, the interaction should take the form of some type of punishment or correction to repress the undesired response.

In a cognitive model of learning, the mobility specialist would be less concerned about the timing of his interaction, believing that the client would perform more satisfactorily once he understood the nature of his error and what the correct response should be. Believing that it is easiest to help the client to understand the nature of a particular problem if the lesson is halted immediately after the mistake has occurred, the instructor might interact with the client without concern for interaction, causing an increase in the problem behavior.

If the mobility specialist feels that learning takes place as a result of classical conditioning he could use his interaction with the client in still another way. For a client who is anxious when disoriented, the instructor's presence may be a calming influence. He might let the client know that he was nearby as the client worked to reorient himself, hoping to pair the calming effect of his presence with the situation of the client being disoriented in the hope of helping the client learn how to remain calm when working out of such problems. For a different client, the instructor's presence and authority may be a source of anxiety. When this client is disoriented, his awareness of the instructor's closeness may generate anxiety which comes to be paired with being disoriented.

These examples illustrate the complexity of the use of reinforcers in learning situations, especially when interaction with the instructor is considered a reinforcer. The mobility specialist should try to understand the reactions of each client to the training situation and gear the use of reinforcers to the particular situation.

Shaping

Another concept in learning theory that has application in mobility instruction is called *shaping*, or the method of successive approximations (Hall & Fox, 1975). It involves the rewarding of behaviors that are somewhat like the desired terminal behavior, gradually applying the reward for behavior which is closer and closer to the desired terminal behavior until the client is performing adequately. In order to use shaping techniques, the mobility specialist must be able to analyze complex terminal behaviors into component parts arranged from the simplest to the most complex. Much of this can be done as part of the curriculum writing. An advantage of writing curriculum content in the form of behavioral objectives is that the breakdown of each skill into its component parts facilitates the use of a shaping procedure. The smaller steps are reinforced when performed properly and the building of the total skill proceeds.

Mobility specialists have used the shaping method in the mobility curriculum as a natural and common sense approach without benefit of research support. The approach is helpful in teaching highly complex techniques such as the touch technique with the long cane or the use of distance telescopes for locating and reading street signs.

The individualized instruction that has characterized mobility services facilitates shaping or teaching by successive approximations. When teaching one-to-one, the mobility specialist is able to control the difficulty and the complexity of any problem that the client will experience by stepping into the situation at a particular point. For example, if a client veers while crossing a residential street, he may cross the intersection diagonally, end up at the wrong corner of the intersection, and proceed in what may seem like the correct direction but is in reality quite wrong. The mobility specialist may allow the client to follow this erroneous course until he discovers himself that a mistake has been made. At that point, if the instructor still remains distant from the client, he is structuring the lesson to include recovery from the error, which will require a high level of skill. However, the mobility specialist can limit the level of difficulty of the task at any of a number of points along the way depending on his objectives for that particular lesson. He can halt the client at the point of stepping up on the opposite curb, telling him that an error has been made, and then leaving him to recover from that point. Or, the mobility specialist can inform the client, while he is still in the street, that he has veered into the parallel street and encourage him to make the necessary corrections. The specialist, observing that the client is lining up for the crossing in such a way as to make a diagonal crossing likely, may ask the client to check alignment before crossing, gearing the lesson to a still different level of difficulty. Ultimately the client will need to be able to perform even the most complex of these tasks, but the mobility specialist is usually able to control the level of difficulty according to what represents the most efficient learning experience for the client during that particular lesson.

Rule Relationships

Another aspect of teaching orientation and mobility is that it must go beyond the teaching of specific techniques and beyond the negotiation of certain types of environments to the learning of critical rule relationships about travel without vision in an environment that has certain consistent features. This is especially important for clients who may lack adequate spatial concepts of the environment, but who are nevertheless able to travel independently by the application of certain rules. Haygood and Bourne (1965) have demonstrated that rule learning in some situations is easier than concept learning, although some rules are harder to learn than others.

Several types of rules are applicable in the orientation and mobility process:

1. Causal rules—events go together because one makes the other happen. In a mobility situation, a client makes the judgment that a traffic light is present at

an intersection because cars are stopping and starting in a systematic way.

2. Probabilistic rules—things may belong together under certain conditions. Since a building is L-shaped, it is probable that the numbering system within the building begins at a reference point at either end of the L, most likely near the main entrance.

3. Spatial rules—areas can be negotiated because one has an understandable relation to the other in space. If a traveler veers into a driveway and, after checking, fails to find the sidewalk with his cane, he knows that he can walk toward the parallel street, trailing the shoreline that has been contacted and will encounter either the sidewalk or the street which are readily distinguishable from one another.

4. Ordinal rules—things belong together in a certain numerical order. The numbering systems of rooms within a building or houses on a block are examples of the application of these rules.

The mobility specialist is constantly gearing his instruction toward helping the client discover and use rules that are made possible by the degree of consistency in the makeup of the environment. Some of the rules tend to be an assist to the client's ability to think logically. Bryant (1973) has devised a written test (Table 1-15) to illustrate and evaluate the use of rules that aid in the identification of certain orientation information at an intersection. Three items of information are very important in orientation decisions that have to be made at corners: the location of the traffic in relation to the traveler, the direction the traveler is facing, and the directional name of the corner. Given two of these pieces of information, the client should be able to deduce the third. For example, if a student is told that he is on the northwest corner of the intersection and that traffic is in front of him and on his left, he should be able to conclude that he is facing south. If he is told he is facing south, and that traffic is in front of him and on his left, he should be able to conclude that he is on the northwest corner of the intersection. In an actual situation where he can hear the traffic in relation to himself, the client who is given one of the other two pieces of information should be able to deduce the remaining fact.

The written test includes 48 possible items in which one of the three points of information in each of the 16 combinations is treated as an unknown.

Exceptions

Once the client has experienced some success in recognizing and using some of the basic rules he is ready for the next step, which is the recognition that rules change. For example, one might learn that in a particular area, odd numbered houses are on the west side of the street. The lessons may then progress to the point where in crossing a major division street the client learns that the rule no longer holds but is actually reversed. In fact, the changeover of even-odd sequences on each side of a division street is fairly common.

An identification of the major rules that are helpful in mobility training, and the development of learning strategies to teach them would be a significant contribution to the profession.

Practice

Another concept related to the implementation of a learning plan in orientation and mobility is the importance of practice. Harrow (1972) pointed out that "A learner's desire to learn any kind of skilled movement is usually more intense if it is based upon the intent to use the newly acquired skill for pursuits he categorizes as worthwhile," Without the opportunity to practice the learned skills, retention

TABLE 1-15.
Drill on Geographic Directions at an Intersection

I	Known	A	The corner one is standing on
		B	The direction one is facing
	Unknown	C	The sides the traffic is on
II	Known	B	The direction one is facing
		C	The sides the traffic is on
	Unknown	A	The corner one is standing on
III	Known	A	The corner one is standing on
		C	The sides the traffic is on
	Unknown	B	The direction one is facing

A Corner	B Direction	C Sounds		I C	II A	III B
1. NW	south	left and front	1.			
2. SE	east	left and behind	2.			
3. SE	north	left and front	3.			
4. NE	west	left and front	4.			
5. SW	north	right and front	5.			
6. SW	east	left and front	6.			
7. NE	south	right and front	7.			
8. NW	north	right and behind	8.			
9. NW	east	right and front	9.			
10. SE	south	right and behind	10.			
11. SW	south	left and behind	11.			
12. NE	east	right and behind	12.			
13. SE	west	right and front	13.			
14. NW	west	left and behind	14.			
15. SW	west	right and behind	15.			
16. NE	north	left and behind	16.			
		Total Correct				

will be very poor, especially for psychomotor skills.

Providing meaningful and sufficient practice opportunities may be difficult in certain programs, especially those in school settings and in residential agencies. Students in residential schools may know the environment so well that they prefer to travel without a cane or they rely only on certain well-formed habits of travel in that situation. It may also be that school administrators and houseparents discourage the use of the cane for fear that the children will not use it responsibly. In a residential rehabilitation center, the layout of the center may not be extensive enough to allow the realistic use of mobility skills, or the center may be located in an area that would require advanced travel skills if the client wished to practice skills in the neighborhood. These realities suggest that special attention be given by the mobility specialist to building in and encouraging whatever could be useful and appropriate in practice opportunities for his clients. This issue also reinforces the importance of building in sufficient lesson times for each client each week.

Another critical factor in the learning of psychomotor skills is the feedback provided by the instructor. In addition to the reinforcing qualities of interaction with the mobility specialist, it is important to provide the client with knowledge of how adequately he is using the techniques that are being taught. Bilodeau and Bilodeau (1961) reviewed studies that showed that feedback or knowledge of results is the strongest and most important variable controlling performance and learning of motor skills. This would seem to be especially true for visually impaired clients who may not be able to perceive the adequacy of some of their techniques. For example, in crossing a street, the client may know that he has arrived at the curb at approximately the right spot, but he may have no way of knowing that his straight line travel was extremely accurate for that crossing unless the mobility specialist provides such feedback.

EVALUATION

Earlier a distinction was made between evaluation and assessment. Assessment was discussed as the fact gathering and diagnosing part of the teaching/learning process. Evaluation, on the other hand, is considered a procedure that comes after some action and makes a judgment about the adequacy of the action, or in the situation of a person, expresses a judgment about the accomplishments of the person.

The evaluation component of the problem solving model that has been suggested is considered as both a separate step in the entire procedure and an ongoing activity of those who are involved in the process. A more recent addition to the problem solving model that Dewey had not included is the concept of a feedback loop. Throughout the process, the mobility specialist and the client should remain open to the possibility that the original assessment about the nature of the problem or the methods of proceeding may be incorrect or insufficient. At that point it becomes necessary to rethink the situation and to develop a new assessment or methodology that takes into account newly discovered information.

Some mobility programs build in periodic evaluations at specified and agreed upon times during the training. This allows both client and staff to consider how effectively they are moving toward their objectives, and whether any modifications are necessary. Without such a procedure it is easy to give in to the daily press of business and to allow problems to slide in the hope that they will work out eventually. The client and instructor then find themselves near the end of the program with unresolved problems and no opportunity to extend the instruction time.

There is a need for a formal evaluation procedure at the end of the program to consider both the accomplishments of the client and the effectiveness of the program. Yeadon (1977) feels that another advantage of a curriculum written as behavioral objectives is that it facilitates a final evaluation and the communication of the results. The client's ability to perform activities that were agreed upon as the objectives of the training should be clearly evident when using such a system. A strict reliance on objectives would be valid to the extent that the objectives themselves were thorough, and comprehensively represented the skills and abilities needed by the client.

Records

A client's growth and accomplishments can be more clearly seen if some type of baseline performance in the different skill areas is recorded at the outset. At the present time, the recording of baseline levels of skill is more characteristic of research related mobility training than of actual service delivery programs.

Usually the mobility specialist will be charged with writing a final evaluation on the student to be reported to the funding source and to become a part of the client's file at the agency. Such reports should be written as accurately as possible and with sufficient detail to clearly communicate the client's accomplishments as well as any limitations that are necessary. These reports are frequently used by other professionals in planning future activities with the client, such as those related to vocational placement or further education. In addition they become an official statement of the services rendered by the agency and the mobility specialist. This information is important in evaluating the overall effectiveness of the agency and in contending with any charges of malpractice or liability that might be brought by a dissatisfied client.

When a client does not reach planned objectives, the conduct of the program and the activities of the mobility specialist must also be reviewed. This is true for each individual case but especially when a number of clients have similar difficulties. Each client represents an opportunity for the program and for the mobility specialist to learn more about what they do that is successful and what needs improvement. Programs and professionals must view themselves as always in a state of development and improvement.

Written records of the training program of each client can play an important role in evaluating both the client and the program. The initial assessment as well as progress notes along the way represent a record of the mobility specialist's thinking about the problems of that particular individual. Often it is useful to review that thinking and the assessments that were made in view of the outcome of the training. The mobility specialist can either come to have confidence in his judgment about clients, or he may notice a pattern to the errors that he has made with a number of clients that may lead to an important change in his approach.

A review and a recording of the successes and failures that are experienced with a number of clients over a period of time may also serve to suggest areas that are in need of research either within the agency or in the field at large.

In regard to all of the types of evaluation that have been discussed, it is important to build in an opportunity for input from the clients themselves. This is necessary throughout the training as well as in the final evaluations of both the client and the program. The client's perspective can suggest areas of strength and weakness that may not be evident to the mobility specialist.

One other type of evaluation important in understanding the long-term effectiveness of the program is the follow-up visit to clients at periodic intervals after training. The mobility specialist should know how well the skills that are learned in the rehabilitation or education setting transfer to a variety of different communities and how skill levels change over time.

TRANSFER OF LEARNING

When mobility training is offered in a central agency to which clients come, the mobility specialist must be concerned with how effectively the client can travel when he returns to his home community. Part of a successful transfer is due to the client's ability to learn. However, other aspects of the transfer relate to how the training experience was structured and whether the client was helped by the program to make the needed transfer of skills.

The basic skills taught in a traditional program are critical, as they provide the background information and principles of skill use which are later needed in more complex environments using the cane. For example, the procedure of trailing with a hand to follow a surface allows the learner to locate specific objectives, determine alignment, and, in familiar environments, determine position in space. When the client moves on to use a cane, he may no longer need to trail with his hand, but he will still use the principles of trailing for the same reasons as before, using the cane instead of the hand to contact the environment.

The same principle can be illustrated with some of the cognitive processes. An indoor numbering system may enable the client to find a room in a building, or later a house on the block, or a building in a downtown area. Principles relating to the ordering of numbers, odd-even sequences, and a central point from which numbers originate in a systematic way all have application in a wide variety of settings. Similarly, the process by which the client solves an orientation problem or deals with offers of help during the indoor lessons will have application again in solving orientation problems and dealing with help in advanced areas.

Because certain principles can be generalized from one area to another, the mobility specialist learns to anticipate which clients are going to have difficulty in using formerly learned skills in new areas. On the other hand, studies of transfer of learning as well as common sense suggest that the more thoroughly a person has learned a particular skill the more likely he is going to be able to transfer it to new areas. Therefore, the effectiveness of the learning process and the intentional use of over learning, where possible, will enhance the possibility of transfer.

The transfer of learning to new areas also relates to the similarity of the stimuli in the new and old situations. If the original learning takes place in an artificial environment that is very different from the actual travel environment, transfer is less likely to occur. For this reason mobility specialists have insisted on the need to conduct lessons in actual environments representing a cross section of the areas through which the typical client will travel independently following completion of training. There have been occasional efforts to develop simulated environments for mobility training, but while simulated environments serve a limited purpose in a training program, they are usually too different from real environments to be considered adequate preparation for travel.

Mobility specialists sometimes rely too heavily on the representative nature of their sample neighborhoods that they overlook the needs of certain clients for support in making the transition from the training to the home area. While many clients are able to make the transfer without assistance, others need the opportunity to work with the mobility specialist in adjusting to travel in their own neighborhoods. In some situations where the option exists, an awareness of a client's difficulty in transferring to new areas may suggest a switch from agency-centered instruction to work in the client's own community. Most agencies currently are not structured to allow staff the time for travel and work in the client's home area, particularly if it is in a distant part of the state.

Clients can be helped to learn to transfer travel skills to new areas through the use of self-familiarization lessons in the program. The client is taken to a new area after acquiring the level of skill necessary for that type of area and instructed to explore the area in a way so as to gather sufficient information to travel independently there. This type of lesson can be used in indoor, residential, and business areas, and can be structured to allow the client to use or not use the assistance of sighted passers-by. The mobility specialist can observe and feedback information to the client about the strategies used in dealing with problems and the conclusions that the client drew from available information.

The transfer of newly learned skills to new areas may also be impeded by the nature of the reinforcers available in the new area. First, the client should learn to monitor his cane technique and not depend solely on feedback from the instructor in determining the adequacy of his cane coverage. After completion of training if the client finds that he brushes objects with his shoulder frequently, he should be able to interpret this deterioration of cane coverage that needs correcting. Unfortunately, or not as the case may be, the environment is structured in such a way that the client does not experience negative consequences every time he is "out of step" with his cane or every time his coverage is deficient. If this was the case, cane skills would not deteriorate as quickly, or perhaps not at all, as a person moved farther away from his training program. Many people, however, develop a tolerance of the occasional bumps and collisions and overstepped curbs that do occur when cane techniques are less than perfect.

The client may also encounter different reactions to his traveling which may serve to diminish a desire to travel. In the training program he was rewarded for learning to use a cane or a distance telescope, and reaching that point in the program was a measure of status. Back home, however, cane travel or use of a telescope may attract negative comment or over-solicitous help which does not tend to reinforce travel skill, and may have the opposite effect.

Also, at home, family members may, for a number of reasons, discourage the client from traveling and transferring his skills to the new environment. Once again behaviors that had been reinforced in the training situation are now being extinguished. The mobility specialist may visit the home area to help orient the client, and at the same time discuss with family members the client's need for encouragement and help in transferring the skills he has learned.

The examples described above reflect a behavioral understanding of motivation and reinforcement that may be applicable to a number of clients. For others who function in accord with the notions of cognitive theory, their own understanding of the importance of learning to transfer skills to a new area, or the sense of accomplishment that comes from success in a training program may provide sufficient incentive to overcome whatever obstacles may be experienced in a new area.

Theories about how man thinks and why he acts as he does are important to the mobility specialist. Equally important is the need for the instructor and the service system to evaluate what is being achieved by the provision of mobility services. Certainly the creation of more effective evaluative instruments and follow-up studies should be high priority items for the profession. In order to meet the needs of all visually impaired persons, revisions in curricula, delivery systems, and instructional methodology may be required. However, the framework on which instruction has developed to date provides a solid base for creation of better and more effective programs.

Bibliography

Allen, W., Griffith, A., & Shaw, C. *Orientation and mobility: Behavioral objectives for teaching older adventitiously blind individuals.* New York: New York Infirmary/Center for Independent Living, 1977.

Armstrong, J. D. *An independent evaluation of the Kay Binaural Sensor.* Nottingham, England: University of Nottingham, 1972.

Bilodeau, E., & Bilodeau, I. Motor skills learning, *Annual Review of Psychology,* 1961, **2,** 243-280.

Bryant, R. *Drill on geographic directions at an intersection.* Unpublished manuscript, Stephen F. Austin State University, Nacogdoches, Texas, 1973.

Dewey, J. *How we think.* New York: D. C. Heath, Co., 1933.

Diggory-Farnham, S. *Cognitive processes in education.* New York: Harper & Row, 1972.

Hall, V. R. *Managing behavior.* Lawrence, Kansas: H. & H. Enterprises, Inc., 1975.

Hall, V. R. & Fox. Changing criterion: An alternative applied behavior analysis research design. In Etzel, B. C., LeBlanc, J. M., & Baer, D. M. (Eds.). *New developments in behavior research theory, methods and applications.* Hillsdale, New York: Lawrence Erlbaum Associates, 1975.

Harrow, A. J. *A Taxanomy of the Psychomotor Domain,* New York: David McKay Company, Inc., 1972.

Haygood, R. C., & Bourne, L. E., Jr. Attributes and rules learning aspects of conceptual behavior. *Psychological Review,* 1965, **72,** 175-195.

Hill, E. & Ponder, P. *Orientation and mobility techniques.* New York: American Foundation for the Blind, 1976.

Hill, W. F. *Learning.* San Francisco: Chandler Publishing Co., 1963.

Ingalls, J. D. A trainers guide to andragogy. Washington, D. C.: U. S. Department of Health, Education and Welfare, 1973.

Koffka, K. *Principles of Gestalt Psychology.* New York: Harcourt, Brace, 1935.

Kohler, W. *The mentality of apes.* Translated from 2nd revised edition by Ella Winter. New York: Harcourt, Brace, 1925.

Lewin, K. *Principles of topological psychology.* Translated by F. Heider and Grace M. Heider. New York: McGraw-Hill, 1936.

Miller, G. A. *Psychology.* New York: Harper & Row, 1962.

Patton, W. E. Research on criteria for measuring mobility readiness of adventitiously blind adults. *New Outlook for the Blind.* 1970, **64**(3), 73-80.

Skinner, B. F. *Science and human behavior.* New York: Macmillan, 1953.

Watson, J. B. Psychology as the behaviorist views it. *Psychological Review,* 1913, **20,** 158-177.

Webster, R. Applying behavior modification techniques to orientation and mobility, *Long Cane News.* 1977, **10**(1), 14-20.

Weisgerber, R. & Hall, A. *Environmental sensing skills and behaviors.* Palo Alto, Ca.: American Institute for Research, 1975.

Wertheimer, M. *Productive thinking.* New York: Harper, 1945.

Yeadon, A. Behavioral objectives—A framework for instruction and management. In W. Allen, A. Griffith, and C. Shaw, (Eds.) *Orientation and mobility.* New York: New York Infirmary/Center for Independent Living, 1977.

Administrative Aspects

Robert J. Crouse

The purpose of this chapter is three-fold. First, organizational guidelines will be presented to assist in the development and implementation of mobility programs in a variety of delivery systems such as public day schools, residential rehabilitation centers, and others. Second, fundamental administrative considerations directly related to mobility programs will be discussed. These topics include accident insurance, third-party liability coverage, report writing and record keeping methods, mobility instruction as an interrelated part of the habilitative or rehabilitative process, and in-service training for non-mobility personnel. Lastly, administrative functions for mobility programs will be presented in the hopes that agency and school administrators can obtain a better understanding of this service and be able to evaluate differing program approaches. These topics include funding, legislation, utilization of mobility staff, appropriate instructor/pupil ratios, determining costs and cost benefits of mobility programs.

The intent of this chapter is not to present a fixed set of approaches in dealing with administrative aspects of mobility programs. Rather, it is intended to discuss relevant and functional topics, and to stimulate attention to the operation of quality mobility services for blind persons.

The development and implementation of effective orientation and mobility programs reaches far beyond competent one-to-one instruction. Successful mobility programs are those that incorporate a number of basic administrative practices in their daily operation. Effective mobility programs are most often well organized, have competent personnel, utilize available resources in the education or rehabilitation setting in which they exist, and are client-centered in their instructional approach. They are also sensitive and responsive to the individual needs of consumers. Careful program planning and design, in addition to effective communication with clients and staff, are essential ingredients in initiating orientation and mobility programs. Mobility specialists may at times fail to take the time to properly organize and implement a carefully designed program for the people they serve. In their eagerness to implement direct services in mobility, some mobility specialists may fail to formulate clear and specific program objectives or to develop precise unit guides and lesson plans. Administrators should also allow appropriate time for their mobility specialists to develop written and specific program objectives and instructional guidelines.

Program planning should be completed before direct services in mobility are rendered. This should include a statement of overall goals and objectives for the mobility services to be delivered, a clear statement of who is to be served, and an indication of where and how the mobility service fits into the administrative structure of the school or program. In addition, all pertinent questions involving insurance protection, transportation, equipment, and necessary facilities should be resolved and set forth in the written guidelines for the program.

DELIVERY SYSTEMS

Program planning including development of unit and lesson plans may vary according to the type of education or rehabilitation setting in which the instruction is given. Specific lessons or routes need to be planned in order to fit into the pattern of scheduling prevalent in the rehabilitation setting or school. Design of actual lessons should take into account not only the rehabilitation setting but the environment in which the center or school exists.

Orientation and mobility services are rendered in a wide variety of administrative and program settings. The majority of mobility services are usually found in one of the three settings: rehabilitation centers, itinerant programs, or residential schools. Each mobility program should be designed to meet the needs of the blind persons served and fit into the organizational structure of the sponsoring agency. Instructional guidelines should be written to reflect the type of delivery system of the particular agency or school. The following paragraphs present a discussion of specific points to be considered in designing mobility services to fit various educational or rehabilitative settings.

Residential Rehabilitation Center

A mobility program within a residential rehabilitation center must take into account the length of time each client will stay at the center, (whether clients will be there for a fixed period of time or allowed to attend the center until they complete skills in various areas). Many rehabilitation centers operate on a fixed time period for the training program averaging from 13 to 18 weeks. In such cases, the mobility program should allow for flexible scheduling of lessons with each client. The mobility program should be designed to allow for either one 50- or 60-minute lesson-per-day, or two lessons-per-day of a similar length. In addition, advanced mobility instruction should take into account the need for longer periods of time in which to teach travel in business areas. Two- or three-hour shopping lessons are often needed in order to give training in a city center. Arrangements in scheduling for special lessons should be made directly with the immediate supervisor and clearly understood by the mobility instructors and administration. The availability of transportaion can be a vital factor in planning and implementing an effective mobility program within the rehabilitation center. Mobility instructors should have available to them the use of a station wagon, van, or other transportation to take clients to areas distant from the center.

The advantages of mobility instruction in a residential rehabilitation center are many. Lessons can be given on a daily basis in a concentrated period of time thereby helping students to develop skills more quickly and with more continuity. Scheduling is less complicated because clients are available at all times during the normal working day. An "esprit de corps" is developed in the training program. Interaction and peer identification can be very positive factors in the rehabilitation process. Disadvantages in this setting are few. Often the biggest problem occurs when training must be completed in a fixed time period by all clients. Shorter programs of 13 to 15 weeks at times do not allow all clients to complete instruction successfully or at their own speed. This can be particularly true for clients with additional disabilities or infirmities. It is recommended that each client be given a minimum of at least one hour of instruction per day and two hours per day if at all possible.

Non-residential Rehabilitation Centers

Transportation and scheduling are two very formidable problems in the non-residential rehabilitation center program. To get clients to and from the center on a daily basis, the easiest solution is for the agency to provide door-to-door transportation. However, with rising transportation costs, this may not be a viable solution. Clients may need to use public transportation, and the mobility specialist will need to work out individual transportation problems with each person. This may involve orienting the client to and from the bus stop near his home, and familiarizing him with all aspects of bus usage before he has actually received a complete training program. Family members, neighbors, and/or friends may be needed to see that the student travels to and from the center safely. While this approach is in opposition to most principles of sequential teaching and learning patterns, it has one distinct advantage; the client realizes from the first day of the rehabilitation program that independent travel skills are necessary, desired, and expected. Another advantage of nonresidential rehabilitation centers is that mobility instruction may take place in areas where the client actually resides. These lessons should be after and in follow-up to training received at or near the rehabilitation center. Many students are self-conscious about receiving initial instruction in their own neighborhood. They should be given instruction in their own neighborhood only when they have reached suitable levels of travel skills so that positive results can be obtained and favorable impressions made.

An important advantage of mobility services in a center-based program whether delivered on a residential or non-residential basis is that specific written unit outlines and lesson plans can be developed and used. They not only give organization to a mobility program but ensure that lessons are given so that clients learn in a sequential pattern beginning with more easily learned basic skills.

Another important consideration in designing a mobility program for a rehabilitation center is a clearly delineated plan as to how clients will be oriented to the center facilities and environment. A clearly written policy must be established and specific assignment of personnel responsible for the orientation and familiarization program for new clients. It must be emphasized that expediency in helping new clients to move independently between classes, to meals, and related office areas is essential but sometimes overlooked by administration and staff. Independence from the first day should be stressed and planned as a program objective.

Itinerant Programs

Itinerant instructional programs serve children in public school settings, adults in local communities, and children or adults in regional and even state-wide programs. In many cases school districts have formal cooperative agreements to purchase special services such as orientation and mobility jointly so as to serve low-incidence handicapped children in sparsely populated regions more adequately.

Community-based or itinerant mobility instruction involves a different set of planning guides to establish services. Itinerant mobility instruction cannot operate on the same basis as center-based or residential-school programs. Whereas center-based instruction uses written lesson plans given in familiar environments, the locale of itinerant instruction changes with each student. Because training areas are always changing, the mobility specialist will not have time to develop written daily lesson plans for each student in each environment. The instructor will need to use more general teaching outlines or unit guides. The unit guides must be developed so that they are competency based in delivering one-to-one instruction to the client. Efforts must be centered on delivering a cohesive pattern of lessons to the client and the instructor must be flexible in the design of daily lesson plans to achieve teaching objectives. There must be concentration on the development of a success pattern in skill acquisition rather than whether one lesson or another has been completed. The most difficult aspect of itinerant mobility instruction is the establishment of a well-organized, cohesive sequence of lessons designed to lead clients from one skill level to another on a graduated performance basis. Planning of itinerant programs should also take into account the need for travel time between clients, and the need for time to be set aside on a daily basis for lesson planning, record keeping, and progress reporting. In effect, the instructor's car will often become the program office.

The advantage of itinerant mobility programs is that adults or children can be served in a wider geographic area by taking the service to where they are, eliminating the need for, and cost of, transportation to centralized locations. One instructor can serve several children in a widely-dispersed school system. A major disadvantage is that instructors usually serve fewer students or clients resulting in higher program costs-per-person served. Frequency of visits in designing student schedules can also be a problem in an itinerant program. In the early stages of intensive mobility instruction in cane use, it is advisable to schedule a minimum of three lessons each week to enhance skill acquisition and retention of principles of orientation. Students receiving instruction less than three days-per-week tend to make slower progress and require more frequent review. In later stages of training when students have firmly established certain successful levels of performance more infrequent scheduling may be planned.

Residential School Programs

Mobility programs within residential schools for the visually handicapped are designed much in the same manner as programs existing in residential rehabilitation centers for adults. One underlying difference is that students often attend residential schools for many years, and become extremely familiar with the residential school campus. Therefore, the design of unit outlines and lesson plans in mobility must stress the need for getting off the residential campus and out into the community in order to obtain a true picture of their orientation and mobility skills. There should be careful coordination with other instruction at the school, such as physical education, personal and home management, and math. Mobility lessons should incorporate not only mobility skills, but should relate to other concepts students have learned.

Mobility instruction for blind and visually impaired students should be a required and scheduled part of the school curriculum for all ages, treated similarly to other subjects and given equal emphasis and priority. Mobility should not be considered an extra-curricular activity.

Mobility programs for children should start at an early age and incorporate provisions for special needs in the areas of concept development, motor development, laterality, and spatial relationships. These important aspects of the total orientation and mobility process are explicitly presented elsewhere in this text.

Parents of visually impaired children must be acquainted with the advantages and objectives of independent travel for their child and to learn to assist in the development wherever possible. Parents should be taught how to reinforce good skills. First hand observation of mobility training by parents insures better understanding of the program.

LEGISLATION AND FUNDING

Delivery of mobility services is affected by local and national legislation. The Rehabilitation Act of 1973 and the amendments that followed contain specific provisions for the delivery of orientation and mobility services through the state/federal program of vocational rehabilitation. Mobility instruction has been provided in past years by funds through state departments of education. Provision of mobility services were also implied in the Older Americans Act of 1975. Because a large proportion of the blind population is composed of elderly persons it is important that local service agencies investigate implementation of mobility services to this special population through its state office on aging. Title XX of the Social Security Act of 1974 contains provisions referring to special services to the blind, and specifically mentions orientation and mobility as a service that could be provided. The Revenue Sharing Act of 1974 administered by local county or city governmental units, is also a possible source of support for rehabilitation programs, including mobility instruction.

The private or voluntary sector is an important source of support for mobility programs and other services that agencies for the blind provide. The largest single provider of voluntary funding is the United Way of America, also known as the United Fund or Community Chest, which has local affiliates in almost every city and county in the nation. Civic organizations such as Lions International have as their primary focus the support of services to the blind, and on a local level, give considerable support to agency services.

Private or corporate foundations sometimes fund the delivery of orientation and mobility services. However, most private foundations would rather fund a short-term project designed to demonstrate a skill, accomplish research, or develop an innovative approach to the delivery of services. They are particularly interested in supporting the purchase of equipment or what is known as "bricks and mortar." Many voluntary agencies use local private foundations to purchase electronic aids for mobility and communication. Private funds and foundation grants are good sources for seed money or matching funds for worthwhile short-term programs but they are seldom interested in underwriting personnel costs of program services on a long-term or continuing basis.

A rather new source of support in the area of mobility and related rehabilitation services has been adult basic education programs most often administered through state departments of education and public instruction. Adult basic education laws in most states provide for the delivery of services which are compensatory in nature. Another possible source of program support is through vocational education programs administered through local community colleges, high schools, or directly from the state department of vocational education. Federal legislation requires that state programs for vocational education spend at least ten percent of their funds in providing services to the disadvantaged and the handicapped. Thus, basic communication skills, math concepts, and related educational services may be offered. Some states such as Florida allow the instruction of mobility as a compensatory skill within its adult basic education program.

Eligibility

There are advantages and disadvantages to most funding sources. Vocational rehabilitation laws specify that each potential recipient of services must meet eligibility requirements that include being classified as able to work. This eligibility criteria may in fact deny or severely restrict services in some states to elderly blind persons who cannot work. Title XX includes regulations concerning eligibility which vary greatly when state regulations are added to federal guidelines. Perhaps the most restrictive eligibility criteria is that of allowed income. Near poverty income guidelines are used to determine eligibility for most Title XX services. Almost every funding source and agency has its own individual reporting regulations. Governmental agencies tend to be more demanding in accountability and reporting requirements.

It is the duty and right of agencies for the blind, administrators, mobility specialists, and consumers to attempt to influence the development of appropriate and effective legislation on the local, state, and national level concerning legislation that will effect rehabilitation of blind persons, including mobility services. Since most states have existing White Cane Laws, their application to actual conditions existing in local communities should be reviewed. Agencies should take an active part in developing legislation concerning vocational rehabilitation, social services such as Title XX of the Social Security Act, and educational services for children and adults. Many federal programs (Title XX) require public hearings so that input from local levels may be obtained. This input can influence and document program changes, policies, and specific services.

PERSONNEL

Administrators have the responsibility for selecting and employing qualified and competent personnel in all areas, and mobility is no exception. In recent years the mobility profession has established college level training programs and certification standards for mobility specialists. Certification standards are consistent with teacher certification procedures in other areas of special education. Current certification is under the auspices of the American Association of Workers for the Blind. Graduates of recognized college training programs are eligible for provisional certification upon graduation. Permanent certification is granted at the conclusion of at least three years of successful teaching experience, but in some cases education is required.

College and university programs are available at undergraduate and graduate levels. Most graduate programs are at least one year in length and lead to a master's degree. Undergraduate programs most often begin the specialization with courses in mobility training and those related to visual impairment in the junior year, if not sooner. All university programs incorporate a student teaching or internship requirement in their curriculum so that graduates have had supervised practical experience.

At present an adequate supply of university trained orientation and mobility specialists is available for employment in schools, and public and voluntary agencies. Hence, potential employers should have little difficulty in hiring professionally trained, competent, and certified mobility specialists. It is important to note that present certification regulations recognize only graduates of university programs with a specialized curriculum and faculty in orientation and mobility. The certification standards do not recognize or make provision for persons trained in non-university settings or for persons attending universities without specialized curriculum and faculty.

PROGRAM PLANNING FOR DIRECT SERVICES

The development of unit outlines and specific lesson plans gives structure to the presentation of mobility techniques and skills to a variety of clients in specific environmental settings. The unit outline begins with the initial evaluation and ends with advanced lessons in skills such as business area techniques presented in an organized manner and in related learning groups, progressing from the most basic skill through the most complex thereby developing a success pattern.

It is extremely important that special instructional units be developed to meet needs of visually impaired persons with additional physical or mental disabilities; for the elderly, for those with low vision, the deaf-blind or other physical disabilities. Special unit guides are needed to instruct educable or trainable mentally retarded children.

Typical unit plans should include the following areas of instruction:

Mobility Skills	**Orientation**
Basic Skills (Pre-cane)	Auditory Awareness
Sighted guide	Sound identification
Protective methods	Sound localization
Direction taking	Sound utilization
Trailing, seating	Masking
Finding dropped object	Olfactory Cues
Diagonal cane	Tactual Cues
Negotiating stairs	Gradients
Touch or Hoover Technique	
Arc	
Rhythm	
Touch	
Outdoor Travel (Initial)	Orientation Cues
Straight-line walking	Sun
Locating intersecting sidewalks	Ambient sounds
	Moving sounds
Residential Travel	Grid Pattern
Street crossings	Environmental Concepts
Block travel	Compass directions
Stop-sign corners	Drop-offs
Locating objects	
Drop-offs	
Light Business	Use of Traffic in Direction Taking
Different sidewalk/settings	Identifying Landmarks
Locating stores	
Stoplight crossing	
Business	Asking Directions
Public transportation	
Advanced stoplight crossing	
Soliciting aid	
Elevators, escalators	
Shopping lessons	

Lesson plans are detailed instructional guides designed to help achieve competencies related to orientation and mobility. Each lesson plan should have a stated goal or objective included in its design. The lesson plan should include:

1. The skill to be presented

2. How it is to be presented

3. The setting where it is to be taught

4. An indication of successful performance

5. The sensory skills to be emphasized along with the mobility techniques.

Instructors must be meticulous in developing both unit outlines and lesson plans. Written lesson plans for a minimum of 100 hours of instruction should be developed for most rehabilitation center or residential school programs. Few instructors are capable enough to ad lib lessons without unit and lesson plans. Flexibility in adapting lessons is a must, and additional remedial lessons may be added if there is difficulty in particular skill areas.

The advantages of written unit and lesson plans are many. First, instruction is delivered in an organized manner so that successful sequential learning occurs. Second, they stress instructor concentration on observing client performance in terms of lesson objectives and unit goals. Performance can, therefore, be measured in a standardized way. Third, the occurrence of having several instructors in one setting teaching clients entirely different skills in varying sequences can be avoided.

It is essential for instructors to become absolutely familiar with the environment in which instruction will be given. The instructors must actually walk through the streets and areas in which they will be teaching students and perhaps don the blindfold themselves. The instructor must assess the environmental characteristics and transportation resources available in the community, including public transportation; prevalent types of sidewalks; patterns of traffic flow; and the nature of the community whether residential, commercial, or a combination. The mobility specialist must also observe and evaluate any environmental hazards in the area of instruction and throughout the community. Street furniture such as signs, support cables for utility poles, types of curbs, design of traffic-light intersections, and whether the city has a right-turn-on-red provision must be noted. A wide variety of environmental peculiarities must be incorporated into the instructional plan and should be updated periodically as environments change.

SPECIAL NEEDS
The Multiply Handicapped

While the multiply handicapped students may not have the potential of other students they still have a right to instruction to help them achieve their highest level of mobility. Working with the multiply handicapped usually requires a team approach and greater communication among the rehabilitation staff. The assistance of other specialists such as audiologists, occupational and physical therapists, psychologists, or special education teachers may be needed to plan appropriate mobility services for multiply handicapped children. It is important to set achievable goals for each child, with programs designed to build on the strengths of the individual to overcome the weaknesses and limitations of various disabling conditions.

Low Vision

Mobility programs for low vision clients should recognize that many of them may not need to learn the traditional orientation and mobility techniques in order to achieve independent travel. A client may function as a low vision person during the day and a totally blind person at night. They may or may not need to use a cane for independent travel. Evaluation of the efficiency of remaining vision of each client is the key to delivery of effective mobility services to low vision persons. Consultation with an ophthalmologist, optometrist, and/or the low vision staff is necessary to understand each individual visual problem. There is need for special lessons in use of monocular distance aids, binocular telescopic aids, sun shields, and other devices prescribed by the low vision staff. Night lessons are essential for proper evaluation and training of some clients. Administrators should provide compensatory time when night work is required. The mobility instructor must observe each client carefully in order to assess efficiency in use of their remaining vision to travel safely and effectively in the environment. The length of the training program may vary greatly from the regular mobility program, and is usually much shorter. Low vision programs require purchase of costly special low vision aids and equipment, which must be remembered in establishing program budgets.

Elderly

Mobility instruction for the aging blind or visually impaired person should take into account the need for careful planning with and for each client. The elderly, more than other visually impaired persons, generally have very definite ideas as to what they need and do not need. The mobility instructor must first have a good understanding of the aging process obtained both from the literature and, to a certain degree, from the person himself. The initial assessment should take into account any allied or related medical or general health problems. The instructor should be particularly alert to problems having to do with auditory, circulatory, or respiratory diseases. Lessons may have to be short to accommodate health problems or lack of stamina. It may be necessary to consult with appropriate medical personnel to design special conditioning programs to supplement instruction in orientation and mobility skills. It is important for the mobility specialist to realize that an older person may feel gratification in achieving even a small amount of success in mobility such as independent travel within his own building or immediate neighborhood.

CLIENT-INSTRUCTOR RATIO

The majority of mobility instruction is given on a one-to-one client-instructor ratio for specific reasons. The one-to-one ratio gives the individual client or student maximum protection during the learning process, particularly in uncontrolled settings such as street and stoplight crossings, business travel, and use of public transportation. It is unsafe and inefficient for mobility specialists to attempt to work with more than one client at a time. Group orientation and mobility instruction should only be given in an inactive classroom setting.

The National Accreditation Council *Self-Study and Evaluation Guide* (1977) recommends that mobility specialists be scheduled for not more than six hours of teaching each day. Administrators should adhere to this guideline so that the mobility specialist has adequate time for record keeping and preparation of instructional guidelines and lesson plans.

IN-SERVICE TRAINING PROGRAMS

In-service training programs for agency staff, personnel from other agencies, or parents of students should emphasize practical understanding and implementation of mobility skills. The format and length of in-service programs will vary and should be designed to meet the specific needs of the group requesting the instruction. For example, nurses and aides in a nursing home are faced with the particular mobility problems of their patients. They also work in a controlled environment where the need to present anything beyond basic skills is unnecessary. Yet, they need special instruction in adapting standard techniques for persons with additional health or physical problems.

Family or friends of the student should be informed of practical, specific activities to be done to reinforce mobility skills learned at school. It is also advisable that they understand the goals and objectives of mobility instruction, and what is involved in training. When possible, the family should be given basic instruction as sighted guides and in direction giving. The mobility specialist should also point out fundamental principles of the technique where problems may occur and where reinforcement may be needed. While attending the rehabilitation center, family members should be invited to observe not only mobility instruction but instruction in all other rehabilitation areas.

Well-planned in-service training programs can be valuable to any community and particularly helpful to related service agencies and organizations. They have public relations value, giving schools and agencies an opportunity to demonstrate the skills they teach and the services they offer to the visually impaired person.

SELECTION AND EVALUATION

Selection of students for mobility instruction should be a process of "screening in" applicants as opposed to one of "screening out" applicants. Ideally, as many people as are interested in achieving some level of independent travel should be accepted for instruction. Many times the criteria for selection is whether a person can complete a *full* course of mobility training. The program should, in fact, be designed to assist each blind person interested in mobility to achieve his highest level of independent travel regardless of physical, mental, or other limitations. Mobility specialists should be flexible and competent enough to work with blind persons who have hearing impairments, physical problems, mental limitations, or psychological problems.

Because administrators and mobility specialists are often faced with long lists of people waiting for mobility services, the selection of recipients is not easy. The process should be a joint endeavor among staff members, and take into account the client's need for the service as related to his overall program objectives. Frequently the applicant needs mobility instruction to attend college or obtain employment, and many programs view these as top criteria for selection. Other factors such as potential for mobility, intelligence, age, and physical health need to be considered too. State vocational rehabilitation departments and similar funding agencies often purchase mobility services for their clients from voluntary agencies or schools. State-federal programs often fund only clients who they consider to have potential for successful vocational placement. The voluntary agency or school can, at best, try to persuade them to provide mobility instruction to all who desire and need the service. Any selection process considered by administrators and mobility specialists should adhere to the Code of Ethics, found in the appendices of this text.

The evaluation process for prospective clients should include the compilation of general and special medical reports, an audiometric report, a concise sociological history, a statement of why the service is needed, and the mobility level desired.

EVALUATION OF CLIENTS

Evaluation systems for mobility students should include both objective and subjective measures. While there are no standardized evaluation measures or procedures in orientation and mobility, several authors have attempted to develop acceptable indications of readiness for mobility and have also designed objective evaluative measures. Patton (1970) suggested several criteria in assessing readiness for mobility among adventitiously blinded adults, including three main criteria for mobility readiness: physiological, psychosocial, and emotional. Angus, Howell, and Lynch (1969) devised twenty questions and answers about mobility designed to supply information to parents of children beginning instruction. Menzel, Shapira, and Dreifus (1967) drew up a detailed test form for mobility training readiness to be used by mobility instructors in a variety of settings. The test is lengthy, but it may be useful in determining mobility potential. However, it is not indicated how the information should be tabulated or used. Bohman, Bryan, and Tapp (1972) developed an auditory quiz board for blind children to test the learning of specific mobility skills and also to establish motivation to learn the skills.

There is a great need for development of pre- and post-evaluation methodology for mobility instruction. At present no research effort has developed reliable statistically significant tools to predict success in mobility or to identify and isolate factors that contribute to learning.

Checklists are used as part of the evaluation technique, and should include enough detail so as to document the level of skills being taught beginning with the basics, such as using a sighted guide, and progressing through business travel. While checklists can be useful in monitoring student progress, they should also be accompanied by comprehensive narrative reports that include description of skills taught and related performance, attitudinal factors, and delineation of student's problems and strengths.

Mobility specialists should develop keen observation habits that will help solve problems encountered by clients, identify strengths and weaknesses, and adapt techniques when necessary.

Many mobility specialists get caught up in a "needs versus potential" dilemma in designing client programs. Should a person receive just enough training to meet basic needs or a challenging mobility program that will develop maximum potential for independent travel? The question is not easily answered and can be frustrating for the conscientious teacher. Although the consumer is often a better judge of his needs than anyone else, the mobility specialist should make every effort to convince clients with high potential for independent travel of the value in completing an entire mobility training course. Many clients stop short of fulfilling their potential in mobility training and take only enough to meet immediate environmental and personal needs.

PROGRAM IMPLEMENTATION

A well-designed mobility program should include:

1. Clearly delineated communication guidelines among administration, mobility specialists, and other staff

2. Assessment and provision of insurance coverage for the institution, staff, and clients

3. Accountability and reporting procedures

4. Public relations and public education activities.

Communication among Staff

Effective communication with clients, co-workers, and administrators is an essential part of any mobility program, as well as the recognition that mobility itself is only one factor in a multi-discipline educational and rehabilitation process. It is important for mobility specialists to be able to communicate with one another regarding the delivery of skills in a coordinated and related manner, each adhering to the same procedures, regulations, and established policies.

Communication with other professionals within the school or rehabilitation setting is extremely important in planning an individual mobility program. Information gathered about the progress of a client in other areas can be helpful in planning for specific goals and objectives in mobility. Development of a mobility plan for any client should be coordinated with the work of the other members of the rehabilitation team.

Effective communications with supervisors and administrators is essential to any program, but is not always easily accomplished. Instructors impatient to design program changes need approval from administrators. The administrator cannot always respond with a satisfactory or prompt response as such decisions often affect more than one individual area of specialty or may involve exceptions to accepted rules or established policies. Approval from a policy-making body such as a board of directors or advisory committee is sometimes necessary, but may be time consuming and frustrating.

Insurance

Adequate insurance coverage should be provided for all participants in a mobility training program. As insurance laws vary greatly from state to state specialists and administrators must investigate local laws carefully to provide appropriate protection. Four parties should be insured: the client; the mobility instructor; the general public, or in insurance terms, the third party; and the agency or school itself.

General liability coverage will, in most cases, provide sufficiently for coverage of everyone involved in mobility instruction. However, the mobility specialists and administrators should explore and delineate the subtle differences in third-party and general liability coverage. In most instances, third-party coverage will be indentured in general liability provisions in a comprehensive insurance policy.

It may be advisable for mobility specialists to carry additional liability insurance beyond that provided by the employer. The employer and the specialist should consider possible exclusions in insurance protection because of negligence and other related acts. A good deal of mobility instruction takes place off the physical premises of the agency, and could be considered an excluding factor in awarding payment of claims by an insurance company. Another potential exclusion involves the direct and proved negligence of the instructor in carrying out assigned duties and tasks in the teaching of mobility skills. A third party or member of the general public involved in an accident with a blind person could claim that the instructor did not exercise care and diligence to prevent the accident.

Further, a former student might claim that improperly taught orientation and mobility skills resulted in deficient skills which caused an accident. It is essential here that mobility specialists keep carefully documented daily progress notes of each student's mobility lessons. The progress notes should document the level of proficiency achieved by each client at each level of instruction. Such notes show whether or not a person had achieved a certain level of travel performance and are, in most cases, reasonable proof of the instructor's competence.

Bina (1976) presents a thorough discussion on the specifics of legal interpretation concerning negligence, and the need to examine liability insurance pertaining to mobility instruction. It is highly recommended that administrators review this article in addition to investigating all aspects of insurance protection with their insuror.

Accountability

Record keeping and report writing are an essential part of any mobility program. Records are maintained for three fundamental reasons: for accountability of services rendered, to evaluate and improve services, and to improve teaching ability of mobility specialists. The record keeping system should document the actual services being delivered and relate specific performance on the part of each and every client. While a wide variety of report writing and record keeping methods may be utilized, the following should be basic to any system: 1) an initial evaluation report, 2) daily progress notes, 3) weekly and/or monthly progress reports, and 4) a comprehensive final summary report.

Written reports should include a description of the planned program and actual delivered services, where the service was delivered, the performance of the client including strengths and weaknesses, the number of lessons given, and hours of training. The final report should be a complete documentation of services rendered and client performance, including a clear statement of the client's highest level of mobility skill achieved and limitations, if any.

Direct and Indirect Cost Benefits

The high cost of delivering orientation and mobility services of good quality and in sufficient quantity cannot be argued as most of the instruction is on a one-to-one basis. Yet, in the long run, the cost benefits of orientation and mobility instruction are more highly cost-effective than almost any service we provide to visually impaired children or adults. In educational or rehabilitation programs, direct and indirect costs are most commonly determined on an annual basis, but mobility instruction is usually given in a time period much less than a calendar year. This is particularly true in adult rehabilitation programs. In residential schools for the blind, orientation and mobility instruction is often given to children in a concentrated manner during the senior high school years. When compared to hours of instruction in other subjects, hours of mobility instruction are relatively few. The true cost-benefit from orientation and mobility instruction lies not only in direct dollar costs for the service itself, but also in benefit derived by the recipient and the positive impact on his family and productivity. Effective and independent orientation and mobility is a directly usable skill in the daily life of a visually impaired person. Good mobility skills may help the blind person to attain a higher level of education, and to obtain and retain employment. More important they impart a sense of accomplishment and independence that few other personal adjustment skills can. Another benefit is that the increased occurrence of blind persons functioning independently creates a positive attitude toward them in the community.

The effectiveness of residential mobility programs versus community based mobility programs is frequently questioned. Delivery of mobility services in a concentrated residential setting is more economical than the less efficient community based or itinerant mobility program. Yet, community and itinerant programs are effective in reaching a wide range of blind persons and are usually capable of meeting specific needs of individuals in orientation and mobility. A residential mobility program achieves most efficient use of personnel, and scheduling of clients and facilities. A residential-setting mobility specialist usually schedules six hours of lessons with an additional hour for program planning and record keeping. Itinerant programs cannot, in most cases, achieve this efficient use of mobility personnel because time must be allotted for travel between clients.

Another question is how often mobility instruction should be given. Most experts agree that mobility instruction for adults should be given in a concentrated period of time, and if possible on a daily basis. The ideal is considered to be one lesson per day, five days per week until completion of the program. Some adults can handle up to two hours of instruction per day, with perhaps an hour in the morning and another in the afternoon. In the beginning, there should not be less than three lessons in any week to prevent loss in the acquisition of skills.

Mobility programs for children are given over a period of years and focus on meeting needs in accordance with natural maturation processes. The best time to start mobility instruction for children is, of course, at birth. However it is most likely that mobility instruction will first be given when the child enters school, as schools and agencies are unable to identify and/or serve preschool children. During the first few years of instruction, mobility training for children should center on basic orientation skills and the development of appropriate spatial and body concepts. The introduction of formal mobility techniques and cane skills will most likely be introduced in the middle or later elementary grades and be continued on through high school. While some children are able to handle cane skills much earlier, most children are not emotionally or physically ready to handle formal cane skills until the later elementary school years.

Follow-up

Client follow-up is without question the biggest deficiency in any mobility program. This is particularly so with residential rehabilitation centers and residential schools for the blind because they serve people from a wide geographic area. Clients are more accessible in local community programs. Follow-up assesses both the degree to which the program was effective and how well clients transferred their skills to local environments.

Effective follow-up will involve additional costs to the normal instructional program in any rehabilitation or educational setting. In establishing a follow-up program, the first step should be to determine the appropriate time interval at which the services should occur, usually three, six, or twelve months after training. Clients should be seen in their normal daily travel activities in order to obtain an accurate assessment of how they are applying and implementing skills in their own environment. It must be noted that some persons suffer a regression in skills shortly after completing a mobility course, because they are no longer in a totally supportive rehabilitation setting. They know that routes traveled in their daily activities are not as carefully selected as those used during training, and that they are now completely on their own without the support or safeguard of a nearby mobility specialist.

Follow-up programs at residential rehabilitation centers are expensive because of travel involved. Therefore, the mobility specialist may have to devise alternate measures, such as a contractual arrangement to use the services of mobility specialists who work in the communities where former clients now reside. Another frequently used, but less desirable method is written or telephone follow-up with clients to attempt to obtain information as to whether they are using their mobility skills at home. This type of consumer interaction should be an important factor in any follow-up program whether community-based or center-based rehabilitation settings. However, it is better for the instructor to observe the overall mobility skills of the client in conjunction with his needs to move about in his environment. Evaluation checklists can be used in conjunction with any follow-up program.

Public Relations

Mobility is a visible outcome of the rehabilitation or educational process of visually impaired persons, so public relations efforts in an agency or school quite frequently involve some publicity regarding mobility as a part of independence. The mobility specialist, therefore, should be aware of how to present mobility training in an understandable, acceptable, and realistic manner. Public relations efforts involve coordination with the public relations officer or administrator of the school or agency. Local news media are almost always anxious to do public interest stories and features. If a school or agency feels it has a good human interest story it should contact the local media and present the concept of mobility and independence versus dependence.

The best public relations program includes year-round scheduling of contacts with newspapers, television, and radio. Most local television and radio stations are eager to have written public service announcements or spots of anywhere from ten seconds to one minute in length. Television stations often use public service announcements projected on the screen along with the station identification logo. Agencies should note that the Federal Communications Commission requires all television and radio stations to schedule a certain amount of time per week for public service announcements and many stations are even willing to help produce slides or related materials for these spots. Agencies should learn who is responsible for public service at each station.

In photographing orientation and mobility techniques it is important that the posture and grace resulting from independent mobility be appropriately displayed. A mobility specialist and public relations officer should ask to see contact prints before publication. Local newspapers often send inexperienced reporters to write public interest stories. It is advisable to request a prepublication draft of an article to review it for accuracy and content and to counter an overly emotional or sensational writing style.

Another form of public education is a verbal and/or audio-visual presentation to civic clubs or other special interest groups. Civic clubs such as the Lions, Rotary, and Kiwanis are particularly interested in learning more about the rehabilitation or education of visually impaired persons. These groups usually have a specific time period during their meetings when programs must be presented. It is advisable to stay within the allotted time period and to use good pictorial presentations of mobility and/or rehabilitation programs. High quality, brief audio-visual presentations are sometimes more effective than a long technical speech.

Brochures and pamphlets should be a part of the public relations effort. Narratives should be brief, to the point, and highlight the message with good photographs of the activities being presented. Some mobility instructors carry "street cards" with them. These are regular business cards with a short but pointed explanation of what is being achieved by mobility instruction printed on the reverse side. It can be effective for instructors to hand the card to someone encountered on a mobility lesson, such as the person who offered assistance and was refused by the client, or to an interested observer.

Summary

High quality effective orientation and mobility services should be the goal of every school and agency. Effective mobility programs are well planned in every respect, from instructional guidelines to evaluation and follow-up of its clients. Administrators are responsible for employing qualified mobility specialists and giving them clearly defined job functions and duties. Few programs can be fully effective without responsive and appropriate supervision or effective inter-staff communications.

The administration should provide support in the areas of program planning, transportation, insurance coverage, record keeping systems, and clerical assistance. Also, the mobility program should be clearly specified within the organizational structure of the agency and be a vital part of its curriculum or overall program.

Mobility services are funded by a variety of public and voluntary institutions and can be offered through widely different delivery systems. Mobility programs should include specific plans for identification, selection, and evaluation of participants, and instructional programs should be individually prescribed and flexible enough to serve persons of wide age ranges and differing abilities. Special programs should be developed to serve persons with low vision, the elderly, and those with additional disabilities. Effective mobility programs should be measured in terms of client or student achievement to each person's optimal level of functioning.

Bibliography

Angus, H. D., Howell, B., & Lynch, J. Twenty questions about mobility. *The New Outlook for the Blind*, 1969, **63,** 214-218.

Bina, M. J. Legal implications of solo experiences in orientation and mobility training. *The New Outlook for the Blind*, 1976, **69,** 225-231.

Bohman, R. V., Bryan, W. H., & Tapp, K. L. The auditory quiz board: An orientation and mobility game for visually handicapped elementary school children. *The New Outlook for the Blind*, 1972, **66,** 371-373.

Menzel, R., Shapira, G., & Dreifus, E. A proposal test for mobility training readiness. *The New Outlook for the Blind*, 1967, **61,** 33-40.

National Accreditation Council. *Self-study and evaluation guide. Orientation and mobility services.* New York: Author, 1977.

Patton, W. E. Research on criteria for measuring mobility readiness of adventitiously blind adults. *The New Outlook for the Blind*, 1970, **64,** 73-80.

Dog Guides

Robert H. Whitstock

Man's relationship with the dog dates back to the Stone Age. In excavations of settlements tens of thousands of years old, the bones of dogs have been found intermingled with those of man. The close relationship between man and dog was always one of mutual assistance; the dog as a household pet is a relatively recent phenomenon. Dog helped man by herding sheep, guarding his home and property, hunting game or fowl, in ancient times and today. He also acted as a guide for blind persons.

HISTORY

Among the murals uncovered at Pompeii, there is one depicting a market scene in which a man, evidently blind, is being led by a small dog. A 13th century Chinese scroll painting shows a blind person with a dog guide moving independently through a crowd of townspeople (Coon, 1959). For a long time, ingenious blind persons have been teaching dogs to guide them using makeshift flexible straps or ropes as a communication link between man and dog.

The systematic training of dog guides for the blind evidently began sometime in the 18th century. One of the earliest blindness "experts," Father Johann Wilhelm Klein (1819), described in his *Textbook for Teaching the Blind*, some approaches to the training of dog guides that were very similar to those in current use. These recommendations probably grew out of his knowledge of blind people who had trained dogs to act as guides. Before the end of the 18th century, a Viennese blind man, Joseph Reisinger, had systematically trained a dog to act as his guide (Coon, 1959). Detailed descriptions were kept of how Reisinger trained his dog guide. He trained the dog to walk in front of him, to stop moving on command, to react to sidewalks, curbs, and obstacles, and then to more complex things:

It was a more difficult job to teach the dog to find doors and other places where the blind man wanted to stop. He solved this by getting someone to help him to take the dog to the proper doorways and when he got in front of the door he would give the signal for a quick stop and then would turn the dog towards the door to indicate his desire. The dog (a Spitz) soon learned what was wanted.

Just so in the house he trained his dog to go right or left by pulling the leash in the proper direction and also he trained him when in a house to walk slowly and keep close to a wall, and then when the right door was reached, a pull on the leash would indicate that he wanted to go in. All of this training was given by the blind man himself, doing the training in his own house or in the house of friends. Often the man knew himself where the doors were and it was a case of training the dog to go to them as directed (Coon, 1959, p. 43).

Reisinger trained three dog guides before he became too old and enfeebled to use this means of mobility.

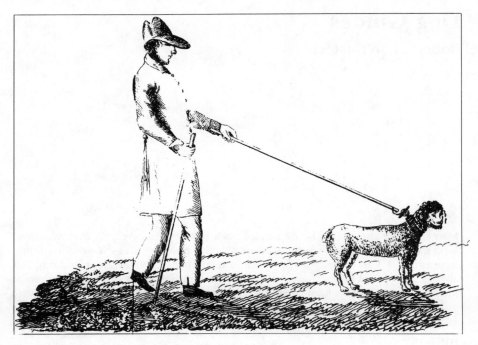

Figure 1-17. Klein's illustration showing early harness.

Klein's key contribution was the concept of a rigid harness handle (Fig. 1-17), markedly improving the ability of a person to detect the movements of a dog more accurately. The developers of the German dog guide program during World War I (the forerunner of all those in existence today), appear to have been familiar with Klein's work (Coon, 1959) and were probably influenced by it.

It was also during the 19th century that major interest in breeding dogs more selectively and for specific traits, and training them more systematically became common. One of the breeds in which selective breeding and systematic training was most successful was the German Shepherd dog (AKC, 1972).

Like so many kinds of human progress, the systematic mobility training of blind persons grew out of war: dog guides out of World War I, and the long cane almost 30 years later out of World War II. During World War I, the German Shepherd began to assume a new role when the first formal dog guide school was established in Germany to train blinded veterans of the German Army. This program developed a systematic process for bringing blind persons and trained German Shepherds together as working units. The veterans were taught how to follow the motions of a trained dog and interpret its actions and reactions through a working harness.

Dorothy Harrison Eustis

Training of dog guides for the blind remained limited to Germany until an American visitor and dog fancier, Dorothy Harrison Eustis (Fig. 2-17), described it in a 1927 *Saturday Evening Post* article called "The Seeing Eye." The response to the article was immediate and eventually led to the establishment of dog guide programs in many parts of the world during the following decades (Ebeling, 1950).

Mrs. Eustis had long been interested in dogs, particularly German Shepherds. In 1923 in Vevey, Switzerland where they were living, she and her husband established Fortunate Fields, a breeding and training station where dogs would be bred for those qualities of temperament, intelligence, and physique that make the ideal working dog (Humphrey & Warner, 1934). The animals bred there were taught a variety of demanding and intricate jobs, and during the 1920s the Fortunate Fields station became internationally famous. The dogs were developed for careers in rescue work, messenger service, prison control, and a variety of military and police work. The procedures developed at Fortunate Fields are still used in the training of working dogs.

It was Mrs. Eustis' search for more information on working dogs that led her to Germany and to her observation of the German dog guide program. Her excitement was evident in her *Saturday Evening Post* article. "To think that one small dog could stand for so much in the life of a human being," she wrote, "not only in his usual role of companion, but as his eyes, sword, shield, and buckler! How many humans could fill these roles with the same uncomplaining devotion and untiring fidelity?" (Eustis, 1927).

The Seeing Eye

When Mrs. Eustis' article was published, there was no systematic method that blind Americans could use to get about freely; a lack which was a major obstacle to their independence and integration into society. Upon learning about the German dog guide program, many blind persons in the United States got in touch with Mrs. Eustis. One of these, a young Tennessean, Morris S. Frank, who had lost his sight as a teenager (Frank & Clark, 1957) persuaded Mrs. Eustis to have a dog trained for him at Fortunate Fields with the understanding that he would go to Switzerland to learn how to use it and then return to the United States to test it under American conditions. The experiment was so successful that Mrs. Eustis decided

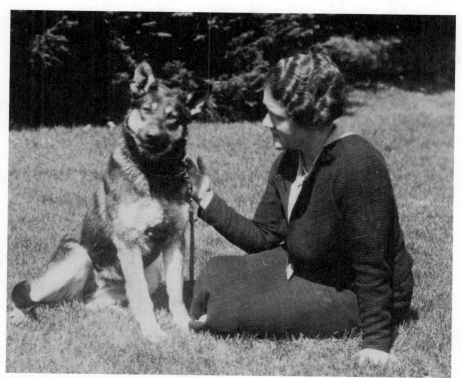

Figure 2-17. Dorothy Eustis at Fortunate Fields.

to devote her full energies to developing dog guide services for blind men and women (Hartwell, 1942). In January 1929 she returned to the United States and formally established The Seeing Eye, Inc., in Nashville, Morris Frank's home town, but in June of that year moved it to Morristown, New Jersey, where it is presently located (Putnam, 1963).

After The Seeing Eye was established, Fortunate Fields trained a number of people from various European countries who later returned to their homes to establish similar programs. Some of these schools, in turn, gave rise to dog guide programs in other nations. For example, the program in Great Britain led to the establishment of a program in Australia. Today, there are nine programs in the United States and schools in a number of other countries including Great Britain, France, Italy, Germany, Denmark, Australia, and Japan (Koestler, 1976).

ELIGIBILITY

The mobility specialist is often the person who counsels a blind client about the choice of a form of mobility. To give counsel to a blind person in this area, the mobility specialist should be knowledgeable about all aspects of dog guide mobility. The specialist should have an appreciation of both the characteristics that tend to make a successful dog guide user and the techniques, activities, and methods of dog guide training from the breeding of dogs through the actual training of dog and person as a working unit.

No profile currently exists that describes the characteristics of a typical dog guide user. The standards and eligibility requirements of schools vary. At The Seeing Eye, which since 1929 has trained more than 4,000 individuals, certain basic patterns have emerged to provide insight into the characteristics of what constitutes a likely candidate for a dog guide program. Most graduates are married and have raised or are raising families; although this does not hold for younger applicants who may obtain their first dogs while still in school or college. Since its inception, the overwhelming number of Seeing Eye graduates have been employed or actively engaged in careers as students or homemakers (Ebeling, 1950).

There are several factors that must be taken into account by a visually impaired client when considering a dog guide: personal preference, life circumstances and activity level, amount of remaining vision, age, health and physical condition, orientation skills, and safety.

Personal Preference

The first factor that must be considered by a potential dog guide user is preferred mode of travel. People are individuals and what appeals to one may elicit a negative reaction from another. For some persons the rapid mobility of the dog guide, who generally walks three to four miles-per-hour, is an asset; for others, this pace is a liability. Some like the companionship of the dog and the providing of necessary care, while others may consider it a burden.

Life Circumstances and Activity Level

Dog guides need a certain amount of systematic use and attention in order to be efficient mobility aids. Thus, a dog should be placed with someone who is relatively active, someone who has places to go and who is motivated to avail himself or herself of such opportunities. On some days, the dog might be used for several miles while on another only sporadically, if at all. Its work should average out, however, and dog guides work most reliably for those who are not sedentary and who enjoy walking.

Likely candidates in terms of activity level and life circumstances are employed persons, students, and people active in civic affairs or who simply enjoy being out of doors for health and exercise (Putnam, 1963). A properly working dog readily accepts the challenge of new situations. A dog guide may be particularly valuable to the blind person who travels to new areas frequently. Because use of a dog guide means a team relationship, the dog is able to assume some of the responsibilities inherent in independent mobility. A blind person with a dog guide in a new and unfamiliar environment can generally handle the challenge with a minimum of stress as well as a minimum of knowledge of environmental detail (Delafield, 1976). Many persons who come to dog guide schools do so because their lives involve travel on unfamiliar routes or in new geographical areas.

Even under familiar travel conditions, the use of the dog guide seems to lessen nervous strain for many individuals. The properly functioning dog guide, for example, tends to maintain a relatively straight line, and an experienced dog will correct its owner at street crossings if they are facing an inappropriate angle for crossing. The dog also negotiates such obstacles as parked cars, truck tailgates, ladders, etc. Sometimes the maneuvers are so skillful that the owner is not aware of the complicated condition through which the dog has just guided him.

Many people who use dog guides enjoy the anonymity that the dog affords. The dog can lessen tension about blindness. It may seem strange to talk in terms of anonymity when a blind person and a dog are striding down a street together. When they are noticed, however, attention frequently seems to rivet on the dog and not on the person and his blindness. Observers may comment, "Look at that beautiful dog," rather than "There's a blind man." This kind of public reaction is a positive reinforcement for some blind people (Pfaffenberger, Scott, & Fuller, 1976) and of no importance to others.

Dog guide users, as a whole, indicate that the presence of their dogs has a positive influence in establishing social contacts and is even, in some circumstances, an ice breaker and opener of conversation. This can be invaluable to the visually impaired person whose circumstances require constant contact with others.

Amount of Remaining Vision

Most visually impaired people have too much vision to be able to work effectively with a dog guide. When a visually impaired person's residual vision is greater than light perception, he tends to depend on his own sight rather than the dog for mobility purposes. As a result he may anticipate stops or turns before receiving such information from the dog guide. Therefore, this dog does not have the opportunity to exercise the training it has received and without appropriate reinforcement may no longer function effectively.

Age

Because potential dog guide users must have the maturity to assume responsibility for the dog, they generally should be at least 16 years of age before they consider this method of mobility. While there is no upper age limit for dog guide users, the training is relatively rigorous and many older people find it too physically demanding. Nevertheless, The Seeing Eye reports that some of its earliest graduates are still physically able to work dogs today (The Seeing Eye, 1975).

Health and Physical Condition

Potential dog guide users should be in good health. Not only is the training rigorous, but once daily activities are resumed, regular and strenuous exercise should be a part of their life. As already mentioned, the average dog guide walks a brisk three to four miles an hour.

The individual should have good coordination and balance, be of at least average intelligence, and have emotional stability.

A group for whom dog guides may be especially well suited are persons who have lost their sight as a result of diabetic retinopathy. Exercise is an important factor in keeping diabetes under control and since dog guides need regular attention and exercise, they tend to help keep owners active. Because dog guides are taught to avoid obstacles and to give owners adequate clearance, the chances of bumping or bruising one's legs or body are negligible. This would be especially attractive to the diabetic who must exercise constant care to avoid minor injuries that can lead to more serious complications. (In recent years, the percentage of Seeing Eye graduates who are diabetics has grown. They now form about 12 percent of each class.)

Orientation Skills

The restrictions cited above tend to explain the result of a study conducted by the New York School of Social Work some years ago (Finestone, Lukoff, & Whiteman, 1960), which indicated that only 1 percent of the population were then using dogs and another 1 percent were interested in obtaining them and had the necessary qualifications to do so. An additional 2 to 3 percent had the qualifications and interest, assuming that there were certain changes in their circumstances that would permit their joining the reservoir of potential dog guide users. Such changes would include receiving appropriate mobility instruction—which has now become available on a much broader scale. A good sense of orientation is necessary for the dog guide user. Today many blind persons who would not have qualified in the past are using dog guides because mobility instruction has improved their orientation skills.

Safety

Many blind persons are, naturally, very concerned about their personal safety when traveling independently. A belief in the increased safety potential of dog guides is a major reason why many blind persons have chosen to use this form of mobility. The dog guide is taught to disobey a command if it appears that such a command may get its owner into difficulties. This is referred to as *intelligent disobedience*. When the dog guide user feels it is safe to cross, based on his evaluation of the traffic conditions, he gives the command, "forward." If the dog refuses to advance, the blind person should not step forward as most often the dog has disobeyed correctly. Such occurrences are not rare as high winds, construction and truck noises, and other circumstances can interfere with the blind person's auditory assessment of what is happening at any given moment.

Dog guides are also taught "respect" for traffic. This is especially reassuring to the many blind persons who suspect that the drivers of motor vehicles do not always pay attention to the street directly in front of them. A dog guide user does not have to count on the driver seeing him, but instead can rely both on his own ability to interpret traffic and on the dog's attention to moving vehicles.

ASSESSING USER POTENTIAL

A good dog guide school serves only those persons who, in its best judgment, can be reasonably assured of benefiting from its program. Therefore, schools take great care in evaluating individuals who apply. The mobility specialist has an important role in the assessment of a client's potential as a dog guide user. After discussing the aforementioned factors with a client, the mobility specialist will usually be asked by the dog guide school to provide a mobility evaluation of the applicant.

The evaluation should include a description of the candidate's coordination and balance, level of orientation skills, and amount of mobility instruction already received. It is also important to have some data on the neighborhood in which the individual plans to function, along with information about his basic ability and capacity to make mature judgments.

After a client has been accepted at a dog guide school, the mobility specialist can also play an important role in preparing the potential student for training. It is helpful for dog guide users to have a clear and accurate picture of their home neighborhoods so that they can introduce the dogs to these environments when training is completed. The client should be encouraged to exercise by walking as much as possible before dog guide training. A student in good physical condition will find it easier to meet the demands of the daily training program.

The mobility specialist who is in a position to recommend a dog guide school to a blind client must have a good understanding of all aspects of a dog guide school program to help the client make a sound choice of school. The dog guide program as a rehabilitation method is unique because several of the component activities take place apart from and before the blind student appears on the campus for the four weeks of training with the dog. The training of the blind person with the dog, naturally, is the aspect of the program that has attracted the most attention in the blindness field itself and among the general public. But a dog guide school is only as good as those aspects in its program that are more or less hidden from public view; that is the breeding, socialization, and training of the dogs themselves, and the selection and training of the instructors.

SELECTION AND BREEDING OF DOGS

Specific qualifications are sought in dogs whether they come from the school's own breeding program or from outside. Regardless of the source, each dog must be judged on its individual merits. Those selected must be healthy, intelligent, and of sound and gentle temperament; this latter trait is an especially important characteristic in a rigorous, stressful, and highly mechanized world. Most dogs selected weigh between 50 and 70 pounds—heavy enough to be felt in harness but not too large to fit comfortably under a workbench or restaurant table. A few unusually small or large dogs must also be selected and trained to meet the unique needs of very tall and very short dog guide users.

The belief that dog guides are taught to be guards as well as guides is a misconception. To be effective, a dog guide must not only work well but must also be sufficiently controlled to fit into all varieties of social and economic situations. Consequently, dog guide users are instructed to discourage protective tendencies in their dogs and the schools themselves select dogs which are inherently gentle and stable. At the same time, there is no question but that the presence of a devoted dog acts in itself as a deterrent to molestation.

Given the temperament, trainability, and size requirements that must be considered in the selection of a dog for a guide program, the breeds that can be used are limited to those that meet these specifications. The German Shepherd dog is, of course, just about synonymous with the term, "dog guide," and for some years was the only breed used. Now, however, Golden Retriever and Labrador Retriever dog guides are as common as German Shepherds and a considerable number of Boxers are used also. Over its long history, The Seeing Eye, for example, has used specimens from at least 29 breeds and has also trained a number of mixed breed dogs. Dogs chosen must also be easy to groom which eliminates very long-haired breeds.

The Seeing Eye uses both female and male dogs, but most are female. A few schools, however, use only females. Females are in general preferred to males because their temperament tends to be more gentle and they are somewhat more easily trained. Dogs are neutered before they begin training.

In its early days, The Seeing Eye received all of its dogs from Fortunate Fields.

As she became totally involved in The Seeing Eye, Mrs. Eustis closed Fortunate Fields in the mid-thirties and, shortly thereafter, the political situation in Europe prevented the importation of any more dogs. In the early forties, The Seeing Eye instituted its own breeding program as did Guide Dogs for the Blind, a school in San Rafael, California founded to serve west coast blinded veterans (Pfaffenberger, 1963). While most schools will accept the donation of sound home-raised grown dogs for training, and a few rely exclusively on them, experience has shown that a good internal breeding program is the best way to assure an adequate supply of sound dog guides.

Socialization of Puppies

The two years in a future dog guide's life between birth and meeting his blind master or mistress make the difference between his success and failure in his work. In recent years, the importance of active handling in the the life of the infant and young child has been proven in study after study. For the puppy, who resembles the young child in so many ways, the same is true. Puppies who are not appropriately socialized to people at the right stages in their lives never form the kinds of bonds to humans that will make them good pets, much less good dog guides (Pfaffenberger, Scott, & Fuller, 1976). That is the reason why dogs accepted as donations are always home raised, never kennel raised, and why good dog guide schools place all potential dog guides in private homes when they are about eight weeks old where they remain until they are a year or so old.

Long before there was scientific evidence of the importance of socialization in a puppy's early life, Dorothy Eustis seemed aware of this need. From the beginning, she placed her Fortunate Fields puppies with neighboring farm families until the dogs were old enough to begin their lessons (Humphrey & Warner, 1934). Thus, as an adjunct to its own breeding program, The Seeing Eye early in 1941 developed a systematic, cooperative program with the 4-H Clubs of New Jersey. This procedure is also used by most other dog guide schools. At about eight weeks of age, puppies already screened as potential dog guides are placed with young 4-H Club members so that they can be raised in normal home surroundings until they reach training age (Pollack, 1954; Latimer, 1976). Along with the crucial socialization, they are introduced naturally to the broad range of experiences they will eventually encounter with their blind owners, experiences they could never get living in a kennel.

Practices vary among dog guide schools as to the amount of supervision given growing dogs. At The Seeing Eye, for example, there are staff members whose sole responsibility is the locating of suitable homes for puppies and the supervision of their development. These staff members visit the homes in which the puppies are placed to check on and record the dog's social and emotional growth. This information is invaluable when used by the instructors who actually work with the dogs when they reach maturity.

All dogs are x-rayed for hip defects (hip dysplasia) before they are placed in training at The Seeing Eye and several other dog guide schools. The dogs also receive periodic physical examinations during the training period to insure that good health is maintained.

Training of Dogs

Dogs generally begin their formal training at about 14 or 15 months of age. This is an age when major growth for dogs of that size has been completed. By this age puppy behavior has been outgrown. While they are living with 4-H Club families, the puppies are, of course, trained in the basics of being a member of a family.

Most dogs like to please their human companions and it is this general desire for affection upon which dog guide training is based. Put differently, dogs are taught their responsibilities as guides through positive reinforcement. The dog is shown by an instructor what behavior is expected of it, and when it carries through the encouraged behavior, the dog receives warm and enthusiastic praise. Praise is used rather than food since the master would find it difficult to have food available at all times. Just as young children do, dog guides must learn which behaviors are unacceptable. A practice commonly used by parents and school staff is the application of a correction, a mild form of punishment to discourage unacceptable behavior. When the dog fails to carry out a command, it is also "corrected" firmly, generally with a jerk on the leash. Great care is exercised to make sure that the correction immediately follows the unacceptable behavior. As soon as compliance with a command is won, positive and delighted praise follows. For example, if a dog fails to give adequate clearance for the instructor as they pass an obstruction such as a parking meter, the instructor, upon impact with the parking meter, will say the word "pfui" (pronounced "phooey"). This is a correction word from the original Swiss training which means, in essence, "very bad." The instructor instantaneously will drop the harness and give the leash a very strong yank. The instructor will then retreat a pace or two and give the dog a command, "forward." The corrected dog guide will then give the offending obstruction a wide berth and will be showered with enthusiastic praise by its instructor for performing the desired behavior.

The learning process for dogs is similar to that for humans. Dogs begin their work in simple uncomplicated settings and move sequentially toward the complex. Instructors work with dogs on a one-to-one basis and seek to win both their affection and respect, without which no learning will take place.

For the first few weeks of formal training, the dogs are taught simple obedience, for example: heel, come, sit, down, rest, fetch. During this part of their training they are also introduced to the positive reinforcement and a mild form of punishment; positive reinforcement through praise for good work and a correction through the word "pfui," issued as a sharp reprimand for poor work. When it is completed, the dog is ready to begin work in harness.

By the end of the training process, which generally lasts about three months, the dog has learned all of the basic methods he will use as a dog guide. He has learned to stop at curbs and steps, to show the instructor their exact location, and to wait for the instructor's command of "right," "left," or "forward." The dog has also been taught to avoid overhanging obstacles such as tree limbs and awnings, and to give adequate clearance to the instructor for obstacles on sidewalks, open manholes, and other dangers that might lie in their path.

The Harness

The leather-covered U-shaped harness (Fig. 3-17) the dog guide wears is the means through which information about the dog's motions—stopping, turning, etc.—is transmitted to its human partner. Much of this communication from the dog is consciously registered by its partner. However, as a result of extensive experience the master learns many of the signals as a conditioned reflex without conscious thought. This communication and teamwork grows and evolves progressively over the months and years a dog guide and his blind master work together.

Along with the basic command and guiding routines, during the three months of training the dog also learns a number of words with specific meanings—for example, "steady," which is used to slow the dog, and "hup-hup," which, said cheerfully, encourages a dog to move at a more rapid pace.

Intelligent Disobedience

The dog learns about traffic progressively. He is worked first in quiet residen-

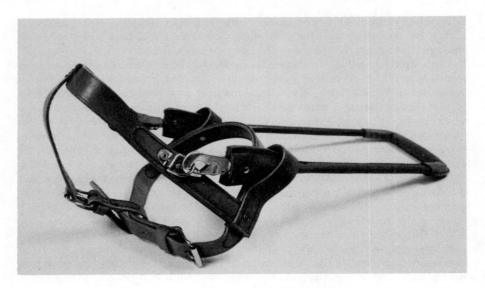

Figure 3-17. Seeing Eye harness. (Photographed by Sally DiMartini)

tial areas and then, progressively moved into areas where the traffic patterns grow more and more complex, and finally into areas where vehicles intersecting the traffic route are encouraged to keep moving rather than to stop for the dog and trainer. It is during this phase of its training that the potential dog guide must learn the concept of *intelligent disobedience,* mentioned earlier. Through repeated experience and conditioning, the dog learns that there are a few exceptions to the rule that obedience is always rewarded with praise, and that he occasionally must refuse to carry out commands that would endanger his owner.

Twice during the 12-week training period, the instructor tests the dog's proficiency in handling responsibilities by wearing occluders and permitting the dog to guide him as it will eventually its blind owner. An experienced supervisor observes the work and steps in if needed. During training the dogs are also deliberately and systematically exposed to a wide range of sounds and conditions and are graded daily on a report card. Factors such as sensitivity to correction, skill in coping with traffic, willingness to work, and overall behavior are evaluated and recorded.

A few dog guide schools use simulated environments to begin the teaching of traffic patterns and "intelligent disobedience." In the experience of The Seeing Eye, however, the actual environment is a much better teacher than any simulated experience.

MATCHING DOG AND MASTER

Generally, an individual instructor will train more dogs in a three-month training class than he expects blind students in his next class, for two reasons. First, not all dogs who go through the rigorous training will complete it as potential dog guides; some may experience difficulty with learning intelligent disobedience, which usually eliminates a number of otherwise superb dogs. Second, this procedure provides a reservoir from which the instructor can select an appropriate dog for each student he will teach.

Because of individual characteristics, matching dog with blind student is extremely important. In this task, the instructor assesses the blind student's coordination, speed, and balance. Also carefully considered are the temperaments of both dog and student.

Another factor that must be considered in matching dog to student is the kind of work the dog will be expected to do in its new life. Some dogs are better suited than others to life in a big city. Others will do better in a small town. Vending stand operators, many of whom have dog guides, would be assigned dogs with a different cluster of characteristics than guides destined for business executives or sales representatives who may have to travel widely in unfamiliar surroundings.

THE INSTRUCTOR

An experienced staff of instructors is essential to a dog guide school. A good dog guide school is as rigorous in its selection of apprentice instructors as it is in its selection of dogs and students. Qualifications vary but most of the larger dog guide schools now train their own instructors through on-the-job training, using the training process that was initiated by The Seeing Eye. The apprenticeship lasts for two or three years during which the instructor-in-training advances gradually from kennel work to the training of two to four dogs under the constant supervision of the training supervisor.

Several factors are considered in selecting apprentice instructors. The main educational requirement at The Seeing Eye, for example, is a high school education but, today, many instructors are graduates of associate or baccalaureate programs. Good physical health and stamina are necessary, as instructors may walk as many as 15 to 20 miles daily in the regular course of their work. Good vision is important because as training progresses, the instructor must be able to fade out of the immediate environment of dog and student yet be able to watch their actions and reactions closely. A crucial quality in a potential dog guide instructor is the ability to relate positively and effectively to other people.

The typical training cycle of a group of dogs limits an instructor to only three classes of students a year. In other words, an instructor works with a group of dogs for three months, or 12 weeks, and with a class of students for another four weeks. Six to eight students in a class are the maximum that can be handled effectively. Thus, in the course of a year, a dog guide instructor has trained from 18 to 24 students. Therefore, it takes a number of years for an apprentice instructor to build up a sufficient backlog of experience from which to draw.

Teaching the Student

At The Seeing Eye and most other schools, the classes for dog and blind student last four weeks. The students are first introduced to the harness and the various commands they will use to direct their dogs. Training itself begins in a quiet residential area. The first lessons are easy ones, for the training like most learning moves from the general and simple to the specific and complex. The initial routes are relatively short but build rapidly in length and complexity as the blind person begins to understand and to interpret correctly the signals communicated by the dog through the harness.

It is the responsibility of the master not to permit his dog's attention to wander from its job; and it is the dog's responsibility to keep its master out of danger. Confidence in the dog is built into the instruction procedures at a dog guide school. Students are exposed early to traffic conditions so that they can have confidence in the dog's ability to "intelligently disobey." The importance of this consideration varies from individual to individual, but for many blind persons who come to dog guide schools, a major motivation is the desire to heighten their personal confidence through improved safety.

By the second week of training, the dog and master team has usually reached a level of efficiency sufficient for them to begin learning to cope with heavy traffic.

The concluding weeks of the course are individualized to meet the particular requirements of each student, such as use of subways or department stores, or traveling in rural areas.

Throughout the course of the training, lectures are given on dog care and behavior. Knowledge about the latter is essential because the blind person must know how to control the dog as well as to work it as a guide. No dog guide is any better than the blind person who gives the unit its directions. Students are also given a perspective on how to help their dogs to adjust to their own life styles and circumstances, such as introducing the dog to their place of work. If they desire it, students are also counselled on how a dog guide affects other aspects of their life such as employment plans.

Unlike most rehabilitation programs, dog guide schools include both new students, and those who are described as replacements, in the same classes. A *replacement* is a visually impaired person who has had a dog guide previously and has returned to the school for a new dog because the previous one had reached the age where it could no longer give effective service. It is estimated that the expected working life of a dog as a guide is 8 to 10 years but dogs who serve as long as 12 are not uncommon. Including replacements with new students has a salutary effect on the blind person coming to the school for the first time. The presence of a replacement student is living evidence that dog guides provide independence successfully (Putnam, 1952).

Students at dog guide schools are also taught to keep their dogs appropriately disciplined and under control. Thus, the dogs are taught to lie for long periods of time so that they can fit into work settings, classrooms, and a myriad of social settings easily. The dogs are, of course, discouraged from barking or whining and are taught not to jump up on people or be a nuisance in other ways. In other words, the carefully selected dog guide placed in the hands of a properly instructed and trained blind person who maintains the dog's discipline becomes a very different type of dog than an untrained pet. The dog becomes instead a happy worker, devoted to its owner.

Some dog guide owners enjoy the constant companionship of their dogs; others keep them with them under most conditions but occasionally leave them at home, in a car, or elsewhere. While this is usually done for the dog's comfort, it must be stressed that a dog guide need not go everywhere its blind owner goes. Dog guides are taught to wait patiently for the return of their owner when he or she is engaged in an activity, such as skiing, in which the dog's presence would be inappropriate.

Life with a Dog Guide

Life with a dog guide can be divided into two parts: the initial adjustment period after the return home, and the remainder of the dog's working life as a seasoned and settled guide.

Like any dog in new surroundings, when the dog guide first arrives home, it requires a greater amount of attention and thought than it will later on. This initial adjustment period may last from a couple of weeks to several months. At first the dog is kept on leash (to facilitate immediate correction of unacceptable behavior) until it learns the rules of the house and the kind of behavior that will be permitted. Attention from family members is discouraged until such time as the blind person has won the full allegiance and respect of his new guide. Airings may require time and thought during this period and the dog should be given as much physical work as its master's schedule permits. Once the dog is settled, however, and relaxed in its new career, the amount of time and care the dog guide requires is negligible.

The cost of maintaining a dog guide, including its routine veterinary checkups, varies from about $12 to about $20 a month. Most dog guides are fed commercial pet foods which require only moments once or twice a day to prepare. The dog must be aired three or four times a day which, with a seasoned dog lasts only a matter of minutes each time. The owner is also asked to maintain at his convenience a daily obedience exercise routine and to groom the dog regularly. These activities take only minutes but pay dividends in good behavior, health, and appearance of the dog. Because of initial careful selection and health maintenance practices, dog guides should require very little medical attention. Should an owner incur inordinate expense or inconvenience because of a dog's chronic illness, schools encourage the retirement of the dog and its replacement with an animal better suited to the rigors of an active life.

The seasoned dog is very much a part of its owner's family. Occasionally, it is appropriate for a family member to feed the dog or take it out for an airing. This insures the dog's flexibility as far as care is concerned and helps to confirm its role as a member of the total family.

Occasionally, working problems develop after a visually impaired person has returned home with a dog guide. Generally, these occur in the early months of their life together. From the standpoint of encouraging self-confidence and independence on the part of the graduate, it is best for the individual to attempt initially to solve any adjustment problems following the detailed instructions he has received during training. However, a dog guide school must be ready to offer advice and, if needed, direct assistance in the home community if there is evidence that the graduate cannot handle the problem alone. The Seeing Eye, for instance, has supervisory personnel available for such trouble-shooting assignments throughout the United States and Canada, and the availability of such ready assistance is essential.

RE-INVOLVEMENT OF MOBILITY SPECIALIST

Once a visually impaired person has returned home from a dog guide school with his dog, the mobility specialist may again become involved. To make a correct decision about exactly what help should be given, the mobility specialist needs to understand the kinds of problems that might arise.

If the client seems to be having problems with the dog's work or behavior, the instructor should encourage him to get in touch with the dog guide school for assistance. However, some visually impaired clients who have returned home with dog guides may need some help from a mobility specialist in familiarizing themselves with the details of an unusually complicated situation.

This may occur when a visually impaired university student needs assistance in orienting himself to the layout of a particular campus. When he is called upon to give such help, the mobility specialist must exercise care not to try to substitute for the dog guide instructor. The mobility specialist should tell the blind person to put his dog at "heel," so that it will be off-duty and relaxed. The specialist then offers his arm to the client using the sighted guide technique, and discusses, at whatever length necessary, the details of the environment. This also allows them to stop periodically without confusing the dog. If the dog were being worked by the visually impaired person while this was taking place, the dog could become confused and the teaching procedure would then interfere with the teamwork between the visually impaired person and the dog guide.

When a specific landmark must be pointed out by the mobility specialist, such as the intersection of two pathways, he and the visually impaired person should stop at the point of intersection while the instructor explains the details of the particular environment—directions of roads, where they lead, etc. It is then up to the dog guide user to let the dog know that henceforth this spot is to be indicated by a stop similar to a curb or street corner. To do this, the dog owner puts his dog at "sit" and indicates the juncture of the walkways by pointing to the ground, and in other ways showing the dog that this is where he wishes it to stop. When the dog shows that he has found the area by himself, praise—positive reinforcement—is lavished upon him by the owner. This process must be repeated several times for the dog guide to become conditioned so that this intersection must be shown to its owner every time they come to it. When the owner feels that his dog guide understands what he is trying to teach, he should then actually work the intersection with the dog in harness and the mobility specialist trailing 10 to 20 feet behind. If the dog fails to stop at the intersection, the mobility specialist calls out to the student who then drops the harness and leads the dog back to the appropriate spot for a repetition of the procedure.

OTHER ASPECTS OF DOG GUIDE SCHOOLS

Philosophy and Policy

While most dog guide schools follow similar training procedures, both for the dogs and for the blind persons, the schools vary considerably in their approach to fees and funding.

The Seeing Eye has a fee policy under which blind persons applying for dog guide training are asked to assume a small portion of the cost of instruction for themselves and their dogs. This fee ($150 for the initial dog) can be paid immediately or spread out over a long period of time. The fee policy was established because through it the visually impaired person demonstrates his willingness to assume responsibility for his own rehabilitation. Many schools, however, charge no fees to the visually impaired person.

Dog guide schools, which are non-profit organizations, obtain funding in a variety of ways. Some organizations use mass mail appeals or rely in large measure on income from service clubs. Some raise money through benefits and similar volunteer activities. The Seeing Eye raises funds by direct personal contacts with past contributors and by soliciting bequests because it believes that the fund raising aspects of the program should be conducted in such a way that it does not embarrass or humiliate the visually impaired person served.

Some of the other areas in which there are differences in policy among the dog guide schools are whether or not there should be a formal graduation; whether title to the dog remains vested in the dog guide school or passes to the visually impaired person; whether there should be contact between the dog guide user and the individual who contributed the dog or raised it in a puppy rearing program.

Education

The dog guide school has a responsibility to educate both the general public and professionals in the blindness field about the value of dog guides.

When The Seeing Eye first opened its doors, the general restrictions on the entry of dogs into most public places in the United States applied to dog guides as well. As a consequence, one of the first tasks was to demonstrate to a skeptical public that dog guides were not pets and that they would not complicate the functioning of public places such as business offices, schools, restaurants, and theaters. Gradually, barrier after barrier disappeared. During the 1930s, railroads and airlines permitted blind persons to be accompanied by their dog guides at no additional cost. Bus lines, subway systems, restaurants, and hotels followed suit, and today dog guides can stay with their visually impaired owners wherever they wish in facilities open to the public. In recent decades, this right, originally won through public understanding, has been reinforced primarily by specific state legislation throughout the United States and in some parts of Canada (The Seeing Eye, 1976).

578

The Seeing Eye educates the professional in the blindness field in a variety of ways, most importantly perhaps through its sponsorship of observation seminars for students in university mobility programs held at The Seeing Eye. Since these trips were established in 1960, more than one thousand students in the university mobility programs have come to The Seeing Eye.

Research

The dog guide school that has a serious commitment to breeding dogs of the highest quality is in a position to make important contributions to veterinary research that will not only benefit dog guides of the future but other animals and humans as well.

For example, two major veterinary research projects, one at The Seeing Eye, and one at Guide Dogs for the Blind, San Rafael, California, were probably possible only in such settings that have long-term breeding programs.

Hip dysplasia, a serious genetic defect that affects a considerable number of breeds including all of those suitable for dog guide work, is a major target of current veterinary research. A recently concluded study of data on 3,025 dogs that passed through The Seeing Eye from 1940 to 1974 (The Seeing Eye, 1977) indicates that there is "a significant genetic correlation between the temperament rating for ear sensitivity in a canine and hip dysplasia." This finding may have important implications for the selection of dogs for breeding.

The importance of puppy socialization and the possibility of determining very early in a puppy's life whether or not it has potential for the kind of training guide work demand were important outcomes of a long-term research project conducted by Guide Dogs for the Blind, San Rafael, and Roscoe B. Jackson Memorial Laboratory, Bar Harbor, Maine (Pfaffenberger, 1963; Pfaffenberger, Scott, Fuller, Ginsburg, & Biefelt, 1976). The findings of this study have had an impact far beyond the dog guide field.

SUMMARY

While the relationship of man and dog is almost as old as man himself, and instances of blind people using dogs as guides dates back centuries, it was not until the 19th century that the systematic training of dog guides was described. In 1929 Dorothy Harrison Eustis established the first dog guide mobility training for blind students in the United States.

There are a variety of considerations in choosing a form of mobility and a variety of individuals who choose dog guides in terms of personal preference, physical abilities, and age.

There are many components of dog guide programs including selection and breeding of dogs, training of dogs, matching dog and master, the instructors, and training the student.

Finally, other aspects of dog guide schools that are important include philosophy and policy, and professional education and research.

Dog guides were the first formalized mobility aid for the blind in the United States and continue to be a valid alternative for some blind individuals.

Bibliography

American Kennel Club, *The complete dog book*. New York: Author, 1972.

Coon, N. *A brief history of dog guides for the blind*. Morristown, N.J.: The Seeing Eye, 1959.

Delafield, G. Adjustment to blindness. *New Outlook for the Blind*, 1976, **70**(2), 64-68.

Ebeling, W.H. The guide dog movement. In P. A. Zahl (Ed.) *Blindness: Modern approaches to the unseen environment*. Princeton, N.J.: Princeton University Press, 1950.

Eustis, D.H. The Seeing Eye. *Saturday Evening Post*, November 5, 1927.

Finestone, S., Lukoff, I., & Whiteman, M. *The demand for dog guides and the travel adjustment of blind persons.* New York: Research Center, New York School of Social Work, Columbia University, 1960.

Frank, M. & Clark, B. *First lady of The Seeing Eye.* New York: Henry Holt & Co., 1957.

Hartwell, D. *Dogs against darkness: The story of The Seeing Eye.* New York: Dodd Mead and Company, 1942. Revised and reprinted, 1960.

Humphrey, E., & Warner, L. *Working dogs.* Baltimore: The Johns Hopkins Press, 1934.

Klein, J.W. *Textbook for teaching the blind.* Wein, Germany: Anton Strauss, 1819.

Koestler, F. *The unseen minority.* New York: David McKay, 1976.

Latimer, H. *Dogs.* May, 1976

Pfaffenberger, C.J. *The new knowledge of dog behavior.* New York: Howell Book House, Inc., 1963.

Pfaffenberger, C.J., Scott, J.P., Fuller, J.L., Ginsburg, B.E., & Biefelt, S.W. *Guide dogs for the blind: Their selection, development, and training.* Amsterdam: Elsevier Scientific Publishing Company, 1976.

Pollack M. These kids raise puppies for the blind. *Saturday Evening Post,* July 24, 1954.

Putnam, P. *Keep your head up, Mr. Putnam!* New York: Harper & Brothers, 1952.

Putnam, P. *The triumph of The Seeing Eye.* New York: Harper & Row, 1963.

The Seeing Eye. *Annual report.* Morristown, N.J.: Author, 1974-75.

The Seeing Eye. Guide for dog selection. *The Seeing Eye Guide,* 1977, **43**(1).

The Seeing Eye, *A Seeing Eye policy.* Morristown, N.J.: Author, 1974.

The Seeing Eye. *A summary of legislation relating to travel with dog guides.* Morristown, N.J.: Author,1976.

Werntz, G., Jr. A living philosophy: Its significance to the agency serving blind persons. In I.S. Diamond (Ed.) *Blindness, 1967.* Washington, D.C.: American Association of Workers for the Blind, 1967.

Originators of Orientation and Mobility Training*

C. Warren Bledsoe

Only the personal is great.
            Disraeli.

During the Christmas holidays of 1786 the children from Valentin Hauy's infant school for the blind in Paris were entertained for eight days at the palace of Versailles by King Louis XVI and Queen Marie Antoinette (Ross, 1966). They played with the royal children and gave demonstrations of what they had learned to astonished royal adults. This included complicated arithmetical calculations done in the head without benefit of tactile aids to thought or memory. The exactitude of results learned were vouched for by the pen and ink calculations of the Duc D'Angouleme, of whom we have the word of his learned uncle Louis XVIII that he was a sharp-witted youth before the Revolution drove him into exile and idleness (Daudet, 1913).

PROLOGUE

This is the first we know of one of the more spectacular skills which was to become the stock in trade of educators of the blind down through the 19th century, eventually termed "rapid arithmetic" in curricula of schools for the blind. Classical education of the blind in those decades included a number of highly developed special arts and techniques, such as touch reading and writing, tumbling, chair caning, and piano playing and tuning, but general competence in living without sight was left to the ingenuity of blind people themselves. This included those functions to which are directed the teaching skill which is termed "orientation and mobility" and was termed during its crude and early beginnings, simple "foot travel."

Formal orientation and mobility training of blind people was first attempted on an organized basis in the United States by the founders of the dog guide school known as Seeing Eye, Inc. (Whitstock, Chapter 17). At that time the teaching of skills for living without sight had been in progress in this country for a century, guided originally by Dr. Samuel Gridley Howe, founder of the Perkins School for the Blind in 1832, whose broad-gauged genius permeated virtually every aspect of social progress from that year until his death in 1876.

Howe's nearest approach to anything resembling structured teaching of mobility was directed by one of his blind teachers during the 1860s. The teacher was Francis Campbell, who later was to emigrate to Britain and become the founder of the Royal Normal College and Academy of Music for the Blind in that kingdom, where he was naturalized and knighted in 1909 for his work as an educator of blind children and youth.

---

*An historical memoir of personal influences in the founding of orientation and mobility, in the writing of which the author has been greatly aided by reading *The Unseen Minority* by Frances A. Koestler. The historian who was there can have no better collaborator than the historian who was not.

Commenting on what he termed "bodily training" at the Perkins School, Howe said it had been carried through with "more or less rigor" as he had been "seconded by assistants who had more or less faith in it" (Howe, 1872). Thus, with his habitual astuteness he stated a principle which subsequently governed everyone who has had success in the teaching of orientation and mobility in this century. Such teachers have found that people have abounded and still abound who are without such faith. Howe went on to reinforce his statement by mentioning Campbell's "system of physical training . . . carried to a high perfection." This was, he said, a form of training which could only be maintained persistently by those who possessed great natural pluck and personal magnetism. He mentioned rowing and swimming and floor scrubbing. But he said nothing which implied, even indirectly, that orientation and mobility were taught as part of a curriculum and stated with unaccustomed resignation that in the absence of such an individual as Campbell, the exercises he had mentioned "fall into comparative neglect." In this also he noted a principle all too familiar to experienced workers for the blind. To promote true self management of blind people involves a never-ending effort. And this is not against inertia alone, for inertia in institutions can keep a thing going once it has gotten started whether it makes any sense or not. The effort combats something far more subtle and complex, a number of sensitivities which not only were to be revealed by the mobility teaching programs, but by resistance to those programs.

On this whole subject uninitiated members of society are often vocal in behalf of "a totally blind man I know who never had any lessons and does beautifully." And so indeed individuals have done down through the ages. The most noted of these was an Englishman named John Metcalf, who in the 18th century was a road builder and performed authenticated feats of getting about by himself on foot and on horseback, once guiding a sighted individual through a bog in dark of night. His doings were regarded by his contemporaries and by succeeding generations as little short of marvelous. To the present they are less so, for an old print shows he had a cane so long it was almost up to his hat. This instrument foreshadowed the principle on which one type of formal instruction was to be built when it finally arrived (Mannix, 1911).

Benign Surreptitiousness

That the long cane was not used earlier was perhaps due in part to what might be termed benign surreptitiousness, its rule being: In order to minimize the impact of blindness on others, do nothing that will make it clear to all that you are blind. This rule may also account for there having been no formal teaching. Those who claim that teachers of the blind have "always" taught orientation and mobility frequently end their protests by saying in effect that they thought at all costs it should be done unobtrusively, indeed in such a manner that the pupil hardly knew he was being taught. Few teachers now talk about such things, but Dr. Edward Allen, Director of the Perkins School (1907-1931), delivered a yearly lecture on what he termed "unconscious tuition" to the graduate students in the Harvard-Perkins course in special methods of teaching the blind.

One can hardly doubt that Campbell (who was extremely mobile himself with a moderately long cane) somehow taught his pupils mobility. His daughter-in-law, Mary Dranga Campbell, hearing an account of the orientation and mobility program of World War II, stated that it "resembled the work of my husband's father, Sir Francis Campbell." A journalist of the period, writing of Campbell's "faithful cane," said it "had brains, could almost talk, and ought to vote" (Willard, 1889).

That he was experimenting in the area of mobility during his Perkins days is revealed in an account of an inglorious mishap for which he was responsible. One of his detractors, Dennis Reardon, wrote of a rope procession which Campbell devised to enable students to go to the beach near the old Perkins School at South Boston. The rope was a long clothes line tied to a lot of broom handles some feet apart. One or two seeing leaders went first, 20 or more blind pupils holding onto handles and following.

The account goes on to say, "Well, one day the teacher who could see partially fell over a bank and brought all the others on top of him. Thereupon they all cast the whole contrivance into the water and left it there. The boys did it. It was he (Campbell) who put it in and we put it out" (Reardon, 1911).

Very much later at least one sophisticated orientation lesson was given by Campbell to a sighted individual. In the *Sunday School Chronicle* of July 8, 1909 he is quoted as saying: "The Duke of Westminster came to see the grounds" (of the Royal Normal College) "when I first planned them, and he told me that, instead of laying out a pleasure ground for my blind students, I had arranged so many death traps for them. But I blindfolded his lordship, and he found his way by signs all around the grounds and back to the house, and he left me a check for a thousand guineas as an expression of his delight at the provision which I had made for my students" (Campbell, 1909).

We may assume that Campbell carefully described the "signs" (present day mobility instructors would say landmarks) and that the Duke who was no ordinary duke was a good listener. Certainly this was the best paid orientation and mobility lesson in history in the days when not only was a guinea five dollars and a quarter, but a dollar was a dollar.

Early Teachers

It may be assumed that other teachers, especially those who were blind, did something in the way of teaching their pupils "signs." Parents also were sometimes adroit in this regard. The noted Italian blind educator of the blind, Augusto Romagnoli, wrote of his father: "He had no training, but at the same time he had not the prejudices of the professional teachers who often make mountains out of molehills. He loved me and made me share his own life. In the workshop I knew how to use the saw, the plane, and the compasses; anything that could not be touched he described to me in a few words. In the country, he taught me to walk beside him and to recognize by ear the proximity of a wall, a hedge, a tree or a ditch. He taught me to swim in the river when we bathed together. If there was a square to be crossed in a hurry, he made me cross it diagonally, explaining that the diagonal is the shortest way" (*Outlook for the Blind*, 1947).

Definitely American teachers in the early 1900s cannot be said to have "made mountains out of molehills" where mobility was concerned. Indeed they did just the opposite.

In 1910 Dr. Edward E. Allen, successor to Howe's successor at the Perkins School, made a survey visit to schools for the blind in Europe. Of German teachers of the blind he wrote: ". . . the German's 'thoroughness or nothing' principle appeared to me to fill and run over. . . . The possession by the blind of the faculty for recognizing objects by the four senses, and the ability to locate themselves at any and at all times in space and to get about readily alone, is deemed by the Germans a too vitally important one to be left to haphazard. We leave our pupils to pick up this sort of thing, and they generally seem to do so" (Allen, 1969).

Dr. Allen each year told his Harvard class that, "the care of the blind from the cradle to the grave," a concept he disapproved, was first said in German. It is significant that in what is the first reference to formal teaching of orientation and mobility in the old *Outlook for the Blind* he was so politely skeptical of a pioneer program of that type. He seems to have transposed Howe's "comparative neglect" to "constructive neglect." For no mobility program was established at Perkins during the ensuing two decades of Allen's administration. And as Perkins went, so went most other schools for the blind in those days.

During the past 43 years, and particularly the last 25, which have been a time of intensive work to develop training programs in orientation and mobility, there has been recurrent speculation about why such action was not taken before.

In this speculation sometimes the obvious is overlooked. For example, the controlled environment of residential schools and other agencies for the blind gave their educators a false sense of achievement. The controlled environment often extended beyond the immediate property of the school or agency to neighborhoods beyond. Trolley cars stopped at spots convenient for the blind pupils. Housewives were careful to keep trash cans and tricycles off sidewalks in adjacent streets. Gradually the institution extended its domain to the community about it, shaping the neighbors' ways to its needs. True, a little beyond that everything was quite different, but very often even the pupil—indeed especially the pupil—was deceived until he went to college or sought a job in an unfamiliar environment. Another factor frequently overlooked is the simple truth that traffic hazards of the days before yesterday were in no way comparable to those of late 20th century America. Vehicles were noisier; sound patterns less sophisticated.

Not so obvious an impediment to the development of mobility training was shyness on the part of sighted individuals at invading the unique preserves of blind people over the barrier, "You'll never know what it is to be blind." This was abetted by doubt on the part of blind people that by *looking* there could be any important observation about what was truly efficient for a blind person. Yet the techniques which depend on the cane when they finally arrived undoubtedly came from visual perception by Dr. Richard E. Hoover. In the 1800s W. Hanks Levy, the noted blind British authority on blindness, seems to have evolved something close to the Hoover methods, yet missed what was to be the most important item of all, that the cane should always touch in front of the trailing foot, rather than the forward foot (Levy, 1872). An observation after World War II of 337 veterans of blindness as well as war, revealed that only three had arrived at a realization that at least in dangerous places some such usage was prudent.

It would be false, however, to paint too bleak a picture of the blind of earlier decades. Very often indeed they got there on their own, sometimes with real skill, sometimes by the stumble and crash method, sometimes abetted by a little vision, frequently by the guidance of a sighted individual's elbow. Newell Perry, the noted California blind educator, managed to go all over the United States and Europe without regular guide or courier. Lord Kenswood, a visitor from Britain during the 1940s, mastered the use of public transportation in New York.

Late one night he alighted on an elevated platform at two in the morning and found himself totally alone.

"Ah," he said to himself, "I am on a high place. I must be careful. I prodded with my cane and felt something soft and pliable. Then it spoke, saying, 'I am blind drunk,' I said, 'I am blind, but I am not drunk. Let us help each other.' "

And they did.

Anecdotes such as that of Lord Kenswood on the elevated platform could be multiplied, for the good grace, capability, and humor of blind people of every age has been, and continues to be a far more reliable resource than is generally realized.

MRS. EUSTIS AND DR. HOOVER

Perhaps it is not too poetic or superstitious to say that the blind people of the

United States were awaiting the arrival upon the scene of two people equal to their needs: Dorothy Harrison Eustis, the mother of the dog guide movement, and Dr. Richard E. Hoover, the father of orientation and mobility with the cane.

Quite different individuals, they never met, although Mrs. Eustis's years in work for the blind overlapped those of Dr. Hoover. She was born in 1886 and died in 1946 two years after Hoover began his training in cane technique at Valley Forge Army General Hospital. At that juncture it is unlikely that they would have communicated very effectively, for in the beginning the dog and cane people saw little need for one another, as is not the case today.

One trait particularly may be noted in both, where blind people are concerned. This is irritation with workers for the blind who want to keep blind people in a prolonged state of gratitude for their rehabilitation. The work of both Mrs. Eustis and Dr. Hoover forever showed a keen desire to remove a lingering feeling of dependency after the cause of the dependency had become a thing of the past. Their greatest satisfaction was to encounter a blind individual using the methods they had devised. But it is unlikely that either was ever tempted to waylay a blind person and introduce him or herself as the inventor of the resource from which the blind person was benefiting. The inward sensitivity and respect for others which this betokens is as real as a cane or a dog. It was part of the open sesame which made it possible to develop acceptance of both dog and cane, and the professional descendants of Mrs. Eustis and Dr. Hoover have succeeded or failed in part because they have shared this sensitivity. But there was an equally important tangible factor in each case.

The most important consideration with respect to any invention is that of *work:* work in the sense of *performing,* if it is a pump, pump, if it is a light, light, and work in the sense of *serving the purpose for which it was designed,* pump enough water for the family or town, put enough light in the lighthouse to warn a ship off the reef. Hoover had always thought a key factor in getting his technique accepted was 300 enormously durable, 6-oz (168 g) canes of thin-walled steel, which toward the end of the war was given an A-1 priority in a steel factory by request of the Surgeon General of the Army.

As well as being practical, Mrs. Eustis and Dr. Hoover were also daring. They took chances which other people cursed, sometimes under their breath, sometimes more loudly, but the curses neither dismayed them nor stopped them. A group of workers for the blind whom Mrs. Eustis had called together to advise her with regard to the inauguration of dog guide training began to argue among themselves vociferously, yet more vociferously, and yet more vociferously. From the edge of the group she and her associates simply detached themselves and went into the hall (it has been said on tiptoe—but that does not sound like Mrs. Eustis), where they agreed that whereas they would be accountable for the success or failure of the venture, they would do it their way. Whereupon they departed from the scene and for many years had little or no association with workers for the blind.

Late in Mrs. Eustis's life an episode which highlighted her point of view and independence occurred when she was offered one of the distinguished service awards in the field of work for the blind. She quite seriously proposed that it be given instead to the dog guides of Seeing Eye, and quite seriously was incensed when this proposal was coldly declined.

Of an equally independent temperament Dr. Hoover as a sergeant in the Medical Corps was asked if it would be beneath the dignity of his mobility instructors to clean the wards.

He replied, "Aside from that, Colonel, they wouldn't have time to teach the blinded soldiers how to get around."

The colonel accepted what he said and promoted him.

When horseback riding was initiated in the War Blind Program another colonel opined that of course it would be necessary to keep the horses at a walk.

"No sir," said Sgt. Hoover, "we're going to start with men who have already ridden and canter the first day."

"But they're blind now," expostulated the Colonel.

"You don't ride with your eyes," said Sgt. Hoover, "you ride with your legs."

"You don't have to tell me," said the Colonel heatedly, "I foxhunt."

And the blind men cantered the first day.

Mrs. Eustis was a woman with an electric nature at the interesting age of 43 when she established Seeing Eye, Inc. in 1929, . . . a divorcee who was in command of the respectful devotion of four adherents, each a strong character in his own right. It would be hard to say which of these was the key figure, but certainly her first blind pupil was indispensable. He was Morris Frank, a Hotspur of a young man. The second key figure was the man who was eventually called "Uncle Willie" by Seeing Eye graduates. Willie Ebeling was a retired business man and dog fancier who was a perfect dynamo for channeling the electric personalities with whom he was associated. His personal advice to other sighted workers for the blind frequently included, "Don't try to be a big shot, and don't crystallize resistance." The third of Mrs. Harrison's associates was a geneticist named Jack Humphrey, who had such a way with animals that he was said to have taught a camel to back up (supposedly impossible) and to have housebroken a horse (thought to have been unlikely).

Arriving on the scene a little later was William Debetaz, a young man from a French canton of Switzerland. A man of abounding energy and native intelligence, he was to become a past master at the art of teaching both dogs and people.

Somewhat later arrivals (1934) were Mary Dranga Campbell and Elizabeth Hutchinson. Mrs. Campbell, a seasoned social worker and librarian, was a daughter-in-law of Sir Francis Campbell. Starting from this base, with a keen intellect she had developed a cold passion for excellence in work for the blind, had been almost everywhere and seen everything in the field. Her addition to the staff of Seeing Eye enabled Mrs. Eustis to maintain her own isolation from the field without losing sight of anything important it had to offer.

Miss Hutchinson had been trained as an occupational therapist. A woman of consummate good feeling, good manners, and common sense, she brought to a high state of effectiveness the social re-training of the clients in such matters as table etiquette, management of wardrobe, keeping track of possessions, those "weak" things of the world, which according to scripture "God has chosen to confound the mighty," and which can loom very large when blindness occurs (St. Paul, A.D. 57).

Before she activated Seeing Eye, Mrs. Eustis had been the founder of Fortunate Fields (see Chapter 17).

At this juncture it should be pointed out that as was the case with the training of children in orientation, German dog guide schools antedated the founding of Seeing Eye. Moreover, during the 1920s dog guides for the blind were an accepted resource for blind individuals in Germany. Over 4,000 were in use.

Dr. Gerhard Stalling, who had been a trainer of search dogs for the German Army during World War I, subsequently directed the opening of a school at Breslau where dogs were trained for the use of the blind. Breslau had long been a center of sophistication where blindness was concerned. In the early 1800s a school for the blind had been founded there by Johann G. Knie, a blind graduate of the University of Breslau, who was the first blind individual to be director of a residential school in Europe and a supreme realist about the senses through which blind children are educated. His school was described as a "melange of bells, rattles, drums, models of animals, machines, buildings," and he wrote a book entitled *A Guide to the Proper Management of Blind Children* which was said to have been "gospel reading" in the world of the blind in the last century (Ross, 1951). This educational realism may well account for the fact that German educators got so much of a head start on the United States in mobility, at least where the dog guides were concerned. Over-preoccupation with the amenities of not "looking blind" can very seriously forestall special use of the fingers and also the nose.

"I smell many people," said a young deaf blind pupil walking into a crowded room.

In the shocked hush of the group his wise teacher said with pioneering tact, "That's his way, folks. Be glad he can smell you."

VALLEY FORGE ARMY HOSPITAL

Social bolts of lightning are sometimes necessary in awakening tyros in work for the blind to the actualities of the situation. One in particular may be said to have set off the orientation and mobility program of Richard Hoover at Valley Forge Hospital.

Dr. James N. Greear, the eye chief at that hospital during World War II, was a past master at holding staff meetings. He had a special gift for putting everyone on one level.

Shortly after the Battle of the Bulge, newly blinded soldiers began to arrive in much greater numbers than they had previously. Seventeen came in one day, all of them much more recently wounded than any who had arrived previously. At the staff meeting that followed this development the staff maintained an exterior calm until close to the end of the meeting when the time came for the colonel to ask if any one had any more questions, but not expecting any more.

"I have an observation to make," said Roberta Wilson, then a social worker at the hospital. "These patients who have just come in to the hospital are a shattered group."

Discussion began all over again turning on the question of what the blinded soldiers needed most, but finally again led to a silence in the face of the large problem under consideration.

This silence was broken by the matter-of-fact voice of Richard Hoover who said, "I think the first thing they need is to know how to get around. We've been working on it, but not enough."

Then came the lightning.

"People say blind people in this country do a good job of getting around. I don't think they do a good job. I think they do a hell of a poor job."

To say that this was felt as an affront by the blind people in the room, both on their own behalf and for those who shared their handicap, would be a monstrous understatement. They ultimately forgave Hoover, became his believers, and one even became his pupil. But at the very time, as work for the blind had been shaped, and in view of what they had been led to believe about themselves, his words amounted to a crowning insult.

Fortunately they struck Col. Greear otherwise. Coming from an experienced teacher of the blind, they seemed to confirm what he had merely suspected, or at least hesitated to say, in his touchy role of ophthalmologist in charge of a program for the blind. He immediately re-opened the question of training the soldiers in what was termed "foot travel," decided to strike while the iron was hot, and, with Hoover and several officers in his wake, set out impromptu for the office of the commanding officer of the hospital.

This was Col. Henry Beuuwkes, a fine old gentleman, who had eagles on his shoulders, and everything handsome in the way of accoutrements about him, for which the blinded soldiers had no respect whatsoever. Indeed he had been through several painful scenes when blinded soldiers had actually gotten into his office and pounded on his desk with their canes, demanding to know what was going to be done with and for them.

Relieved to have something practical offered that afternoon, he forthwith put all he had learned in the way of military administration into following out a prescription which Sgt. Hoover offered, and which the eye chief endorsed. This was not merely training in foot travel with the cane, but a large number of specially chosen, highly qualified instructors, a sufficient number to spend hours and hours teaching on an individual basis.

To accomplish this, Col. Beuuwkes persuaded Major General Hayes to send Valley Forge Hospital panels of picked men, thirty at a time, from which the War Blind Service was allowed to choose "orientors." Regrettably the formula for this selection does not survive. However, it is reasonably certain that since Hoover had a hand in it, the words "common sense" found their way into whatever document was drawn up. Its product was a flow of excellent medical corpsmen whose very presence buoyed the atmosphere. This was the real beginning of what has been called "foot travel."

To avoid confusion, the term "orientation and mobility" will be used hereafter in this chapter, but this is a good place to say that the term was not common until the 1950s. Hoover and his associates adopted the term "foot travel" because it was believed that the term "orientation," which had previously been used, had gotten off to a sour start. "Foot travel" was chosen for its unpretentious, self-explanatory simplicity which it was hoped would be a point in its favor with the G.I.s. "Mobility" did not come into use until the initiation of a program at the Catholic Guild for the Blind after the war. It was at that agency the term "peripatology" was coined. The more sophisticated terms have accompanied the maturing of the art. The term "foot travel," however, was curiously appropriate to the almost Homeric atmosphere of Valley Forge.

The quality of the Valley Forge program was one of those paradoxes in human experience which those who shared in it find difficult to explain. Colonel Elliot Randolph, who succeeded Greear as eye chief, once shocked a roomful of Federal Security officials by saying that those who had worked on the war blind program at Valley Forge had had "fun." He himself was one of those lucky men to whom his work (ophthalmology) was "fun." This may well have been because he was always on the patient's side, not the kind ever to use his knife out of ambition or curiosity.

Despite many tragic factors which brought Valley Forge Hospital into existence, there is no doubt that it had about it an unaccountable "happy ship" quality. This has been described by Hoover himself in terms of the unusual talents of doctors and the community surrounding the hospital.

Other hospitals had somewhat similar resources, but did not have Hoover. He found a way not only to get the right men together to teach the soldiers, but knew how to handle both patients and corpsmen to get the best out of them. Also, by the time the selected panel of instructors came to the hospital, he had evolved both the idea of the light cane and the technique for making the most of it. This had come not only of observing with his eyes, but of blindfolding himself and experimenting, as have many of the gifted sighted pioneers, including Howe (Ross, 1951). It should be added that such pioneers are made of the stuff to ignore the protests of blind people who rush to tell them that they will never know what it is to be blind. But when results are good, the protesters forget they ever protested. Such was the case with respect to Hoover's system, but only after years of controversy.

RIVALRIES

Rivalries played their curious roles in the events which ultimately led to widespread acceptance of mobility training programs. The interested spectator from a good vantage point could not fail to observe what reminded him of a miniature war with a long series of skirmishes and battles. Animosities, affinities, egos, ids, and an occasional superego all played their parts. The intensity caused a good deal of comment among bystanders inexperienced in the ways of the human spirit consecrated to the improvement of life for blind people. To them it was unbelievable that there should be such heat for or against formal mobility training for the blind.

Part of the heat undoubtedly was generated by the fact that it was an impassioned time. The program began in a war and because of a war; a sort of holy war against Hitler, Mussolini, and the Japanese. This gave people who wore the uniform in those days a basic self-assurance for the time being with respect to their ways and doings. According to the law of the land, the war blinded until discharge belonged to the armed services.

Before they had lost their sight the word "belong" applied to them had carried no sinister connotation. But in the United States in this century as soon as you mention any blind person belonging to any agency whatsoever you are in trouble. Those who see blind people forever threatened by domination of the sighted are particularly sensitive on this point. At least one conversation between an ophthalmologist in uniform and the head of an agency for the blind got off to a bad start when the agency head told the ophthalmologist the blinded soldiers belonged to themselves. By World War II, work for the blind had reached such a point of strain on this subject that no one with any delicacy would use the term "belong," with regard to a client, in any sentence which could possibly be misconstrued.

But with World War II, lo and behold! here were some blind people who actually did *belong* to the Army, the Navy, and the Marine Corps. And deep down in their hearts workers for the blind felt the glamorous war blinded should belong to them from the moment they were blinded. It should be taken into account that the people involved were in fact dedicated people, and that they were not contending for the riches of the world, but for the tough job of helping blind people learn to deal with their blindness. There were a number of armed camps which had been working and reworking uneasy truces with each other over the decades.

In one camp was the American Foundation for the Blind, commanded by its executive director, Dr. Robert Irwin, the champion of public school education for the blind. In the U.S. Office of Education was another camp commanded by Joseph Clunk, the architect of the national program of vocational placement of the blind, then in its infancy. In the education field Dr. Gabriel Farrell of the Perkins School had his camp, and Dr. Merle Frampton, principle of the New York Institute for the Blind, another. Farrell regarded Frampton as an archrival, Irwin regarded Frampton as an archenemy. A novice in work for the blind, though not at wheeling and dealing, Frampton was a long term stormy petrel, an impassioned promoter of residential schools, sometimes called the Admiral Rickover of work for the blind.

This was not the end of the personality clashes among the influential. Irwin and Joseph Clunk turned deaf ears to each other. For two decades Irwin had been cultivating the Foundation's position of national leadership, and lately Clunk had been speaking for the blind of the nation from his ranking position in the federal government. Clunk had hopes that Congress would bestow the program for the rehabilitation of veterans on his office. This was a disturbing thought to Irwin.

There was, however, a rather loose-jointed confederation of opinion in the various camps which occupied the field, and there was one subject on which nearly everyone agreed. It was outrageous that the cream of challenges to their skill, the war blinded, should be where they could not be got at immediately and taken in hand by experienced practitioners. Indignation over this was heightened by the fact that, as in other wars, the Surgeon General of the Army had made ophthalmologists responsible for the rehabilitation of the war blinded, and the field of work for the blind had been telling itself for two decades that ophthalmologists had made the war blind program of World War I a disaster.

This had been said so often that even the people who did not believe it had given up putting in a word to the contrary, except to say the World War I program had forced the field to take a look at how it was organized nationally. This had produced a brief era of rare harmony during which the American Association of Workers for the Blind had joined forces with the American Association of Instructors of the Blind to found "a national clearing house for problems of the blind," and for this purpose established the American Foundation for the Blind.

When war clouds gathered in the early part of 1940, certainly it was time for another era of rare harmony, and at first it appeared one might ensue. With professional aplomb the American Association of Workers for the Blind had appointed Irwin chairman of a distinguished committee to advise the government about the "Care, Training and After Care of Persons Becoming Blind as a Result of the United States Defense Program and Possible Participation in the Present World War."

Responsibility

Frances Koestler in *The Unseen Minority* describes how the committee went about its business sagaciously, issued a public warning against exploitation of the war blind, favoring the federal government's assumption of responsibility for the rehabilitation of the war blinded and, when Congress placed the responsibility with the Veterans Administration (VA), offered a clearcut plan for rehabilitation which theoretically could fit into the framework of Public Law 78-16, which authorized the VA to provide rehabilitation for disabled veterans.

But very shortly Irwin was writing, "We have complications, growing out of the fact that the Veterans Administration, which is responsible for the rehabilitation of disabled veterans, has no jurisdiction over the men until they are discharged from the Army. Blinded men who may be kept in hospitals for months are under the Surgeon General of the Army or of the Navy" (Koestler, 1976).

For the orientation and mobility program this was a godsend. Not a single leader in the field at that time would have backed Hoover's teaching the way Col. Greear did. The only one who came anywhere near having the connections and nerve to ask for so much manpower was Dr. Frampton. He had stolen a march on everyone and had himself put in charge of the Navy's program for rehabilitation of the handicapped at Philadelphia Naval Hospital. Yet visiting Valley Forge Hospital, he viewed the mobility training, and showed no sign of being impressed. In this he was no different from most other heads of agencies for the blind in the 1940s.

For a time one of the major points at issue between the Army and its critics, especially in the Office of Vocational Rehabilitation, was the emphasis put on orientation and mobility, and taught by sighted instructors!

It is strange to think in retrospect that many very fine leaders of the blind should have objected to the practice, still thinking as did Dr. Allen that the blind were best left to "pick up" mobility "on their own." (With perhaps a few pointers from some experienced blind person.) To be too hard on them for this would be equally benighted. Even the workers for the blind who had seen the war blinded of World War I had not seen what the staff at Valley Forge saw, soldiers flown back to the

States within a few days of being abruptly and completely blinded. One of their few advantages was that they knew nothing about being blind and knew that they knew nothing, and were therefore amenable to early training as no large group of blind people had ever been before.

The numbers and situation of the war blinded not only produced the setting for simple experimentation and the organization of method. The needs of the men made them willing to submit to them. It was strange and ironic that as it was being developed, a systematic approach to problems of blindness was criticized as the "army way" of doing things, which of course meant ineptly. Indeed certain prominent state directors, some of whom were blind, "dug in" and were little fortresses against such practices until death or retirement parted them from the field. It should be said in fairness, however, that many of them had neither the experience nor the connections to obtain a clear idea of what was going on inside the service programs.

A good deal of confusion existed at the time, and continues in retrospect, over how the three army hospitals for the war blinded differed. Their differences were in theory quite clearcut, but practicalities blurred them. Valley Forge Army General Hospital at Phoenixville, Pennsylvania, and Dibble Army General Hospital at Menlo Park, California, were designated early in the war as centers for eye care, Valley Forge to serve eye casualties from the European Theater of Operations, Dibble those from the Pacific Theater. The need for giving them basic rehabilitation while in the hospital was almost immediately apparent, since many of them had disabilities which necessitated long-term hospitalization. Both programs grew by leaps and bounds through necessity, and many observers thought that no other installation for the blind was needed, although the committee Irwin had headed called for a rehabilitation center. Public Law 78-16 indicated that such a center should be operated by the VA.

The VA, however, was reluctant to involve itself. Its administrator, General Frank T. Hines, was against such a center on principle, based on his personal experience with the program for the war blinded of World War I. According to Dr. Irwin, it had been "a headache, and all the VA officials were a bit leery . . ." (Koestler, 1976). General Hines and his assistants were even more leery of various agencies for the blind, which began to make plays for a contract to operate such a center, funded by the VA. This possibility was deeply disturbing to those who believed that the rehabilitation of the war blinded must be shouldered by the federal government. Such harmony as there had been on that subject was at an end. Opposing forces neutralized each other in conversations with VA officials, leaving them even more reluctant to run a rehabilitation center.

Meanwhile one agency was not in a position to wait on indecision and debate. This was the Army, which had a sizeable number of eye casualties, some of whom had become the "war blinded" by late 1943, and were clamoring to be discharged from the service with or without rehabilitation.

AVON

The situation was taken in hand by Col. Derrick T. Vail, chief consultant in ophthalmology in the European Theater of Operations. He had exactly the temperament and capabilities the deadlock demanded. He was a very impatient man, very intelligent, had an impregnable reputation as a professor of ophthalmology at Northwestern University, and he stood in awe of no one. He came back from Europe to push for a center for the war blinded, and when he found the VA unwilling to budge, before anyone knew quite what was happening, he had persuaded the Surgeon General's office to assume responsibility for operating it. President Roosevelt signed an agreement authorizing the Army to operate a center.

591

Other signatories were the Secretary of War, the Secretary of the Navy, the Chairman of the War Man Power Commission and the Adminstrator of Veterans Affairs.

Thus the program at Avon, Connecticut came into existence. In time it was to receive almost as much criticism as had the War Blind Program of World War I. Its stated purpose was the social adjustment of the war blinded prior to discharge from the service. This was to include "mental adjustment as may be necessary to develop a proper attitude and a will to overcome the handicap" (Koestler, 1976). The staff at Avon took on this awesome charge with gusto, but there were certain immediate realities which hampered them from the start. The last program to be activated, it served trainees many of whom had spent long months at one of the two general hospitals and often felt rightly or wrongly they had learned to manage their blindness. It was a moot question, moreover, from the beginning whether any lasting "adjustment" to blindness would take place before the men were out of uniform and while still at Avon.

Avon was like no setting most of the men had ever encountered before, or were ever likely to encounter again. A masterpiece of medieval academic architecture, idyllic, on a 2,000 acre estate, it would have offered the mystic or scholar an ideal retreat in which to while away eternity. But it was not ideal as a launching pad back to common daily living in the United States. Dr. Vail, while in England, had been exposed to the world-renowned, British war blinded institution, St. Dunstan's. He saw its American counterpart in Avon, but he was soon to discover the British model required very drastic modification to meet American concepts of rehabilitation. St. Dunstan's was monolithic, paternal, and there was not the slightest chance the American G.I.s would allow such an institution to be built around them.

It is a natural goal of virtually every severely handicapped American to mingle with the world. Certainly this was part of the philosophy of President Roosevelt, whose authorization of the Avon program limited the stay of the blinded service man to eighteen weeks. At the end of this time he would be discharged from the service. His further rehabilitation training and treatment would be provided by the VA, preferably in programs with the sighted. He could also if he chose elope from rehabilitative programs and institutions forever.

Avon's defenders, of whom there were a number, claimed that this was what they were promoting, but at least in one area their program took an unfortunate course toward that end. The training officer made the serious mistake of failing to recognize Hoover's work in orientation and mobility. Going even further, the Avon program espoused an old legend that a cane was unnecessary and insisted that trainees discard their canes on arrival at the installation.

In actual fact, to get about the premises of Avon without a cane was no great accomplishment. Its uneven floors and passageways offered many orientation cues, but more significantly it was a controlled environment, as much as any residential school for the blind. In lieu of cane training Avon invested heavy belief in the ability to detect obstacles through the sensation which has rather fancifully been called "facial vision," but which present day mobility experts term "obstacle perception." This phenomenon has been demonstrated to be associated with hearing. Objects intercept sound waves and this absence of sound transfers itself to an illusion of cutaneous sensation.

More than the program at Valley Forge, the program at Avon was a program of entrepreneurs, who had somehow convinced themselves that teachers of the blind had been too steeped in tradition to exploit a God-given radar, available to blind people for the tuning in. This was in total disregard of common knowledge of the experienced—that "facial vision" only works for certain individuals, better on days when they are feeling well, that it is just not as reliable as touching an object with a cane and never, never warns of objects below the knees or drop-offs such as curbs or the Grand Canyon.

With wasted fortitude, therefore, the Avon program undertook to persuade the blinded service men to dispense with their canes altogether, or if not that, to use them minimally away from Avon. Moreover, having considerable influence with the Surgeon General's office, for a time Avon personnel were able to convince the chief consulting ophthalmologist that this was correct policy and that it should prevail at Dibble Hospital.

At Avon the policy gave way in the face of opposition from the blinded soldiers themselves. This came to a head when the uses of "facial vision" were exalted beyond measure in a *Saturday Evening Post* article "They Learn to See at Avon Old Farms." Several hundred copies of the magazine lay unbought upon the counter of the Post Exchange at Avon, a grim admonition from the blinded soldiers. Those in charge of the program took the hint, and modified their position to the extent of having some token advanced cane training in downtown Hartford. This was hardly more than a gesture, but it accompanied an increased realization both at Valley Forge and the Surgeon General's office that Hoover's method was valid. As a result, in the summer of 1945 the Surgeon General's office dispatched an orientor from Valley Forge to Dibble to teach the cane method.

DIBBLE ARMY HOSPITAL

The Hoover method could hardly have been taken to a more unfriendly environment. Reliance on obstacle perception was virtually the religion of the staff, antedating the establishment of the Avon program. The anti-cane doctrine had been accepted as gospel by the eye chief, Colonel Norman Cutler, a brilliant ophthalmologist, whose responsibility for rehabilitation of the blind had been thrust upon him in the fortunes of war. He had quite naturally and sincerely begun by relying on the advice of his staff, confirmed by the sanction of the Surgeon General's office. However, following a visit to Valley Forge, he had begun to have doubts. After the *Saturday Evening Post* fiasco, he struck his colors and asked for a Valley Forge orientor to teach his staff the cane method.

When the Valley Forge orientor arrived at Dibble, the Colonel was much bedeviled by his blind staff members. Having heard it was correct practice to hire the visually handicapped, he had hired a number in quick succession, only to find that each thought he or she should be in charge of the program. All were unalterably opposed to the teaching of mobility as it was going forward at Valley Forge Hospital.

The Colonel also had on his hands a cadre of sighted instructors, not particularly well screened as they had been at Valley Forge. The blind staff had shown little inclination to share with them the facts of living as blind persons.

In conference with the Valley Forge instructor, they complained that one or more blind members of the staff had a habit of coming behind them, while they were in dealings with a blind soldier, and telling him he didn't have to do anything sighted people told him to do. This, they said, made teaching by facial vision uphill work. The Colonel himself had entered on his duties with a relatively fresh point of view toward the integrating of blind people into society. But he confessed to the Valley Forge instructor that he wondered if he should not persuade some of his wealthy friends to endow an institution like St. Dunstan's for their lifelong care.

By all this the blinded soldiers were relatively undamaged because of the mother wit God gave them. However, one of them had sat next to a congressman on a train and raised a curtain on the goings-on at Dibble as he had experienced them. The congressman had broken a story about this in the newspapers, and this was one of the factors which had led Dibble to seek help from Valley Forge.

For two months the Valley Forge mobility instructor gave lessons under the blindfold to the sighted corpsmen of Dibble. He also chose one soldier to teach. And one of the blind staff members did indeed shadow these lessons with some heart-to-heart talks, the nature of which could only be surmised. The blind soldier, a Kansan, did all that was expected of him, was competent with the cane, but kept his own counsel about his long term intentions with regard to the mode of foot travel he would use. On this subject there were conflicting reports in after years.

Simultaneously with the Kansan's training, the head mobility instructor at Dibble undertook to train a blinded soldier by the obstacle perception method for comparison with the cane method. This was a very impressive performance, which at least made the two instructors friendly journeymen in their trade. It is a curious fact, however, that several years after the war the Valley Forge instructor met the soldier (now a veteran) who had been trained by the Dibble method and discovered that the obstacle perception lessons had totally faded from his memory. This might seem to betoken the perfect job of rehabilitation which leaves no dependency whatsoever, had not the veteran in the intervening years adopted the use of a rather inadequate cane and technique for using it.

The war ended during the second month of the Valley Forge instructor's assignment to Dibble, and relatively little time remained for a program of training with the cane to develop momentum. George Gillispie, presently Chief of Service for the Blind in the central office of the VA, was a patient at Dibble at the time. He was given the task of showing the Valley Forge instructor what could be accomplished by the Dibble method. This he did extremely well. However, he now reports that he was given some lessons with the cane before leaving the hospital and that after leaving he paid for a course of lessons with the cane and has used one ever since.

The manner in which the Valley Forge method was received at Dibble Hospital was prophetic of the reception which was to greet subsequent efforts to offer it to the field, giving those who were interested in promoting it an inkling of what might be expected from the adult blind of the United States who had grown up in the school of hard knocks, won their way on their own and were proud of it. Both extremely hot and chillingly cold opposition came not merely from blind people who went without canes. One of the least sympathetic ridiculers of the Hoover method was the admirable, redoubtable cane user, Joseph Clunk. Wearing well-earned laurels for getting the federal program of vocational rehabilitation of the blind under way, he himself was a totally blind individual who could get anywhere he wanted to go, and he was absolutely dedicated to the cause of the blind. But he was very jealous of the prerogatives of blind individuals, and increasingly as the years went by could hardly bear to think of a sighted person having any say about the working of his program. His style early alienated him from doctors in charge of the war blinded, who kept him at arm's length. Offended at this, he regarded it as a real impertinence that foot travel was being taught to blinded soldiers by Hoover and his sighted helpers, including the author of this chapter.

Hitherto it has not seemed important in this narrative to say it was I who was the Valley Forge instructor at Dibble Hospital. However, the editors of this book have suggested that I must find some way of backing up my account of persons and scenes by identifying myself and the role I played in the evolving program of orientation and mobility. And I feel no compulsion in my retirement to withhold any of my experiences which may be of use to those who are now more active.

A CONGENITAL WORKER FOR THE BLIND

One of the most important of those experiences was being the son of my father, John Francis Bledsoe. He was just at the point of retirement when World War II came, having had a long career as an educator of the handicapped (1893-1941). As a young man, he had studied at the Harvard graduate school of education under Michael Anagnos, who had also taught principles of education of the handicapped to Anne Sullivan (Macy). With Anagnos my father read in the archives of the Perkins School, especially the theories of Samuel Gridley Howe. He was made superintendent of the Maryland School for the Blind in 1906 and immediately set about reorganizing it and rebuilding it according to Howe's "cottage family plan." The purpose of this was to make friends of teachers and pupils, give the pupils constant social acceptance and training and de-institutionalize the school. For many years it was a model for educators updating their systems. In the war years he was perhaps the most venerable figure in the field of work for the blind, whose good will was sought by such diverse personages as Irwin, Farrell, and Frampton.

Thus I inherited some influence in work for the blind from my father. During World War II, I tried to put it to use, as had my father, for the good of the blind. And it is only fair I should give my version of what it did and how it worked.

A Transfer

The first evidence I had that I might have some force in the war blind program came in a letter, which I received in 1944 when I was a sergeant in the Air Force. It came from Major M.E. Randolph, Chief of the Ophthalmology Branch in the Office of the Surgeon General. It was a gracefully worded invitation to acquiesce in a transfer from the Air Force to the War Blind Program.

I had no doubt this letter was written more to my father's son than to me. Dr. Randolph had conversed with him and discovered, I think, that they had similar views on life and work.

Among other things Dr. Randolph was seeking the names of workers for the blind in the Army, in order to secure their transfers to his program. My father gave Dr. Randolph my address, but discouraged him from arranging the transfer in my case, because be felt his influence had unconsciously worked beyond its due to draw me into work for the blind. I was out and away, having just published a novel before going into the Air Corps, was working in a public relations office, was getting articles published in *Yank,* and my father was enjoying the fact that I was doing things on my own. He also was human enough to hope I could be kept out of the brewing squabbles over the war blinded, his experience with such contention having been the part of his work which he had enjoyed least. In actual fact I had grown more interested in work for the blind than either of us had expected, particularly in the squabbles and what caused them.

A Teacher

When I graduated from Princeton in 1934, my father had rather cautiously and temporarily allowed me a teaching job at the Maryland School for the Blind. He was not averse to giving members of the family employment if he could get them at a good price. It was common practice in the past for schools for the blind. But he made it clear I must be out and away on my own in a reasonable time. In the meantime I had four very happy years coaching dramatics and teaching English as part of a superlative faculty.

One of my father's most fortunate professional accomplishments was the recruitment of Richard Hoover as mathematics teacher and athletic coach the school year of 1938-9, during which I was away taking the Harvard course of special education of the blind. On my return Hoover and I got to know each other. It would be hard to overestimate the importance of the experience Hoover had with blindness in the setting of the school. He was with blind boys around the clock, living in the cottage with them, eating meals with them, teaching them and coaching term in athletics.

But at the school, as in every other school for the blind in the United States, we did not teach mobility, nor did it then appear necessary on a hundred acres of controlled environment in which the pupils spent as much as twelve years.

A lifetime in and around work for the blind was only half of my preparation for the war blind program. Equally important were two years of picaresque adventures in the Army after war broke out. As an enlisted man I found out at first hand something about soldiers, from whose lips I learned to appreciate the beauty and force of bad grammar, spoken by experts.

I at least learned enough about the Army to know what to do when I received Dr. Randolph's letter. I wrote to him immediately saying I was agreeable to the transfer. In about a month I received orders transferring me to Valley Forge Hospital.

On my train journey from Alabama to Pennsylvania I read in the newspapers that for the first time an enlisted man was being transferred from the higher priority Air Corps to the lower ranking Medical Corps. As the Air Corps had until them been the next thing to holy when demanding personnel, this gave me an inkling of the authority which had been generated in behalf of the war blinded. Afterwards I learned from Dr. Randolph that he had invoked Lt. General George H. Brett, commanding general of the Caribbean Air Force to get the transfer accomplished.

THE USE OF INFLUENCE

Here, if my self-revelation is to have any value at all, it is important that I give some personal experience and views with regard to the use of influence. Though I had not discussed my transfer at Craig Field, I had talked with some of my friends in work for the blind when on leave in Baltimore.

"Don't take it," said a surprising number of them, "unless they make you a _____." (Here various ranks above captain were mentioned.)

I was amazed at the naivete of these suggestions both about the Army and influence where programs for blind people are concerned. You may be able to do that kind of bargaining where atomic physics is concerned. But any confidence man would have known this would be the sure way to lose the ears of perplexed officials who were seeking guidance in so delicate a side of the national catastrophe as blindness. It was also obvious in the situation described in Dr. Randolph's letter, as new and strange to me as to everyone else, the place to start was as near the bottom as possible and at the the operating level.

It so happened that in the Valley Forge war blind program, when I was first assigned to it, rank was almost a disadvantage. The chief of the eye service, Lt. Col. James N. Greear, was far more eager to pick the brains of his non-commissioned specialists on blindness than his commissioned ophthalmologists. He listened to both Hoover and me, but better to Hoover, which I early detected, and from then on depended on Hoover to pass on my ideas to the Colonel or not, as he saw fit. He had arrived at Valley Forge before me, already absorbed a great deal of information about what had been done up until then, and had sized up the personalities involved shrewdly.

One of the the first things Hoover and I had to get straight between us was what we thought of the budding fascination with obstacle perception. We gave it secondary rating. That was done together. I recall exactly when. In his open-minded way Hoover was giving it every opportunity in a long discussion we were having in a restaurant after all the patrons were gone. He said one of the authorities on obstacle perception would claim that an individual trained by the facial vision method could make his way through that room full of jumbled chairs without touching one. The chairs were hardly waist high.

I said this went against everything I had ever seen, and he had ever seen.

He said, "You're right. We're going to have to use canes."

The next day he blindfolded himself and started working on his cane technique. I did not perceive what he did about its use until he went over it a number of times, as he was afterwards to do with hundreds of others, both sighted and blind. I did not see the advantage of the light cane until he explained it to me. Nor did I have anything to do with its manufacture, which, according to legend, he arranged by getting somebody to stop making part of a battleship for half an afternoon. However, when he had gotten the practicalities in hand, I learned to teach his technique, and taught it to the soldiers at Valley Forge. I also shared in teaching it to new instructors and gave several classes of them basic indoctrination in the ways of work for the blind before going out to Dibble Hospital.

Attitudes

One knotty question which we had to deal with early in our efforts was the extent to which you can train sighted people to be more graceful and considerate in their dealings with the blind. We found that you can, and there is very little doubt that our attention to this was one of the things which gave the Valley Forge program its happy ship quality. One of the tools we used in training the instructors was a short etiquette pamphlet, which spiced its message with a certain amount of surgical humor.

This was the forerunner of subsequent leaflets on guiding in which I had a hand at the VA and other agencies.

Colonel Greear was a staunch supporter of everything Hoover did, as was Col. Randolph later when he came to Valley Forge as chief of the eye service. Randolph's return to the role of physician and surgeon in the eye service there was a reward for yeoman service warding off axe grinders in the Surgeon General's office. It was not easy to tell them from the good citizens who could also be trying, at times, in their own way. Eventually the Surgeon General's office concluded that the best course was to pay formal attention to this latter category, who in many ways resembled the "hard core altruists" of the Harvard sociobiologist, Edward O. Wilson (Wilson, 1978).

Two such staunch souls were Dr. Irwin and Dr. Farrell. Irwin loathed all residential schools for the blind, based on a childhood aversion to the manure pile next to the athletic field at the Washington School for the Blind, where he had been a pupil. He had, nonetheless, managed to overcome this aversion to the extent of making friends with Farrell, who was a member of his board at the American Foundation for the Blind.

Though director of the Perkins School, Farrell was far from a dyed-in-the-wool residential school man. Having been appointed to his job with no experience whatsoever in work for the blind (he had been a canon in the Episcopal Church, was a scholar, publicist, and organizer), he wore the scars of welcoming scorn from old timers in the field. But he wore them stoically, having managed to master his job, as he put it, by giving Perkins an organization, which it badly needed. By 1942 he was, on the whole, objective about subjects in work for the blind (with the exception of Dr. Frampton), and he had a sense of responsibility which went beyond his immediate domain, as is a tradition with directors of the Perkins School.

Correctly or incorrectly Irwin and Farrell regarded Avon as an extension of Frampton's power because its training officer, Capt. Blackburn, had once worked at Frampton's New York Institute.

Farrell had briefly aspired to be put in charge of the Army program as Frampton was of the Navy program, and when this did not materialize, he took up the role of *éminence grise*, joining forces with Irwin to influence the federal government at the highest possible levels.

Before he had become director of the Perkins School, Farrell had been a clergyman too, and had the ear of Laura Delano, President Roosevelt's cousin, who was in the special confidence of the President, was in fact one of those in the room with him when he died. By managing this pipeline to the top prudently, Farrell gained entry to the programs for the war blinded.

At Valley Forge, Farrell was one of the first heads of a residential school to see an orientation and mobility lesson given, becoming thereby one of the first civilian workers for the blind to say kind words about it.

Undoubtedly it did not hurt the cause of the cane with Farrell that Avon had foolishly attempted to close its doors to him, and when he had to be admitted, kept what he dryly called a "bodyguard" with him when he went about. At Valley Forge he was much freer. I had gotten to know him quite well during the year I spent taking the Harvard course at Perkins, and he looked me up and aired his dissatisfactions with the war blinded program, telling me he was thinking very seriously of taking his views to the President through Miss Delano. I told him that I thought instead he should attempt to find out more about what the Army was trying to do, that I thought he could accomplish much more by making friends with the ophthalmologists and that Hoover's work was so valuable it should be a part of the Perkins program after the war. He nodded, but did not give himself away as to his intentions. I reported this conversation to Col. Greear, who took it with some irritation. I also told him I had heard there was a movement afoot to get the Surgeon General to appoint a citizens advisory committee on the war blinded and from my experience such a committee would be a good means of explaining the Army's good points to the field of work for the blind, which could not be ignored forever. He did not say "aye, yes, or nay." But not too long after that the committee was appointed and Farrell was made a member of it. It was almost a disaster.

Citizens Advisory Committee

The brainchild of Irwin, who chose its membership, included blue ribbon men and women. It was especially well laden with shining examples of successful blind people: Irwin himself, Philip Harrison, a World War I blinded veteran, who was head of the Pennsylvania program for the civilian blind, Peter Salmon, whose strong points were low vision and diplomacy, and at least one international status figure, Col. Edward Baker, in charge of Canada's blind program. The executives from agencies included at least two who had been hewers, haulers, fetchers, and carriers in their youth (Eber Palmer of the Batavia School for the Blind and Dr. Richard French of the California School). There was even that very necessary ingredient, the stormy petrel or radical, Father Thomas J. Carroll of the Catholic Guild for the Blind in Boston, pro tem chaplain at Avon.

The first meeting of the committee could hardly have had a more inauspicious beginning. Dr. Derrick Vail, who spoke for the Surgeon General, began by scolding the committee for interagency rivalries and lack of cooperation with the Army (Koestler, 1976). He was particularly irritated that Frampton had flatly refused to honor the Navy's commitment to make use of the program at Avon and made his refusal stick by invoking the influence of his friend Admiral Ross

McIntyre, the President's physician. Dr. Vail was unaware that the members of the committee he was addressing, which included Irwin and Farrell, to a man or woman were hardly on bowing terms with Frampton. None had the slightest influence with him, nor cared to. Years later Vail told me ruefully he afterwards learned it was one of his brother ophthalmologists, Dr. Norbert Wiener, who had innocently encouraged the Navy's high ranking officers to take their wayward course with respect to Avon.

Nevertheless, Vail was right in thinking the committee had some negative views about the Army program, based not alone on vague rumors, but reports of a highly qualified emissary of Irwin's.

MISS GRUBER

Dr. Irwin never made the mistake of thinking he could get along without extensive vicarious use of eyesight, and for several months before the committee met he had had one of his representatives looking at the program of the war blinded. Early in 1945 he had appointed Kathern Gruber as director of the War Blind Service of the American Foundation for the Blind.

When he engaged her he wrote, "I am not quite sure what is needed. For quite a while your job is to find out what the government is not doing and why not. You can then accumulate the facts which we can lay before the proper government officials and get things going the right way" (Koestler, 1976).

Events were to show that Irwin's talents were at his best when he employed Kathern Gruber, but very soon he began to wonder if he had gotten more than he bargained for by saying to one of his assistants, "Miss Gruber would give the Foundation to those boys, and I love her for it, but you hold her down."

Moving into the war blinded scene, she was not merely an arresting and charming personality. She had brains and was a power in her own right by force of her overwhelming energy and absolute concentration on the good of the blinded service men. She was a seasoned professional in education of the blind, having been a resource teacher for blind pupils in the Minneapolis public schools, for whom she had managed to get summer jobs in the impossible job market of the depression.

Looking like a European queen in exile, she made her appearance at all the military hospitals where there were blinded military personnel. Elegant yet durable in war worn conveyances and inns, she made friends wherever she went, but no one in those days ever called her by her first name. She was "Miss Gruber," so much a part of the war blinded years by that appellation that even those of us belonging to her own generation who have known her a long time have difficulty remembering to call her "Kay."

Helen Keller was at the time the Foundation's international representative, and she opened Miss Gruber's way into the military hospitals by paying visits to them first, explaining that Miss Gruber was to follow. Miss Gruber when she arrived had with her a notebook which sopped up information like a sponge. And if a blinded soldier, sailor, or marine had a need nobody knew how to deal with, she was sure to get wind of it, after which she would not rest, nor let others rest until a remedy had been found.

On her first visit to Valley Forge she saw the importance of the orientation and mobility program there, in the promotion of which she was to take a leading role. To start with, she described it to Irwin, persuaded him to keep an open mind on the subject, and finally give it active support. Also, she was highly effective in giving Irwin the information he needed to fence with the Surgeon General's representatives and make the citizens advisory committee effective, for despite its bad beginning the committee went into action successfully. This was due in large part to the discerning participation of Father Carroll, of whom she had made a friend, and whom she introduced to Irwin.

FATHER CARROLL

Much has been written about Father Carroll. Frances Koestler (1976) describes him at the time of World War II as a "tall, Hollywood handsome young cleric endowed with a logical mind, a fighting spirit, and so deep a capacity for empathy with problems of blindness that the men in the rehabilitation centers fondly called him 'Father Tom,' while others, disregarding the fact that he was sighted, spoke of him as 'the blind priest.' "

Father Carroll had entered work for the blind at the command of the Church. He often told of standing in a line of newly ordained priests and experiencing the quality of trauma he associated with loss of eyesight when he was assigned to the Catholic Guild for the Blind. A great parish priest was lost when he was assigned to the Guild. But the blind people of the United States acquired a priest who spent his life trying to serve them. Ecumenized long before the time of Pope John, Father Carroll was the deadly enemy of sanctimonious pity for blind people. He worked very hard at his job at the Guild, and he also burned the midnight oil studying blindness in all its phases. These lucubrations he was fond of calling "typhlology" after the definition in the Oxford Dictionary—"the science that deals with blindness." For years he wrote and re-wrote his careful book, *Blindness: What It Is, What It Does, and What To Do About It.*

An intense, not very pleased young man in the Avon days, his Irish sense of humor mellowed as the years went on, but he never lost his basic intensity, and in his later years kept a plain wooden coffin in his study, which his devoted secretary did her best to disguise as a couch. His spirit asserted itself in a tiny rugged cross which he left to be put in his hand when he was dead. On it was inscribed, "Everything must be built new."

When Irwin had him appointed to the Surgeon General's advisory committee, he became the driving force that would not let the committee be blocked from effectiveness by courtesy and protocol. He had been at the grass roots as Avon's chaplain, and he was armed with facts. To some extent he had Vail's confidence, in part because he was clearly in favor of the Avon program, and indeed of continuing some form of federally controlled center for the war blinded after the war, a concept to which Vail was deeply committed.

Father Carroll persuaded Irwin and Vail to arrange for three members of the committee to visit and inspect the Army installations for the war blinded, and also persuaded the committee to accept their invitations to go. The three were very well chosen: Peter J. Salmon, whose Industrial Home for the Blind was a model for agencies of its kind; Mrs. Lee Johnston, executive director of the Missouri Commission for the Blind, who had managed to make peace between social work and rehabilitation in her state; and Henry P. Johnson, executive director of the Florida Council for the Blind.

These solid citizens came back with a report which mollified Vail by its understanding of what the Army was trying to do. At the same time Peter Salmon, who was noted for being able to put plain facts in acceptable terms, pointed out that the Army program was alienating the war blinded from civilian organized work for the blind on whom they might one day need to depend. He also admonished those who were in charge of the vocational training program at Avon for building "grandiose hopes."

Neither Father Carroll nor Vail wholly agreed with this latter criticism, but a new climate for exchange of opinions had been generated, and the committee was invited to make a second visit to the installations early in 1946. This they did, but to discover an entirely new set of problems, because with the war over, it was now in the wind that the Army was about to divest itself of all its programs for the war blinded. This was concomitant with a widespread determination to reform the VA and force the agency to face up to its responsibilities. Toward this end, President Truman had replaced General Hines with General Omar Bradley and appointed Maj. General Paul Hawley chief medical director. At the time, General Bradley had the type of charisma which is in eclipse in the world today. Just by going into the building and sitting down at his desk, he gave the country a feeling things were better at the VA. In the world of medicine General Hawley was also inspiriting. As an old army doctor he had accomplished the exceptional feat of giving civilian specialists in uniform a chance to work unhampered by military tradition, making of them an echelon of consultants in the European theater. In the VA one of his first measures was to negotiate the same arrangement between that agency and the same top flight specialists as they went back into civilian life. Vail, Greear, and Randolph, all were to serve the VA in this capacity in the next several years, and it is a fact of history that without their support orientation and mobility would never have found a place to take root when the Army program was discontinued. And, without the cultivation afforded by the VA, it is almost certain it would have fallen into Howe's "comparative neglect."

In the face of these new developments, Irwin's advisory committee took the unusual, strategic step of disbanding, but not before volunteering itself intact to advise General Bradley. Against the advice of holdovers from the Hines administration, he accepted the offer. A VA Advisory Committee on the Blinded Veterans was appointed in March 1946. This gave Father Carroll as a member of the committee, and Miss Gruber at Chairman Irwin's elbow, the opportunity to use their brains, information, and zeal to sway the course of the VA program for the blind. They were not slow to go into action, which I observed at first hand, having been appointed special consultant to the VA Department of Medicine and Surgery a little earlier.

The previous summer Col. Vail had offered to have me commissioned in the Medical Corps as a reward for my labors. This I saw fit to decline. I had gotten to be a staff sergeant on my own in the Air Corps, and what I was doing in the Medical Corps I thought I could do as well or better in that grade. Col. Randolph did not dispute this, but kindly advanced my pay by giving me another stripe. Turning down the commission was to affect both my own fate and the fate of orientation and mobility. Enlisted men were mustered out of the service more rapidly than officers when the war ended. I was discharged from the Army in January of 1946, and thus the first person from Valley Forge or Avon to whom the new VA talked. It goes without saying that I did my duty by Hoover's "foot travel" program, and I can vouch for the fact that no one else from the Army program (except Hoover) would even have seen fit to mention it.

THE NEW VETERANS ADMINISTRATION

I found the iron hot. Dr. Donald Covalt was just then establishing a new medical rehabilitation program in the VA Department of Medicine and Surgery, with the full backing of General Hawley. I was assigned to look into the situation of 337 aging blind veterans of earlier wars, and see what should be done to bring service programs for them into line with up-to-date theory and practice.

I spent six weeks traveling to nine centers, where I interviewed all 337 blinded veterans and made notes on their ways of getting about. This left me more than ever convinced that it is a sad waste of good intentions and human power for the average blinded individual to work out his own methods of getting about without benefit of systematic instruction. Only three of the 337 men had worked out any approximation of Hoover's method of touching the cane to the ground in front of the trailing foot. All the old blind men seemed to be acting out a visual memory of how the cane was carried as a walking stick, exploring a little in front tentatively at dangerous points, but then bringing the cane back to the side. Suggestions that the cane should be wielded in an arc were greeted with objections about how this would "look." This is so natural a reaction that I decided it would take a lot of teaching, not only with the veterans of past wars, but of future wars to overcome it.

It was fortunate that it was Dr. Covalt to whom I reported this idea. No other official in Washington at the time who had authority in the rehabilitation of the blind would have thought they were important. Clunk at Federal Security had shown his utter scorn of what was going on at Valley Forge by destroying an entire consignment of 1,000 copies of the Valley Forge cartoon brochure. Covalt, however, as an expert in physical medicine, was extremely interested in body mechanics and how they needed retraining because of a disability. He was in natural agreement with what might be called Hoover's basic premise: that if common physical problems of self-management can be mastered by a newly handicapped person, most Americans have a basic philosophy to do what is known as "adjusting." He read my report promptly, and presented it favorably to General Hawley. Both of them approved my recommendations that the nine centers I had visited be revitalized by the introduction of orientation and mobility. For a start I had urged that each have a blind chief and one mobility instructor. I recruited chiefs for the homes which did not have them, and we arranged for them to go to Valley Forge Hospital for a two week indoctrination with the hope of recruiting instructors from among the corpsmen about to be discharged.

The Meeting

With the help of ophthalmologist friends from the Army, now civilian consultants to the VA Department of Medicine and Surgery, I was able to interest Covalt in establishing a new program at a hospital away from the other nine centers, unhampered by previous routines, which would serve newly blinded service men when the Army and Navy programs were closed out. This was the genesis of the program at Hines Hospital. Whether or not such a center should be operated was one of the major points at issue when Irwin's advisory committee met on May 25, 1946. Our accomplishments thus far gave Covalt and me seats at the meeting by request of Irwin, although the committee was actually the affair of the Vocational Rehabilitation Service of the VA.

Father Carroll took the initiative by asking 51 specific questions which he and Miss Gruber had developed with respect to the program for blinded veterans. The ensuing eight hours of discussion were a revelation with respect to the skill with which the old guard of the VA had learned to fence with critics. Some answers to questions were forthcoming, some promised another day, some made to appear irrelevant, some beyond the agency's mandate. All was said with bureaucratic ceremony and correctness. But nothing was said which gave Father Carroll, Miss Gruber, or me encouragement that the agency had any intention of coming to grips with one major responsibility: coordinating its entire program. And certainly there was a strong undercurrent of opposition not only to running a center in the Vocational Rehabilitation Service, but also in the Department of Medicine and Surgery. The VA officials were already mustering support for the idea of contracting for services with private agencies, including substitutes for blind rehabilitation centers, since, in fact, there were no centers in the present day sense.

The Report

None of this was wholly unexpected by Father Carroll. Taking all the documents furnished by the VA, he composed a 21-page report which pushed hard for coordination of blinded veterans affairs, and for a basic rehabilitation center. But beyond that he set forth vigorously and succinctly what the agency had done and left undone; which it should not have. With the concurrence of the other members of the committee it was dispatched to General Bradley on Oct. 3, 1946. On Oct. 10th a polite acknowledgement was sent from General Bradley's office. Then further communication was not forthcoming for weeks.

In September, Irwin had employed me at the American Foundation for the Blind to edit the *Outlook for the Blind* and perform other functions. At the behest of Covalt he had allowed my other functions of assisting with plans to establish a VA hospital program for blinded veterans which he had decided to go ahead with. On visits to Washington I very soon concluded that the VA had buried the advisory committee's report. Then I heard from a knowledgeable source that the report was "dead." I also learned that those who had given the report this fate were opposing the idea of establishing a center according to Covalt's plan.

I asked Covalt if he minded if I took our copy of the report to General Hawley with a message that it was important. Almost as unorthodox as I, he gave his blessing.

GENERAL HAWLEY

It was a quarter of five in the afternoon, but I went immediately to one of the general's secretaries and had a parley with her explaining the circumstances. She took the document from me, went in to see the General and came back in a few minutes saying he would read the report that night and see me in the morning.

When I saw him that morning, he had indeed read the advisory committee's report, and it was quite clear to him what people inside the VA were up to. Also, he had made up his mind what to do about it, which was to go straight ahead with the plan to establish a blind program in a VA hospital, no matter what anyone thought about it. He spoke as though, naturally, I would help him, and naturally I did, though in the end it meant the finish of my career as an editor.

In 1969, I wrote an article for the *Blindness Annual*, which minutely dissected the happenings that culminated in the opening of the Hines Rehabilitation Center on July 4, 1947. Titled *From Valley Forge to Hines* with the sub-title *Truth Old Enough to Tell*, it gives in detail the agonies through which we put ourselves in getting the program established. Reviewing this document after another decade, seeing in sharp focus forgotten scenes in which I participated, is a little like looking on a distant scene through a telescope. And as various contentions are seen in relation to each other, along with the thought, "How shocking!" comes also the thought, "How necessary!"

One of the reasons why the Hines Center emerged and has endured is because it was a polished bone of contention. It was justified and rejustified, and re-rejustified both in spoken and written words countless times. Every check and balance which General Hines had left as his legacy to the VA was used against it. I will not tell this tale again in this chapter, since it is available for those who care to study altruistic politics, and it had very little to do with orientation and mobility itself.

However, there was one practical question and one philosophical one which are significant in retrospect. Philosophically Irwin objected to all centers for the blind, because he was totally committed to the idea of integrating blind people with the sighted. Like Howe he was eternally mistrustful of any program which might evolve into a home or asylum, "charitable tyranny . . . the consequences a clannish spirit, a defiant disposition, restlessness and discontent" (Bledsoe, 1964). Irwin gave in to Miss Gruber and supported the center, also giving me a leave of absence to help set it up. But he never felt easy with it.

In the practical area, when I had my conversation with General Hawley, Father Carroll was still holding out for the center to be a continuation of Avon, and along with that he and I differed over the emphasis which Hoover and I put on orientation and mobility.

During the war Father Carroll had been steeped in Avon philosophy and was indeed one of its best influences. But no one at Avon had an attitude which was much more than patronizing toward the Hoover method. When eventually Father Carroll became a believer, he summed up his early doubts by saying the Valley Forge approach to rehabilitation had been to the psyche through the body, whereas it came natural to him to approach the body through the psyche. He always remained doubtful about one of the basic tenets of Hoover and Valley Forge, namely that the great majority of the war blinded had enough philosophy dormant in them to manage their souls if they were given the practical help they needed to function on a practical basis. At bottom it was not basic to Hoover's profession, either as an educator or later as a doctor, to pry into the soul. It was a requirement of Father Carroll's, to which he adhered in a decidedly unorthodox way, but to which he adhered. In any case, when he saw the effect of Hoover's work on the whole human being, he became a staunch supporter, though at times a wayward one. Once the Hines program was established, he became one of the indispensable influences which helped to keep it alive, and later to transplant its method outside the VA.

Not to go into the intricacies of the controversy over whether or not the VA should have a center, suffice it to say that it involved not only the VA Departments of Medicine and Surgery, the Vocational Rehabilitation Department, as main contenders, but all the outside ophthalmological consultants, the heads of several residential schools, including Frampton, the Administrator of Federal Security, the professor of ophthalmology at Johns Hopkins, who had his own plan for a civilian-veteran center, the Blinded Veterans Association, the Solicitor of the VA, the Bureau of the Budget, Father Carroll, who at one point denounced the VA to the press, and finally President Harry Truman, who transferred all responsibility for rehabilitation from the Army back to the VA on an ordinary business day (May 31, 1947).

General Bradley and General Hawley had only agreed to give the VA two years of service, and they were both due to retire Dec. 31, 1947. Hawley, having viewed the shilly-shallying over the blinded veterans program for two years, sent for me in early September and told me Bradley had asked him to straighten out the blind program. He said that if I would take on a specially created job as coordinator of blinded veterans affairs, which would cut across medical and vocational rehabilitation, he would use all the influence he had to see that I could act, that Bradley wanted the position in the Vocational Rehabilitation Department, but he would see to it that I had freedom to set up the center in medical at Hines Hospital. To get me started immediately he would give me a slot in the Department of Medicine and Surgery until the position was set up in Vocational Rehabilitation. I had very little faith in H.V. Stirling, the director of Vocational Rehabilitation who was "old VA," and I knew opposed to the establishment of the center, but I had great faith in Hawley and events proved I was justified. I agreed to his plan.

I was sworn in to the position in medical on Sept. 15, but my first weeks on the job established the fact that I would have no cooperation whatsoever from Vocational Rehabilitation. There was endless parleying between the personnel staffs of medical and vocational rehabilitation; efforts of the latter to eliminate my responsibility for establishment of the center from my job description; their suggestion that the original proposed grade and salary be cut in half; my acceptance of this while refusing to give up an iota of authority promised. To this there was no reply. Before I had agreed to take the position, Hawley had introduced me to Stirling, gone over the terms laid down by Bradley for my hiring, and he had concurred with everything the General had proposed, but now it was as though this had never been.

While these developments were occurring I did what I could to get the Hines center going, went out to Hines, started getting a building put in readiness, got equipment in process of procurement, seven positions set up and had suitable personnel available, but the fact that everyone knew I was in administrative limbo made them anxious, to say the least, about doing my bidding.

In December I set all these facts forth in a memorandum to General Hawley, expressing my anxiety over what would happen to the center when he and General Bradley were gone. I took the memorandum to the General and he read it at once.

After a pause to reflect, he said, "Well, I'm awfully sorry."

And I never heard anybody say these words as though he were more truly sorry.

Then he said, "I could go to Mr. Stirling and say, 'Jesus Christ!' and 'God damn it!' But it wouldn't do any good. Stay here in the Department of Medicine and Surgery and get the center going."

Which is what I did. In the end it was necessary for the General himself to stay on after January 1st as a special assistant to the new administrator.

Then he issued a classic memorandum on January 14, 1948:

To: Deputy Chief Medical Director
From: Special Assistant to the Administrator
Subj: Reassignment of Mr. C.W. Bledsoe
1. The Administrator has directed me to straighten out the difficulties which have been threatening the agreement made by General Bradley with the representatives of welfare organizations for the blind.
2. This memorandum will, therefore, relieve Mr. C.W. Bledsoe from further duty in the Department of Medicine and Surgery and will assign him to my office.
3. You will continue to furnish Mr. Bledsoe with office space and clerical assistance.

General Hawley had seen the new administrator, Carl Gray, and made this highly unorthodox arrangement. Thus for a few months the blinded veterans had an unusually privileged chain of authority, and suspended upon it, the center was hoisted into position.

HINES VETERANS ADMINISTRATION HOSPITAL

General Hawley perceived very readily that the crucial factor in setting up the Hines center was the leadership of the chief, and was one of the few doctors in the VA who did not demur over the first principle which I laid down: that it must be a blind person and a veteran.

General Hawley said he would take care of money for supplies and equipment, but I must take care of personnel. However, he read, amended and approved the job description I wrote for the chief of the center, which I think in retrospect was the key to its success. It said:

The Chief of Physical Medicine and Rehabilitation of the Blind at Hines Hospital will have charge of the key operation in the training program offered blinded veterans of the Veterans Administration. He is in immediate charge of a staff of seven of whom he is one, all of whom are assigned to Hines Hospital.

The importance of his position and of the training operation is not to be measured by its size in relation to other programs in the Veterans Administration. It should be stressed that insofar as there is an operating unit for training blinded veterans inside the Veterans Administration, the unit at Hines will be that unit, and whoever is responsible for the training there will be responsible for the training of all blinded veterans who wish to receive training from the Department of Medicine and Surgery of the Veterans Administration. The Chief of Physical Medicine Rehabilitation for the Blinded at Hines will be responsible for the training of these men, for everything that happens to them from their arrival to their departure, for actually putting into effect all that we know, and all that is discovered with regard to this type of social adjustment.

No matter what is offered a blind person from a martini to braille, it is likely to be compared with sight. It has to be good, and it runs a little better chance of acceptance if it is offered by a blind person. This is something which workers for the blind can very easily forget, and it is a fatal form of forgetting. It is an evil decade when sighted people forget to listen to the way blind people feel about what is done for them. Blind people are then likely to listen with only half a disbelieving ear to what sighted people tell them they see.

One of the subjects I had repeatedly discussed with the doctors in the VA was the importance of having a blind chief of the center. Physicians have a hard time with this thought because they are so habituated to the principle that the patient must not treat himself. However, one of the services which St. Dunstan's did the American war blinded was to get Vail used to the idea that the program should have a blind leader. Now, as we were setting up the Hines program, he had recently become chief consulting ophthalmologist to the VA, and he came to our assistance. During the long suspense over whether or not we were to have a center I had been able to canvass people still close to the blinded veterans about who would make a good chief, and, almost invariably, the name of Russell Williams was mentioned. The single most inspiring recollection I can call to mind from my working life is the thought that I implemented a recommendation from Hoover and others, sought Russell Williams out, and persuaded him to take the position as chief of the program at Hines if and when it was available.

Dr. Kelso Carroll was the manager of Hines Hospital in 1947 when we established the center. After the publication of "From Valley Forge to Hines" in 1969 he wrote me:

> Of course there will never be another blind center such as we had, and there will neve- be another Russ Williams. For my money Russ is one of the really true Americans— accomplished and dedicated to his work, family and country. Do you know the only information and direction I gave him when he first reported for duty? I told him how to get to the center, but probably insulted him by offering him a car to get there. Speaking thus of Russ is not to take anything away from you, Miss Gruber and others who did organize the center.

Carroll himself was the ideal doctor-administrator of a hospital, one of the best of the pre-war VA employees, who had served in the Army Medical Corps during World War II, and returned to the VA in the company of General Hawley. His temperament was in fine balance between the sanguine and the saturnine. His heart was not one "too soon made glad." But he knew what was good, and his retrospective praise of the center gave Williams and me better assurance than any other we ever received that the Hines program had done what it was intended to do. Since this is the case, despite Carroll's thought that there never will be another blind center like Hines, I think it is worth while recording the principles under which we activated the program.

THE WILLIAMS PRINCIPLES

The first principle was realism with respect to the fact of blindness. This was stated very clearly by Williams many years later when he was asked what he thought of the term "blind center."

To this he replied, "I'm not very fussy about whether you call it a rehabilitation center for the blind or a blind center: I don't mind either of these terms. I can't think what else you might call it and use the *term* blind, and I think the *term* blind should be used. To me blindness isn't an ugly word at all, and it seems to me that the people who think it is have very little faith in the ability of blind people to meet the conditions of life with all the resources at their disposal. I can't really involve myself very seriously in arguments over whether a center or a school can be blind in fact. This seems to me a classic time-waster around meetings and conventions" (Williams, 1965).

Along with realism a second principle which Williams and I held above every other consideration was the principle that a program for blind people depends on the steadiness of the personnel who make it up. Especially in a training period the vicarious use of the eyes of the sighted is crucial. Not only outstanding willingness, but outstanding dependability is required.

Williams and I made it clear from the beginning that we did not want an imposing center built for the program, that we wanted adequate, unpretentious quarters for it, but that we would settle for nothing but what we thought best in the way of personnel.

Concerning this we had some very "square" ideas, about which I will again let Williams speak for himself, "The formula is rather simple: someone who really gets a sincere pleasure out of the growth of someone else and who just seems to have good standards—good level-headedness about him. There are certain guiding factors which are followed by people who have respect for other people. These are not the people who seem to live to depreciate other people, and seem to get a real satisfaction out of it . . . I don't think the center should be made up of people who are very far out in any direction" (Williams, 1965).

Speaking for myself in retrospect, I wanted everybody connected with the center to be a little better than I was—at everything except the kind of palace politics I had to learn to get the center approved. I wanted them all to be above that sort of thing, practicing the really high calling of teaching the blinded veterans how to get around. I was looking for the best type of supporters for a leader I regarded as indispensable. And in order to give double insurance to his leadership, remembering my experience at Dibble Hospital, I insisted that he be the only totally blind staff member to start with. This was my decision, based on my own worldly wisdom, for which I made it understood Russ Williams was not to be blamed, perhaps the only decision about which I did not even ask his opinion.

It was in implementing our ideas with respect to personnel that we made full use of the unusual authority which General Hawley had secured for us. For the time being we ran into very little opposition of any kind. Everyone seemed to be standing back and giving us room, our friends not to hamper us, our opponents hoping we would fall on our faces. In fact the opponents were making one more stand in the VA Solicitor's office, trying to block a technical bulletin announcing the opening of the center, but Williams and I decided to leave this to Hawley and Carroll, who at the last ditch went to Washington, defended the idea of the center roundly and got the technical bulletin released. In the long run the delay was to our advantage, since it gave us time to recruit and train personnel.

Recruiting

In view of the way the question of the center had been debated publicly and heatedly, recruitment possibilities were not promising at the beginning of 1947. The Valley Forge orientors had by then almost all been mustered out of the Army and had no difficulty finding jobs for themselves or getting admitted to college and universities under the G.I. Bill of Rights. During the war I had lost many of my personal contacts in work for the blind, and in any case most teachers of the blind adhered to the philosophy that what we were doing was unnecessary. However, I had one staunch friend at the Maryland School for the Blind, Stafford, "Charlie" Chiles, a manual training teacher. Our first piece of recruitment luck was inducing him to take on the initiation of whatever manual training we were to have.

From then our recruitment was inside the VA with two exceptions. General Hawley had met Miss Gruber and decided forthwith to invite her to be a consultant to the program. Somewhat later Hoover was also appointed. From the time I left Valley Forge I had attempted to persuade the VA to associate Hoover with the orientation and mobility program. However, even before leaving Valley Forge, encouraged by Randolph, Hoover had decided to study medicine. There-after, although both the VA and I would have preferred to have him do the things I had been doing, he was no longer available and resisted all our enticements to draw him back. In the years since, blind people in the United States have had in him an ophthalmologist who can interpret their needs to his brother physicians with acumen, compassion, and first hand knowledge. He has perhaps served as consultant on blindness to more agencies for the blind than any other ophthal-mologist in the world. However, his first appointment was by no means a shoo-in. It fell to me to ask a distinguished doctor in the VA to appoint him, when he was a medical student, consultant to the Department of Medicine and Surgery. Fortu-nately, the doctor was E.H. Cushing, a man of vision, but I will never forget his face as he said, "A medical student!"

I said, "All I ask is that you interview him."

He did, sent for me, and simply nodded.

We also appointed Harry Spar, of the Industrial Home for the Blind in Brooklyn, as consultant on manual training, and he, Hoover, and Miss Gruber were the only representatives of work for the blind, looking over our shoulders, and at times taking an active part in the setting up of the center. Miss Gruber spent weeks at Hines assisting both in the selection process and training of the staff.

How we did this has been described twice elsewhere, both in "From Valley Forge to Hines" (Bledsoe, 1969) and from the instructor's point of view in "The First Fifteen Years at Hines" (Malamazian, 1970). It is worth reviewing, however, be-cause it illustrates the effect of Williams's leadership qualities, which made the most of opportunities the rest of us put in his way.

At the time when I became associated with the VA, Dr. John Davis was fathering and bringing into the world the paramedical specialty of corrective therapy, a phase of physical medicine and rehabilitation nicknamed "the coach approach" and defined more formally as "exercise therapy." Davis was a psychologist who had been associated with Dr. Adolf Meyer, the psycho-biologist, who when heading the psychiatric service at Johns Hopkins gave as much attention to training ward personnel as he did to his residents. Many of Davis's concepts were similar to those of Hoover, and he suggested that some of his corrective therapists could be retrained as orientation and mobility instructors. He further disclosed that the corrective therapists at Hines Hospital were a blue ribbon group, their nucleus having been formed by an elite unit trained in the Army medical corps by Dr. Allan Stinchfield. All were soldiers who had been wounded, reconditioned for combat and then selected to remain at the center, reconditioning other wounded soldiers. Obviously this gave promise of rather staunch and likeable personality traits. The chief of the corrective therapy section at Hines, Carl Purcell, had been one of Stinchfield's unit.

Williams was able to accomplish the very delicate bureaucratic maneuver of persuading him and his chief, Dr. Louis Newman, to allow us to interview the Hines corrective therapists and offer them the opportunity to be trained as orientation and mobility instructors. This was similar to our having a choice of the panels of specially selected men sent into Valley Forge Hospital, but even better since the corrective therapists had already proven themselves in many areas of importance to orientation and mobility. They had had education and experience in physical education, kinesiology, anatomy, psychology, remedial exercise, posture and gait training.

THE HINES PATTERN FOR INSTRUCTORS

Twelve men applied for the five orientation and mobility positions which had been established. All were interviewed by Williams, Miss Gruber, Stafford Chiles, and myself. Williams interviewed candidates by getting each to guide him on a long walk about the hospital. My interview consisted of giving each candidate a lesson in orientation and mobility blindfolded and then getting them to give the same lesson back to me while I wore the blindfold. Miss Gruber, always a superlative listener, then had a long talk with the candidate during which she extracted quantities of information both about him and the hospital. Stafford Chiles by contrast interviewed by talking man to man and, if the candidate was boastful, finding out what he was boastful about. After this we four spent hours discussing the candidates together, after which Williams meditated and made his decision. Some attention was paid to the papers of the candidates, but far more to our mere knowledge of humanity.

The names of the first six mobility specialists chosen suggest that the interviewers had something like divine guidance. They were John Malamazian, Stanley Suterko, Alfred Dee Corbett, Edward Thuis, Lawrence Blaha, and Edward Mees, each one almost apostolic in character, Malamazian as the St. Peter and Suterko as the St. Paul. All became past masters at the art of teaching orientation and mobility to blinded veterans and to other instructors. Malamazian became to Hines what Debetaz was to Seeing Eye, the preserver of its integrity year in and year out, eventually to be its first sighted chief without the slightest objection from anyone, including myself. Suterko was to become the missionary of the Hines methods to the outer world, first at other VA hospitals, then at Western Michigan University, and later outside the United States. Lawrence Blaha activated the training program for instructors at Los Angeles State. But before that, the six trained the first 80 blinded veterans to go through the Hines program, set in motion constant refinement of the Hoover method, and established an esprit de corps which was to make the staff perhaps the most stable unit in the entire VA and the most admired. In the 1950s more instructors were selected and trained to meet the needs of the Korean War blinded. The original six assisted Williams in recruiting and training this group who for the next decade worked out methods which in the sixties were to become the substance of the master's degree university training programs, described in Chapter 19.*

Williams had, and has, an extremely easy-going way of relating to people and the art of finding something in common with almost everyone he meets. Like Abraham Lincoln and King George V, he gives the deceptive impression that he is an ordinary man, whereas in fact he is most uncommon. Behind his unpretentious dignity is a very carefully thought out philosophy of rehabilitation, with principles and practices, which he hammered out on his own anvil and which he imparted to his staff day by day rather than in formal statements. The philosophy was never more active than when he chose personnel. He never made the mistake of employing an individual to serve the interests of anyone but the blinded veterans. He never made the mistake of employing an individual to rehabilitate him. The center was for the blinded veterans, not to rehabilitate its own personnel. But after hiring them Williams was constantly teaching his staff and learning from them. He

---

*The names of these men, who deserve to be recorded, are Lee Farmer, Edward Polfus, Richard Russo, Richard Bugielski, Franklin Wood, James Lassen, James Enzinna, Cecil Miller, Raymond Brooks, Oscar Olivia, Norman Roche, Jack Henschen, Walter Olenek, Everett Bjork, Lloyd Widerberg, Berdel Wurzberger, Robert Gochman, Clovis Semmes, and Robert Smith.

had a real gift for choosing the creatively innovative and excluding the brilliant rebel program smasher. He had the great advantage of tapping the resources of corrective therapy at a stage which Alan Gregg described as "healthy adolescence" (Gregg, 1951). Working for Williams, boys became adults.

One of his happiest personnel choices was Donald Blasch, who went to Hines in 1951 as a counseling psychologist. Destined to his present position as chairman of the Department of Blind Rehabilitation at Western Michigan University, he very soon became Williams's philosophical sounding board, as well as a practical and profound psychotherapist for the blinded veterans in training. Blasch was very gifted in perceiving signs of mental health and strength which manifested themselves without the aid of therapy and not tampering with them.

RUSSELL WILLIAMS

Williams himself was a prime example of an individual whose handling of blindness a therapist would have been much put to it to improve. A technical sergeant in the artillery, he was blinded after the Normandy invasion, knew he was blind immediately, and was told in the hospital that he would be blind. He took it in such a way that the doctor who told him asked him to bolster the courage of a blind soldier in the next bed who the doctor did not feel was yet ready to be told he was blind. This Williams did.

The burden of another blinded veteran was put upon Williams within a few days of being told of his own prognosis. Whatever mystique is, he has it, which Greear, Randolph, and particularly the ward officer, Dr. Linus Sheehan readily perceived as he passed through Valley Forge and Avon.

He had been an Indiana school master and basketball coach before the war and they decided these were ideal qualifications to do the kind of counseling the other soldiers needed—a decision more pleasing to soldiers he served than to the personnel office, but the kind the eye chiefs had the authority to make if they chose, and they did so choose.

Though he had no degree in psychology or social work, and never would, he had observed everything the training programs had to offer at Valley Forge and Avon, where he was one of the soldiers who managed to acquit himself well without a cane. Back at Valley Forge, after conferring with Hoover, he took it up again and became a master at the art. In addition to learning the techniques of managing life without sight he had been observing the rehabilitation processes seething about him shrewdly, quietly, and compassionately. He had more than his share of people who saw possibilities in him and wanted to steer his career in one way or another. It was providential for the other blinded veterans that he chose the job at Valley Forge which took him back to the source of the war blind program and gave him an opportunity to see how it affected individuals and groups while no longer a part of it himself. In later years it was a recurrent phenomenon for trainees to want to emulate Williams's career. His reply to this was, "Not until you learn a good deal more about yourself, and all those people you want to help."

I believe it was at Valley Forge that he learned one of the most important lessons a blind leader of the blind can learn: to objectify beyond his own experience, not to think his way is the only way or that because he overcame a particular obstacle all blind people can, to determine in fact what it is reasonable to expect of all, or most, blind people.

By the time Williams came back to Valley Forge the staff there had more to offer in higher learning about blindness than any graduate school in the country. Not only was he associated with Hoover, but Martha Miller, a blind social worker, whom Irwin had been educating since her school days, became one of his colleagues, devoted to teaching him everything she knew. Paul Conlan, on leave from his position as head of the Michigan rehabilitation program, was his immediate supervisor. Louisa Walker, principal on leave from the South Carolina School for the Blind, and James Moxom, a blind graduate of the Maryland School for the Blind, both braille teachers, made friends with him, and were two more people who wanted to tell him what they knew, as was Ilah Oja, a typing teacher. These people organized themselves into a kind of morning seminar discussing with each other, case by case, what was emerging with respect to blindness in war. Miss Gruber was a frequent visitor, already sure in her own mind that Williams's fate was with the other blinded veterans. She formed a friendship with him that led to a remarkable correspondence which helped to build the Hines program.

Williams's philosophy of rehabilitation was best recorded in a series of statements he made for an interview on centers, which was published in the *Blindness Annual,* 1965.

There are some extremely difficult conditions imposed upon the staff of a center. It is a group of people interposed between two groups of doubters. On the one side of this staff is the client group who come in to this relationship without sufficient experience to realize that blindness can be lived out in quite a wholesome fashion.

They are entering blindness for the most part, since we are talking about centers, after having seen. They have come from a seeing society and bring into blindness many of the attitudes which are generally found to exist among seeing people. So that's why I call them doubters, and they come to the center to have their doubts removed.

Williams's faith in his principles was put to the test many times, but never more than when the chief of physical medicine wanted to deny a blind epileptic patient the use of a wood lathe. Williams put his job on the line in this case because in his opinion the lathe was the only thing holding that particular veteran to his rehabilitation, and he said no one had the right to deprive him of the privilege of getting hurt.

Ever since Valley Forge we have been drawing to the attention of medical men the fact that it is as important to save a personality as to save a life, and this to me was very complete support of this idea (Bledsoe, 1952).

ORIENTATION AND MOBILITY BOTTLED UP AT HINES

It will doubtless puzzle the present day reader that the practices and principles developed in the Hines program should have remained almost exclusively resources of the veterans for a number of years. As an official responsible for the program, I have been reproached for this of late years almost as much as I was reproached for being one of the godfathers in the beginning.

Certainly VA officials had no desire to keep the art exclusively for their clients. Efforts were made in the 1950s to share the skills of Hines instructors with the field of work for the blind. But none of us realized then how time-consuming this would be. A few instructors whom Hoover trained in his spare time while he was at Johns Hopkins medical school were a mere handful. Curious agencies sent representatives to Hines for periods of two weeks, but this did little more than confuse them about what was going on.

The Film

In 1952 the VA went to considerable trouble and expense to make a film, *The Long Cane,* depicting the Hines program. It was in one respect an enormous success, in another the next thing to a disaster. It was realistic. (Blinded veterans reenacted scenes from their lives in it.) It was so great an artistic success that it was shown at the Edinburgh Festival. It is one of the few training films of the 1950s which is still shown today. It proved a sure-fire mechanism to make converts of intelligent *sighted* public officials, including *sighted* workers for the blind. But the force of the message was so visual it was a dud as far as the blind population was concerned. This included important blind workers for the blind in positions of influence, whose minds were already made up that the Hines program was an impertinence because it was sprung from Valley Forge.

The makers of the film took too literally the "normality" of blind people and their "enjoyment" of movies. Quite a few years after the film had been made and shown I discovered that Hiram Chappell, one of the most knowing of Clunk's blind staff members, simply did not take in the basic action of Hoover's method, though he had sat through the film at least twice. A man of very fixed opinions, but also totally honest, he heard me say something one day which made him wonder if he had understood what the Valley Forge method was. When I demonstrated it to him by touch, he admitted he had never really understood it, and indicated he would have adopted it if he had been at the beginning of his career instead of at the end.

What we were up against with die-hard civilians, including those working in the rehabilitation field, became clear in 1953 when Father Carroll made an attempt to organize mobility instructors at what has always been referred to as "the Gloucester Conference." Though it was described in *Time Magazine*, no formal report was ever published. An informal gathering which had great charm, it was actually sponsored by Father Carroll's family, who entertained 30 key people in work for the blind and kindred professions in summer cottages at Gloucester, Massachusetts. Father Carroll's purpose was to persuade the few mobility specialists then in existence to form a sort of association or union and thus persuade agencies for the blind to accept them as a legitimate part of rehabilitation services.

It was quite clear to the mobility specialists after a few days that they could hardly hope for more than janitor or valet status from the agencies for the blind at the time. Russell Williams, Stanley Suterko, and I were all at the conference and saw this plainly. We decided that the only thing to do was let the Hines program prove itself under the protection of the VA without entangling alliances, at least for the time being. Elizabeth Hutchinson from Seeing Eye was also at the conference and she agreed with us. Father Carroll sent her and Williams out of the room three times to form a union. But they came back three times without a report.

Father Carroll was furious with all of us the night the conference broke up. But early the next morning, having been to mass, he told us goodbye with authentic forgiving grace. I thought then, and I think now, that we would have done harm had we followed the course he was promoting before expertise had been sufficiently perfected or demonstrated.

Punted Down The Field

Not until Joseph Clunk had been succeeded by another chief of services for the blind, and another, and another did the hazards of bureaucracy produce a *succes fou,* which some might regard as an act of God. After the center at Hines had been set up, and at the end of the year I had agreed to give the project, I had resigned, intending fully to try my hand at novel writing again. Almost immediately, however, I was asked to take consultant status in the VA, was called upon more and more when the Korean Conflict broke out, found myself interested as well as engaged, and finally was sworn in once again, this time as chief of services for the blind in the Department of Medicine and Surgery. In that position I conducted a survey of the status of the war blinded in the post war setting, a joint undertaking with social service. Within three months 386 social workers visited 1,949 blinded veterans of World War II and Korea with service connected disabilities, which was more than 98 percent of the entire group. I found things which needed to be done. Once again I was prodding people into action. My proddings wore out my welcome. Eventually a tight budget enabled officials to abolish my job with great regret and punt me down the field to the Office of Vocational Rehabilitation, a little uneasy about what I would do there.

This was in August 1958 and General Hawley wrote me a letter which said, "the situation is very different from the days when General Bradley was administrator. He is a man completely immune to political pressures; and his only objective was to do well what was to be done. The only order he ever gave me was to make the best medical services possible. He never disapproved any recommendation I made to him and he gave me full authority to issue instructions in his name. This perfect atmosphere in which to do a creditable job disappeared on 30 November when he closed his desk and left the Veterans Administration" (Personal communication, Hawley, 1958).

How right the general was we had already found when Dr. Carroll retired and Hines had a new manager, a congenital tamperer with everything God and man had ever created. On one of my visits to Hines before I left the agency I was startled to have him ask why I did not find a better job for Williams. This was about the time when the manager's own right hand man said publicly that the blind center had brought Hines Hospital more authentic good will than all the rest of the hospital's programs put together.

It was plain to me as it was to others that the manager was dangerously ambitious to leave his mark by doing startling things, and along this line he would like to damp down the reputation of Williams and the center.

He was matched in central office by the coterie which was going about the business of ousting me by taking advantage of the shortage of funds to say that the blind program was in such good shape that my job was no longer necessary, especially in view of the small number of blinded veterans (a perennial bureaucratic bugbear to blind programs).

Some well-meaning friendly advisers in central office urged me to attempt to save my job by going to my congressman. This I declined to do, instead writing a letter to go up through the VA hierarchy to my superior and his and his, protesting against the abolition of the position, but stating that if it were retained I would under no circumstances occupy it. Imperviously the VA officials let my protest go through at all levels. I therefore continued my protest in a letter to President Eisenhower, asking for the privilege of an interview.

At this juncture apparently someone in the President's office called Sumner Whittier, newly appointed administrator of the VA, and suggested that he give personal attention to the blind program. He summoned me to an interview. In our conversation it was apparent that up to then he had been told very little about the story of the blinded veterans.

He said, however, that he had looked into the whole subject of my central office position and that "everything had been done wrong," that dealing with doctors was like beating on a soft pillow. Then he said he understood I was leaving the organization no matter what he did about the position, and I assured him this was the case. Then he asked me what I thought he should do. I had regained amateur status as a counselor of state.

Successors

I told him that in my opinion workers for the blind would never let him rest unless he retained the position and filled it, and if he appointed Williams to it the old guard in the VA would never dare touch him. Whittier had at least heard what a good job Williams was doing and protested that this would be a great sacrifice for the Hines program. I agreed, but told him there were 1,949 other blinded veterans with service connected disabilities, that some of them were rising in the rehabilitation field and Williams could find a replacement for himself. I suggested Loyal E. Apple as an example.

This parting advice was my legacy to the old guard in the VA. Miss Gruber and Hoover backed it up vigorously, as did the Blinded Veterans Association, and Whittier actually followed it. Williams became as universal a favorite in central office as he had been at Hines, and from there was able to fend off the meddling of the Hines manager until he learned what not to tamper with. Apple was appointed to succeed Williams, and almost immediately there was a battle with the manager over whether the blinded veterans should be allowed to fill their own cigarette lighters. It ended in a compromise of sorts, however, which left the manager somewhat unnerved about the program, and thereafter he busied himself with other things and let his assistant deal with the blind center. Apple acquitted himself extremely well. He had been chosen for having some of the same characteristics as Williams, but distinct individuality, which subsequently found its way into the establishment of the center for blinded veterans at the Palo Alto Veterans Hospital. At that time John Malamazian became chief of the Hines center, a clear case of a man being chosen for his qualifications without regard to whether he was blind or sighted.

During the interregnum after Williams went to central office and before Apple was appointed, Donald Blasch came to the fore in the role of something more than a counseling psychologist. He was acting chief of the center for a number of months, and during that time acquitted himself with judgment as a stabilizing force which foreshadowed the major role he was to play in establishing the graduate program at Western Michigan University.

There is no doubt in my mind that the people in the VA who set up the chain reactions which moved several of us about on the chess board were trying to contain and restrain our creative spirits. That they should unwittingly have had an opposite effect accounts to some extent for what might be regarded as my superstition about the good auspices which governed the fate of orientation and mobility. It was extremely important that it be given time to mature unhampered by careless innovation for a decade, but equally important that it emerge to stand the test of general consumption at the end of that time. Events decided this in a way which strongly suggest the idea that, "There is a destiny which shapes our ends, rough-hew them as we will." This is sometimes a little hard to see in a time which glories in its rough hewing.

One of the unrecognized problems with American institutions is a national prejudice against anyone doing his job with easy comfortable grace as though he liked it, the assumption that without tension to the breaking point an individual is not earning his salt. We do not seem to want anyone to stay in any one spot long enough to get a firm grasp upon his situation. During my time in the VA there were four people in the hierarchy above me up to the president, making sixteen people with other things to do who could make or mar the program. Not one of the four in office knew what to do when we developed the crisis over my leaving. This is not so surprising when you consider they were short termers with the entire medical and VA program to learn about during the short term.

In the VA I began to learn how difficult it is to give even the most willing co-professional in the helping professions a grasp of what work for the blind is all about. One unlucky administrator of the VA emerged from viewing a training film about Hines to say in the presence of reporters, "Well, I guess that will put the guide dog out of business."

After Seeing Eye had gotten the congressman from New Jersey to enlighten him, he was somewhat wiser, but not enough to refrain from boasting to a visiting blinded veteran that the VA was doing everything possible for the blinded veterans. This was at a time when the doctors were blocking the publication of the survey of blinded veterans which we had made, the familiar excuse being a shortage of funds, and the veteran, a sociologist from Harvard knowing this, drew it to the administrator's attention. The result was that the study was published, largely through force of the embarrassment, which has been the unfortunate motivation for a great many measures taken by the VA in behalf of blinded veterans. Most of the in-and-out administrators in my time were well-meaning men caught with want of knowledge about blindness, who never met their own specialists on the subject until they were in dire trouble.

MARY E. SWITZER

In the Office of Vocational Rehabilitation of the Department of Medicine and Surgery I found myself in an entirely different world from the VA. Mary Elizabeth Switzer was director of the agency, and a management improvement firm had just made a survey of her program which had summed up its report with "What Mary wants, Mary gets."

Fortunately what Mary wanted was "the good of the world," toward which she said she "connived," and she did night and day, seven days a week, with courage, stamina, salty common sense, lively, idealistic imagination, and, she said, "above all, hope."

Her excellent mind was in a head which seemed to have been sculpted for public appearances. Like the old Shakespearean actresses, she had large features. A fine fleece of silver white hair came to her beautifully modeled forehead in a widow's peak. She had a strong jaw and clear blue eyes. Her features which may have been formidable in earlier years had a weathered grace which both individuals and crowds found arresting and appealing. About the time I went to her organization, reporters had begun to write about her as a "grande dame." Certainly she had all the better elements that the term implies. Yet she was anything but a snob. "Great commoner" would have been a better description of her than "grande dame."

The first staff meeting at which I saw her preside was on the budget. Dwight Eisenhower was president and Maurice Stans was director of the Bureau of the Budget.

Miss Switzer sat for a long time listening to the croaking of her misanthropes. One of her legs was crossed over the other, and she was swinging her foot as though she were kicking Plato's "large and sleepy horse, the State."

When the lugubrious finally stopped talking she spoke, saying, "Well, if I were in Mr. Stans' position, I might do as he does. Everyone knows there is a double standard. One for the military and one for the rest of us. But I've decided not to get emotional about it, because when we get into Congress, *we've got the votes*."

The votes she did indeed have. As time went on her prestige at hearings in Congress was unique. Her skill at extracting money from the legislators for her thousands of research and demonstration grants for the good of the physically handicapped was proverbial.

Presiding over the grants, she wore grandma half-moon glasses and knitted, but could keep track of the cash approved from grant to grant better than those with pencils in hand. It almost goes without saying that, after her early years understudying and supporting individuals who were at the top, when she first emerged as head of an agency, there was some unrest among the males about her, who at first mistook her style for weakness and fretted themselves unduly over her knitting at meetings. They would have estimated her more wisely, as they afterwards learned to do, if they had spent a little less of their lives reading about statistics and a little more about Elizabeth I of England, the Empress Maria Theresa of Austria, and Catherine the Great of Russia. Like the strong queens in history, Mary Switzer was feminine in her speech, in her surroundings, in personal dealings. And gradually she got people to see there was nothing wrong with her ways, no deficiency in logic, nor on occasion unalterable resolution.

Like the above-mentioned women heads of state, she had long-term trusted supporters, including the secretaries of Health, Education, and Welfare, as they came and went.

"She always weeps when they go," said Joseph Hunt, her right hand man, "but ends up by practically marrying the next one."

Her devil's advocate was Samuel Marta, an old Bureau of the Budget man, whom she dispatched to the VA to see what we were up to when we did the social work follow-up study of blinded veterans. The chasm between the VA and HEW was so great I cared very little about his criticism, which we had not invited, and which had to do with our not attempting to pry into the personal incomes of the veterans with service-connected disabilities. Apart from this I had an impression he acquired a reluctant admiration for the work we had done. I believe it was on the strength of this with strong backing from Miss Gruber and Father Carroll that Miss Switzer welcomed me into her agency.

I had had two encounters with her before that. One was over the abortive attempt made by Dr. Alan Woods, the professor of ophthalmology at Johns Hopkins, to establish a joint civilian-veteran center for the newly blinded. The other was over the spending of $25,000 left in the care of an ophthalmologist to be spent for the benefit of the blind. Mary Switzer and I had tried to get him to set up revolving loan funds to make it possible for truculent promising young blind people to buy and pay for psychiatry without benefit of agency supervision. But the ophthalmologist was all surgeon, said there were no good psychiatrists in his city, and gave the money to the agencies.

When I went to HEW, Mary Switzer had just persuaded Louis Rives to take the job of acting chief of services for the blind, and I was put on his staff. I had met him only once before, at an American Association of Workers for the Blind convention. He had made a statement at one session concerning the VA, some detail of which I disagreed with, but I was sufficiently impressed by him not to take the floor and correct him on the spot. After the meeting we had had a brief pleasant exchange, and I thought he gave hope of better things with respect to orientation and mobility in HEW. But, this was dashed when I heard he was not interested in being chief of services for the blind permanently, and was only acting at the convenience of Miss Switzer. But there is an old rule of institutions that there is nothing so permanent as the temporary, and he remained a reluctant, but superlative head of the unit for almost ten years. During that time rehabilitation of the blind had a kind of golden age. Ten million dollars was spent on 183 research and demonstration projects of wide diversity.

LOUIS RIVES

Rives was, and is, an accomplished negotiator with the better traits of a southern gentleman and a Yankee horse trader. He has a not unbecoming cloak of cynicism, which he can wear against the chill of the world, but I very shortly discovered he was a warm-hearted, spacious man, with a magnificent brain. And I never had a difference with him over what was worth a good laugh, or what a good laugh is worth. I suppose it is necessary to mention that he is blind, but in no one that I ever knew did it seem more incidental. A graduate of the William and Mary Law School, he had worked in the Office of General Council of Health, Education, and Welfare and then had done a great service for the Office of Vocational Rehabilitation in designing the state-federal agreements to implement the Vocational Rehabilitation Act of 1954.

Rives had a real gift for using whatever personnel he had under him. His indoctrination in rehabilitation had been through a course in vocational placement given by Clunk, where he had heard little good of the VA program, but he listened to what I had to say about orientation and mobility, and I presume also to Hiram Chappell, with whom I became great friends, having lunch with him every day, and thereby disabusing him of the misconceptions he had gotten from seeing "The Long Cane." I do not know whether Rives would recall that I pressed the subject of orientation and mobility too enthusiastically, but in any case it was clear in time he was making ready to invest.

During the weeks of my getting acquainted with Rives and Hiram Chappell, I saw little of Miss Switzer, but it was her habit to find some means of getting personally acquainted with every member of her staff and communicating with them directly at will. One day she asked for a copy of my novel, which I furnished her.

It so happened that one of the most sympathetic characters in the book is a spinster librarian with a great sense of civic responsibility, a heart of gold, and a caustic tongue. It was almost a portrait before I met her of Miss Switzer's lifelong friend, unofficial consultant and sounding board, Isabella Diamond, who was Treasury librarian for twenty-five years. My book has brought me many more friends than work for the blind has, and such was the case with Miss Diamond and Miss Switzer, whom it gave the feeling that I understood their mission and purpose in life. Miss Switzer then began to consult me directly on many subjects, including orientation and mobility.

At this juncture Rives revealed how broad-gauged he was. He told me frankly he saw this situation developing, and though it sometimes bypassed him, he knew I would keep him informed and communicate with Miss Switzer for the good of the blind. This I can honestly say that I did. Rives himself had an excellent relationship with her. His predecessors had foolishly tried to exclude her from decision making with regard to services for the blind. He made use of her brain and powers of persuasion to the full. When Miss Diamond retired as Treasury librarian he brought her also into the fold by making her editor of the newly established *Blindness Annual* of the American Association of Workers for the Blind, which was to become the organ through which orientation and mobility got a hearing nationally. Miss Diamond's focus on blindness was an extremely important pipeline into Miss Switzer's consciousness. They were on a par intellectually. Miss Switzer had a Radcliffe trained brain, and Miss Diamond had gone to Bryn Mawr. They had a house together and forever pooled their wits against ignorance, superstition, and every other kind of skulking evil which might impede the flourishing of the human race. Rives and I saw to it that rehabilitation of the blind had a regular place on the agenda, and orientation and mobility came into its own as will be seen by the following letter of June 30, 1960 written to Sumner G. Whittier, Administrator, Veterans Administration, with its "great commoner" postscript.

Dear Mr. Whittier:

For several years we have watched with interest the development of the Veterans Administration program of physical re-training of newly blinded veterans at the Veterans Administration Hospital at Hines, Illinois. Our advisors agree that in improving methods and techniques in this important aspect of a blind person's life, the system established by Mr. Russell Williams and his group of orientation therapists at Hines Hospital, has no counterpart elsewhere.

At the same time, the Office of Vocational Rehabilitation has become increasingly aware of the need for basic training of blind people in general competence, especially in the management and handling of themselves as blind persons. With this in mind we have made a training grant to Boston College to enable that institution to train mobility instructors of the

617

blind, not only in motor skills, but in some depth concerning the psychological implications of what they are doing and the nature of social responsibility entailed in rehabilitation.

I have long had a very real concern that our two agencies use the resources available to blind people in a cooperative way. I see clearly a need for exchange, both of ideas and people, and I would like to make this possible. It is very clear that on a country-wide basis there will have to be more courses and different kinds of courses in mobility, not only for blind people but for their instructors. Though the authorities on the subject so far have tended to avoid refresher courses for instructors, we see this as one of the primary needs of the present. This possibility and others I would like to have freely and cooperatively discussed between our two agencies.

In my opinion this would best be accomplished if we could arrange for responsible group action by members of our staffs most familiar with these matters, both in theory and in detail. It seems it would also be wise to draw into in these counsels persons from Boston College and other training institutions as they entered the field.

I understand a real respect exists between your Chief of Blind Rehabilitation, Mr. Russell Williams, and our Chief of Services to the Blind, Mr. Louis H. Rives, Jr., each of whom is blind and each of whom contributes a different type of experience to rehabilitation.

Without our mutual action I am afraid a skill which is really useful will not reach the great majority of blind people for many years to come. This is something so important to the future of blind people that I think you and I should get together personally and see to it that the machinery is set up and the policies are carried out which will make sure that something good and lasting is accomplished.

Sincerely yours,
Mary E. Switzer
Director

Hon. Sumner G. Whittier
Administrator
Veterans Administration
Washington 25, D.C.
cc: Mr. Hunt
     Mr. Garrett
P.S. A fascinating effort but we need to bring the boys together.*

Orientation and Mobility Grants

The grant to Boston College which Mary Switzer mentioned in her letter to Sumner Whittier inaugurated the use of Vocational Rehabilitation during the decade of the sixties to fund a massive constellation of orientation and mobility grants which were vehicles for much of the progress described by Wiener and Welsh in Chapter 19. In *Blindness* 1971 under the title "Orientation and Mobility Fans Out" the remarkable break-through which occurred has been delineated succinctly with impressive statistical detail. In this national and then international movement Donald Blasch proved to be an indispensable pivot figure in conjunction with Dean George Mallinson at Western Michigan University. Blasch now knows more orientation and mobility instructors and more about them than anyone in the world who is not one. Unfortunately in work for the blind it is simply not true that no one is indispensable. Many good services come to a halt when people die, and would never have existed without them in the first place. In my opinion Blasch is one of the elements without which orientation and mobility would not have spread as it has.

Wiener and Welsh (Chapter 19) show that the spur which was to set so many people in motion was a conference held in June 1960 at the American Foundation for the Blind. Out of the conference came support of the graduate courses at Boston College, Western Michigan University, and California State of Los Angeles. Out of

---

*Written by hand by MES on original

the graduate courses came the instructors who put into operation demonstrations of orientation and mobility teaching in 30 communities in 22 states. Paid for by the Vocational Rehabilitation Administration, it was these demonstrations which finally convinced agencies for the blind that mobility instruction was a basic and legitimate part of rehabilitation service for the blind.

An important lesson in public administration would be lost if it were not recorded that at the time Miss Switzer made these grants they were regarded by respected experts on blindness as a most dubious investment. Indeed it was still a rather unpopular dubious investment, and it would have helped to solidify her popularity with some heads of state agencies for the blind if she had turned her back on orientation and mobility altogether. It was only through the skillful diplomacy of Louis Rives and H. A. Wood that the idea of endorsing orientation and mobility was given approval by the National Council of State Agencies for the Blind as "something Mary and Lou want."

Miss Switzer was a firm believer in putting money into her causes and talking about them in language that could be understood. She was tireless both in making speeches to skeptical audiences and keeping guardianship of her budget at every stage. She never lost sight of the fact that most audiences, including Congressional committees needed to learn the ABCs of rehabilitation over and over and that you cannot run services for the severely handicapped without cash.

"You can't get people behind causes," she often admonished her staff, "by talking to yourselves."

After she had acquired a certain number of honorary degrees (she had twenty-two), she declined to accept any more unless she were invited to accept with a speech about rehabilitation. The speeches were simple, to the point and practical, drawing attention to such facts as the income taxes paid by rehabilitants after receiving rehabilitation services.

"Nothing turns Mary on like a budget," said her successor John Twiname.

"She's tough. That means we respect her over here," said James Hyde, a blinded veteran who had risen high in the councils of the Bureau of the Budget.

The remarkable thing about such a statement from a budget man was that Mary Switzer often frightened her own staff by the originality and scope of her programs, such as dance therapy for the deaf at Gallaudet, appreciation of art for the blind, and when she first began to support it, orientation and mobility undoubtedly seemed rash to some of her veteran staff. Fears of her in fiscal matters were generated in part because she was the first big spender in the federally financed rehabilitation program, following frugal beginnings in the 1920s, the depression, and World War II. Roosevelt himself had been remarkably skeptical about money spent on rehabilitation. To one of the rehabilitation experts of his time is attributed the dictum, "Nothing large, expensive, or technical."

Accounting

This was not Mary Switzer's policy by any means. To some people she seemed extravagant in administering public funds. In my opinion she was generous, but prudent and I paid close attention over the course of more than ten years to money she spent on research and training programs for the blind. In fact, this became one of my particular functions in Services for the Blind along with being the guardian of orientation and mobility and optical aids projects. Beginning in 1965 Miss Switzer made me co-author of a yearly account of where and how vocational rehabilitation money was spent on programs for the blind. This was published each year in *Blindness Annual*. Services for the Blind was the only unit in Vocational Rehabilitation which published such reports, separated from material on other categories of the disabled, and in a publication which reached a large number of workers in the specialty reported.

From these reports it is a matter of public (and easily available) record that from 1960 until 1970 Mary Switzer's administration paid $3,200,000 as matching funds to universities for salaries of faculty and fellowships for students learning to teach orientation and mobility in the master's degree programs. This was at Boston College, Western Michigan University, and California State.

In the same ten years the Vocational Rehabilitation Administration paid $1,113,298 to thirty communities as seed money to pay the salaries of instructors in demonstration programs. It fell to me to draft the guide lines of these projects and follow their progress.

During the demonstration period approximately 1,500 blind individuals, including blind children, were given an average of 30 lessons each in orientation and mobility, making the cost per lesson about $25 at the demonstration stage. Extravagant this may appear to some people, but, if you believe, as I do, that orientation and mobility is one of the secrets of preserving the personality of the individual who loses his sight, the cost is on a par with psychotherapy, and not excessive. An overwhelming demand for mobility instructors which followed the demonstration projects seemed to confirm this emphatically.

The very first day at Valley Forge talking with the first World War II blinded veteran to whom I was assigned, to get things straight in my own mind, I asked him if he minded the fact that I had not been in combat, and was not blind.

He said, "No. I'm glad you haven't been in combat, haven't been hurt, and if you're going to teach me, I'm glad you can see."

There was nothing whatsoever I had to add to that man's philosophy or management of his emotions, or his grace under pressure.

But other instructors and I did teach him orientation and mobility. He was grateful, and I think it kept him from becoming a handicapped person.

Defenders

Nevertheless, all such experience notwithstanding, hardly had the training grants at universities been approved before their opponents began to suggest that if they were a success, federal aid should be phased out. And when they were a success this thought was spoken more loudly. To this kind of talk, when everyone had had their say, Mary Switzer paid no attention, perceiving that in the face of the obstacles to be overcome only an unremitting attack over a long period of time would answer. In continuing to support the graduate programs both she and blind people were fortunate in the lieutenants she had who were immediately responsible for her programs for the blind. Louis Rives, her assistant, Joseph Hunt and Cecile Hillyer, in charge of training grants, whether or not they were believers in Miss Switzer's ideas, carried them through with vigor and efficiency as though they were. Both Hunt and Rives, who were superb public officials, became staunch defenders not only of orientation and mobility, but of the standards of the graduate schools.

But it was Mary Switzer who was its champion defender, both with words and money.

Once when she was lunching with a group of educated bureaucrats, none but she was able to translate the second motto on the back of the American dollar bill.

She freely rendered into English: "Annuit coeptis novus ordo seclorum," as: "A new order of the ages favors our undertakings."

No one ever spent the federal dollar toward such a hope more devotedly than she. Her support of orientation and mobility continued to the very end of her life, both with power and discernment. Indeed it seemed to have become a prime example for her of what she wanted to give handicapped people, as can be seen from the following memorandum which she wrote to her successor John Twiname on February 1, 1971, a few months before she died.

> I have been thinking almost constantly about our conversation the other day concerning the cuts in the training programs and what it will mean for our handicapped people and those we have the responsibility for training to serve them.
>
> As I told you, I feel the most telling evidence of the effectiveness of the vocational rehabilitation training programs is the record of where the students go after they are trained. One of the most graphic studies is in the field of mobility instruction for the blind and visually handicapped. The attached copy of an article, which appeared in the January 1971 issue of *Long Cane News*, contains just the type of data that should be available for every single specialty. The sooner it is available the more effective can be the case for not cutting away this important program at a time when we are trying to bring more effective and efficient services to everyone.
>
> You will note from this article that there is practically no slippage at all in the graduates of mobility programs away from work with blind and seriously visually handicapped people. You will note also that the distribution of these instructors is about what you would expect and what you would think would be right. The largest percentage are in public schools, state agencies serving the blind, and private agencies serving the blind—these would be, of course, lighthouse, rehabilitation centers (many of which are under private auspices), etc. Residential schools have another 18 percent which is excellent and probably should be higher. I would suggest that you ask people in other fields to get you similar documentation. Naturally, I will be glad to help in any way possible.

No one knew better than Mary Switzer that the acceptance of the programs she offered to blind people came very largely from interpretation of them by Rives. His ability to make use of even the most unorthodox methods in gaining his ends made collaboration with him exhilarating in the extreme. A case in point was a device we used to promote the orientation and mobility program after he had sold the idea to the higher echelons in the National Council of State Agencies for the Blind and we wanted to reach the House of Commons, so to speak, as well, many of them blind, who had heard unsettling rumors about feats of foot travel they might be called upon to perform.

The Skit

In discussing how we might reach them, I pointed out to Rives that I thought the film *The Long Cane* had produced some opposite results from those intended, because its message was so visually conveyed. In presenting our case to workers in the field through the American Association of Workers for the Blind, we should do it entirely orally and tactilely. A presentation was to be made at the association's 1960 convention. I wrote a humorous skit entitled "Propaganda for Living" in the manner of an Alfred Hitchcock movie, based on the realization that the audience would be overwhelmingly seasoned workers for the blind, half of them blind, and unsentimental about blindness. The skit was recorded on a disc, to be followed by a question and answer session in which Hoover, Father Carroll, and Rives participated. We then arranged for Hoover and half a dozen mobility instructors to give individual demonstrations to the blind members of the audience. The audience reacted from the start as we had hoped. Doubtless they were the only audience to be found anywhere who would have laughed heartily when a blind man who refused to use a cane landed under a train. The punch line came after sound effects of a train whistle, a train chugging into the station, and then silence, broken by the words, "Inasmuch as it has pleased God to take unto himself our beloved brother, at least he *went his own way*." The record did what *The Long Cane* had not because it was in a medium which depended on vision not at all. As soon as the meeting broke up, flocks of blind people came forward for demonstrations which continued through the day.

It should be said, however, that *The Long Cane* continued to be an enormous success in letting sighted people know what orientation and mobility is all about. With the sighted, "Propaganda for Living" was often found to produce an adverse reaction, even among audiences presumably sophisticated with respect to rehabilitation. The record cost seven dollars, the film thirty-two thousand. It would be hard to say which did most to promote orientation and mobility. In my opinion the record marked an important turning point in the acceptance of orientation and mobility. But Miss Switzer and Miss Diamond, who liked the movie very much, and undoubtedly espoused mobility in part because of it, could not bear the record, even though they granted it had the desired effect on the audience for which it had been written. Laughter at blindness as a rule is best left to blind people themselves. But seven years after the Gloucester Conference, with no appreciable progress in the outer world, and an excellent program bottled up at Hines, it seemed time for a desperate ill to be overthrown by a desperate remedy.

The lengths to which those with an antipathy toward the orientation and mobility program would go in opposition were demonstrated the night before the session at which "Propaganda for Living" was played. A hardened scoffer at the emphasis put on orientation and mobility training, much given to convention antics and buffoonery, undertook to keep Rives at a very lengthy symposium, in fact kept him talking until five in the morning, hoping he would beg off from presiding the next day and giving his very necessary blessing. But Rives proved as staunch as Socrates, at dawn took a dip in the ocean instead of going to bed, and managed the morning session with panache. Hoover was his guide swimming, one of the countless times he has stood by the cause of orientation at every level, from sitting among the elders of the land to giving a lesson to one of his patients who needs it then and there, the only ophthalmologist in the country capable of doing this, and probably the only one willing. He also understands resistance to his methods as well as anyone alive today.

It will never be safe to assume that controversy over the very fundamentals of work for the blind will be over. To be outdone with this circumstance, to say that people "ought not to be that way" is one of the common reactions of "rookies" and "tyros" in the field.

EPILOGUE

To understand why people have been, are, and are likely to be with respect to problems of blindness is one of the many reasons to study the history of human experience with regard to this particular phenomenon. It is also basic to resolutions of current controversies. There are certain very important lessons workers for the blind have at hand for the learning from the long internecine war waged over orientation and mobility. It is the second war of its kind the field has experienced in this century, the first having been over punctography, the great contention between the promoters of braille and the promoters of New York Point, termed "The War of the Dots" by Robert Irwin in his memoirs.

The first lesson from both wars is that people who deal with human problems should not expect to have calm sailing. In retrospect, it is rather surprising that anyone should have expected tranquil waters for such an innovation as the long cane used not to whack passing tree stumps, but to locate curbs off which the bearer was expected to step onto a street he was then expected to cross. On this subject I would like to bring out of anonymity a statement I made for Hoover to publish in the *Blindness Annual* of 1964:

> It is hard to please me, I confess, with anything written about methods of teaching blind people mobility. What might be termed an "executive" or "administrative" view of this part of work for the blind frequently finds its way into print full of statements that tell nothing at

all. Almost never is there a real impression of pupil and teacher working their way, minute by minute, quarter hour by quarter hour, foot by foot, rod by rod, fighting a hard battle which is part of the so-called adjustment to blindness, by which is meant also getting on top of rage, jealousy and frustration which are brought forth and dealt with by pupil and teacher. I *object* to bland language and pretense that it is no trick to master the art of seeming a gracious being under these circumstances, much less actually becoming one. Too often language used to describe all that goes into the struggle of blind people to be mobile is far too tender. Blindness is not a tender thing, nor are most of the means to surmount it. They are for the brave and the faithful, who are rather difficult to describe in official or scientific language.

Many years later Dr. Hoover gave a retrospective prescription for dealing with these complex difficulties at one of the many meetings which were held in the U.S. Department of Health, Education, and Welfare for the perpetuation of his work. This unpublished document of six pages reveals as well as any other what is required in theory, strategy, and tactics for surmounting these difficulties.

It is only when the trainee feels secure and comfortable in the instructor-trainee relationship that he will do his best and the instructor be the most helpful to him.

The most ideal combination for this type of therapy is when there is a collaboration between the instructor and trainee, each learning from the other. Many times he cannot be patterned after a preconceived plan but must always be modified and adapted to the particular needs of a particular life situation . . .

You might say that we must give the trainee a series of opportunities to gratify certain basic needs which are present in varying degrees in all types of inability or struggles.

If one were to outline the basic needs I think you could do it in five attempts.

The best method of alleviating tension is known to be bodily activity. Next to this is the need to talk. I include those both in the same category because they both afford an opportunity for an individual to discharge pent-up feelings and can provide a companion upon whom the individual depends for understanding and guidance.

There is nothing unimportant, so particular attention must be paid to everything that is done and everything that is heard. It is impossible to set down any general rules but one might say, (a) listen patiently, (b) do not interrupt, (c) think along with the patient, (d) show a real interest and personal warmth to what is going on, and (e) avoid criticism and argumentation.

The second basic need is the need to be told what to do. If one suffers from an inability, a discomfort, and is in emotional distress, he needs definite support and guidance. He would like to depend on someone who is certain of himself and knows just what to do to alleviate our misery and suffering and at the same time provide him with methods of carrying on by himself. The value of routines and schedules of exercise, rest, and recreation may be attributed in part to this basic human need. Sometimes we want to be freed from having to think for ourselves.

The third need is the need to be accepted. One who has just recently been maimed or handicapped is tense, worried and uncomfortable, and anxious.

We should evaluate the trainee thoroughly, then discuss why it is thought certain methods should be learned or taught. Do not allow ourselves to portray we feel he is foolish, stupid, or unscientific with his questions or his attempts to use his own methods. He may be testing our interest in him as a person as well as seeking further reassurance. Make the patient feel that he is a collaborator. Tell him how he is doing. Use his own words as much as possible in order to tell him what it is he needs and what it is he is accomplishing. He will be impressed by our sincere interest and feel that we consider him worthwhile and intelligent. Do not make the mistake of trying to minimize his difficulties. He knows he has difficulties, and we cannot change this by minimizing them.

We must not be afraid to speak the truth, if it seems indicated. Probably the individual will be complimented by our personal interest in his illness, in his troubles and feel encouraged to do his best and to tackle other problems.

The fourth basic need is the need to be oneself. Encourage him to do what he really wants to do. Also guide him into doing some of the things that we know will be necessary for him.

He will gradually learn to think of himself and for himself, and with it will come a sense of freedom of action and a feeling of well being.

The fifth and final basic need is that of the need for the trainee to finally emancipate himself from the influence of the instructor, because he must at some time leave the controlled protective environment and finally face even more stark reality. Lessons and routine should be reduced and finally discontinued. Be sure he is not exchanging one set of problems for another which will limit his activities and keep him a semi-invalid continuing to rely on someone to tell him what to do and to be with him. One might emphatically state that the patient is not a good traveler until he is completely capable and comfortable in doing this on his own, feeling free to act like any other healthy emotionally secure individual, in keeping with his personal needs and social interest.

Bibliography

Allen, E. Impressions of institutions for the blind in Germany and Austria. *Blindness*, 1969, 220-224. (Originally published *The Outlook for the Blind*, February 1910, & Spring 1910.)

Bledsoe, C. W. The "blind center": Ideal or spectre. *Blindness*, 1965.

Bledsoe, C. W. From Valley Forge to Hines: Truth old enough to tell. *Blindness*, 1969, 97-142.

Bledsoe, C. W. *Survey of World War I blinded veterans in hospitals and homes.* Unpublished report in archives of Veterans Administration and Bledsoe papers.

Campbell, F. J. Statement by in the *Sunday School Chronicle*, July 8, 1909. An Apostle to the Blind. Sir Francis J. Campbell Papers, Library of Congress, Box 34.

Carroll, T. Blindness: What it is, what it does, what to do about it. Boston: Little, Brown and Co., 1961.

Daudet, E., & Stawell, Mrs. R. translator. *Madame Royale.* New York: George H. Doran and Co., 1913. 235-6.

Gregg, A. Corrective therapy, the adolescent profession. Unpublished lecture, 1951.

Howe, S. G. *Forty-first annual report of the trustees of the Perkins Institution and Massachusetts School for the Blind.* Boston, 1872.

Howe, M. de Wolfe. (Ed.) *The correspondence of Mr. Justice Holmes and Harold J. Laski.* 1916-35. Cambridge, Mass.: The Harvard University Press. 1953. Vol. 2.

Irwin, R. *As I saw it.* New York: American Foundation for the Blind, 1955, 173.

Koestler, F. A. *The unseen minority.* New York: The David McKay Co., Inc., 1976.

Levy, W. Blindness and the blind, London 1872. Reprinted in the *New Outlook for the Blind*, April 1949, 106-10.

Malamazian, J. The first fifteen years at Hines. *Blindness*, 1970, 59-75.

Mannix, J. B. John Metcalf: Blind Jack of Knaresborough. In *Heroes of Darkness*. London: S. W. Partridge and Co., 1911. (Reprinted in *Blindness Annual*, 1976.)

Outlook for the Blind, Medice, Cure te Ipsum. Author, **41**(5), 142.

Reardon, D. Statement in Campbell Papers at the Perkins School Library. Unpublished.

Ross, I. *Journey into darkness, The story of the education of the blind.* New York: Appleton-Century-Crofts, Inc., 1951. 103.

St. Paul, First Epistle to the Corinthians. Chapter I, verse 27, King James Version of the Bible. London: Robert Barker, 1611.

Saturday Evening Post. They learn to see at Avon Old Farms, Author, 1945.

Willard, F. *Glimpses of 50 years.* Boston: Women's Temperance Publication Association, 1889.

Williams, R. C. How a blind center can be run for the rehabilitation of blind people. An interview. *Blindness*, 1965, 32-48.

Wilson, E. O. Altruism. *Harvard Magazine.* Nov.-Dec. 1978, 23-28.

The Profession of
Orientation and Mobility

William R. Wiener and Richard L. Welsh

Orientation and mobility as a profession is relatively new. Like several other occupations, it has participated in the twentieth century phenomenon of professionalization. Although this development has been chronicled in various places (Ball, 1964; Bledsoe, 1969; Malamazian, 1970; Blasch, 1971), no comprehensive treatment has appeared in a single source. This chapter is an effort to present a coherent picture of the profession's emergence, current status, and future directions.

Carr-Saunders (1928) has defined a profession as an occupation requiring specialized study and training for the purpose of supplying skilled service or advice. A profession is generally considered to develop around a specific body of specialized knowledge and is practiced by persons trained in its application. Practitioners with common interests come together in professional associations to develop and share information, establish minimum qualifications, certify practitioners to possess certain competencies, and determine and enforce standards of professional conduct. Greenwood (1957) has identified five elements of a profession as:

1. A body of systematic knowledge
2. Authority granted by the clientele of a particular service
3. Community sanction of this authority
4. A code of ethics to regulate the relations of practitioners with their clients and colleagues
5. A professional culture encouraged by professional associations.

The profession of orientation and mobility can be analyzed as it corresponds to these criteria.

Bledsoe (Chapter 18) described the Army and Veterans Administration Rehabilitation Programs in which the techniques to systematically teach blinded veterans to travel were first developed. As articles describing these programs began to appear, and veterans from these programs began to disperse to their home communities around the country, agencies and schools for the blind became very interested in what was being taught at the Hines Veterans Administration Hospital. The Hines staff began to receive requests to train people to teach mobility and to provide literature and materials dealing with orientation and mobility techniques (Malamazian, 1970).

During the 1950s, the Hines staff tried to respond to these requests and to share as much information as they could. According to Malamazian (1970), visitors to Hines came for varying amounts of time ranging from several days to a few weeks to observe the program and learn how to teach the techniques that were developed. In addition, Hines staff members sponsored by agencies for the blind gave short-term courses for groups of workers for the blind around the country. The effect this sharing of newly developed knowledge had was expressed by Malamazian thus, "In most cases, all we imparted was a hearty respect for street crossings, a frustrating respect for ourselves and a desire on the part of the would-be instructor either to have a lot more training or have nothing to do with it himself because he thought there was too much risk" (Malamazian, 1970, p. 72).

In 1952 the Rev. Thomas Carroll, Kathern Gruber, and Russell Williams, individuals described by Bledsoe (Chapter 18), and Hines staff members met to develop guidelines for "mobility technicians." According to Koestler (1976) this group developed a memorandum stating that the mobility specialist's responsibility went beyond instruction in the proper use of a cane or dog, and extended to helping the blind person make use of his remaining senses, working with the blind person's intelligence by providing knowledge of objectively evaluated methods of travel, and working with the blind person's will by stimulating his confidence in his ability to move without dependence.

In 1953 Carroll assembled a group of people in his home in Gloucester, Massachusetts, to discuss the dangers involved in allowing untrained persons to set themselves up as mobility experts (Koestler, 1976). The group included practitioners in work with the blind along with specialists in physical education, physical medicine, general rehabilitation, ophthalmology, clinical psychology, and psychological research. The report of this meeting, referred to as the Gloucester Conference, was never published because, according to Koestler (1976) it was felt that many in work for the blind did not believe that such formal instruction was necessary and were not yet ready to accept the kind of standards some of the participants recommended.

In June, 1958 the Office of Vocational Rehabilitation identified the training of mobility specialists as its second highest priority in the area of training rehabilitation personnel (Voorhees, 1962). To implement this, the American Foundation for the Blind (AFB) was funded for a national conference on orientation and mobility, held in 1959, to establish criteria for the basic selection of mobility personnel, to develop a curriculum, and to recommend length of training and appropriate sponsorship.*

This conference was a significant step in the establishment of orientation and mobility as a profession. A major decision was to establish the minimum training period for mobility specialists as one year of graduate study. The greatest support for this provision came from mobility instructors attending the meeting, especially those with the longest experience, who were unwilling to support short-term training because their own experiences had proven it to be ineffective. They believed that, "Necessary emotional conditioning was so intricate a process, the ingraining of principles through time-consuming laboratory experience so necessary, that the needs of the situation could not be met in a compressed teaching

---

*Papers and other materials were prepared by Richard Hoover, Rev. Thomas Carroll, and Frederick Jervis. Participants included practitioners and administrators in work for the blind. Those in attendance were: Georgie Lee Abel, program specialist in education, AFB; Oliver Burke, chief of orientation and mobility, Arkansas Enterprises for the Blind; William Debetaz, The Seeing Eye; Irving Kruger, rehabilitation instructor, New Jersey Commission for the Blind; Harold Richterman, director of rehabilitation services, Industrial Home for the Blind, Brooklyn; Ed Ronayne, resource teacher, Denver, Colorado; Keane Shortell, mobility instructor, Industrial Home for the Blind; Frederick Silver, mobility instructor, St. Paul's Rehabilitation Center for the Blind, Newton, Mass.; Stanley Suterko, supervisor of orientation and mobility, Hines Veterans Administration Hospital; Russell Williams, chief, Physical Medicine and Rehabilitation Division, Veterans Administration, Washington, D.C.; and Charles Woodcock, principal, Oregon State School for the Blind. The conference coordinator was Arthur Voorhees, program specialist, AFB, and the recorder was C. Warren Bledsoe, assistant chief of the Division of Services to the Blind, Office of Vocational Rehabilitation. Two others who addressed the conference were M. Robert Barnett, executive director of AFB and Kathern Gruber, director of the Division of Research and Specialist Services, AFB(*American Foundation for the Blind*, 1960).

program of two weeks, two months, or even four months" (American Foundation for the Blind, 1960).

This conference also established the principle that mobility specialists should be sighted rather than blind. Although this point went against the thinking of many in the field, it was felt necessary to allow an instructor to move away and still provide for the client's safety. This further reinforced the need for extended training in order that the instructors could habitually think about how to manage the problems of living without sight. Other standards related to the academic prerequisites of students and personal and physical characteristics that were thought necessary. These will be discussed later in this chapter.

Areas of Study

The conference also recommended that five areas of study be included in the training program curricula. These were:

1. Physical orientation and mobility, taught through learning the essential skills and techniques of orientation and mobility under a blindfold, by observations of personnel in a variety of settings such as schools, agencies, and hospitals, and by supervised teaching of blind persons. In this area information about the special needs of different clients, for example, totally blind, partially seeing, the newly blinded person, the experienced blind person needing remedial work, congenitally blind children, those with multiple handicaps, and the aging would also be included;
2. Dynamics of human behavior related to blindness, focusing on the need to modify certain actions in the presence of blind people, for example the instructor's own feelings about blindness and ways of relating to blind people, as well as skills in observation and description;
3. The functions of the human body as they relate to blindness, involving the study of anatomy and physiology, hygiene, kinesiology, orthopedics, and remedial exercises;
4. Sensorium, including the study of the senses, their use and coordination, and an understanding of advances in knowledge in this area;
5. Cultural and psychological implications of blindness, closely related to the second topic and dealing with attitudes toward blindness and changing attitudes, as well as ideal methods of dealing with the problems of blindness and the successes and failures of methods used. This area was also intended to provide an opportunity for mobility specialists to learn about the other disciplines related to blindness. (American Foundation for the Blind, 1960).

University Training Begins

The conference participants also addressed the question of appropriate settings for this training. A university in a metropolitan setting with a medical school and nearby clinical facilities was recommended. Such facilities were intended to provide exposure to the full range of types of clients, including those who were newly blinded. The opportunity to draw upon instructors from other departments of the university as needed, strength in research, especially in neurology and electronics, and an ongoing program of rehabilitation counseling sponsored by the Office of Vocational Rehabilitation (OVR) were also suggested as requirements for universities considered.

A favorable review of the conference report by the National Council of State Agencies for the Blind, led Louis Rives, then chief, Division of Services to the Blind of the OVR, to announce implementation plans. The first OVR grant to establish an orientation and mobility university training program in orientation and mobility went to Boston College; the program began in June, 1960. The Rev. Carroll had been instrumental in bringing the program to Boston and made members of his staff available as faculty. The first coordinator was Joseph Runci; the orientation and mobility components were developed by Frederick Silver and Bernard Hickey. In 1962, John Eichorn was appointed coordinator (Blasch, 1971).

The second university training program was established in 1961 at Western Michigan University (WMU), Kalamazoo. Dr. George Mallinson, dean of the WMU College of Graduate Studies had been working closely with OVR and the Veterans Administration to establish such a program. Donald Blasch, a counseling psychologist, and former acting director of the Blind Rehabilitation Center at Hines was selected as director of the WMU program. Stanley Suterko and Larry Blaha of the Hines staff were selected to develop the orientation and mobility content of the program (Malamazian, 1970; Blasch, 1971).

The graduates of the new programs were in great demand. Further stimulating this demand was the initiation of a number of research and demonstration grants by the Vocational Rehabilitation Administration (VRA) (formerly the OVR) as a method of demonstrating the value of skills in orientation and mobility training and the effectiveness of instructors trained in these techniques. Beginning in 1962, VRA awarded 30 grants in 22 states which essentially paid the salaries of mobility specialists hired by participating schools and agencies. The success of these projects inspired enthusiasm about this specialty and increased the demand for the services of mobility specialists. Unexpectedly, demand for mobility specialists also came from residential and other school programs for visually impaired children (Blasch, 1971, and Mills, Chapter 12). Since the methods had been developed in work with adults, it had not been anticipated that they would transfer so readily to work with congenitally blind children.

When Blasch, Suterko, and Blaha left Hines for Western Michigan University, one concern was that the university training programs would be short-lived. The original grants for the training programs were for five years, but Malamazian (1970) and others felt that the two programs at Western Michigan and Boston College would meet the nation's need for mobility specialists in three to five years. By 1966, recognition of the value of trained mobility specialists by agencies and schools led to such a great demand that another conference sponsored by the Vocational Rehabilitation Administration and the School of Rehabilitation Counseling, Richmond Professional Institute, was held in Washington, D. C. Forty people representing the Vocational Rehabilitation Administration, the Office of Education, the Veterans Administration, private and state agencies, residential schools, and others were called the Ad Hoc Committee Concerned with Mobility Instruction for the Blind. Spurred on by the perceived need to come up with the greatest number of well-trained mobility specialists in the shortest time, the Committee reviewed the existing training programs and explored other possibilities of increasing the number of mobility specialists. While some questions were raised concerning whether or not mobility specialists needed to be trained at the graduate level, a general respect for the existing programs was expressed. In addition, it was concluded that even if programs were developed on an undergraduate level, mobility instructors could not be mass produced in less time. As a matter of fact it was reported that summer sessions held by Western Michigan and Boston College for teachers working with blind children and for certain agency personnel were not successful in producing contributing personnel to the field. Of the 50 trainees enrolled in such programs, only four remained as instructors (Ad Hoc Committee on Mobility Instruction for the Blind, 1966).

As a result of this conference, the existing programs were encouraged to double their student enrollment and the VRA to continue its support for these programs and to consider supporting new graduate and undergraduate programs. A number of research studies to provide more empirical information about the need for mobility instruction and the actual knowledge and skills needed by mobility specialists were also suggested. The necessity of studying the mobility needs of partially sighted persons also received attention. Finally, representatives of the Office of Education indicated their intention to support a new orientation and mobility graduate program at San Francisco State College under the direction of Georgie Lee Abel and a pilot program for mobility instructors at the undergraduate level at Florida State University coordinated by Gideon Jones. The Office of Education entry into this area reflected the increased demand for mobility specialists in school programs. In the meantime, the Vocational Rehabilitation Administration decided to support another program, this time at California State University at Los Angeles. Larry Blaha left Western Michigan to develop the California State program beginning in September, 1966.

As the need for mobility specialists increased, so did training programs. In 1969, the U.S. Office of Education funded two programs, at the University of Pittsburgh and the University of Northern Colorado. Pittsburgh began taking students in fall, 1969, and Northern Colorado in 1970. These programs attempted to produce mobility specialists who could be certified as mobility specialists and as classroom teachers of the visually impaired to meet a perceived need in some areas, for example the western and mountain states, where school systems might have too small a visually impaired population to justify two separate specialists. Dual certification was thought to be a solution. The continually increasing demand for mobility specialists, however, did not allow much opportunity for this experiment to be evaluated since graduates of these programs gravitated toward traditional mobility positions.

Three undergraduate programs began in 1972. One was at Stephen F. Austin University in Nacogdoches, Texas, to meet the mobility needs of Texas and surrounding states; another at Cleveland State University in response to the expressed needs of agencies in Ohio and surrounding states which felt that they were unable to attract enough graduates of the existing programs to meet their needs. These two programs on the undergraduate level shared another similarity, establishment in departments oriented toward social services rather than special education as had been the case previously. The Cleveland State program functioned initially with the support of the Cleveland Society for the Blind, but in 1974 a grant was obtained from the Cleveland Foundation which sustained the program for two years. The third undergraduate program was established at Talladega State College in Alabama.

Two graduate programs were begun in 1975 again largely as a result of the encouragement of private agencies in the area. One was established at Hunter College of the City University of New York, and the other at the University of Arkansas, Little Rock, in conjunction with the Department of Counselor Education. These were on the graduate level and associated with education programs. This brought the number of programs to twelve, eight graduate and four undergraduate.

The university training programs have become the primary means of articulating and delivering the body of knowledge that has come to be the core of the profession of orientation and mobility. The first programs were guided in curriculum development by the report of the 1959 Orientation and Mobility Symposium. Later programs following the model set by the first programs as well as the suggested content of programs published as part of the COMSTAC Report (to be discussed later). While individualized learning experiences under the blindfold, supervised teaching opportunities, and information about diseases of the eye seemed to be the most consistent parts of all of the programs; there were differences in the amount of background information provided and the course structure in which it was delivered (*Long Cane News,* 1975). This was true among programs and within the same program over time. In the beginning, the programs tended to provide background knowledge in areas such as kinesiology, audiology, and psychology through courses in these subjects given by other university departments. Over the years, however, orientation and mobility faculty have taken on responsibilty for providing the basic information in these areas through their own courses or seminars to make the content in these areas more relevant to the mobility specialists' needs. Material related to blindness and services for visually impaired persons was offered either as seminars or as courses. General professional information in education, rehabilitation, or social services was provided along with some background in research.

At present, no specific standards for the accreditation of programs have been developed nor has an accreditation procedure been implemented. The certification committee of the Orientation and Mobility Interest Group of the American Association of Workers for the Blind (AAWB) has functioned in a capacity similar to that of an accreditation body since it has certified persons as mobility specialists based on the similarity of the content of the university programs to those programs in operation when certification standards and procedures were developed in 1968. The Orientation and Mobility Interest Group has struggled with this problem since its 1975 meeting at the AAWB Convention in Atlanta. While the need for standards is clearly recognized, no comprehensive and explicit set of program standards has yet been developed and adopted by the profession.

In Other Countries

The body of knowledge that has been developed in relation to orientation and mobility for the visually impaired has also spread to other countries. Blasch (1971) discussed how this began in the 1960s as a result of interaction between American and British programs. British specialists visited American programs, and American mobility specialists visited Great Britain for extended periods of time to initiate mobility training programs for visually impaired people and to train mobility specialists.

Similar extensive exchange visits were also made to programs in Australia, and shorter programs were concluded for persons interested in orientation and mobility in Paris, Japan, Brazil, South Africa, and elsewhere. Students from other countries studied in the United States and returned to establish mobility programs in their own countries (Blasch, 1971).

The profession's development is also indicated by the rise of a body of literature. The *Long Cane News,* originally a newsletter for Western Michigan and Boston College graduates (Blasch, 1971), has developed into a basic source of practice information, with a mailing list that far exceeds the number of mobility specialists who have graduated from the various programs. In addition, beginning in the 1960s, more and more articles related to orientation and mobility steadily began to appear in the *New Outlook for the Blind,* now the *Journal of Visual Impairment and Blindness,* the *Blindness Annual, Education of the Visually Handicapped,* and in *Low Vision Abstracts.*

For some time there was a reluctance to publish the actual techniques taught by mobility specialists. There was a fear, typical of new and developing professions, that if the techniques were easily available in print they might be used incorrectly by those who did not understand them completely or that the need for mobility specialists might lessen. As the profession has matured, however, these fears related to the publication of methods and techniques have been replaced by the recognition of the need to put the present body of knowledge of the profession into print as a necessary step toward the standardization and further development of the field. The American Foundation for the Blind published the first techniques book, by Everett Hill and Purvis Ponder, in 1976. This was followed in 1977 by a Center for Independent Living publication of the techniques of orientation and mobility in the form of behavioral objectives (Allen, Griffith and Shaw, 1977).

This text represents another significant stage in the growth of the profession, the first effort to bring together the wide range of background information needed by mobility specialists.

PROFESSIONAL ASSOCIATIONS

Carr-Saunders (1928) and Greenwood (1957) identified another characteristic of professions: the development of associations of members of the profession who come together to share information and to act collectively to advance the profession's goals. The first national organization of mobility specialists developed as divisions within the American Association of Workers for the Blind (AAWB) and the Association for the Education of the Visually Handicapped (AEVH), formerly the American Association of Instructors for the Blind (AAIB).

At the 1964 AAWB Annual Convention in New York City, an informal meeting was held for all individuals interested in orientation and mobility. Sixteen persons attended and discussed forming an association through which mobility specialists could exchange ideas, discuss common interests, receive current information, and provide for professional growth. A petition was presented to the AAWB Board of Directors requesting a new interest group devoted to orientation and mobility. The Board approved the petition and appointed Rod Kossick the first chairman.

The first meeting of the new interest group (Group IX) took place at the 1965 Denver AAWB meeting, with much of the initial meeting devoted to organizational activities. Loyal E. Apple was elected chairman, reaffirming the continuing influence of the Hines Blind Rehabilitation Center which Apple directed, and Robert Whitstock of The Seeing Eye was elected secretary. Interest Group IX gradually became the chief policy-making body of mobility specialists, destined to play a significant role in the development and implementation of certification standards and procedures and a code of ethics for the profession. The AAWB structure unfortunately prevented the group from developing into a true professional organization. Like other Interest Groups, Group IX could not restrict membership to professionally trained or certified mobility specialists. Rather, membership was open to any AAWB member who wanted to join. While most members have always been professionally trained mobility specialists and the actions of the Interest Group have always reflected the priorities of the profession, this membership policy prevents the organization from being as strong and as effective as it might otherwise be.

A similar group interested in orientation and mobility emerged in the Association for the Education of the Visually Handicapped. Following a general session presentation at the 1966 Utah Convention on the development of the orientation and mobility training programs, a call was made for anyone interested in forming an orientation and mobility group within the association. This group first met during the AAIB meeting in Salt Lake City, Utah, in 1966. Donald Blasch was the first chairman of the group. While the group was composed largely of persons who taught in schools, many issues and many members were the same as in AAWB. Efforts have been made recently to promote collaboration and mutual action between AAWB and AEVH mobility interest groups. Consultation and input has been sought by the AAWB group from the AEVH group in the development of certification standards and procedures. Currently the AEVH group appoints two official members to the AAWB-AEVH certification committee, the certifying body in orientation and mobility, although the actual certification is granted by the Board of Directors of AAWB.

While seeking and incorporating the input of AEVH mobility specialists in the deliberations of the committees of AAWB insures the broadest possible representation of mobility specialists in the decisions of the Interest Group, the process also tends to delay the work of both organizations. There is a two year lag between meetings of each of the larger organizations, since AEVH has a national meeting one year and AAWB the other. If an AAWB committee takes action on which it would like collaboration from AEVH, that organization cannot take up the matter until its convention the following year. Another year lapses before the AAWB committee can receive and incorporate input from AEVH. The current structures of the two organizations simply do not lend themselves to efficient action on matters facing the mobility profession.

In recent years organizations of mobility specialists have developed at the state and regional levels to more effectively exchange ideas and share information. Some of these developed as interest groups within state AAWB chapters and have similar organizational structures and membership requirements. Others have developed independently, motivated in part by the desire to establish organizations limited in membership to professionally trained mobility specialists. This movement began in 1966 with the establishment of the California Association of Orientation and Mobility Specialists (CAOMS). As a professional association, CAOMS published proceedings of annual meetings and lists of mobility specialists and agencies providing mobility services throughout the state. CAOMS hoped to promote professional growth among its members, upgrade the quality of mobility services provided, maintain a code of ethics, provide public education, promote research, and encourage the employment of professionally trained mobility specialists.

The New York State Association of Orientation and Mobility Specialists (NYSAOMS) was begun in 1970, because of the need for an organization that would take a strong stand on professional training for mobility specialists certified in accord with nationally established standards. This was particularly necessary in New York State where a large number of mobility personnel were being trained on-the-job in agencies without regard for the standards that had been established. The NYSAOMS group evolved two levels of membership, one for professionally trained and certified mobility specialists with the privileges of voting and holding office. Another type of membership for those not professionally trained but interested or involved in orientation and mobility was also offered so that such personnel could be involved and benefit from professional growth activities. It was thought, however, contradictory to the organization's purposes to allow such persons the opportunity to hold office and to vote.

A group established in Pennsylvania in 1972 closely followed the model established by the New York group and called itself the Pennsylvania Association of Orientation and Mobility Specialists (PAOMS). This group was developed largely in response to action taken by the Penn-Del chapter of AAWB which contradicted the position taken by the national AAWB on the issue of certification of mobility specialists. As a result of the efforts of PAOMS, agreement was reached between AAWB and the Penn-Del chapter on the importance of and need for unity in the support of standards of excellence in the certification of mobility specialists. PAOMS went on to promote the sharing of ideas and information about mobility specialists throughout the state. Similar organizations have begun in Illinois and in Washington. In other areas, more broadly based organizations of mobility specialists have sprung up. The Northeastern Orientation and Mobility Association (NOMA) draws its membership from throughout New England. The Southeastern Orientation and Mobility Association (SOMA) draws mobility specialists from the southeastern states. Most recently regional mobility interest groups have developed within the regional structure of AAWB to provide additional stimulation and opportunities for action supplementary to the national mobility group.

DEVELOPMENT OF STANDARDS

One reason why professionals come together in formal associations is to develop standards of education and training to insure that those entering the area of service are of high calibre by developing a method of identifying and recognizing those persons who have the necessary amount and type of training. Orientation and mobility became involved in this process early in its history as a result of the widespread attention to accountability and certification issues current at the inception of the profession.

The medical and the teaching professions were first to begin certifying that their members possessed certain personal and professional qualifications which made them particularly suitable for service as doctors or teachers respectively. Efforts to accredit institutions such as hospitals and schools often required that the professionals who staffed them met certain prescribed standards, usually those established by recognized professional organizations.

Similar efforts to develop and upgrade standards appeared in the professions serving visually impaired people as early as 1940 when AAIB initiated a nationwide certification program for teachers of the visually impaired. In 1943, AAWB launched a comparable certification program for teachers of the adult blind. Moving toward accreditation of agencies, AAWB, in 1954, adopted a code of ethics and began to award a seal of good practice to agencies operating within it. While commendable, the program lacked the organizational machinery and strength necessary to affect standards significantly in the field.

Influenced by these precedents and increased concern for accountability, AFB, in October 1961, began a study "to project the method, scope, and structure necessary to carry out an accreditation program in the field of work for the blind" (COMSTAC, 1966). The study recommended the formulation of standards for agency administration and service programs, and an organization to administer a nationwide system of voluntary accreditation based on them. From this the Commission on Standards and Accreditation of Services for the Blind (COMSTAC) was created. This study also initiated the process which led eventually to the development of standards and a process for certifying orientation and mobility specialists.

COMSTAC appointed a Committee on Standards for Orientation and Mobility Services to conceptualize and express the role of these services in agencies and schools, the skills to be taught in relation to both cane and dog guide programs, the physical, personal, and professional qualifications of mobility specialists, and similar concerns.*

This Committee outlined principles for some of the program aspects of orientation and mobility services and standards for physical, personal, and professional qualifications for mobility specialists. These standards reflected most of the points made at the 1959 conference which led to the establishment of the initial university programs. Most notably, the standards called for the mobility specialist to have vision correctable in each eye to 20/20, no restrictions in visual field, and no evidence of visual pathology which would contribute to progressive deterioration. This strong insistence on good vision reflected the same concern of the 1959 conference that the mobility specialist had to be able to insure the client's safety during travel while distancing himself from the client physically. The other

---

*The Committee was composed of George Werntz, chairman, Donald Blasch, John Eichorn, Richard Hoover, William Johns, A. Ryrie Koch, Russell Williams, Louis Rives, McAllister Upshaw, and Arthur Dye.

physical and personal standards called for normal hearing, good physical health, a personality capable of meeting the demands and stresses of the job, the ability to develop professional relationships, good observation skills, work organization skills, the ability to accept supervision, and a number of other characteristics.

The professional qualifications formulated by the committee also reflected back to the 1959 conference in that they called for graduation from an accredited graduate level program in orientation and mobility. While the standards did not go so far as to stipulate the content and structure of such programs, the report from the committee did allude to the existence of differences in opinion about the preparation required for the profession and included in an appendix a description of the content of graduate level training programs (Appendix A). At this stage, the early 1960s, the description presented information mostly about the content of such a training program, but relatively little about other aspects such as the number of hours of supervised practice required, course structure, and faculty qualifications.

Finally, the Committee recognized that a certifying body would be needed to implement standards developed, especially since there were already a number of practicing mobility specialists who had not graduated from a university program but who were performing well and had a right to recognition. In another appendix to the report, the Committee called for an "appropriate body" to be established to develop and implement standards for certification of mobility specialists, both those trained in academic programs and those trained in non-academic settings currently serving as mobility specialists.

Certification Process

While COMSTAC was formulating its criteria and methods for evaluating and upgrading work for the blind, the orientation and mobility interest group within the American Association of Workers for the Blind was emerging and taking form. When the Interest Group met for the second time in 1966, the intent and standards of the COMSTAC group were known, and the challenge to an appropriate body to develop and implement a certification process for mobility specialists was accepted by the group. In July, 1966, at the AAWB Convention in Pittsburgh, C. Warren Bledsoe moved that "Whereas it is a major concern of this Interest Group to insure safe and effective mobility instruction by licensing, registering, certifying, or a like process, it shall be the primary objective of the Interest Group during the ensuing year to study means of reaching this goal for which purpose the chairman is empowered to appoint a committee" (AAWB, Group IX, Minutes). The resolution was passed, and the first certification committee, Gerald Mundy, Wilma Spake-Seely, Stanley Doran, John Malamazian and James Doyle was established.

Before the 1967 convention, the certification committee formulated standards based heavily on the standards recommended in the COMSTAC report. There was a reiteration of the physical and personal qualifications of COMSTAC, including the requirement of vision correctable to 20/20 in both eyes. The professional qualifications called for graduation from an accredited graduate level program that meets the standards outlined in the COMSTAC report, as well as membership in good standing in at least one professional organization in the field. In addition, a grandfather clause was developed to allow for the certification of individuals who had been teaching as mobility specialists for a minimum of five years, and who met the physical and personal qualifications established. The grandfather clause required that such individuals had learned mobility techniques with a cane while working under a blindfold in an agency that met COMSTAC standards, and submitted evidence of background knowledge or course participation in anatomy, physiology, and disease of the eye, kinesiology, hearing, mobility devices, dog guides, electronic devices, and low vision aids. In lieu of this, such applicants would have to pass a written examination in these areas. This avenue of certification was time-limited.

The certification standards also established two levels of certification, permanent and provisional. Provisional certification was for those who had completed an approved graduate program. Permanent certification was to be granted to those who had completed three years of satisfactory work experience following the completion of their university training program.

A report of the certification committee was presented to and accepted by the Interest Group at its 1967 meeting in Miami Beach and a committee selected to investigate methods for implementing certification. The committee, Martha Rosemeyer, Larry Blaha, Monica Cain, Robert Long, Stanley Suterko, William Walkowiak, and Marvin Weesies, had to decide upon the appropriate body for actually bestowing and overseeing the certification, the election of the certifying committee as well as the responsibilities, duties, and operating procedures of the certifying body.

It was first decided that the certification process should be under the auspices of AAWB, but that since a number of mobility specialists were associated with AAIB, the committee decided to investigate the possibilities of joint AAWB/AAIB certification. After encouragement by both parent organizations, the certification committee recommended a joint committee to both organizations, at their separate annual meetings in Toronto in July, 1968. The proposal presented by the certification committee included physical, personal, and professional qualifications, a grandfather clause, an inactive provision (calling for loss of certification for those completely out of the field), and stipulations for provisional and permanent certification. It was presented first to the AAIB Interest Group, and passed, with some revisions, notably the addition of a provision which recognized that graduates of undergraduate mobility programs could be certified during the following two years, receiving permanent certification if they had been employed for three years and were enrolled in a master's degree program. Otherwise, such applicants would receive provisional certification. AAIB, however, decided to allow the actual certification to be done by AAWB.

The document, with the changes recommended by the AAIB Group was then presented to the AAWB Group and passed along with the recommendation that another five person committee continue to study the document and recommend further changes that might be needed. The passed document also recommended that the National Accreditation Council (NAC), the implementation body for COMSTAC, also incorporate the use of certified instructors as an integral part of its requirement for mobility personnel in agencies and schools seeking accreditation. The Interest Group then presented the following resolution to the AAWB Board of Directors: "Whereas, the AAWB and AAIB Orientation and Mobility Interest Groups have passed and thereby adopted the following procedures and requirements for certification of Orientation and Mobility personnel, and Whereas, this certification process has been studied for the past two years, the Interest Groups highly recommended implementation of this resolution as soon as possible. Now, therefore, be it resolved that the Board of Directors of the AAWB approve the attached procedures and requirements for certification of Orientation and Mobility instructors."

Certification Begins

The passage of this resolution by the AAWB Board of Directors in October, 1968, officially marked the beginning of certification in orientation and mobility. This certification would be granted by AAWB on the advice and recommendation of the Certification Committee of mobility specialists. AAIB was invited to appoint a non-voting member to the committee. The first certification committee to be involved in the actual implementation of certification consisted of Stanley Suterko, John Malamazian, Robert Whitstock, Paul McDade, Robert Hughes, and Gary Coker (the non-voting member from AAIB). This committee drew up applications for certification and mailed them to all known practitioners of orientation and mobility. In July, 1969, the first mobility specialists were certified by AAWB at the Chicago convention. At this same meeting, the certification study committee made several recommendations including continuing study of the possibility of joint AAWB-AAIB certification.

The membership of Interest Group IX continued to evaluate the effect of the certification procedures and to consider difficulties that arose with the intention of developing the most fair and comprehensive set of standards. Following the 1969 convention, a Certification Review Committee (CRC) was appointed to deal with some of the concerns that had been raised. The chairman was Bruce Blasch and other members included Robert Crouse, Everett Hill, James Kimbrough, Dave Koper, and Robert Mills. This committee reported its recommendations to the Interest Group in Richmond at the 1971 meeting.

In response to concern that the original vision requirement was unrealistic, the committee recommended that the vision requirement be changed to 20/40 in the best eye with correction and a contiguous field of vision no less than 120°, and no evidence of pathology contributing to progressive eye deterioration. These standards were based on research on the amount of vision necessary to safely operate a motor vehicle in the belief that there was some similarity between the latter and the necessity of assuring the safety of a visually impaired client in traffic. This change was adopted by the Interest Group as a part of the certification standards, as it was thought to be preferable to the seemingly arbitrary requirement of 20/20 vision in each eye and no restriction in the visual field. In 1976, the technical committee on mobility instructor qualifications appointed to advise NAC on possible changes in NAC's standards for mobility specialists reaffirmed the action taken by the Interest Group on this question. In recognition of the mobility specialist's need to separate himself physically from the client as the training progressed, and still be able to observe the client's reactions to situations both to insure his safety and to better discuss with the client the events of each lesson, the technical committee determined that a visual acuity of 20/40 was needed to assure the safety of a client at a distance of 500 feet (150 m) and to observe a client's actions and gestures at shorter distances.

The grandfather clause and the undergraduate provision, both time-limited in the first standards, were due to expire in 1973. The CRC recommended that the grandfather clause be allowed to expire, although it was eventually decided to extend it for another limited period in view of the change in the vision requirement, since some of those eligible for certification under the grandfather clause might not have applied under the more restrictive visual standards. The CRC recommended and the Interest Group approved a revised undergraduate provision that continued to allow the graduates of the Florida State program to receive provisional certification. It was stipulated, however, that these individuals would have to apply for permanent certification within five years. Permanent certification would be granted provided the applicant could furnish evidence of three years of satisfactory employment as a mobility specialist and evidence of having obtained a master's degree in special education or rehabilitation.

The CRC also brought to the Interest Group's attention at the 1971 meeting the fact that a discrepancy existed in the COMSTAC standards implemented by NAC. In the section dealing with orientation and mobility, the standards called unequivocally for the training of mobility specialists in university training programs. In a later section of the report, dealing with standards for rehabilitation centers, the standards seemed to allow the training of mobility specialists to continue in on-the-job programs in agencies. The Interest Group voted to communicate its own support of the higher standards and to ask NAC to clarify which set of standards it could support.

On-The-Job vs. University Training

Finally, it was recommended that individuals from non-university mobility training programs not be considered as qualified for certification under the present criteria. This issue reflected the fact that there continued to be some dispute concerning the proper level of training for mobility specialists (Kimbrough, 1969). Some agencies had established on-the-job training programs for mobility instructors and wanted to continue them to be assured of a continuous supply of personnel attuned to their own agencies, and available at a lower cost than university trained and certified mobility specialists. In addition, there was a feeling that mobility specialists did not need to be trained at a master's degree level. There was concern that such specialists would not continue to work as practitioners but would rather move into administrative positions.

Blasch and Wurzburger (1971) attempted to deal with these concerns through information they collected about the location and status of graduates of orientation and mobility training programs. Of the 332 graduates of university mobility training programs covered in the survey, 87 percent were still in services to the visually impaired, 83 percent working in orientation and mobility, and 75 percent offering mobility instruction directly to visually impaired persons. Only 13 percent of the graduates from these programs were no longer working with the visually impaired. Approximately 3 percent of these were women not working due to family responsibilities. Another 2.5 percent had returned to school to obtain advanced degrees. About 2 percent were unaccounted for, leaving approximately 3 percent who were known to have left work for the visually impaired. Of the 87 percent of the graduates who were still involved in work with visually impaired persons, 95 percent were still involved with orientation and mobility either as instructors or supervisors.

In the early years of the Nixon administration, when so many rehabilitation personnel training programs were threatened by cutbacks, Mary Switzer used the Blasch and Wurzburger findings to argue for the effectiveness and the continuation of these programs and encourage other professional training areas to develop similar documentation of the success of their efforts.

Many agencies that insisted on continuing on-the-job training programs, in spite of the increase in university programs and the development of certification standards, assumed that university programs were not producing enough mobility specialists to meet the needs. Welsh and Blasch (1974) collected information to provide a more factual basis for such judgments. They asked respondents to discuss their actual and theoretical needs for mobility specialists. In other words, they differentiated between the number of actual positions open for mobility specialists and the administrator's projection of how many he might need if he had sufficient funds to serve all the clients who needed such service from his agency. The actual number of positions turned up by the survey was 50. When these were projected to the entire population of agencies and school programs based on the percentage of response to the questionnaires, it was concluded that slightly more than 100 actual positions for mobility specialists were probably open, a figure very close to the total number of mobility specialists being graduated each year at the time. Thereafter the argument that a shortage of personnel justified the continuation of on-the-job training lost credibility.

The same study also provided information about the employment and use of mobility specialists; one aspect is relevant here. Scott (1969) pointed out that one negative aspect of agency training was that such personnel were usually "locked into" those agencies that had trained them. The study verified Scott's contention: respondents indicated their strong preference for recruiting new mobility staff from university programs and their avoidance of individuals trained in agencies. This indicated support for the efforts to professionalize mobility instruction and for the impact of professionally trained instructors on the field of work with the visually impaired.

By the time the AAWB Orientation and Mobility Interest Group convened in Cleveland in 1973, three new undergraduate training programs had developed, and there was a need to examine again and possibly change the certification criteria to reflect new developments. The professional standards called for graduation from a graduate program or from the undergraduate program at Florida State University. Graduates from the Stephen F. Austin University, the Cleveland State University, and the Talladega State College programs would apply for certification, and the Interest Group had to consider how it would react. Another Certification Review Committee (CRC) was appointed to consider whether and in what way the criteria would have to be changed and to recommend specific curriculum standards which could be used to evaluate new and developing programs. This committee soon realized that similar detailed standards were not even available for graduate programs, and felt that they could not complete their charge prior to the next meeting in 1975. At the 1975 meeting in Atlanta, the CRC proposed a temporary solution, certification of graduates of new training programs to the extent that the committee judged that content of the new programs was comparable to those whose graduates were currently being certified. This was approved. In the meantime, an augmented CRC was directed to further develop a draft curriculum proposal submitted to the committee by William Wiener.

STANDARDIZATION OF TRAINING

With this action, mobility as a profession moved toward the type of accountability and standardization needed in view of the continuing expansion of the field. For two years the augmented CRC, under Wiener's leadership, worked as subcommittees across the country developing components of the certification standards proposal. The proposal finally presented to the Interest Group at the 1977 AAWB convention in Portland was a comprehensive document that contained four distinct sections. The first section suggested standards for university programs which for the first time discussed: type and number of faculty members needed for an adequate program; addressed some of the instructional requirements of a training program, including the kind and quality of clinical teaching experiences provided for students; considered questions of admission standards and evaluation procedures; and provided a detailed list of the curriculum content thought necessary. Not only were subjects related directly to orientation and mobility discussed, but also the areas related to general background in blindness, professional concerns, and research.

The second section of the 1977 CRC proposal addressed the need for an accreditation process to review and approve orientation and mobility training programs in universities. A formal review process was recommended to help programs meet the proposed standards and to assure the certification committee that graduates had been exposed to the information and learning experiences deemed necessary for entry into the profession.

The third section of the proposal called for a revision in the standards for certification including a revision in the categories of certification offered. Instead of provisional and permanent certification, the proposal called for a change to baccalaureate and graduate certification, with both requiring periodic and ongoing continuing education and professional development as is customary in most other professions. These changes were motivated in part by the fact that permanent certification contained no incentive for continued professional growth, particularly unfortunate in a profession so new and developing so rapidly. These changes also made it possible for persons entering the profession from the undergraduate level to continue to serve as certified mobility specialists without getting a master's degree, provided they participated in professional growth activities similar to those proposed for graduate mobility specialists. A final section of the CRC proposal suggested a special certification in the teaching of electronic travel aids.

While there was general support for the concepts contained in this proposal, the document's comprehensiveness and wide-ranging implications led the Interest Group to decide to take more time and to solicit more input from practitioners about the changes. The document would form the basis for soliciting input from mobility specialists at regional and state meetings of AAWB before the national meeting in 1979.

Use of Paraprofessionals

Two other issues germane to a discussion of standards and certification for mobility specialists need additional elaboration. These are the role of paraprofessionals and/or mobility aides in mobility services, and the certification needed by mobility specialists to work in public schools. The issue of paraprofessionals or mobility aides is confused by a lack of consistency in terminology. When these terms are used to indicate mobility instructors who are trained through programs conducted by agencies, the issue is clear. Such agency-trained instructors do *not* meet the criteria currently established for mobility specialists by the profession. On the other hand, there is a category of personnel variously referred to as mobility aides, paraprofessionals, and other titles, whose training and responsibilities are limited. Despite attention to this issue by ad hoc committees of Interest Group IX of AAWB during the past several years, no clear consensus of opinion has emerged.

Some mobility specialists have trained aides to assist them in some of the learning activities that precede formal mobility instruction, for example concept development, exposure to different environments, sensory training, and basic physical conditioning. Others have trained aides to provide instruction in basic skill areas such as sighted guide and protective techniques and indoor orientation skills. Still others have trained aides to teach some of the cane skills to provide orientation services and to provide supervision of mobility lessons as part of the regular mobility training. Obviously a point is reached where the duties and responsibilities of some workers called "aides" parallel those of mobility specialists. Some would say that the difference is that those considered aides work under supervision, while mobility specialists can work independently. However, a wide range of opinions exist in regard to which duties might be appropriately assigned to mobility "aides," Scheffel's (1975) study illustrates this range.

Scheffel reported on a project to train "rehabilitation aides" to assist in mobility instruction and in rehabilitation teaching. The project was operated by the Virginia Commission for the Visually Handicapped and funded by the New Careers in Rehabilitation Program of the Rehabilitation Services Administration. Scheffel indicated that he originally intended to train the aides to provide basic skills in orientation and mobility and especially to work with older blind persons. However, agencies sponsoring students and providing internship and employment opportunities suggested that the aides' functions should be:

1. To provide sighted guide and reader services

2. To provide instruction in basic orientation and mobility and daily living skills, including the techniques of using a sighted guide, hand and forearm, trailing, direction takers, cane techniques including the diagonal, touch, and stairs techniques, familiarization, independent orientation, block travel, rote street crossings, locating lost objects, seating, entering and exiting automobiles, home management, personal management, and limited communications

3. To provide familiarization services

4. To provide transportation services

5. To construct and repair canes

6. To assist with recreational and leisure time activities

7. To assist with in-service training programs

8. To provide on a rote basis instruction in methods of safe and independent street crossings in rural or uncongested urban areas

9. To conduct on a prescription basis follow-up evaluations to determine if additional training is necessary; and

10. To conduct on a prescription basis drop-off or independent lessons with advanced travelers.

Scheffel indicated that these suggestions from agencies led to changes in the original concept of the functions of aides, but did not reveal the direction or the extent of the changes. Obviously, the functions listed by agency administrators would challenge the abilities of professionally trained mobility specialists as well as those of rehabilitation teachers. To attempt to prepare individuals whose educational qualifications did not have to exceed a high school diploma for this wide range of functions in a six month training program does not seem to consider the needs of visually impaired clients for quality services. Such shortcuts to quality training are frequently justified by citing the needs of multiply handicapped blind persons and older blind persons. It seems, however, that these clients might require the skills of the most capably trained instructors rather than the services of minimally trained "aides."

Employment in Public Schools

Mobility specialists who have applied for positions in public school programs have sometimes encountered another certification problem. Most states require that teachers in public schools qualify in one of the categories of certification as a teacher. Yet only six states, California, Colorado, Hawaii, Michigan, New Hampshire, and Rhode Island (Smith, Dickerson and Liska, 1978), have developed separate categories of certification for mobility specialists which reflect their particular role and background and education necessary for this position. Many school systems require that the mobility specialist meet the requirements for certification as a classroom teacher of the visually impaired. Some who attend a university program which prepares for dual certification as both classroom teachers and mobility specialists meet such criteria. Others meet the criteria as a result of previous education or work experience as teachers before participating in a mobility training program. Most mobility specialists, however, do not meet such educational criteria and are not able to qualify to work in the public schools.

One challenge facing the profession is to work with state departments of education to develop appropriate categories of certification for mobility specialists based on criteria appropriate to mobility instruction as developed by the professional organization. Lack of such criteria not only excludes mobility specialists from working in the schools, but means that persons certified as classroom teachers but not trained as mobility specialists, can be assigned the duties of a mobility specialist without the training needed. Recently, the Orientation and Mobility Interest Group of AAWB has appointed a committee to gather data about this situation in various states, to develop a position, and suggest appropriate actions to remedy this situation.

The mobility profession will have to continually monitor and be a part of all efforts to develop standards related to services for the visually impaired. Part of the obligation of the profession is to guarantee that its expertise in the area of orientation and mobility is reflected in whatever standards are promulgated. This is another way in which the professional demonstrates commitment to provide the highest quality services to visually impaired persons.

REGULATING THE PROFESSION: A CODE OF ETHICS

Most discussions of the hallmarks of professions include the activities that guarantee society that its members will use their specialized knowledge in a way that will benefit people who must avail themselves of members' services. As certification became more firmly established, mobility specialists realized that it was insufficient to establish such a process without some mechanism to assure society that those who have entered the profession with the appropriate preparation also practice it in accord with acceptable and respected principles. In 1972 the Orientation and Mobility Interest Group appointed an ad hoc committee to investigate the feelings of the membership concerning the need for a code of ethics and to pull together some of the principles that might become a part of it.

Under the chairmanship of William Wiener, the committee composed of Richard Welsh, Everett Hill, Robert LaDuke, Robert Mills, and Gerald Mundy examined codes of ethics of other professional organizations and considered the rationale for such a code. Once established, a code could benefit four groups of people. Clients would benefit from the existence of an explicit statement of what was considered acceptable practice in orientation and mobility. Such a statement could encourage and reinforce the type of service that reflected the worth and dignity of clients and their right to confidentiality, safety, objectivity, participation in the decision making, and the highest quality services available. The community would benefit from having an explicit statement of the profession's intent to deliver services worthy of the investment and services that would be available to all members regardless of race, sex, age, severity of disability, or other characteristics. Administrators and employers could benefit from having a clear indication of what was considered acceptable practice in the profession against which they could evaluate the practice of their employees in mobility. The principles expressed in the code might also stimulate administrators to upgrade their mobility services when necessary.

The code of ethics was also potentially of benefit to mobility specialists themselves. With a consensus statement of what was considered acceptable practice, the mobility specialist could operate in difficult situations with some assurance that his actions would be supported by his peers. Such assurance is particularly necessary today when malpractice is a concern in all professions. A code of ethics would provide a set of criteria against which disputed actions might be judged when claims of malpractice are brought against a mobility specialist. Such principles would protect the professional from having his actions evaluated against criteria formulated by an opposing party in a court of law as a result of a particular claim. In addition, mobility specialists would have some support when they have to resist pressure from employers to participate in actions that are outside the scope of acceptable practice. This step in the profession's development would also promote acceptance of mobility specialists among other disciplines which in turn can lead to greater and more effective teamwork and collaboration.

With these goals in mind, the code of ethics committee surveyed mobility specialists for their input to insure that whatever was developed would represent the thinking of a wide range of members of the profession. Those surveyed were asked whether a code of ethics was necessary, and to react to a selection of principles culled from the codes of other professions which the committee thought might be applicable. Respondents were asked to suggest other principles that they thought should be considered and to relate specific incidents that they had experienced or knew about which they felt suggested ambiguous or unethical practice in need of clarification.

The responses indicated very strong support among mobility specialists for the concept of a code of ethics. Based on the material received from mobility specialists, the committee drafted a sample code which was published in the June, 1973, *Long Cane News*. The proposed code was discussed at the Interest Group meetings during the 1973 AAWB convention, reactions to various principles and sections were discussed, changes made in the code and it was officially adopted at the final meeting of the Interest Group (Appendix B). The membership present at this meeting, however, failed to approve the suggested procedures for implementing the code of ethics and for processing reports of unethical practice. These procedures were referred for further study and discussion. Some felt that the profession was not yet ready to take on the difficulty and expense of a national process for reviewing reports of unethical behavior. Others felt that the process was moving too quickly and that the membership was not keeping up with these changes. At the 1975 meeting, the code of ethics committee reported again to the membership. It was felt that if a review procedure was to be implemented, the ultimate sanction would be the revocation of certification. However, since the Interest Group was issuing permanent certification to members after three years of successful practice, it was unclear whether such certification could be revoked. Further consideration of this issue became linked to the ongoing process of certification review and the review of categories of certification underway.

In the meantime, the application for certification was modified to include the new applicant's pledge of support for the code. It was also recommended that a national registry of mobility specialists who support the code of ethics be established and published periodically. An ethics committee was established as a standing committee within the Interest Group and assigned to continue to study the possibility of a formal review procedure, to be responsible for publicizing the code among mobility specialists, employers, and consumers, to encourage an understanding of its principles, and to continue to update the code when necessary (Welsh & Wiener, 1977).

FUTURE DIRECTIONS

In spite of and perhaps because of the rapid development of orientation and mobility in recent years, a number of critical issues still face the profession and will precipitate difficult decisions about future directions. One such issue has to do with the level of training for mobility specialists. Most of the mobility training programs are on the graduate level in accordance with the recommendations of the 1959 conference that led to the establishment of the first programs. While this approach as stated before was suggested as the best way to provide a sufficient amount of concentrated time to allow beginning mobility specialists to develop the in-depth sensitivity about the problems of blindness and the possibilities for adaptation thought necessary, it should be remembered that most professions were using graduate level programs and that federal support for such programs was tied to the graduate level. In addition, it was thought that the kinds of students who would participate in such programs at the graduate level would be more mature and more settled and, therefore, more likely than undergraduate students to stay with the profession they were entering, and better able to work with adults. This was particularly important in relation to mobility since the program structure that was being proposed and used was an expensive operation compared to other types of graduate programs.

Undergraduate Program

As in many other human service professions, there have more recently been efforts to develop entry level education programs at the undergraduate level. Part of the reasoning for these efforts in orientation and mobility is the expanding demands for the amount and type of knowledge that is becoming necessary for mobility specialists to acquire, particularly in the areas of low vision, electronics, geriatrics, multiple handicaps, and other disabilities. This is making it increasingly difficult for the one year graduate programs to include all of the information needed and still maintain the same amount of blindfold and supervised teaching experiences. Undergraduate programs would permit students who begin on this level to broaden their backgrounds and obtain additional knowledge in the expanding areas as they do their graduate studies.

The continuation of two levels for entry into the orientation and mobility profession is desirable because it provides maximum flexibility in terms of attracting the variety of types of people who can contribute to the growth of the profession in various ways. However, orientation and mobility, along with professions such as social work and rehabilitation counseling, has to define a coherent hierarchy of program structures so that those who begin on the undergraduate level will be in a position to continue to add to their knowledge base while pursuing the next higher degree.

Low Vision

A second critical issue concerns the growing involvement of many mobility specialists in low vision. More and more mobility specialists are finding themselves in situations where the best way to help their clients become more proficient travelers entails lessons designed to help them learn to use their remaining vision more efficiently. With some clients this involves vision stimulation; with others, work with low vision aids and other optical devices. For many it is a combination of both approaches. Perhaps mobility specialists are filling a temporary gap in services that will be filled by vision specialists as the need for this type of direct instruction and stimulation is more generally recognized. However, it may be that these changes in emphasis constitute a more fundamental and permanent change that will endure even as vision specialists such as ophthalmologists and optometrists respond to the new emphasis on low vision.

Electronic Devices

Still another issue relates to electronic mobility devices and the expertise needed to teach clients how to use them. Currently, this expertise is obtained only through short-term training programs available to mobility specialists after graduation. It is not yet clear whether this training should be part of regular training or should continue to be provided on a more limited basis. Those who oppose the expansion of the training programs for all mobility specialists to include electronic devices, cite the fact that currently relatively few clients can afford to purchase electronic devices and therefore comparatively few mobility specialists need training. Others have some doubt about the devices' usefulness and think that the expansion of the training programs is not justified at present. Some feel that electronic training devices should not be integrated into the university programs since it appears that a certain amount of experience as a mobility specialist is needed before an individual can learn how to teach the use of electronic devices. This argument is difficult to evaluate since only a couple of programs have experimented with integrating this training in the regular program. Until these programs have had some experience, there is no alternative against which to measure the current practice of short term programs for experienced mobility specialists.

Related to this issue is the proposal that manufacturers of these devices train mobility specialists in their use. This would relegate an important component of the training of mobility specialists to private companies which would not fall within the purview of the standards and processes of accreditation that would be developed for universities. There is also debate about whether a special category of certification should be established or whether all mobility specialists should be proficient in teaching the use of these devices.

Still another trend that has implications for the profession is the extension of mobility instruction to persons with other disabilities but who are not visually impaired. (See Blasch and Welsh, Chapter 13.) This trend has already begun and is gathering momentum. It is an idea that has the force of logic and is perceived by many as overdue. Reflecting these feelings, the Office of Rehabilitation Service has funded the first university training program for mobility specialists to work with persons with all disabilities. It began at the University of Wisconsin at Madison under the direction of Bruce Blasch in 1978. Mobility specialists must consider how they are going to alter their training curricula, their certification criteria, and their identities to respond to this trend.

One implication of this trend is the growth of orientation and mobility beyond the confines of the professional organizations that deal exclusively with blindness and visual impairment. What might be needed eventually is a professional mobility association that relates to all types of clients. Even though orientation and mobility began in work for the blind, it may come to resemble other professions such as rehabilitation counseling and occupational therapy in which members are identified by their discipline but serve a variety of types of clients.

Given the continuing emergence of new issues facing the profession, two general challenges take on the most importance in the long run. First, there is an urgent need for professionals to become much more active than they have been in the development and verification of knowledge related to the discipline. Like many professions, the knowledge and skills of orientation and mobility have grown largely from the practice experiences of the early practitioners, but there has been relatively little effort to demonstrate and document the validity of this knowledge and move the profession ahead. Mobility specialists must do more writing and research than they have in the past, and the profession must stimulate and reward such activity.

The second general challenge facing the profession concerns efforts to continue to upgrade the knowledge and skills of those who have already entered the profession. Most human service professions require members to demonstrate that they have continued to study and learn about their area of expertise. The mobility profession's choice of the terminology "permanent certification" when categories of certification were first established was unfortunate. This has complicated efforts to require upgrading of those individuals who have already become permanently certified. Unless some provision for continuing education is established, there is a risk that the differences in preparation between those entering the profession and those practicing for several years will widen and have a negative effect on the standardization of services available for clients served by different mobility specialists.

Appendix A

Content of Graduate Level Programs for Professional Training of Orientation and Mobility Teachers*

SETTING
Programs to train teachers of orientation and mobility are on the graduate level and are administered by departments, schools or colleges of education.

SELECTION OF CANDIDATES
Students are selected from candidates who meet the physical and personal qualifications outlined in Standards 1.4 and 1.5.

Academic prerequisites are an undergraduate degree in behavioral or biological sciences. At the discretion of the program director, students from other areas of specialization may be accepted when the students' records and college curricula suggest that prerequisites are made up.

CURRICULUM CONTENT
The curriculum includes the following:

1. Course work and experiences which identify and describe sensory deficiencies.
2. A study of complications which may develop out of visual and accompanying sensory impairments.
3. Course work and clinical experiences which help students to learn about the emotional climate which surrounds the blind or visually impaired individual.
4. A study of the etiology, incidence, care and treatment of visual impairments and blindness.
5. A historical review of the care, treatment, education and rehabilitation of those who are blind or visually impaired.
6. A study of the special programs and services which have evolved for the benefit of people who are affected by complications arising out of visual impairments and accompanying impairments, if any.
7. Information about various administrative frameworks and agency settings of the aforementioned special programs and an understanding of how those who teach orientation and mobility fit into and contribute toward the larger objectives of these programs.
8. Information regarding such specialized agency functions as public relations, fund raising, etc.
9. Course work and experiences which reveal the dynamics and objectives of education, rehabilitation and other services of special benefit to those who are blind or visually handicapped.
10. A study of the special state and federal laws and regulations relating to the blind and visually impaired.
11. A historical review of orientation and mobility, including a study of the role of

*COMSTAC Report

human guides, dog guides, canes and all other related prostheses and sensory aids; also consideration of pertinent current research.

12. Use of low vision aids as they relate to orientation and mobility.
13. Correlation of theoretical work with a continuous program of practicum, clinical training, internship or residency.

Appendix B

Code of Ethics for Orientation and Mobility Specialists

(Adopted by Interest Group IX of the American Association of Workers for the Blind, July, 1973.)

PREAMBLE

Orientation and mobility specialists (peripatologists) recognize the significant role that independent movement plays in overall growth and functioning of the individual and are dedicated to helping each individual attain the level of independence necessary to reach his full potential. Orientation and mobility specialists gather, develop, and utilize specialized knowledge in accomplishing this goal. As with all professions, the possession of special knowledge obligates the practitioner to protect the rights of the individuals who must avail themselves of the particular service. To assure the public of our awareness of this obligation, we commit ourselves to this code of ethics.

In order to fulfill this obligation orientation and mobility specialists pledge themselves to standards of acceptable behavior in relation to the following five commitments:

> Commitment to the Student
> Commitment to the Community
> Commitment to the Profession
> Commitment to Colleagues and Other Professionals
> Commitment to Professional Employment Practices

It is the duty of each orientation and mobility specialist to adhere to the principles in the code and encourage his colleagues to do the same.

1. COMMITMENT TO THE STUDENT

1.1   The orientation and mobility specialist should value the worth and dignity of each individual.

1.2   It is the responsibility of the orientation and mobility specialist to strive at all times to maintain the highest standards of service by providing instruction in accord with procedures indicated in section S-3 of *The Comstac Report* and in accord with the physical, personal, and professional qualifications accepted as the criteria for certification by Mobility Interest Groups of AAWB and AEVH.

1.3   The orientation and mobility specialist should take all reasonable precautions to insure the safety of his student and to protect him from conditions which interfere with learning.

1.4   The orientation and mobility specialist should respect the confidentiality of all information pertaining to the student. He must not divulge confidential information about the student to any individual not authorized by the student to receive such information unless required by law or unless withholding such information would endanger the safety of the student or the public.

1.5   Before beginning lessons with the student, the orientation and mobility specialist should make every attempt to obtain and evaluate information about the student which is relevant to the orientation and mobility training.

1.6   The orientation and mobility specialist should respect the right of the student to participate in decisions regarding his training program.

1.7   Decisions regarding continuing or discontinuing training should be made with the student and should be based upon objective evaluation of the student's needs, abilities, and skills. These decisions should be made independent of personal or agency convenience.

1.8   The orientation and mobility specialist should provide sufficient information regarding the various types of orientation and mobility guidance devices and should explore with the student which device will best meet his needs.

1.9   The orientation and mobility specialist should seek the support and involvement of the family in promoting the student's training goals and in advancing his continued success. This should include sharing information with the family that will facilitate the student's welfare and independence, but not communicating information which violates the principles of confidentiality. The orientation and mobility specialist should not change training objectives upon suggestion of the student's family if the specialist's professional judgments would be compromised.

1.10   The orientation and mobility specialist should ask the consent of the student before inviting others to observe a lesson or before arranging to have the student photographed or tape recorded.

1.11   The orientation and mobility specialist should make all reports objective and should present only data relevant to the purposes of the evaluation and training. When appropriate, he should share this information with the student.

1.12   It is good practice to consult with another orientation and mobility specialist when assistance is required in evaluating students.

1.13   The orientation and mobility specialist should endeavor to provide all individuals involved with the students with sufficient knowledge, training and experiences relative to orientation and mobility so as to facilitate the goals of student.

1.14   The orientation and mobility specialist should not dispense or supply orientation and mobility equipment unless it is in the best interest of the student.

1.15   The orientation and mobility specialist should not allow consideration of his own personal comfort or convenience to interfere with the design and implementation of necessary travel lessons.

1.16   The orientation and mobility specialist should be responsible for services to students referred to him and should provide adequate ongoing supervision when any portion of the service is assigned to someone else. He should not assign to a less qualified person any service which requires the skill and judgment of the AAWB-certified orientation and mobility specialists. Such duties or services may properly be assigned to interns or student teachers who are enrolled in orientation and mobility university programs with the understanding that each individual will function under strict supervision.

1.17   The orientation and mobility specialist should make every attempt to see that follow-up service is provided at the completion of training.

2. COMMITMENT TO THE COMMUNITY

2.1   The student should not be refused service by the orientation and mobility specialist because of age, sex, race, religion or national origin.

2.2   The student should not be excluded from service because of the severity of his disabilities unless it is clearly evident that he cannot benefit from the service. The orientation and mobility specialist should attempt to influence decision making which establishes the rights of individuals to receive service.

2.3   The orientation and mobility specialist should contribute to community education by defining the role of orientation and mobility in the community, by describing the nature and delivery of service, and by indicating how the community can become involved in the educational and rehabilitation process.

2.4   The orientation and mobility specialist should not engage in any public education activity that results in exploitation of his students. Exaggeration, sensationalism, superficiality and other misleading activities are to be avoided.

2.5   The orientation and mobility specialist should strive to remedy those deficiences in services that exist in the community.

2.6   The orientation and mobility specialist should encourage and participate in agency or school accreditation.

3. COMMITMENT TO THE PROFESSION

3.1   The orientation and mobility specialist should seek full responsibility for the exercise of professional judgment related to orientation and mobility.

3.2   To the best of his ability, the orientation and mobility specialist should accept the responsibility throughout his career to master and contribute to the growing body of specialized knowledge, concepts and skills which characterize orientation and mobility as a profession.

3.3   The orientation and mobility specialist should interpret and use the writing and research of others with integrity. In writing, making presentations, or conducting research, the orientation and mobility specialist should be familiar with and give recognition to previous work on the topic.

3.4   The orientation and mobility specialist should conduct his investigations in a manner which takes into consideration the welfare of the subject, and report research in a way as to lessen the possibility that his findings will be misleading.

3.5   The orientation and mobility specialist should strive to improve the quality of his service and promote conditions which attract suitable persons to careers in orientation and mobility.

3.6   The orientation and mobility specialist should, whenever possible, support and participate in local, state, and national professional organizations.

3.7   The orientation and mobility specialist should comply with professional practice in making known his availability for professional services.

3.8   The orientation and mobility specialist should accept no gratuities or gifts of significance over and above the predetermined salary or fee for professional service.

3.9 The orientation and mobility specialist should not engage in commercial activities which result in a conflict of interest between these activities and his professional objectives with the student.

3.10 The orientation and mobility specialist involved in development or promotion of orientation and mobility devices, books or other products, should present such products in a professional and factual way.

3.11 The orientation and mobility specialist should expose incompetence, illegal, or unethical behavior.

3.12 The orientation and mobility specialist should strive to provide fair treatment to all members of the profession and support them when unjustly accused or mistreated.

3.13 Each member of the profession has a personal and professional responsibility for supporting the orientation and mobility code of ethics and maintaining its effectiveness.

4. COMMITMENT TO COLLEAGUES AND OTHER PROFESSIONALS

4.1 The orientation and mobility specialist should engage in professional relationships on a mature level and should not become involved in personal disparagement.

4.2 The orientation and mobility specialist should communicate fully and openly with his colleagues in the sharing of specialized knowledge, concepts, and skills.

4.3 The orientation and mobility specialist should not offer professional services to a person receiving orientation and mobility instruction from another orientation and mobility specialist, except by agreement with the other specialist or after the other specialist has ended his work with the student.

4.4 When transferring a student, the orientation and mobility specialist should not commit a receiving specialist to a prescribed course of action. The receiving specialist should take the student's former training into consideration when developing a continued plan for training.

4.5 The orientation and mobility specialist should seek harmonious relations with members of other professions. This should include the discussion and free exchange of ideas regarding the overall welfare of the student and discussion with other professionals regarding the benefits to be obtained from orientation and mobility services.

4.6 The orientation and mobility specialist should not assume responsibilities which are better provided by other professionals who are available to the student.

4.7 The orientation and mobility specialist should seek to facilitate and enhance a team effort with other professionals. In such situations where team decisions are made, the orientation and mobility specialist should contribute information from his own particular perspective and should abide by the team decision unless the team decision requires that he act in violation of the code of ethics.

5. COMMITMENT TO PROFESSIONAL EMPLOYMENT PRACTICES

5.1 The orientation and mobility specialist should apply for, accept, or offer a position on the basis of professional qualification and should conduct himself with integrity in these situations.

5.2 The orientation and mobility specialist should give prompt notification of any change of his availability to the agency or school where he has applied.

5.3   The orientation and mobility specialist seeking to hire other specialists should give prompt notification of change in the availability or nature of a position.

5.4   The orientation and mobility specialist should respond factually when requested to write a letter of recommendation for a colleague seeking a professional position.

5.5   The orientation and mobility specialist should provide applicants seeking information about a position with an honest description of the assignment, conditions of work, and related matters.

5.6   The orientation and mobility specialist should abide by the terms of a contract or agreement, whether verbal or written, unless the terms have been falsely represented or substantially changed by the other party.

5.7   The orientation and mobility specialist should not accept positions where proven principles of orientation and mobility practice are compromised or abandoned, unless he accepts the position with the intention of amending or modifying the questionable practices and providing that he does not participate in the behavior which violates the code of ethics.

5.8   The orientation and mobility specialist should adhere to the policies and regulations of his employer except where they require him to violate ethical principles indicated in this code. To avoid possible conflicts, the orientation and mobility specialist should acquaint his employer with the contents of this code.

5.9   The orientation and mobility specialist who intends to resign from his position should give his employer sufficient advance notice and leave his work in such a way as to allow his successor to continue effective service.

5.10   The orientation and mobility specialist may provide additional professional service through private contracts, as long as these services remain of the highest quality and do not interfere with the specialist's regular job duties.

5.11   The orientation and mobility specialist should not accept remuneration for professional instruction from a student who is entitled to such instruction through an agency or school, unless the student, when fully informed of services available, decides to contract privately with the specialist.

5.12   The orientation and mobility specialist should establish a fee for private contracting in cooperation with the contracting agency or school that is consistent with the reasonable and customary rate of that particular geographic region.

5.13   When providing additional service through private contracts, the orientation and mobility specialists should observe the agency or school's policies and procedures concerning outside employment including the use of facilities.

Bibliography

Ad Hoc Committee on Mobility Instruction for the Blind, Report of the National Conference. Vocational Rehabilitation Administration, 1966.

Allen, W., Griffith, A. & Shaw, C. *Orientation and mobility: Behavioral objectives for teaching older adventitiously blinded individuals.* New York: New York Infirmary/Center for Independent Living, 1977.

American Foundation for the Blind. Mobility and orientation—A symposium. *New Outlook for the Blind, 1960,* **54**(3), 77-94.

Ball, M. J. Mobility in perspective. *Blindness,* 1964, 107-141.

Blasch, D. Orientation and mobility fans out. *Blindness,* 1971, 9-18.

Blasch, B. & Wurzburger, B. Mobility instruction: A professional challenge. *Long Cane News,* 1971,**4** (3), 1-5.

Bledsoe, C. W. From Valley Forge to Hines: Truth old enough to tell. *Blindness,* 1969, 96-142.

Bledsoe, C. W. Manual for orientors. *Outlook for the Blind and the Teachers Forum,* 1947, **41**(10) 271-279.

Carr-Saunders, A. M. *Professions: Their organization and place in society.* Oxford: The Clarendon Press, 1928. Reproduced in *Professionalization,* H. M. Vollmer and D. L. Mills (Eds.) Englewood Cliffs, N.J.: Prentice-Hall, Inc., 1966.

Commission on Standards and Accreditation of Services for the Blind. *The COMSTAC Report.* New York: The Commission on Standards and Accreditation of Services for the Blind, 1966.

Greenwood, E. Attributes of a profession. *Social Work,* 1957, (May), 45-55.

Hill, E. & Ponder, P. *Orientation and mobility techniques.* New York: American Foundation for the Blind, 1976.

Hoover, R. E. Foot travel without sight. *Outlook for the Blind and the Teachers Forum,* 1946, **40**(9), 244-251.

Hoover, R. E. The Valley Forge story. *Blindness,* 1968, 55-78.

Kimbrough, J. A. Concerning certification of orientation and mobility specialists. *New Outlook for the Blind,* 1969, **63**(9), 275-279.

Koestler, F. *The unseen minority.* New York: The David McKay Company, Inc. 1976.

Long Cane News, Orientation and mobility programs, 1975, **8** (1).

Malamazian, J., The first 15 years at Hines. *Blindness,* 1970, 59-77.

Scheffel, R. R. The rehabilitation aide project. *New Outlook for the Blind,* 1975 (March), 116-120.

Scott, R. A. *The making of blind men.* New York: Russell Sage Foundation, 1969.

Smith, T., Dickerson, C. & Liska, J. Availability of orientation and mobility services in public schools. *Journal of Visual Impairment and Blindness* 1978, **72**(5), 173-176.

Voorhees, A. Professional trends in mobility training. *The New Outlook for the Blind,* 1962 **56**(1) 3-9.

Welsh, R. L. & Blasch, B. B. Manpower needs in orientation and mobility. *New Outlook for the Blind,* 1974, **68**(10), 433-443.

Welsh, R. L. & Wiener, W. R. The code of ethics for orientation and mobility specialists: A progress report. *Journal of Visual Impairment and Blindness,* 1977, **71**(5), 222-224.

Wiener, W., Welsh, R., Hill, E., LaDuke, R., Mills, R., & Mundy, G. The development of a code of ethics for orientation and mobility specialists. *Blindness,* 1973, 6-16.

Research and the Mobility Specialist

William R. De l'Aune

Would it not be far better to let things go on as they are and hope that somehow something will emerge, while we create a valuable impression that we are really trying to solve the problems of blind mobility and in the process satisfy all sorts of personal needs? Put in this underhand way I do not suppose anybody would answer the question in the affirmative. And yet, broadly speaking we are apparently and quite cheerfully prepared to let things go on as they are, using as excuses that we do not really know what blind mobility is all about, that it is some mysterious craft at best, and that almost anything is worth trying regardless of rationale, cost, raising of false hopes, and the rest. All this would just about be all right if there were unlimited resources in manpower and finance, if there were not urgent problems crying out to be solved to make life just a little bit more tolerable for all or some of our users rather than provide a haven for just one or two.

J. Alfred Leonard, (1973)

Don't be afraid of this chapter. The topics covered will be primarily concerned with the way research fits into the field of orientation and mobility and the role you, as a practitioner, play in this grand scheme. It is hoped that you will have had lectures, readings, and classroom experiences with statistical procedures. Assistance in statistics is obtainable through books, mathematically oriented friends, and the new cheap statistical calculators. As a result this once insuperable hurdle to nonresearch specialists is not the problem it was. Readings and lectures on details of research design and methodology are also available and should be consulted to expand the cursory coverage of this fascinating area attempted in this chapter.

Research can be thought of as a rather ritualized way of organizing and understanding the superficially chaotic world around us. The information gained by this process should be shared with others who might benefit from it. Because of the access mobility specialists have to observations in a greater variety of situations than could ever be hoped for in the laboratory, it is not unreasonable to expect them to share in the task of expanding the state of knowledge about their work. By going through the effort of structuring situations so that the practitioner is provided with more reliable events to observe, making the commitment to process these observations and then relaying the resultant information to fellow professionals, the instructor can make such a contribution. This undertaking will serve not only to help others, but will sharpen the individual's skills in assessing the validity of information generated by others.

DIFFERENT RESEARCH APPROACHES

"You get what you pay for," is a common expression. In research the entity purchased is knowledge and the payment is extracted through the effort and skill of the investigator in the currency of the control he is able or willing to exert on the subjects and their environment. Although the more elegant research designs are "better" in the sense that they provide more secure information, they may not prove to be practical in the everyday world of the mobility specialist because of too narrow a focus, ethical ramification, or irreconcilable problems of control.

A number of different research approaches should be examined before any study is undertaken. The investigator must make the decision of which one to use on the merit of the design in the specific situation and not on the basis of what method is "best" in a more abstract sense. Although it might be assumed that an $1,800 bicycle is "better" than a discount store special selling for $59.95, it may not be desirable for you to spend the money for such a machine or even appropriate for your needs. How long, for example, would this extraordinary means of transportation last chained to the bike rack in front of your office?

Naturalistic Observation

In this approach, the researcher observes things in a natural setting in as unobtrusive a manner as possible and records and interprets his observations. This can be done as casually as a mobility specialist recording the progress of a group of clients, or in as rigidly structured a manner as the actuarial tables generated by insurance companies. The effort expended by the investigator to integrate and report on relevant features of a large number of observations, and the skill with which these efforts are expended determine the quality of the descriptive information derived.

One of the cardinal tenets of this approach is that the information gained must remain descriptive. Because the researcher has chosen to remain detached from the situation there are simply too many variables out of his control for him to make any statements of causality. You may note, for example, that all of your clients seem to have trouble learning to cross a certain intersection, and may suggest or hypothesize reasons for the difficulty. These can be the subject of another, more in-depth study, but you can make concrete statements that describe only the difficulty and the peripheral events.

Correlational or Psychometric Analysis

In this type of study the naturalistic techniques of observation are processed at a more formal level. Once again, while not extensively intervening in the situation, the researcher might want to test the hypothesis that the reason for the difficulty in learning to cross a specific intersection is the density of traffic. The records of clients' progress could be scoured to ascertain whether intersections with less traffic tend to give clients less difficulty. The mobility specialist/researcher might even want to inject more effort and skill into the enterprise by taking a random sample of his clients and observing their difficulty (as measured by some wonderfully quantifiable factor such as the time it took them to learn independent crossing successfully) and the traffic flow (perhaps measured in cars-per-minute). From this data a graph such as the one shown in Fig. 1-20 might be generated, and a correlation of .800 between learning time and traffic density might be computed.

The computed correlation of .800 indicates that 64 percent of the total variation in learning time can be explained by the covariation in the traffic density, a highly significant amount. Although enthusiastic about the findings, our hero is careful to report the correlation between traffic density and learning time as simply a relationship. Because of previous readings he knows that a statement indicating that the increase in learning time was caused by the increase in traffic density is unwarranted. Once again, too little control was exerted on all of the extraneous influences to justify such a statement.

The real cause may have been the complicated signal systems which go hand in hand with highly trafficked intersections. It may have been the low blood-sugar levels of the clients at the 5 PM exposure to the more dense rush hour traffic. It could have been due to countless other things that were simply linked to the density of traffic variable. Although none of these possible contributing factors make the statement that there is a relationship between learning time and traffic density any less valid, they do make the causal statement false. Because we are not in the position to rule them out logically, we cannot logically make the causal statement.

The Experimental Method

The basic rule of the experimental method is to keep all factors, except two, constant and then observe the effects of varying one (the independent variable) on the behavior of the other (the dependent variable). If the change in the independent variable is associated with a statistically significant change in the dependent variable, and if the assumption that all factors except the two variables in question have been held constant (or neutralized by random sampling techniques) is true, then the change in the dependent variable can be concluded to be caused by the change in the independent variable. This approach provides the strongest case for causal statements available to the researcher, but it still must be tempered. A lot of scientists and philosophers would argue about the validity of the notion of causality in the first place, but that is another story.

If our intrepid researcher/mobility specialist now wishes to go whole hog and test his hypothesis that traffic density does increase learning time by the experimental approach he would find himelf very busy. First an indoor intersection would have to be created so that factors like temperature, level of pollution, level of noise, and lighting could be held constant. He would then set up a formal

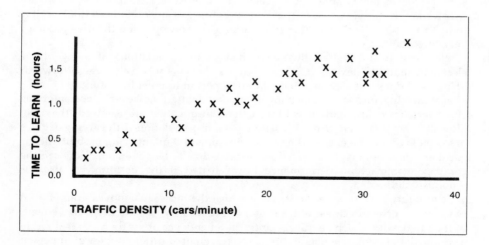

Figure 1-20. Learning time-traffic density correlation.

hypothesis such as, "A heavy traffic rate, as defined by a flow of 20 or more cars a minute, will result in an increase in learning time to successfully cross the intersection without sight when compared to a light traffic rate, as defined by less then 20 cars a minute."

After securing a random sample of subjects to neutralize potential confounding factors in the population such as level of anxiety, hearing problems, intelligence, motor disabilities, he would record the time required for instruction when traffic rates (which were under his control of course) were more than or equal to 20 cars-per-minute or less than 20 cars-per-minute.

If his statistics allowed him to reject his null hypothesis (a statement that there would be no differences between the two conditions of traffic density), he could then accept his alternative hypothesis and assume causality.

The three basic types of behavioral research are not nicely separated, and you can find examples of studies which straddle these arbitrary divisions. It might be more productive to think of research approaches as lying on a continuum in which *the amount of certainty we attribute to the results is proportional to the amount of experimental control exerted by the researcher.*

EXAMPLES OF MOBILITY RESEARCH

This question of control is central to our discussion of research and its place in orientation and mobility. While good research and experimental design are worthwhile goals, a lot of our research questions present both practical and ethical problems in exerting this control. Examples of how several major research centers have dealt with this consideration may illustrate the variety of solutions possible. It should be noted that these examples do not represent any attempt at fairness in sampling of the research. They were chosen because they fit the needs of this chapter.

George Psathas's article "Mobility, Orientation, and Navigation: Conceptual and Theoretical Considerations," is an example of an extreme lack of effort at experimental control. It shows a theoretical framework which is laid almost independently of organized real world observations. Much loved by the classic Greeks, this approach exhibits a concern with semantic clarity and the minute details of task description that help researchers to formulate their thoughts in a much more precise manner than otherwise possible. While easy to dismiss this sort of effort as mere "armchair speculation," it must be remembered that we are involved with studying an area that is as ill-defined as any other I can think of. It is in just this type of situation that rumination over concepts and theories becomes very important.

Nowhere is this better illustrated than in the evaluations of many of the electronic mobility devices. The question asked seems relatively straightforward: "How well does this device assist a blinded person to meet his mobility needs?" The answering of such a question is another matter, however. Even after the characteristics of the particular blind person in question are resolved (they are, after all, members of an incredibly heterogeneous population with varying degrees of visual loss and travel needs) a way of defining and quantifying mobility needs and performance must be devised for testable data to be generated. How can the complex man/machine performance be evaluated if the performance itself is tenuously defined?

Is mobility performance the speed at which the individual moves from point *A* to point *B*, or the directness of his route, or the security he feels in his movement, or the safety with which he travels, or the independence of his travel, or is it rather a composite of a lot of separate things, each weighted differently for each person based on individual needs? If this is so, professionals have to sit back and piece the bits of this puzzle together so that the framework of a testable theory of mobility will have a firm foundation upon which to build. The significance of the "armchair" contributions brought by Psathas and others like him to this cause will be judged by the magnitude of the response it precipitates from researchers and practitioners in the field, and how well it lends itself to and stands up under empirical testing.

Observational

Research, undertaken by Weisgerber and Hall (1975) under contract from the Veterans Administration, serves as an example of a more observational approach to this same problem of clarification and definition. The compendium was developed by filtering the opinions and observations of researchers and practitioners in the field of orientation and mobility into logical subdivisions of the overall "mobility task." The authors divide the environmental sensing needs of the blind into four major sections, each of which is further divided into topical areas. The topical areas are each given a working definition, a rationale, examples of effective and ineffective behaviors, and a listing of those requisite behaviors which are thought to be components of that particular topical area. These behaviors are observable and as such lend themselves to the quantification researchers lust after.

Although significantly less lively reading than most best selling novels, the mobility specialist who plunges into this work is afforded a glimpse of his profession from an angle he may not even have thought existed. At worst, the nit-picking nature of a system such as this provides a forum through which debate can take place on the appropriateness of the inclusion of various tasks. The compendium might also provide material for the preparation of skill area "checklists" to be used in measuring the progress of clients. But the most exciting potential contribution coming from an endeavor of this sort is to provide an objective, quantifiable basis for understanding and improvement of the mobility needs of the blind. As such, even considering its self-avowed untested nature, it should be reacted to by professionals in this field, either positively or negatively.

Multivariate Analysis

De l'Aune and Needham (1977) in the Proceedings of the Fifth New England Bioengineering Conference illustrated one of the products of a multivariate analysis approach used by the research program of the Eastern Blind Rehabilitation Center of the Veterans Administration. The computer coding of a large array of patient characteristics (the basic data profile consists of 113 demographic, physical, and psychological variables from each veteran) makes it possible to "observe" the characteristics of a large number of blind clients. Among other things, it is possible to compute mean values for different variables on the center's clients. Histograms can be plotted to illustrate characteristics such as age distribution of the client population. The computer also can easily compare the depression scores of nondiabetic blinded veterans to the scores of diabetic blinded veterans. Correlations can be generated between age and depression scores, if this type of information is desired. Indeed, it is possible to compute correlations between every variable and every other variable (6,328 correlations), which at the .05 level of significance should randomly provide the investigations with 316 statistically significant relationships and a lot of publications!

It should be obvious to the reader that such a system is vulnerable to abuse, but it should be equally obvious that in the absence of significant prior research attacking characteristics of this large a variety, such a method has tremendous power to define relationships and major factors involved with blind rehabilitation and all of its component parts. This is especially evident when performance on a device is added to the variable list and analyzed for relationships with the items on the data profile. This allows the researchers to make some sense out of the mysterious catch phrase, "Some people just seem to do better than others." The initial correlative studies can be used to identify major predictive factors and direct the investigators into studies of a more specific nature. They also provide data valuable to the design of screening, pretraining, and lesson plans for the device or skill.

Three-factor Measurement

A similar, although much more narrowly focused technique was employed in the assessment of mobility performance by a group at the University of Nottingham (Armstrong & Heyes, 1975). By concerning themselves with three factors assumed to be linked to the illusive "mobility skill," and monitoring these factors, the researchers were able to construct performance profiles of blinded individuals using dog guides, long canes, ultrasonic spectacles, and the Swedish laser cane. The first factor, safety, is measured by recording the "frequency of unintentional physical contact with various parts of the environment and the frequency of unintentional departures from the sidewalk, both midblock and at the end of the block." The second factor, efficiency, is measured by both the walking speed and the smoothness or continuousness of the walking. Smoothness is defined as "the ratio between the length of time taken by the person to cover a specific distance and the proportion of that time during which he was actually physically moving forward." The final factor, psychological stress, is measured by monitoring the average stride length of the subject. All of this data is gathered while the subject travels on a standard outdoor route.

It should be noted that even with all of the computer coding mentioned in the previous study and the sophisticated videotaping used by this group, we are still dealing with observational and correlative techniques. There has been no attempt made by any of the researchers to intervene actively in an experimental sense except, perhaps, in the skill-measuring tests.

Heightened Controls

The Department of Electrical Engineering, University of Canterbury, Christchurch, New Zealand (Kay, 1976) goes even further and controls such things as lighting and temperature as their subjects are electronically tracked in a 60 ft x 40 ft (18 m x 12 m) enclosure. As the subject moves, signals can be generated by a computer under the command of the experimenters. These are presented to the subject as indications of imaginary objects in the laboratory. Through their investigations of the optimum signals for effective perception of the imaginary objects, the researchers can design mobility devices employing these signals. In this case the investigators are not only observing the behavior of their subjects while they travel in a highly controlled, standardized environment, but they are also presenting controlled stimuli to them. The resulting data is therefore capable of being much cleaner than that obtained in any of the methods previously cited.

The tight focus, the very aspect of this work which makes it so methodologically attractive, also makes it essential that all of the other "human factor" variables which are not considered explicitly in the design are cancelled out by random sampling techniques. As a chain's strength is defined by the strength of its weakest link so is the strength of a research project defined by its weakest aspect. Because of the difficulties encountered in samples from the visually impaired population this factor usually provides the truest test of a study's worth. The sophistication lavished on the instrumentation could be lost if poor sampling techniques were used in subject selection.

One must also keep in mind that the results from laboratory settings such as this one are not automatically applicable to the universe outside. If a display proves to be significantly more effective in this setting we cannot assume that these results will generalize into the highly variable environment of the real world. However, this approach does provide us with the best estimate we can obtain.

Cratty's study (1967) provides us with another example of a tight research design executed and reported in a terse, economical manner. The subjects are many and are blind, encompassing a wide range of ages, etiologies, and levels of impairment. The information obtained from such a project can be regarded as very high in quality.

We still face the problems of generalizability of the data, and one could explain that such a narrow focus contributes little to filling in the large gaps of knowledge in the mobility field. However, the response that if complex mobility problems were broken down into such manageable chunks they could eventually be solved seems difficult to dispute.

Up to this point I have not cited any examples of studies in mobility utilizing a classical experimental design. This is not because of a lack of such studies (most research projects done in partial fulfillment of master's level degrees are of such a design), but because of the lack of any ''major'' research being carried out in this manner. The focus of such studies is by definition very narrow, and this makes the results much less interesting to practitioners. This, added to the difficulties in sampling which limit the reliability of the results anyway, makes the studies less than exciting.

De l'Aune, Scheel and Needham (1974) exposed an experimental group to an acoustic training experience for approximately 300 seconds and then their performance in detecting lateral openings in a corridor was compared to the performance of a control group not exposed to the training. The statistical analysis of the results indicated that the performance of the experimental group was significantly higher than that of the control group.

This design provided very high quality information about the efficacy of this particular training technique for the analysis of lateral openings in the hallway used in the experiment, but no information could be generated as to the generalizability or durability of the training effect. Further evaluation was required for this. But we could conclude that the increase in performance was brought about by the exposure to the training session.

YOUR RESEARCH APPROACH

In the course of reading this chapter you have been exposed to a wide range of research being done in mobility. All of the different designs have their advantages and disadvantages. They all have problems which compromise the reliability of the information they provide. You will have the same sorts of problems, and like the researchers cited, you must not let them keep you from undertaking the projects in which you are interested.

Because one of the most pervasive trouble spots is the sampling of subjects from our population, I will spend some extra effort in expounding upon it. Our blind subjects bring to our research projects a multitude of variables that are not under our control. The best method of getting around this is through the use of random sampling techniques in the hope that the differences between clients will cancel themselves out. This, unfortunately, requires that we have fairly large samples, a luxury of which not many researchers in this field can boast.

In a given geographic area the blind population is not always numerous enough to provide a good subject pool from which to draw a random sample. In addition, some of the potential subjects may not be willing to participate in research projects.

This factor gives the investigator the additional concern of having his few subjects come from a non-random sample. This problem is especially apparent in some device evaluations, where one suspects only the very device-oriented segment of the blind population participates.

Even if good sampling opportunities present themselves, we run into confounds caused by the lack of standardization in the visual condition of the blind. If we compartmentalize visual abilities into subgroups we further reduce our sample size and emphasize the aforementioned problems. If we impose standardization by blindfolding all of our legally blind subjects we expand our sample but overlook the effect of useful residual vision on the task in question by a majority of the blinded individuals. The problem of varying levels of novelty in the sightless experience also becomes a matter of concern. Of course, we can solve most of our sampling problems by using sighted subjects in our studies made artificially blind by the use of blindfolds or low vision simulators. We are now confronted with all sorts of additional questions such as abnormally high anxiety levels induced by the blindfolds, prior experience advantages of the "real" blind people, ad infinitum. The generalizability of data generated from such a study becomes a matter of great concern.

If all of these basic problems are added to the difficulty of designing or finding tests appropriate to the dimensions about which assessment is desired in the first place, we have what seems to be a hopeless situation. It seems patently impossible to eliminate all of the problems.

Compromise

The remedy is not very satisfying, but is the same as used by researchers in other, more traditional, scientific fields—compromise. The researcher must try to do the best he can with the situation he has.

The ideal of an experimental design should be approached as closely as possible, but valid investigations should not be deferred simply because the ultimate in scientific rigor is unobtainable.

When the work of others is read, this must be kept in mind. It is permissible to utter a sad, "tsk, tsk," when a methodological "error" is spotted, especially if the reader can visualize a way in which the source of the flaw is minimized without adding additional problems. This should be brought to the author's attention, but in the meantime the study should still be read and the information believed in terms of the level of work. All studies are flawed. A responsible investigator will call these flaws to the attention of his audience and explain the reasons for their presence and the consequences they have on the results.

This all boils down to a reassertion of the validity of the variety of ways in which cat skinning is possible. The practical applications of this pragmatic research philosophy may be made more apparent if we examine possible solutions to a problem with which you might be faced.

If we can assume that some sort of follow-up is desired to assess the effectiveness of your services, what would be the best way to accomplish this? The answer, as you might expect, is a resounding, "It depends."

Follow-up

The "best" way would probably be to observe the client in his home environment at various times after the delivery of the services in question and ascertain the effectiveness of the services directly. The ideal would include pre-intervention observations against which the post-intervention observations could be compared. To this, a control group for whom no services had been provided should be added. For example, a group of randomly sampled clients may have been observed indulging in independent travel an average of 15 minutes a day before mobility training. After training this group may have averaged four hours a day of independent travel contrasting sharply with the 15 minutes a day average maintained by the control group. This data would indicate a spectacularly effective mobility program.

Not only would this experiment be marginally ethical because of the unannounced observation and the arbitrary withholding of services for the control group, but it would be incredibly costly and difficult to do. A lot of time and effort could be saved by simply visiting the client after the delivery of services and asking him how much he traveled now as opposed to the amount of traveling he did immediately before training.

This method would give us the same general information we had in the previous example, but would force us to assume that the client had an accurate knowledge of this information and that he was providing us with undistorted answers. We could never be certain if he was trying to please the agency by reporting an excessive improvement, or was attempting to pay back an instructor who made him do all those dumb things by mimimizing the benefit of the training. The interviewer could make note of corroborative evidence such as the condition of the client's cane (especially tip wear), the client's physical condition, and the comments of his family, in an attempt to make the data more reliable.

If a personal visit is not possible because of time or distance involved, a phone follow-up could be a viable alternative. All of the problems involving reliability that were present in the preceding method would remain with no possibility of improving this factor by corroborative clues. It would be possible, however, to speak to the client after the formal part of the interview and attempt to verify the statements conversationally.

Another alternative is that of a mail follow-up. In addition to the normal problem of questionnaire reliability, we face, with the blind, varying degrees of difficulty in independently answering the questionnaires. If sighted assistance is required, then new social pressures may act to influence the responses. We also now have a problem of a significant number of individuals not responding at all. This may bias the sample and give data only on a selected number of the clients.

As you can see, there are, indeed, ways to attack this rather simple problem. Each method has inherent levels of confidence in the information gathered. One thing remains certain, even the method giving us the least information provides more information than that which would be obtained if no type of follow-up had been attempted.

SUMMARY

The stated purpose of this chapter was to encourage you to become personally involved with research. The bulk of the material presented, however, has covered little but the difficulties encountered in doing this. You have been shown that the research of the "professional researchers" in mobility is far from being without fault or beyond criticism. And now, to pile insult onto injury, I expect you to enter into this arena of ambiguity.

The crux of this chapter is the opening quote by J. Alfred Leonard. We cannot afford to turn our backs on the gaps in our present knowledge of mobility. Information is needed and practitioners have the best access to it.

The products of your research should be well thought out and carefully executed, but not considered immune to criticism. Because all of the systems have flaws, valid comment on these flaws is desirable. Comments in the paper coming from the author are the most desirable of all, but constructive criticism from others should be welcomed.

Methodological criticism, if valid, can be used to improve future research efforts.

The results may not mean what you had originally thought they meant because of a design flaw, but they will undoubtedly mean something.

The opposite comment concerning not the exquisite nature of your design but the trivial nature of your results should bother you a little. Trivial findings are not as nice as big Nobel Prize level findings, but there aren't enough of those kinds of findings to go around. The determination of the importance of a research result is usually through hindsight in a historical perspective so you may even have the last laugh, albeit posthumously. The normal function of "trivial" findings is to serve as a piece of a jigsaw puzzle involving a "major" problem.

This chapter was not intended as a work to which you would refer as you design your research. There are other books available and other individuals to consult who can serve much more adequately in this mission than I. You should expect to read and talk a lot about research design and statistical methods before you get seriously involved with research. Ask your favorite teachers for their recommendations.

This chapter was intended as an encouraging agent, a sort of cheerleader for research. If you still feel shaky about the project lying dormant in your head, talk it over with a teacher or an experienced researcher. You will find that very few of us have unlisted phone numbers.

Bibliography

Armstrong, J. & Heyes, A. The work of the Blind Mobility Research Unit, *Proceedings of conference, Devices and systems for the disabled.* Philadelphia: Temple University, 1975.

Cratty, B. The perception of gradient and the veering tendency while walking without vision. *American Foundation for the Blind Research Bulletin,* 1967, **14,** 31-51.

De l'Aune, W. & Needham, W. *Proceedings of the Fifth New England Bioengineering Conference.* Michael Cannon (Ed.) New York: Pergamon Press, 1977, 111-115.

De l'Aune, W., Scheel, P., & Needham, W. Methodology for training indoor acoustic environmental analysis in blinded veterans. *Journal of the International Research Communications System,* **2,** 1974, 1212.

Kay, L. *Sensory Perception Laboratory Newsletter.* Department of Electrical Engineering, University of Canterbury, Christchurch, New Zealand, 1976.

Leonard, J. A. The evaluation of blind mobility, *American Foundation for the Blind Research Bulletin,* 1967, **26,** 73-76.

Psathas, G. Mobility, orientation, and navigation: Conceptual and theoretical considerations. *New Outlook for the Blind,* 1976, **9,** 385-391.

Weisgerber, R. & Hall, A. *Environmental sensing skills and behaviors.* Palo Alto, California: American Institutes for Research, 1975, VA Contract No. V101 (134) P-163.

About the Authors

L. Eugene Apple is executive director of the American Foundation for the Blind. He has served as chief of the Western Blind Rehabilitation Center of the Veterans Administration in Palo Alto and of the Central Blind Rehabilitation Section in Hines, Illinois. He is the author and co-author of numerous articles on rehabilitation, mobility, and low vision.

Marianne May Apple has a master's degree in orientation and mobility from Western Michigan University. She is an author and co-author of articles on low vision, mobility, and kinesis.

Adrienne M. Difrancesco is a mobility specialist for the New York State Commission for the Blind and has been a physical therapist. She has a bachelor's degree in psychology, a certificate in physical therapy and a master's degree in orientation and mobility from Western Michigan University.

Billie Louise Bentzen is coordinator of the dual program for teachers of the visually handicapped and orientation and mobility, Division of Special Education and Rehabilitation, Boston College. She has a master's degree in peripatology from Boston College and has written many articles focusing on the design of graphic aids for visually impaired persons.

Donald Blasch is chairman of the Department of Blind Rehabilitation, Western Michigan University. He has a master's degree in psychology from the University of Chicago and has served as counselor and acting chief of the Central Blind Rehabilitation Center, Veterans Administration Hospital, Hines, Illinois. He has written many papers on various aspects of blindness with an emphasis on the role of professional training.

C. Warren Bledsoe is retired from service as principal consultant on blindness to the Rehabilitation Services Administration of the United States Department of Health, Education, and Welfare, where he also served as chief of services to the blind from 1958 to 1966. In the Veterans Administration, he served as chief of blind rehabilitation, coordinator of blinded veterans affairs and consultant on blindness following his service as a mobility instructor in the United States Army War Blind Service. He has written much on blindness and orientation and mobility.

Nancy W. Bryant is superintendent of the Michigan School for the Blind. She has held other administrative positions in programs for the multiply handicapped and

663

served as the director of the graduate program in visual disabilities at Florida State University. She has a master's degree and doctorate in special education for the visually impaired, mentally retarded, and in psychology from George Peabody College for Teachers.

Robert J. Crouse is executive director of the Maine Institution for the Blind, Portland, Maine. He has served as the executive director, Atlanta Area Services for the Blind, as an instructor of special education and rehabilitation, University of Northern Colorado, and as principal of the National Mobility Centre, Birmingham, England. He has a doctorate in vocational rehabilitation from the University of Northern Colorado and a master's degree in orientation and mobility from Western Michigan University.

William R. De l'Aune is research supervisor, Eastern Blind Rehabilitation Center, Veterans Administration, West Haven, Connecticut. He has a master's and a doctorate in experimental psychology with a minor in audiology from Florida State University. He has published and spoken widely on audiology and research related to the needs and characteristics of blind people.

A. James Enzinna is a supervisor of orientation and mobility at the Central Blind Rehabilitation Center, Veterans Administration Hospital, Hines, Illinois, where he has served since 1949 as a corrective therapist and a mobility specialist. He has a bachelor's degree from North Central College, Illinois, and has published papers on mobility for a blind bilateral hand amputee.

Leicester W. Farmer is an orientation and mobility research specialist at the Central Blind Rehabilitation Center, Veterans Administration, Hines, Illinois. He has a bachelor's and master's degree from The University of Iowa. His publications and research have focused on the evaluation of electronic travel aids and sensory systems.

Sandra J. McCloskey Gamble is a consultant physical therapist at the Valley Infant Development Service in Springfield, Massachusetts. She served previously as the chief physical therapist at Children's Hospital in Pittsburgh and as a mobility specialist at the Oak Hill School in Connecticut. She holds a certificate in physical therapy and a master's degree in orientation and mobility from Western Michigan University.

Verna Hart is an associate professor in the early childhood program in the Department of Special Education and Rehabilitation at the University of Pittsburgh. She was assistant professor in the multiply handicapped program at the George Peabody College. She has a master's degree and a doctorate from Wayne State University and has written a number of publications in the area of education of severely handicapped, multiply handicapped children.

Everett Hill is on the faculty of George Peabody College for Teachers. He received a doctorate in Special Education, Western Michigan University, and has been on the faculties of the Department of Blind Rehabilitation, Western Michigan, University and the Department of Special Education, Florida State University. He was the co-author of *Orientation and Mobility: A Guide for the Practitioner* and has also written a number of articles on concept development of visually handicapped children.

Wayne A. Jansen is a mobility specialist for multiply handicapped students at the Michigan School for the Blind with previous experience as a mobility specialist in Maryland, Utah, and Illinois. He is a graduate of the mobility training program at Western Michigan University.

Robert O. LaDuke is assistant professor, Department of Blind Rehabilitation, Western Michigan University. He served on the faculty of the Stephen F. Austin State University in Texas and holds a doctorate in special education and administration from the University of Northern Colorado.

Denis A. Lolli is head of the orientation and mobility department at the Perkins School for the Blind, where he has taught orientation and mobility to deaf-blind students. He is a graduate of the peripatology program at Boston College and a project consultant to the orientation and mobility program for multiply handicapped children at George Peabody College.

Robert J. Mills is chief peripatologist and director of the orientation and mobility program of the Ohio State School for the Blind. He is a graduate of the peripatology program at Boston College and the author of articles on sensory stimulation and mobility for teachers.

Herbert L. Pick, Jr. is professor of psychology and child psychology at the Institute of Child Development, University of Minnesota and a former director of the Center for Research in Human Learning, University of Minnesota. He has written extensively about perception and learning. His current research activities center on perception and perceptual development with a focus on the spatial orientation of people in general, and a special interest in the spatial orientation of the visually handicapped.

Kent Tyler Wardell is an associate professor in the orientation and mobility training program, Department of Special Education, California State University, Los Angeles. He has served on the Committee on Architectural Barriers of the Los Angeles Mayor's Commission on the Handicapped and was co-author of *Guidelines: Architectural and Environmental Concerns of the Visually Impaired Person.* He is a graduate of the mobility training program at Western Michigan University and has also written other articles on orientation and mobility.

Robert H. Whitstock is vice president for programs, The Seeing Eye, Inc. and a graduate of Harvard Law School. He has written many articles on mobility and on public relations and blindness. He is a past president of the American Association of Workers for the Blind and a past chairman of its orientation and mobility interest group.

William R. Wiener is associate professor and coordinator of blind rehabilitation at Cleveland State University. He served as supervisor of orientation and mobility at the Syracuse Association of Workers for the Blind. He has a master's degree in orientation and mobility from Western Michigan University and a master's in audiology from Cleveland State University. He has written a number of articles on the professional development of orientation and mobility and various aspects of mobility training.

Index